CHALONES

Chalones

Editor:

John C. Houck

Department of Child Health and Development,
George Washington University Medical Center,
Research Foundation of Children's Hospital,
Washington D.C. 20009, U.S.A.

1976

NORTH-HOLLAND PUBLISHING COMPANY – AMSTERDAM · OXFORD
AMERICAN ELSEVIER PUBLISHING CO., INC., NEW YORK

North-Holland ISBN: 0 7204 0600 5
American Elsevier ISBN: 0 444 11202 2

QP
572
.C47C47

PUBLISHERS:
NORTH-HOLLAND PUBLISHING COMPANY – AMSTERDAM
NORTH-HOLLAND PUBLISHING COMPANY, LTD. – OXFORD

SOLE DISTRIBUTORS FOR THE U.S.A. AND CANADA:
AMERICAN ELSEVIER PUBLISHING COMPANY, INC.
52 VANDERBILT AVENUE, NEW YORK, N.Y. 10017

Printed in the Netherlands

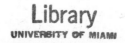

Contents

Chapter 15.   Lymphocyte chalone, by A. M. Attallah and J. C. Houck . 355

Contents

CHAPTER 1

Introduction

JOHN C. HOUCK

Scientific Director, Research Foundation, Children's Hospital,
Washington, D. C. 20009, U.S.A.

The word 'chalone' (from the Greek, meaning 'to slacken') was originally proposed by Sir Ernie Shafer to stand in theoretical contradistinction to 'hormone'; namely a material which would slow down rather than stimulate biological events. The world of science was completely underwhelmed by 'chalone' and it was not again to enter the literature until the middle 1950's when some workers studying the secretion of gastric and intestinal hormones used the word 'chalone' to refer to a tissue-derived inhibitor of the secretion of these hormones. It was not until Professor Bullough of Birkbeck College decided that the inhibitory principle which he had found in the epidermis of rodents for the proliferation of the epidermis was both cell-specific and not species-specific that 'chalone' was resuscitated. Professor Bullough was consumed with the intuition that most cells would be controlled mitotically by a specific and endogenous negative feedback inhibitor of mitosis. Subsequently, in a discussion with the Master of Birkbeck College, he was reminded that there was such a word as 'chalone'. Noting that the word was still carried in the dictionary, he thereby applied the generic term of chalone to a whole series of putative specific and endogenous mitotic inhibitors. His concept of the cell, then, was one in which the cell was actively restrained from entering the mitotic cycle, rather than the previous concept that the cell needed to be actively pushed into the mitotic cycle via a 'wound hormone'.

Within a period of less than ten years, chalones had been suggested for a number of other cells and had been confirmed by workers all over the world to be involved in the control of epidermal, lymphocytic, granulocytic, and melanocytic proliferation, both in vitro and in vivo. Further, it was also found that these crude tissue extracts containing the putative chalone could inhibit the proliferation of the tumor variety of the cell. It was this type of finding, plus the internal intellectual elegance of the theory of an endogenous cell-specific mitotic inhibitor which lent a certain 'cachet' to the search for the isolation, purification, characterization, and application of chalones to the clinical situation. This attitude probably reached its zenith in mid-1968 with the publication of a series of papers on epidermal, granulocytic, and melanocytic chalones in Nature.

The simplicity of the idea, the claim of cell-specificity, and the ability to use tissues from other species for application to the human situation all combined to raise great expectations which, as Iversen justly pointed out, were extremely premature and hence foredoomed. About this time, Mohr discovered that his extracts of melanoma, which had demonstrated a melanocytic effect in vivo, were contaminated by bacterial spores. The biological effect of these clostridia spores in vivo would more than compromise the results obtained using these extracts to effect the regression of melanoma in vivo in experimental animals. Subsequent production by other workers, notably Dewey, of melanoma extracts which were sterile, yet were still able to inhibit the proliferation of melanoma cells in culture, did not restore the confidence which had been lost by the interested portions of the scientific community as a result of Mohr's bacteriological explanation of his findings in vivo.

Enormous technical difficulties are involved in establishing beyond doubt the validity that a crude tissue extract, even though partially purified, contains a cell-specific noncytotoxic inhibitor of the proliferation of a given cell type. Technically the two primary methods for studying mitotic activity and proliferation of cells in vitro involve either trapping these cells in metaphase or by determining by either direct counting or autoradiography the amount of radioactive thymidine which has been incorporated into the acid insoluble DNA of the cell. More rarely used and yet effective is the determination of the proliferation rate of cells in culture by actually counting the numbers of cells at various periods of time after seeding the culture. The primary criticisms of these methods are, a) cytotoxicity, and b) alteration or catabolism of the thymidine label. Add to these already formidable experimental difficulties the very real probability that most extracts of crude tissues prepared in most laboratories will be contaminated by bacteria. In our own laboratory, we have found that a peculiar strain of bacteria will grow in the ultrafiltrates prepared from spleen at 4 °C. This particular bacterium contains a material which, after lyophilization, can be removed from the surface of these cells and which will inhibit the PHA-stimulated transformation of lymphocytes on an apparently cell-specific basis. Thus, the bacterial contaminant which grows only in the cold and only in tissue-extracted media can mimic many of the effects of leukocyte chalone in vitro.

These experimental problems and potential artifacts in the interpretation of data were discussed at the Brook Lodge Chalone Conference in 1972 which involved almost all of the workers interested in pursuing the elusive chalone. As indicated in a number of chapters in this book, these criticisms have been acted upon and for the most part dealt with quite effectively by the appropriate control experiments. The reader's attention should be directed to the discussions by both Verly and Paukovits of the artifacts in using thymidine to determine cell proliferation and to a summary of the criticisms of chalone experimental problems in the terminal chapter of this book.

Another difficulty in establishing the credibility of the chalone concept experimentally has been the lack of any totally purified chalone to date. In the late 1960's, an attempt was made to purify the epidermal chalone, which certainly resulted in highly concentrated and much more purified biologically active preparations than had hitherto been available; unfortunately, since the source of the epidermal chalone was the epidermis from scalded pit skin, the final preparation was found to contain (by calculation from its amino acid analysis) at least 40% gelatin. Although this material would have no biological activity as a chalone, the fact of this large degree of contamination did not reassure the biochemical world as to the material composition of chalone.

In 1970, the Growth Control Panel of the Medical Research Council in London held hearings and made a detailed study of the experimental data supporting the reality of the chalone concept in general and various specific chalones and their application to the control of tumors in particular. It is the author's opinion, derived as a consequence of extensive conversations with a number of the members of this panel and with those 'chalonists' who were involved in this study, that most biomedical scientists felt that if a name were granted to a functional material, than that material should be completely in hand, i.e., isolated, reasonably purified, and certainly characterized as far as to its composition. These expectations were obviously not satisfied by the data available. The artifactual problems of cytotoxicity, thymidine destruction, and bacterial contamination were thus colored by this sense of disappointment. It is the writer's opinion that these feelings are very widespread among biomedical scientists *marginally* knowledgeable about published work on chalones.

The proceedings of the Brook Lodge Conference were published as a National Cancer Institute monograph in 1973. These proceedings were attented by a number of rigorous and highly knowledgeable biomedical scientists who were not themselves directly involved in chalone research but who brought their sophisticated expertise to bear in the discussions of these papers presented at the Brook Lodge meeting. The results of this dialogue between the workers in the field of chalones and experts in the various disciplines brought to bear upon this study area is, to some extent, demonstrated in the following chapters of this volume. The reader must make up his own mind as to how rigorous in experimental design and how critical in interpretation these various authors have been in coming to grips with the chalone concept in general and in their particular tissue of interest. The editor bears total responsibility for the selection of these contributors.

Two lines of research currently being conducted in the editor's laboratory might bear discussion in this Introduction. Firstly, we believe that much of the difficulty in the isolation and purification of chalone activity stems from the considerable degree of biological sophistication required to assay chalone (in view of all the various artifacts possible) and the considerable degree of biochemical sophistication required to effect the actual isolation and purification of the chalone molecule itself. The major difficulty with the latter process is that most tissue extracts are contaminated with large amount of RNA. Even after ultrafiltration, there is still a considerable amount of RNA small enough to move through a 50,000-dalton restraining filter and to which is adhered the biologically active chalone molecule. Since this RNA–chalone complex appears to be fairly stable, it is extraordinarily difficult to fractionate this material in the usual fashion. Thus, isoelectric focusing is fruitless, since the anionic polyelectrolyte character of the RNA is maintained even after the partial neutralization of its secondary phosphate charges by interaction with the basic amino acids of the chalone molecule itself. It is a characteristic in the RNA research field that the anionic polyelectrolyte is extremely difficult to purify because of its ability to adsorb to a number of different materials. We hope that the judicious use of trypsin-free ribonuclease may permit a rapid acceleration of the purification of the larger molecular weight chalones which may not be as large a molecular weight as hitherto indicated by ultrafiltration and exclusion chromatography studies.

Secondly, we are of the opinion that the application of chalones to the clinical situation will not be a direct one, with the possible exception of the unique cytotoxic effects of spleenic extracts containing lymphocyte chalone upon leukemic lymphocytes, as described subsequently. Rather, we believe that since a large number of chalones apparently work in the G_1 phase of the cell cycle, the major clinical use of chalones will be as an adjunct to chemotherapy in terms of the synchronization of cancer cells. Specifically,

CHAPTER 2

An analysis of the epidermal chalone control mechanism

WILLIAM S. BULLOUGH and EDUARDO MITRANI

Mitosis Research Laboratory, Birkbeck College, University of London, U.K.

2.1 Introduction

Any analysis of the mechanism of cellular homeostasis in the mitotic tissues of adult mammals must take into account a pattern of interrelated problems: the way in which in normal circumstances a perfect balance is maintained between the number of new cells gained and the number of old cells lost; the way in which an episode of tissue destruction is countered by an episode of tissue regeneration; the way in which control is maintained when the tissue mass shrinks into hypoplasia or increases into hyperplasia; and the way in which control is lost when a tumour develops.

There have been many theories of growth control. The most important earlier models were those of Osgood (1957) and of Weiss and Kavanau (1957), while the most important later model, which concerned epidermis, was that of Iversen and Bjerknes (1963). The history of the cybernetic approach to the problem of growth control has been reviewed by Iversen (1965).

Almost all attempts to explain cellular homeostasis have been based on the simple proposition of a negative feedback mechanism by which the rate of new cell production is inhibited by tissue-specific feedback information emanating from the cell mass. Such a mechanism would obviously imply that each tissue must contain a diffusible messenger molecule that inhibits mitotic activity specifically within that same tissue. The existence of such a substance, the epidermal chalone (Bullough, 1962), was demonstrated by Bullough and Laurence (1960a, 1964a) in mouse epidermis, while a similar substance, the granulocytic chalone, was found by Rytömaa and Kiviniemi (1964, 1968a) in circulating granulocytes. Today some twenty tissue-specific chalone systems have been described (see Bullough, 1975). A new system of chemical messengers has been discovered.

However, new information now emerging, especially from studies of epidermis (see Bullough, 1972, 1975), has shown that the mechanism of cellular homeostasis is by no means as simple as the earlier models had suggested. There is always a continuing necessity 'to bring cybernetic philosophy down to earth by proper experimentation' (Iversen, 1965), and the present paper develops a new model of cellular homeostasis that is consistent with the latest information. One assumption has been made, namely that each tissue synthesises only one chalone, although it is evident that there may be two (see p. 22). This simplification of the argument does not affect the form of the model.

The present analysis derives both from a survey of the known or suspected biological facts and from a series of computer analyses of the interrelationships of these facts. The details of these analyses will be given elsewhere.

It is a particular pleasure to acknowledge our indebtedness to Johanna Deol for her constant help in the production of this manuscript.

2.2 The steady state

The steady state is illustrated by any type of epidermis in which the number of cells gained by basal mitosis is balanced by the number of cells extruded from the basal layer to be lost by distal keratinisation. It is seen equally in chronic hypoplasia, in normal epidermis, and in chronic hyperplasia; it is, however, not seen when the epidermis is in the process of change from one of these states to another (Bullough, 1972; see p. 18).

2.2.1 Cell gain and cell loss

Most epidermal models have proposed that the steady state is assured when the distal cell mass (the epidermal thickness) is great enough to produce sufficient negative feedback information, or chalone, to prevent further basal mitosis; then as distal cells are lost by keratinisation the chalone concentration falls and mitosis begins again. Obviously a feedback mechanism of this type can only function if the rate of cell loss is independent of the rate of cell gain; only if this is true can a change in the rate of mitosis lead to an equivalent change in the tissue mass. This point has commonly been disregarded since cell loss has been thought of as a 'wearing out' process which, accidents apart, continues at a relatively constant rate. Analysis has, however, shown clearly that the ageing and death of post-mitotic cells is a dynamic process, which is as closely controlled as is mitotic activity itself (Bullough, 1967, 1972). The rate of post-mitotic cell ageing depends on the same factors that determine the mitotic rate; in normal human epidermis the post-mitotic cell lifespan is 14–21 days, while in hyperplastic epidermis it is only 4–5 days (Scott and Ekel, 1963). A post-mitotic cell shows two separate, probably gene-controlled, activities: that leading to tissue function (which is not relevant) and that leading to cell death (Bullough, 1967).

In epidermis the evidence is that the lower the chalone concentration (as after tissue damage) the higher the mitotic rate in the basal cells and the faster the ageing process in the distal cells; and that the higher the chalone effectiveness (as during chronic stress; Bullough and Laurence, 1961, 1964a) the lower the mitotic rate in the basal cells and the slower the ageing process in the distal cells (Bullough, 1972). Furthermore, the rate of cell gain and the rate of cell loss are affected in equal degree, so that:

rate of mitosis : rate of post-mitotic ageing $= R$, a constant, which also means that:

number of mitotic cells : number of post-mitotic cells $= N$, another constant (Bullough, 1972).

From this it is clear that tissue mass, which in epidermis means thickness, is determined not by the mitotic rate but by the tissue-specific value of R. This alone disposes of the concept of epidermal homeostasis achieved solely by a simple negative feedback mechanism.

2.2.2 The role of the epidermal chalone

Although the most obvious action of the epidermal chalone is its inhibition of mitosis and of post-mitotic ageing, it is probable that its basic action is to divert the epidermal cell from synthesis for mitosis to synthesis for ageing and keratinisation (Bullough, 1967). A basal intermitotic cell (see p. 15) has two possible fates: below a critical chalone level it will re-enter mitosis, while above this critical level it will enter post-mitosis. The lower the sub-critical chalone level the faster the cells re-enter mitosis; the higher the supracritical chalone concentration the slower the post-mitotic cells pass to their deaths.

2.2.3 Chalone control; a model

Using these various basic facts and assumptions an attempt was made to build a theoretical computer model of cellular homeostasis that did not depend entirely on a negative feedback mechanism. This new model was based on the assumption that, in the steady state, chalone action is not constant throughout the whole epidermis but that it exists in the form of a gradient. The chalone influence is weakest in the basal layer, which is therefore mitotic, and strongest in the distal layers, which are therefore post-mitotic.

A preliminary model showed that if it is assumed that one action of the chalone is to dictate deterministically the mitotic cycle length (the weaker the chalone action the shorter the cycle) then an initially unsynchronised cell population will eventually become synchronised with all mitoses occurring simultaneously. This is because those cells which are initially in the same phase of the mitotic cycle and which happen to have a slight numerical advantage will have that advantage continually reinforced. Whenever they divide it is their neighbouring cells in some other phase of the mitotic cycle that will be extruded from the basal cell population (see p. 15). Thus the cells with the original numerical advantage will ultimately come to dominate the basal layer; all cells will then be synchronous. This is contrary to observation.

To avoid such synchronism it was found necessary to introduce the assumption that cell cycle time, or at least intermitotic time, is not fixed but includes an element of probability. This finds support from the work of Smith and Martin (1973, 1974), who from an analysis of cell behaviour in vitro have concluded that the transition into the mitotic process is determined by probability. At any given mitotic rate, an intermitotic cell, however long it has been in that state, always has a constant probability of re-entering the mitotic process. It is this probability that is chalone-dependent (see p. 24).

The work of Smith and Martin has concerned only the simplest of in vitro systems. The new control model therefore not only introduced this probability concept (which has remained a basic feature of all the later models) but also took account of the more complex situation in vivo in which an intermitotic cell may not only re-enter mitosis but is in constant risk of being extruded from the basal layer into a region of higher chalone effectiveness. This significantly alters the age distribution function of the intermitotic cells as calculated by Smith and Martin.

When run in the computer the new model proved to be stable not only when the gradient of chalone action was itself stable but also when perturbations, simulating sudden reductions in overall chalone concentration, were introduced.

It was therefore concluded that, given a stable gradient of chalone action within the epidermis, cellular homeostasis can be achieved without a negative feedback loop. The concept of a gradient in the chalone concentration due to chalone loss into the dermis was introduced into some of the earlier negative feedback models to account for the fact that mitosis is basal; the theory that the gradient is not of chalone concentration but of chalone effectiveness created by the opposing action of a mitotic stimulant, or 'antichalone', emanating from the dermis is given below; it is also possible that both these situations co-exist.

2.2.4 The role of the mesenchymal factor

There is extensive evidence from many tissues, including skin, that a mitotic stimulant, the mesenchymal factor, is produced by connective tissue cells, and that it acts to counter chalone effectiveness in any immediately adjacent epithelial tissue cell. This evidence, reviewed by Bullough (1975), comes from studies of both embryonic and adult tissues and organs, and relates especially to skin and gizzard, to lung and prostrate, and to salivary, pancreatic and mammary glands. The most extensive data is from the skin.

When epidermis is separated from dermis and placed in vitro, basal mitotic activity ceases and all the cells die, sometimes with keratinisation spreading down to and involving the basal cells (McLoughlin, 1961; Brigga-man and Wheeler, 1968). Evidently, in the absence of the dermis, the chalone is so dominant as to force the whole epidermis into post-mitosis, keratinisa-tion, and death. If the separated epidermis is replaced on dermis, basal mitosis is re-stimulated and the tissue remains normal; this also occurs if the dermis is inverted, or if other types of connective tissues are substituted, or if fibroblast culture medium or fresh serum or embryo extract is used (Bullough, 1975).

The conclusion is that the mesenchymal factor is a chemical messenger synthesised by connective tissue cells, that it acts as a non-tissue-specific antichalone, and that its influence is normally felt only in those epithelial cells that are in actual connective tissue contact. In the skin it may originate from the dermal fibrocytes, or it may reach the dermis from the blood, or both. The reason for its short-range action is not known; it may be held in a solid substrate (Yaoi and Kanaseki, 1972; Igarashi and Yaoi, 1975). Its action on epidermis only extends to the suprabasal cell layers when the chalone concentration is reduced in hyperplasia (Bullough and Deol, 1975a; see p. 18).

Thus mitotic control in the epidermis depends on the low basal layer chalone effectiveness (i.e. the chalone concentration *plus* the stress hormone concentration *minus* the mesenchymal factor concentration) and the high distal layer chalone effectiveness (i.e. the chalone concentration *plus* the

stress hormone concentration). In this situation any change in either the
chalone concentration or the stress hormone concentration affects cell gain
and cell loss in equal degree.

It is important to emphasise that these conclusions apply to epithelial
tissues in general, the 'basal cells' being those that are connective-tissue-
adjacent and the 'distal cells' those that are not (Bullough, 1975; see p. 30).

2.2.5 Epidermal homeostasis

The perfection of the balance between cell gain and cell loss is now explained.
An epidermal cell is mitotic or post-mitotic according to its position within
the tissue. The pressure caused by each basal mitosis forces the extrusion
distally of an adjacent cell which, entering the zone of high chalone effectiveness, must then become post-mitotic, acquire a particular life-span, and so
die. Epidermal cellular homeostasis is ensured by a 'positional effect'. So
long as the chalone concentration in the distal cells remains above the level
needed to ensure post-mitosis this positional mechanism is stable, and this
is the situation over the wide range from hypoplasia to extreme hyperplasia.
Problems do however arise at both ends of this scale (see below and p. 28).

2.2.6 Phase 1 epidermis

In theory, if the basal chalone effectiveness reached that critical level at
which mitotic activity is completely inhibited, an all-mitotic basal layer
would be abruptly transformed into an all-non-mitotic basal layer. In fact,
this does not happen; as the chalone effectiveness rises the basal layer comes
to contain a mixture of mitotic-cycle cells and early post-mitotic cells. This
is phase 1 type epidermis (Bullough, 1972).

In man this state is abnormal and is termed hypoplasia; in mouse it is
normal. Such epidermis is characterised by a lower mitotic rate and a longer
post-mitotic ageing process (higher chalone effectiveness), by a relatively
thin structure, and by the fact that epidermal thickness (mass) is independent
of the mitotic rate (Bullough and Ebling, 1952).

Each mitosis usually occurs in the horizontal plane so that both daughter
cells remain basal (Bullough and Laurence, 1964b); the pressure so produced
causes the extrusion distally of a closely adjacent early post-mitotic cell
(Mackenzie, 1970; Christophers, 1971). Evidently a post-mitotic cell has a
weaker dermal grip than a mitotic cell. The result is that, throughout phase 1,
the greater (or smaller) the number of mitoses, the greater (or smaller) the
number of post-mitotic cells that are forced distally, and the faster (or

slower) these cells keratinise and die. However low the mitotic rate may fall the epidermis does not become thinner; the epidermal mass is determined simply by the N ratio, which in phase 1 must be rewritten as:

number of basal cells : number of distal cells = N, a constant.

The justification for this is that the basal post-mitotic cells, which are recognised by early keratin precursors (Christophers, 1971), evidently differ fundamentally from the distal post-mitotic cells. The post-mitotic ageing process does not seem to begin until the cells leave the basal layer.

Since epidermal homeostasis depends on the positional effect, the problem that now arises is how this mechanism can continue to function when the basal layer consists of a mixture of mitotic and post-mitotic cells. The theoretical answer is that these two cell types must form a stable pattern so that the state of any cell depends on its position within this pattern. This theoretical necessity is in fact met by the mitotic pattern imposed on the basal layer by the phenomenon of distal cell stacking (Mackenzie, 1970; Christophers, 1971, 1972a). Each stack overlies some 10 basal cells and it is those cells that lie under the edges of the stacks that tend to be mitotic. The reason for the existence of this pattern has not yet been established, but the fact that it is there ensures epidermal stability.

When in phase 1 the mitotic rate rises, the proportion of mitotic-cycle basal cells increases while that of post-mitotic basal cells decreases. Phase 1 ends and phase 2 begins when all the basal cells are in the mitotic cycle.

2.2.7 The components of the mitotic rate

This leads to an important conclusion. The epidermal mitotic rate (number of mitoses per unit area of skin per unit time) has two components: the duration of the mitotic cycle and the number of basal cells that are involved in the cycle. An increase in the mitotic rate results both from a shortening of the cycle and from an increase in the number of mitotic-cycle cells per unit area of skin.

2.2.8 Phase 2 epidermis

This rule does not change when epidermis enters phase 2: with an increasing mitotic rate the number of mitotic-cycle cells per unit area of skin continues to rise because the mitotic activity spreads into the distal layers.

In pig and man both normal and hyperplastic epidermis are in phase 2; in mouse phase 2 is seen only in hyperplasia. It is characterised by a higher mitotic rate and a shorter post-mitotic ageing process (lower chalone effectiveness), by a relatively thick structure, and by the fact that, although the R ratio is still operating, an increasing mitotic rate results in increasing epidermal thickness (hyperplasia; see p. 18). This is because the increasing number of basal mitotic-cycle cells per unit skin area results in an increasing number of distal cells (according to the N ratio), even though these cells are ageing and dying more quickly.

2.2.9 Conclusions

The main conclusions arising from the above considerations are as follows:

The mass of an epithelial tissue such as epidermis is determined basically by the R ratio, which is tissue-specific; the lower the value of R the greater the tissue mass. This is a critically important safety mechanism; any change in the rate of mitosis is immediately countered by an equal change in the rate of post-mitotic ageing.

The perfect balance between cell gain and cell loss in steady state epidermis is ensured by the positional effect. There is a gradient of chalone effectiveness with its low point in the basal layer where the chalone influence is neutralised by the mesenchymal factor; mitotic activity therefore occurs only in cells that are dermis-adjacent; any cell forced from this basal position into a distal region of high chalone effectiveness must become post-mitotic, survive only for a particular life-span, and then die.

An important component of the epidermal mitotic rate is the number of mitotic-cycle cells per unit area of skin; the higher the mitotic rate, the more mitotic-cycle cells there are. In phase 2 epidermis this leads also to more distal cells (the N ratio) and so to an increased tissue mass. This is the basis of hyperplasia, whether induced by injury, or in hormone-dependent tissues by a mitogenic hormone.

2.3 Dermo-epidermal adhesion

In phase 2 epidermis the increasing number of mitotic-cycle cells per unit skin area that are produced during a period of increasing mitotic rate is accommodated mainly by the spread of these cells into the suprabasal layers (Bullough and Deol, 1975a); in addition, as in pig and man (Bullough and Deol, 1975b; Braun-Falco, 1971), the superficial dermis may expand to provide an increasing area for basal cell anchorage (p. 19). The first impression is that these responses may be the outcome of rising pressure generated by the rising mitotic activity of the cells in the basal layer, and this introduces the question of the grip of the basal cells on the dermal boundary.

2.3.1 The epidermal grip

This has been studied almost entirely in terms of the force needed to detach a relatively large area of human epidermis from its dermal bed and so to raise a suction blister (see Kiistala, 1972; Leun et al., 1974a, b). The evidence is that, over a wide range of suction pressures, $pt = A$, where p is the pressure, t the time taken to blister, and A the adhesion strength; and that the value of A decreases exponentially with increasing skin temperature. These relationships indicate that the epidermis is held to the dermis mainly by the viscosity of a fluid interface.

In a physical system the force taken to break a viscous bond is time dependent; in the skin this is also true except that at low pressures the rule ceases to apply and the epidermal–dermal bond is able to resist detachment apparently indefinitely. This has led Leun et al. (1974a) to postulate the existence of another weaker adhesion mechanism, such as a system of fibrous connections between the bases of the epidermal cells and the dermis, or a process of re-adherence by which the basal cells constantly repair the damage being done to the dermo–epidermal junction. Fibrous epidermal–dermal connections, that could provide a weak elastic adhesive force, have been described (Brody, 1960; Kobayasi, 1961; Palade and Farquhar, 1965); a repair process for the regeneration of epidermal adherence certainly exists (Leun et al., 1974a); and both systems may operate together.

Another important point is that the adhesive strength, whether due to the viscous bond or to the other systems, must also depend on the area of contact between the epidermal cells and the dermis. The data are inadequate, but at least in pig and man, Winter (1972) and Schmidt et al. (1974) have shown how deeply the proximal surface of each basal cell may be inter-digitated into the dermis. The consequent enormous increase in the area of dermo–epidermal contact must greatly increase the cell grip.

2.3.2 The cell cycle and basal cell extrusion

Although studies of suction blisters have been invaluable in defining the nature of dermo–epidermal adhesion, they do not explain the manner of separation of a single basal cell in response to a neighbouring mitosis. In analysing this the first conclusion is that, since the mitotic daughter cells retain their basal grip while some adjacent cell is forced out, not all basal cells are equally liable to be displaced.

The mitotic cycle of the basal epidermal cells is divisible into the following sequence of phases: G_{1c}, or prosphase, which is the first phase of the mitotic process; S phase, in which the DNA is duplicated; G_2, in which the cell prepares for mitosis; M, in which mitosis occurs; G_{1a}, or apophase, which is the final phase of the mitotic process; and G_{1b}, or dichophase, or interphase, in which the cell 'rests' before re-entry into G_{1a} or entry into the post-mitotic state (see Bullough, 1975).

Evidence from normal mouse epidermis (Bullough and Laurence, 1964b) and fore-stomach keratinising epithelium (Frankfurt, 1967) shows that S phase cells (and therefore also prosphase cells) are always basal, as also are cells in mitosis (and therefore also in G_2) and in apophase. Thus throughout the whole mitotic process a cell does not lose its basal grip, and the only cells lost during this time are the distal daughter cells of those few mitoses that are angled vertically (Bullough and Laurence, 1964b; p. 20).

Any cell forced distally by the pressure of an adjacent mitosis must therefore be in the dichophase or, in phase 1 mouse epidermis, in the early post-mitotic phase. Since it may be assumed that the degree of viscosity of the interface fluid is uniform over wide areas of the skin it follows that the weaker grip of a dichophase cell, or of an early post-mitotic cell, probably depends on some structural difference in its basal cell membrane. This could result from a change in the connecting fibres or in the degree of dermo–epidermal interdigitation.

2.3.3 *Dermal grip and normal hyperplasia*

It follows that in considering the relationships between basal layer pressure, cellular homeostasis and epidermal structure it is the grip of the post-mitotic (phase 1) and dichophase cells (phase 2) that is significant. To date these relationships have been studied only in the mouse by contrasting the situation in the thin ear epidermis with that in the thick sole-of-foot epidermis (Bullough and Deol, 1975a).

The degree of basal cell pressure was estimated by measuring the height/width ratio of the basal nuclei and by determining the number of basal cells per unit baseline area. The ear epidermis has a nuclear ratio = 1 which means that it is under equal pressure from all directions; the cell number per unit area is that typical of an unpressurised cubical epithelium. Each mitosis produces a thrust of pressure that is adequate to extrude a neighbouring dichophase cell, which implies that this cell must have a relatively weak dermal grip.

The sole-of-foot epidermis is markedly different. The nuclear height/width ratio approaches 4, and the basal cell layer is obviously under strong lateral pressure. In the centre of each footpad the baseline is folded. The crowding of the basal cells combined with the folded baseline means that the number of mitotic cells per unit area of skin is unusually high and it follows from the N constant that the number of distal post-mitotic cells must be equally high. Thus the epidermis is thickened in what may be regarded as normal hyperplasia.

The reason why in sole-of-foot epidermis a basal dichophase cell requires a higher pressure before it is extruded must lie with its stronger dermal grip. When the thrust of pressure produced by a mitosis is not strong enough to detach a neighbouring dichophase cell within the time available (the dichophase half-life), no cell can escape from the basal layer. This leads to cell crowding which has two consequences: the cells are compressed from a cubical to a tall columnar form, and the rise in pressure leads to a shortening of the time required to detach a dichophase cell. A point is finally reached when the thrust of extra pressure produced by each mitosis becomes great enough to detach a neighbouring dichophase cell within the time available. The system is then stable.

It must be emphasised that this type of hyperplasia develops independently of the mitotic rate, which in mouse sole-of-foot is not high. This is in marked contrast to the situation in pathological hyperplasia (p. 18).

2.3.4 Regional epidermal characteristics

This analysis sheds light on the question of the different types of epidermis seen in the different regions of the body.

In each such region the number of basal cells per unit baseline area is fixed by the dermal grip; the number of distal cells is therefore also fixed, and so too is the epidermal thickness. It is interesting to recall that, in a series of important experiments, Billingham and Silvers (1968) showed that when mouse ear epidermis and sole-of-foot epidermis are transposed, each changes its thickness and structure to that typical of the graft site. They concluded that the epidermis is 'equipotential' and that the maintenance of each regional epidermal type 'turns upon the persistent influence of . . . the underlying dermis'.

The explanation of their work is now clear: the epidermal mitotic rate is partly dependent on the concentration of the mesenchymal factor, while the epidermal thickness is a function of the epidermal grip which, at least in the dichophase, must be determined not by the epidermal cells but by the nature of the dermal surface.

2.3.5 Conclusions

The grip of the basal epidermal cells depends primarily on the strength of the viscous bond at the dermo–epidermal interface, and secondarily on such other factors as the fibrous dermo–epidermal connections, the active movement of epidermal cells to retain their dermal proximity, and the interdigitation of the basal cell membrane into the superficial dermis. Only post-mitotic (phase 1) and dichophase cells (phase 2) lose their dermal grip, perhaps because in these phases the basal interdigitation is weakened.

The grip of a dichophase cell may be relatively weak or strong. If it is weak the cell is readily detached, the unpressurised basal layer is cubical, (according to the N ratio) the epidermis is relatively thin. If it is strong the basal layer is pressurised, the epithelium is columnar, and (according to the N ratio) the crowded basal layer is balanced by a relatively thick epidermis. This is normal hyperplasia and it develops irrespective of the mitotic rate.

In each body region the characteristic epidermal thickness is determined by the regional strength of basal cell grip, which is dermis-dependent.

2.4 The changing state

In any type of normal epidermis the probability that a dichophase cell will re-enter the mitotic process is equal to the probability that it will be forced distally to enter post-mitosis. However, after any form of damage, when the mitotic rate is increasing, the probability that a dichophase cell will re-enter the mitotic process temporarily exceeds the probability that it will become post-mitotic; the number of mitotic-cycle cells therefore increases. This leads to the production of the pathological form of hyperplasia which, when chronic, regains the steady state.

2.4.1 Pathological hyperplasia; epidermis

The explanation for the increase in the number of mitotic-cycle cells during an increase in the mitotic rate is simple: the fall in the chalone concentration allows the promitotic influence of the mesenchymal factor to extend further into the epidermis so that the suprabasal cells tend to become mitotic. Then with an increase in the number of mitotic-cycle cells there must be an equivalent increase in the number of post-mitotic cells (even though these are ageing and dying more rapidly), and the result is a thickened hyperplastic epithelium.

After epidermal damage the initial increase in the mitotic rate is due to the reduced length of the mitotic cycle. In man this reduction may be from approximately 308 to 37 h, which is mostly due to the reduction in the length of G_1 (the greater part of which is dichophase) from approximately 284 to 24 h (Flaxman and Chopra, 1972). Since in normal human epidermis about 90% of all basal cells are in the dichophase, this drastic dichophase shortening results in these cells entering the mitotic process en masse. There is then a wave of mitosis (Christophers, 1972b) which is presumably followed by an increase in basal cell crowding since not enough dichophase cells remain available for extrusion. However, any such cell crowding must be only transient; it is quickly relieved when the post-mitotic cells re-enter the dichophase en masse and when large numbers of cells are seen to be forced distally (Christophers, 1972b). Certainly no extra pressure builds up in the basal layer; no change has been found in either the nuclear height/ width ratio or in the number of basal cells per unit baseline area (Bullough and Deol, 1975b).

The whole process is then repeated as the cells, still in the form of a wave, pass through a second mitotic process, the numbers being augmented by extruded dichophase cells that remain in the mitotic cycle.

The return to the steady state occurs in one of two ways. If the damage heals, the chalone concentration rises to its normal level, mitosis is again confined to the basal layer, and as the number of mitotic-cycle cells is reduced, the epidermis again becomes thinner. Alternatively, if the damage is chronic, the steady state is attained as soon as the increase in the post-mitotic cell number comes to equal the increase in the mitotic-cycle cell number. By this time the wave of cells passing round the mitotic cycle has been damped out of existence and the flow of cells round the mitotic cycle is again uniform (the reason for this rapid damping is considered on p. 24).

2.4.2 Pathological hyperplasia; dermis

When the skin is damaged the mitotic response of the epidermis begins after only about 24 h (Bullough and Laurence, 1960a); in contrast the mitotic response of the dermis does not begin until after some 5 or 6 days (Bullough and Laurence, 1960b). Thus full hyperplasia is reached in two steps: the first leading to epidermal thickening and the second to dermal thickening. Dermal hyperplasia, which is mostly confined to the superficial dermis, depends on an increased number of dermal cells (see p. 31), an increased production of connective tissue, and a pronounced oedema.

As a result of the dermal thickening the hyperplastic epidermis is lifted upwards. In pig and man, but not in mouse, the basal epidermal layer retains at certain points its connexion with its original baseline, so that, with part of the epidermis lifted up and part remaining where it was, the dermo–epidermal junction becomes deeply folded. This greatly increases the dermal surface area and therefore the number of basal epidermal cells per unit area of skin. However, the number of cells per unit area of baseline remains unchanged (Bullough and Deol, 1975b).

This phenomenon needs further study. The expansion of the dermal surface could be due solely to changes in the dermis; these could lead either to a potential negative pressure that would be countered by a temporary lack of basal cell extrusion after mitosis or to a softening of the superficial dermis such that the mitoses would be unable to cause cell extrusion. Alternatively it could be epidermis-dependent, the dermal surface being forced to expand under the mitotic pressure as the basal epidermal cell layer lengthened and folded. It is also not known whether the redistribution of the mitotic-cycle cells that is brought about by the folding of the dermo–epidermal junction involves any change in the numbers of these cells per unit area of skin, and therefore any change in the degree of epidermal hyperplasia.

2.4.3 The release of pressure; vertical mitosis

The absence of any increase in pressure in the basal layer of hyperplastic epidermis is surprising. In particular, since an increased mitotic rate is accompanied by such a dramatic reduction in dichophase duration, it might be expected that the number of dichophase cells available for extrusion would become inadequate. Accurate figures are lacking but it can be roughly estimated that the ratio, dichophase cells : mitotic-process cells, which is normally about 10:1, changes in hyperplasia to about 1:1 or even less (derived from Flaxman and Chopra, 1972). Even a ratio of 1:1 does not mean that each mitosis will always find a dichophase cell locally available to be extruded.

Another factor, so far unexplored, that could contribute to a shortage of extrusible dichophase cells is the possibility that when, in hyperplasia, the dichophase half-life is reduced beyond a certain point the time available for dichophase cell extrusion may become inadequate.

If a shortage of locally available dichophase cells leads to basal layer pressure then this pressure is not countered by basal cell crowding, since such crowding is not observed (Bullough and Deol, 1975b); it may, however, be countered by vertically angled mitosis (when one daughter cell is directly extruded), which has been observed. In normal mouse epidermis the number of vertical mitoses is about 10%, while in the same epidermis made hyperplastic it rises to about 24% (Bullough and Deol, 1975b).

This problem was examined by computer, it being assumed that a cell in dichophase can be extruded 'instantaneously' (i.e. in less than the dichophase half-life), that the baseline is non-expandable, and that of the two daughter cells of each mitosis one occupies the space belonging to the parent cell while the other searches for a local extrusible dichophase cell. The biological validity of this last point is not certain. The extra space needed for the two daughter cells is claimed suddenly (in approximately 10–15 min) when the mitotic cell expands in early metaphase; the search for a local dichophase cell would have to be completed within less than the metaphase duration (1 h in man to 2–4 h in mouse; Flaxman and Chopra, 1972; Bullough and Laurence, 1966); and the dichophase cell would have to be recognised because it is flaccid or because it can be extruded before the end of the metaphase. Both these suggestions are speculative.

The computer analysis tested the relationship between the potential pressure (represented by the vertical mitoses) and the mitotic rate (represented by the dichophase half-life and by the duration of G_{1c}-S-G_2-M-G_{1a}). Over a wide range of real values for the dichophase half-life and for the duration of the mitotic process, it was found that the potential pressure due to the lack of extrusible dichophase cells remains low, but that when the dichophase half-life shrinks sufficiently (to about 15 to 10 h) the pressure rises extremely rapidly (at about 7 to 5 h). Over this short span the system passes from stability to potential instability as the increasing number of new cells produced markedly decreases the probability that sufficient extrusible dichophase cells will be locally available.

Two systems have been described that are near, or actually in, this extreme condition. The first is hyperplastic ear epidermis: using the recorded mitotic rate the computer predicted a vertical mitoses rate of 15–30%; the measured value, as mentioned above, was about 24% (Bullough and Deol, 1975b). The second more dramatic example is the active hair bulb which has the highest mitotic rate yet recorded in any mammalian tissue: the whole mitotic cycle is complete within about 12 h (Bullough and Laurence, 1958; Cattaneo et al., 1961) and the dichophase half-life must be less than 3 h. The potential pressure must therefore be maximal and all the mitoses should be vertical. Observations have shown that this is indeed what happens (Bullough and Deol, 1975b).

2.4.4 Conclusions

The loss of chalone after epidermal damage leads to an increase in the number of mitotic-cycle cells per unit skin area; according to the N ratio there must then be a similar increase in the number of post-mitotic cells; and the epidermis therefore thickens. This is the essence of pathological hyperplasia.

This is also evidently the essence of target-tissue hyperplasia in response to the appropriate mitogenic hormone. Such a hormone may act by specifically neutralising the chalone of the target tissue (Bullough, 1967).

With a high mitotic rate the supply of basal extrusible dichophase cells becomes inadequate. The potential rise in basal layer pressure is then countered by an increased number of vertically oriented mitoses. In a hair bulb, with no dichophase cells available, all mitoses are vertical.

Evidently a sequence of responses exists for relieving mitosis-generated basal layer pressure. In order of increasing resistance they are: extrusion of basal post-mitotic cells, extrusion of dichophase cells, and vertical orientation of mitosis. To these may be added the effect of dermal hyperplasia which, in pig and man, increases the area of the superficial dermis.

2.5 Outstanding problems

There are a number of important problems relating to the present argument for which adequate explanations are lacking.

2.5.1 The G_2 inhibition

The epidermal chalone, the first to be discovered was recognised by its power to inhibit the mitotic process in the G_2 phase (Bullough and Laurence, 1960a, 1964a). Later, with the development of the tritiated thymidine technique for labelling S phase cells, evidence began to accumulate that epidermis may contain two different chalones, the one acting in late G_1 and the other in G_2 (see Hall, 1969; Elgjo, 1973). This still needs confirmation; the apparently differing molecular weights of the epidermal G_1 and G_2 chalones, like those of the various tissue chalones (see Houck and Daugherty, 1974), could be due to the binding of the chalone molecule, specifically or non-specifically, to other molecules.

The role of a G_1 chalone is obvious; it is part of the mechanism whereby the choice is made between mitosis and post-mitosis. The role of the G_2 chalone is obscure. Indeed the ability of this chalone to inhibit in the G_2 phase can only be demonstrated by the injection of extra amounts of the substance; the normal chalone concentration in the epidermal cells provides no obvious impediment to the passage of a G_2 cell into mitosis. The naturally occurring impediment at this point is provided by the stress hormones, and especially by adrenalin, which acts in association with the chalone (Bullough and Laurence, 1964a) perhaps via the cyclic AMP concentration (Elgjo, 1975).

This involvement of the stress hormones is the basis of the diurnal mitotic cycle. When an animal is awake the high adrenalin concentration prevents those epidermal cells that arrive in G_2 from entering mitosis, and consequently the longer sleep is delayed the greater is the number of arrested cells. When sleep begins and the adrenalin concentration falls, the accumulated G_2 cells enter mitosis in a wave (Bullough and Laurence, 1961).

Thus in normal epidermis there is a rhythmic production of new cells, a rhythmic rise in basal layer pressure, and a rhythmic extrusion of basal post-mitotic cells (mouse) or dichophase cells (pig and man).

The significance of this phenomenon is unknown. However, it could be suggested that in normal epidermis the basal layer pressure is so low that the extra pressure produced by isolated mitoses would be inadequate to force the extrusion of any dichophase cells; Leun et al. (1974a) have shown that below a certain pressure the basal epidermal cells can never be separated from the dermis however long the pressure is applied. If this is so then two possible solutions exist: the basal layer cells, being unable to leave, would become increasingly crowded until the pressure reached a high enough level, but this would lead to the thickened epidermis of normal hyperplasia (p. 16); or the mitoses could be synchronised so that the surge of mitotic pressure reaches a high enough level to cause the extrusion of the dichophase cells.

One conclusion is, however, certain: neither the adrenalin alone nor the chalone alone can inhibit in the G_2 phase. In some unexplained way they operate together (see Laurence et al., 1972). The consequence is that, as the chalone concentration falls and the mitotic rate rises towards hyperplasia, the diurnal mitotic cycle begins to fade out; in hyperplastic epidermis, as in all tissues with an especially high mitotic rate, there is little or no diurnal variation (Bullough and Laurence, 1957, 1961).

2.5.2 The duration of the dichophase

The data published by cell kineticists give the impression that, for any particular mitotic rate in any particular tissue, the duration of each phase of the mitotic cycle is fixed. However, in epidermis the duration of G_2 depends on how long the animal remains awake (Bullough and Laurence, 1961), while the duration of the dichophase can be expressed only in terms of its half-life so that at any moment there is 'a constant probability that DNA synthesis will commence during the following minute' (Cattaneo et al., 1961).

Recently Smith and Martin (1973, 1974), following Bürk (1970), have re-examined the problem of the intermitotic period and have also concluded that cells re-enter the mitotic process at random 'in the sense that radioactive decay is random'. At any given mitotic rate the probability of a dichophase cell re-entering the mitotic process is constant; any change in the mitotic rate is the result of a change in the value of this probability.

Applied to epidermis this concept provides stability in the present model of cellular homeostasis (p. 9). It also explains the rapid damping of the mitotic wave that follows any form of damage (p. 19). The first wave has a spread of about 10 h (Christophers, 1972b), which reflects the greatly shortened dichophase half-life; the second wave then flattens in relation to the half-lives of the first generation of dichophase cells which already show the 10 h spread; the third wave is damped almost to extinction.

2.5.3 The chalone trigger mechanism

Once a cell enters the mitotic process the decision is irreversible; entry is controlled by a trigger mechanism (Bullough, 1965, 1967). The concept of a dichophase half-life suggests that a low chalone concentration (or effectiveness) does not itself trigger the dichophase cell into the mitotic process, but rather that it acts by increasing the probability that the cell will be so triggered.

Smith and Martin (1974) conclude that there must be a single triggering event which occurs at random. They speculate on the joint problems of how the randomness of the event is generated and of how its frequency of occurrence is controlled. For the present model these problems have no great significance but one possibility does arise. The fate of a dichophase cell may depend on the number, or proportion, of receptor sites that are occupied by chalone molecules; these sites may be in the cytoplasm or on the cell surface. If the occupation of a site is unstable so that the situation is constantly changing, entry into the mitotic process could depend on a small enough number of sites being occupied for a long enough period for the trigger to operate. Post-mitosis, which for a time is reversible, would then depend on a large enough number of sites being constantly occupied.

2.5.4 Conclusions

The main conclusion from this evidence must be that the present model of epidermal mitotic control and cellular homeostasis is incomplete. The unsolved problems are important and must now be studied further. When new data are forthcoming and fitted into the framework of the present model, this framework may well need significant modification.

2.6 Pathological conditions

There remains to be considered the response of the tissue homeostatic mechanism during wound healing and tissue regeneration, and also the state of the chalone mechanism in cancer cells. Except in the case of wound healing, most of the available evidence comes from tissues other than epidermis, and it is therefore necessary to widen the discussion.

2.6.1 Wound healing

The two main problems in tissue regeneration concern the reactions of the affected cells and the manner in which the lost tissue is replaced in spite of the fact that an increase in the rate of cell gain is always matched by an increase in the rate of cell loss. There are two situations to consider: small-scale tissue loss leading to wound healing, and large-scale tissue loss leading, but only in some tissues, to compensatory hypertrophy.

The reaction to a wound is strictly local: in epidermis the first response is the migration of epidermal cells from the wound edges over the exposed dermis (Winter, 1972); the second response is the local increase in the mitotic rate (Bullough and Laurence, 1960a).

In theory, all that is necessary to re-establish the epidermis is epidermal migration. The normal epidermal structure and thickness would then be re-created as the normal mitotic activity produced new distal cells that aged and synthesised keratin at the normal rate. However, this would be a slow process with the first keratin squames being formed only after some 14–21 days (in man) and with the build-up of the stratum corneum taking much longer.

In practice, the high mitotic activity that develops both in the wound edges, and in the re-surfacing cells once they have ceased migrating, results in the rapid production of new distal cells that quickly age to produce keratin. This high mitotic rate is caused by a fall of about 50% in the chalone content of the affected cells (Bullough, 1969), which is evidently due to cell membrane damage. The mitotic activity may reach about 17 times the normal maximum sleep level (Bullough and Deol, 1975a), which means that it must be even higher since it is not subject to a diurnal rhythm (Bullough and Laurence, 1957, 1961).

This greatly increased rate of cell production is matched by the greatly reduced life-span of the newly-forming post-mitotic distal cells; in human epidermis, from approximately 14–21 days to approximately 4–5 days (Scott and Ekel, 1963). However, epidermal recovery is normally complete within this reduced time limit, the cell membranes recover, the chalone concentration rises, the mitotic rate and the rate of post-mitotic ageing both fall, and the newly-formed distal cells acquire the normal post-mitotic life span. Cell gain is achieved without cell loss.

If the wound is wide so that wound closure takes longer than the reduced time limit, the mechanism still works efficiently: the high mitotic activity, in the form of a wave, follows the advancing edges of the sheet of migrating epidermal cells (Bullough and Laurence, 1960a) so that in each successive area healing is complete within the reduced life-span of the newly-formed distal cells.

When epidermal damage is chronic this shorter post-mitotic life-span operates as a safety mechanism. The high rate of cell production is offset by the equally high rate of cell death and the situation stabilises in hyperplasia.

This type of local response to local damage may or may not be regarded as a form of chalone-controlled negative feedback mechanism. The basic control evidently lies in the cell membranes. It is only when these return to normal that the chalone concentration, and therefore the mitotic rate, can follow suit.

2.6.2 *Compensatory hypertrophy; the plateau phenomenon*

In massive tissues, but not in small tissues, large scale loss or damage leads to a pattern of response called compensatory hypertrophy. This cannot be studied in epidermis since large-scale epidermal destruction is fatal. The main information comes from hepatocytes, kidney cells, granulocytes and erythrocytes (see Bullough, 1975).

Local liver damage leads to the local mitotic response typical of wound healing, but large-scale liver damage, or partial hepatectomy, produces a general mitotic response throughout the whole remaining hepatocyte population, including liver tissue implanted at a distance or situated in a parabiotic twin (Bucher et al., 1951; Leong et al., 1964; and see Bullough, 1965). This general mitotic response begins only when 10% of the liver has been excised, from which point onwards the increase in the mitotic rate is in direct proportion to the amount of liver removed (Bucher, 1963; Bucher and Swaffield, 1964). The response continues until the hepatocyte mass is again normal, when it ceases. The reactions of the kidney, erythrocyte, and granulocyte systems are essentially similar, although in the last two the reactions are more complex (Bullough, 1975).

With tissues whose mass is great in relation to the total body mass there is evidently a considerable systemic chalone concentration; this results in the establishment of a dynamic balance between the higher chalone concentration within the tissue cells and the lower chalone concentration in the body, especially the blood. In such a system a sudden reduction in chalone synthesis following large-scale tissue loss must lead to an equivalent fall in the systemic chalone concentration, and consequently to an increased rate of chalone loss from the remaining tissue fragment. There is therefore a general rise in the mitotic activity which is proportional to the degree of tissue loss.

The recovery of the normal tissue mass then differs from that seen in wound healing only in degree. The newly-formed post-mitotic cells have a reduced life-span (in rat hepatocytes from the normal 200–450 days to approximately 26 days; MacDonald, 1961) but they are not lost since the normal tissue mass is regained within the time available. The chalone concentration then returns to normal and the post-mitotic cells acquire their normal life span. If the damage is chronic (as in liver cirrhosis; MacDonald, 1961) the short post-mitotic life span acts in the usual way as a safety mechanism to prevent excessive tissue growth.

This type of response is a simple negative feedback mechanism. The tissue mass plateaus at a point relative to the systemic chalone concentration; even if the damage is chronic the tissue mass still plateaus but at a higher level that is termed hyperplasia.

Clearly such a situation can only exist in massive tissues. With small tissues the systemic chalone concentration must be negligible, its reduction will be imperceptible, and compensatory hypertrophy cannot occur.

2.6.3 Tumour formation; the plateau phenomenon

Recent studies of a wide range of tumours from several animal species, including man, have indicated that tumour cells continue to synthesise the chalone of their tissue of origin and continue to respond by mitotic inhibition to that same chalone (see Bullough, 1975). The basic abnormality of these cells is evidently that they fail to hold the chalone they produce, whether inside themselves as originally suggested by Bullough (1971), or on their cell membranes as later suggested by Houck and Daugherty (1974). The chalone loss is so great that the 'distal cells' do not retain enough to ensure that they will enter post-mitosis; this breaks the homeostatic mechanism and ensures that cell gain exceeds cell loss.

The excessive chalone loss from the tumour cells (it may reach 90%; Bullough, 1975) leads to an excessive chalone concentration in the blood (Rytömaa and Kiviniemi, 1968b); the larger the tumour the higher the systemic concentration (Bullough and Deol, 1971a).

The progressive growth of a tumour should therefore have two consequences: first, it should cause a progressive inhibition of the mitotic activity of its tissue of origin, and second, it should progressively inhibit itself. The first point is illustrated, for example, during the growth of an epidermal carcinoma when the mitotic activity of the entire epidermis is steadily reduced, the other body tissues being unaffected (Bullough and Deol, 1971a). Epidermal mitotic activity may ultimately almost cease, but the epidermis, being then in phase 1, does not become thinner.

The second response, beginning later, is that of the tumour itself. It is well established that tumour growth typically follows a sigmoid curve (Laird, 1964, 1965, 1969; Burns, 1969; Bichel, 1972), which has commonly been explained in terms of deteriorating conditions due, for instance, to the failure of the blood supply or to the accumulation of toxic byproducts. Certainly such factors may play a part (Bullough and Deol, 1971b), as may also an immune response, but the dominant factor is commonly the chalone itself. Bichel (1973) has explained the sigmoid curve as exponential growth limited by an exponential retardation caused by the increasing systemic concentration of a mitotic inhibitor produced by the increasing number of tumour cells. From a series of experiments with a number of chronic ascites tumours, he has provided clear evidence that each tumour inhibits its own growth in a tumour-specific manner by the synthesis of a substance with the characteristics of a chalone (Bichel, 1970, 1971, 1972, 1973).

A chronic tumour is one that reaches a plateau that the animal can support; a lethal tumour is one in which the plateau level is too high for the animal to survive. A chronic tumour at the plateau level may at any time begin to grow again if any of its cells suffer further damage of a kind that reduces its chalone content to a still lower level. This is the phenomenon of progression (Foulds, 1969), which may make the plateau a receding goal until finally it cannot be reached before the animal dies.

2.6.4 *Conclusions*

The abnormal mitotic activity adjacent to wounds, during compensatory hypertrophy, and in tumours is in all cases related to excessive chalone loss from the affected cells.

Wound healing is a local event. The higher mitotic rate is matched by a shorter post-mitotic life span. However, since healing is normally completed within this shorter period, the post-mitotic cells, before they can die, acquire the normal longer life span. Thus cells gained are not lost.

Compensatory hypertrophy is similar except that the mitotic response is general throughout the tissue, evidently because of a general chalone loss in response to a reduced systemic chalone level. Only a tissue massive enough to create a significant systemic chalone level can be regenerated in this way. Again, the cells gained are not lost.

Tumour cells synthesise and respond to their tissue chalone, but they lose it at such a high rate that not enough remains to ensure distal post-mitosis. The homeostatic mechanism therefore breaks down. As the tumour grows the systemic chalone concentration rises until it reaches a level that is high enough to inhibit any further tumour growth; a chronic tumour plateaus without killing its host; a lethal tumour would have reached a plateau if its host could have survived.

Thus in compensatory hypertrophy the tissue mass plateaus at the normal systemic chalone level, while in tumour growth the cell mass plateaus at a higher than normal systemic chalone level.

2.7 *General conclusions*

The main question arising from this analysis of the epidermal chalone mechanism, and of its ramifications, is whether this method of cellular homeostasis is specific to the epidermis or whether it is also typical of the other mitotic tissues of the adult mammal.

2.7.1 The chalone mechanism

This may be taken to comprise not only the chalone itself but also the antichalonal mesenchymal factor; acting together they maintain the permanent gradient of chalone effectiveness on which cellular homeostasis depends. Chalone systems have been described in some 20 tissues, that is in every tissue in which they have been sought; the promitotic action of the mesenchymal factor has been described in some 10 tissues, again in every tissue in which it has been sought (Bullough, 1975).

The gradient model of cellular homeostasis also seems to be generally applicable to the epithelial tissues. Mitotic activity tends to be confined to cells that are connective–tissue–adjacent, as is particularly obvious in the various tissues of the skin. The fate of a cell is determined by its position, basal or distal, within the tissue. In all cases the original chalone message is tissue-specific but in all cases it is probable that the ensuing sequence of cellular responses, leading to the activation of either the genes for mitosis or the genes for post-mitosis, shows no tissue-specificity.

Without the chalone the cells of a tissue remain mitotic and will explode into a tumour (see below); without the mesenchymal factor all cells will become post-mitotic and the tissue will disappear (as in the dispersed tissues; p. 31).

2.7.2 The plateau phenomenon

Chalone control is normally exercised locally within each tissue but when the tissue is massive it also exercises a systemic effect. This is because such a tissue produces enough chalone to create a significant blood concentration; a dynamic balance then develops between the intra- and extra-tissue chalone levels; and since the tissue chalone concentration is then dependent on the systemic chalone concentration, the tissue mass can only plateau when the systemic chalone concentration reaches a 'normal' level.

A similar conclusion applies to any large tumour. The general rule is emerging that cancer cells synthesise, and respond normally to, the chalone of their tissue of origin, but that because of their abnormal cell membranes they are unable to retain their chalone. The growth of a tumour is therefore accompanied by a rising systemic chalone concentration, which inhibits, first, the mitotic activity of the tumour's tissue of origin, and later, the mitotic activity of the tumour itself. Again a dynamic balance develops between the tumour chalone concentration and the blood chalone concentration, and tumour growth reaches a plateau and ceases when the blood chalone concentration reaches a high enough, but now abnormal, level.

2.7.3 Non-epithelial tissues

These comprise three main groups: the non-mitotic nervous and muscular tissues, the various dispersed tissues, and the connective tissues.

The non-mitotic tissues were, of course, all mitotic at an early stage of development, and although no studies have been made, it may be reasonably presumed that, at that time, they were controlled by typical chalone mechanisms. The initial loss of mitotic activity may have been due to the increasing power of the chalone within the cells, but in the adult the loss of mitotic potential has become permanent. Evidently the mitotic genes have been silenced in the same way as were all the other alternative genetic potentialities of the cells during embryonic differentiation. Whether the one remaining genetic programme, post-mitosis-with-ageing, is still under the influence of a chalone system is not known; there is some evidence that it may be (Bullough, 1973).

The dispersed tissues, such as the erythrocytes and granulocytes, are particularly interesting because, although they possess typical chalone systems (Rytömaa and Kiviniemi, 1968a; Kivilaakso and Rytömaa, 1971), they are evidently not connective-tissue-based. Without the mesenchymal factor they should quickly disappear, and this in fact they would do were they not able continuously to recruit new cells from a relatively undifferentiated stem cell population by means of an embryonic-type differentiation. This stem cell population is connective-tissue-based within the bone marrow and is therefore self-supporting.

A similar stem cell system may provide for the replacement of the various connective tissue cells, which clearly poses a special problem. Although these cells may continually synthesise the promitotic mesenchymal factor they typically show no mitotic activity; when, after damage to the skin, mitotic connective tissue cells appear in the area to contribute to dermal hyperplasia and regeneration, these cells have evidently come from a relatively undifferentiated stem cell population that exists somewhere else in the body (Winter, 1973; Sumrall and Johnson, 1973). The type of connective tissue cell into which these immigrating stem cells are transformed depends on the type of connective tissue that they encounter on arrival. An extensive study of cell replacement in the various connective tissues is now needed; it is already known that fibroblasts have their own specific chalone system (Houck et al., 1972, 1973).

2.7.4 Tissue mass

The mass of the epidermis is determined by the area of the dermo–epidermal boundary and by the epidermal thickness, which is itself a function of the R and N ratios. This conclusion applies to epithelial tissues in general, whether the epithelial–mesenchymal boundary is flat, as in any typical lining epithelium, or whether it is folded into a complex network, as in a solid tissue such as the liver.

Variations in the basic tissue mass also occur commonly giving rise to either hypo- or hyperplasia. Thus in normal circumstances a weak mesenchymal grip produces the uncrowded cubical cells typical of a thinner epithelium, while a strong mesenchymal grip produces the crowded columnar cells, sometimes on a folded baseline, typical of a thicker epithelium.

In abnormal circumstances hypo- and hyperplasia are the results of changes in the mitotic rate. Such hypoplasia occurs in chronic stress and in old age; such hyperplasia occurs to a greater or lesser degree after any form of tissue damage. Similar responses also occur in hormone-dependent tissues: hypoplasia due to a low mitotic rate is seen in the thin epithelium of an unstimulated vagina or in the small mass of an unstimulated prostate; hyperplasia due to a high mitotic rate is seen when these tissues are stimulated by the appropriate hormones.

Both normal and abnormal hypo- and hyperplasia depend on the N ratio; any increase in the number of basal mitotic-cycle cells, by whatever means it is achieved, leads to an equivalent increase in the number of post-mitotic cells; this response is then always countered by an increase in the speed at which the post-mitotic cells pass to their deaths.

There are a number of specialised variations on this theme. Thus, for example, in the duodenal lining epithelium the high mitotic rate is offset not by epithelial thickening but by the facility with which the post-mitotic cells slide sideways along the mesenchymal boundary to their deaths in the duodenal lumen.

2.7.5 Generalisations

It is becoming clearer that all mammalian tissues maintain cellular homeostasis by the same type of chalone mechanism, although some of them, for specialised reasons, have developed their own variations on the common theme. It is also becoming clearer that when cellular homeostasis breaks down the cells of the resulting tumour typically show a reduced chalone concentration while retaining their ability to respond normally by mitotic inhibition to the chalone of their tissue of origin.

References

Bichel, P. (1970) Tumor growth inhibiting effect of JB-1 ascitic fluid. Europ. J. Cancer 6, 291–296.

Bichel, P. (1971) Autoregulation of ascites tumour growth by inhibition of the G_1 and G_2 phase. Europ. J. Cancer 7, 349–355.

Bichel, P. (1972) Specific growth regulation in three ascites tumours. Europ. J. Cancer 8, 167–173.

Bichel, P. (1973) Self-limitation of ascites tumor growth: a possible chalone regulation. Natl. Cancer Inst. Mon. 38, 197–203.

Billingham, R. E. and Silvers, W. K. (1968) Dermoepidermal interactions and epithelial specificity. In: Epithelial-Mesenchymal Interactions (eds. R. Fleischmajer and R. E. Billingham), pp. 252–266. Baltimore: Williams & Wilkins.

Braun-Falco, O. (1971) Dynamics of growth and regression in psoriatic lesions: alterations in the skin from normal into a psoriatic lesion, and during regression of psoriatic lesions. In: Psoriasis (eds. E. M. Farber and A. J. Cox), pp. 215–237. Stanford: University Press.

Briggaman, R. A. and Wheeler, C. E. (1968) Epidermal–dermal interactions in adult human skin: role of dermis in epidermal maintenance. J. Invest. Derm. 51, 454–465.

Brody, I. (1960) The ultrastructure of the tonofibrils in the keratinization process of normal human epidermis. J. Ultrastructure Res. 4, 264–297.

Bucher, N. L. R. (1963) Regeneration of mammalian liver. Int. Rev. Cyt. 15, 245–300.

Bucher, N. L. R. and Swaffield, M. N. (1964) The rate of incorporation of labeled thymidine into the desoxyribonucleic acid of regenerating rat liver in relation to the amount of liver excised. Cancer Res. 24, 1611–1625.

Bucher, N. L. R., Scott, G. F. and Aub, J. C. (1951) Regeneration of the liver in parabiotic rats. Cancer Res. 11, 457–465.

Bullough, W. S. (1962) The control of mitotic activity in adult mammalian tissues. Biol. Rev. 37, 307–342.

Bullough, W. S. (1965) Mitotic and functional homeostasis. Cancer Res. 25, 1683–1727.

Bullough, W. S. (1967) The Evolution of Differentiation. London: Academic Press.

Bullough, W. S. (1969) Epithelial repair. In: Repair and Regeneration (eds. J. E. Dunphy and W. van Winkle), pp. 35–46. New York: McGraw-Hill.

Bullough, W. S. (1971) The actions of the chalones. Agents Actions 2, 1–7.

Bullough, W. S. (1972) The control of epidermal thickness. Brit. J. Derm. 87, 187–199; 347–354.

Bullough, W. S. (1973) Ageing of mammals. Zeitschr. Alternsforsch. 27, 247–253.

Bullough, W. S. (1975) Mitotic control in adult mammalian tissues. Biol. Rev. 50, 99–130.

Bullough, W. S. and Deol, J. U. R. (1971a) Chalone-induced mitotic inhibition in the Hewitt keratinising epidermal carcinoma of the mouse. Europ. J. Cancer 7, 425–431.

Bullough, W. S. and Deol, J. U. R. (1971b) The pattern of tumour growth. Symp. Soc. Exp. Biol. 25, 255–275.

Bullough, W. S. and Deol, J. U. R. (1975a) Dermo-epidermal adhesion and its effect on epidermal structure in the mouse. Brit. J. Derm. 92, 417–424.

Bullough, W. S. and Deol, J. U. R. (1975b) Unpublished.

Bullough, W. S. and Ebling, F. J. (1952) Cell replacement in the epidermis and sebaceous glands of the mouse. J. Anat. 86, 29–34.

Bullough, W. S. and Laurence, E. B. (1957) A technique for the study of small epidermal wounds. Brit. J. Exp. Path. 38, 273–277.

Bullough, W. S. and Laurence, E. B. (1958) The mitotic activity of the follicle. In: The Biology of Hair Growth (eds. W. Montagna and R. A. Ellis), pp. 171–187. London: Academic Press.

Bullough, W. S. and Laurence, E. B. (1960a) The control of epidermal mitotic activity in the mouse. Proc. Roy. Soc. B 151, 517–536.

Bullough, W. S. and Laurence, E. B. (1960b) The control of mitotic activity in mouse skin. Dermis and hypodermis. Exp. Cell Res. 21, 394–405.

Bullough, W. S. and Laurence, E. B. (1961) Stress and adrenaline in relation to the diurnal cycle of epidermal mitotic activity in adult male mice. Proc. Roy. Soc. B 154, 540–556.

Bullough, W. S. and Laurence, E. B. (1964a) Mitotic control by internal secretion: the role of the chalone-adrenalin complex. Exp. Cell Res. 33, 176–194.

Bullough, W. S. and Laurence, E. B. (1964b) The production of epidermal cells. Symp. Zool. Soc. Lond. 12, 1–26.

Bullough, W. S. and Laurence, E. B. (1966) The diurnal cycle in epidermal mitotic duration and its relation to chalone and adrenaline. Exp. Cell Res. 43, 343–350.

Bürk, R. R. (1970) One-step growth cycle for BHK 21/13 hamster fibroblasts. Exp. Cell Res. 63, 309–316.

Burns, E. R. (1969) On the failure of self-inhibition of growth of tumours. Growth 33, 25–45.

Cattaneo, S. M., Quastler, H. and Sherman, F. G. (1961) Proliferative cycle in the growing hair follicle of the mouse. Nature 190, 923–924.

Christophers, E. (1971) Cellular architecture of the stratum corneum. J. Invest. Derm. 56, 165–169.

Christophers, E. (1972a) Correlation between column formation, thickness and rate of new cell production in guinea pig epidermis. Virch. Arch. Abtl. B Zellpath. 10, 286–292.

Christophers, E. (1972b) Kinetic aspects of epidermal healing. In: Epidermal Wound Healing (eds. H. I. Maibach and D. T. Rovee), pp. 53–69. Chicago: Year Book Medical Publishers.

Elgjo, K. (1973) Epidermal chalone: cell cycle specificity of two epidermal growth inhibitors. Natl. Cancer Inst. Mon. 38, 71–76.

Elgjo, K. (1975) Epidermal chalone and cyclic AMP: an in vivo study. J. Invest. Derm. 64, 14–18.

Flaxman, B. A. and Chopra, D. P. (1972) Cell cycle of normal and psoriatic epidermis in vitro. J. Invest. Derm. 59, 102–105.

Foulds, L. (1969) Neoplastic Development, Vol. 1. London: Academic Press.

Frankfurt, O. S. (1967) Cell proliferation and differentiation in the squamous epithelium of the forestomach of the mouse. Exp. Cell Res. 46, 603–606.

Hall, R. G. (1969) DNA synthesis in organ cultures of the hamster cheek pouch. Exp. Cell Res. 58, 421–439.

Houck, J. C. and Daugherty, W. F. (1974) Chalones: A Tissue-Specific Approach to Mitotic Control. New York: Medcom.

Houck, J. C., Sharma, V. K. and Cheng, R. F. (1973) Fibroblast chalone and serum mitogen (antichalone). Nature New Biol. 246, 111–113.

Houck, J. C., Weil, R. L. and Sharma, V. K. (1972) Evidence for a fibroblast chalone. Nature New Biol. 240, 210–211.

Igarashi, Y. and Yaoi, Y. (1975) Growth enhancing protein obtained from cell surface of cultured fibroblasts. Nature 254, 248–250.

Iversen, O. H. (1965) Cybernetic aspects of the cancer problem. Prog. Biocybern. 2, 76–110.

Iversen, O. H. and Bjerknes, R. (1963) Kinetics of epidermal reaction to carcinogens. Acta Path. Microbiol. Scand. Suppl. 165, 165–174.

Kiistala, U. (1972) Dermal–epidermal separation. Ann. Clin. Res. 4, 236–246.

Kivilaakso, E. and Rytömaa, T. (1971) Erythrocytic chalone, a tissue-specific inhibitor of cell proliferation in the erythron. Cell Tiss. Kin. 4, 1–9.

Kobayasi, T. (1961) An electron microscope study on the dermoepidermal junction. Acta Derm. Venerol. Stockh. 41, 481–491.

Laird, A. K. (1964) Dynamics of tumour growth. Brit. J. Cancer 18, 490–502.

Laird, A. K. (1965) Dynamics of tumour growth. Brit. J. Cancer 19, 278–291.

Laird, A. K. (1969) Dynamics of growth in tumors and in normal organisms. Natl. Cancer Inst. Mon. 30, 15–28.

Laurence, E. B., Randers Hansen, E., Christophers, E. and Rytömaa, T. (1972) Systemic factors influencing epidermal mitosis. Europ. J. Clin. Biol. Res. 27, 133–139.

Leong, G. F., Grisham, J. W., Hole, B. W. and Albright, M. L. (1964) Effect of partial hepatectomy on DNA synthesis and mitosis in heterotopic partial autografts of rat liver. Cancer Res. 24, 1496–1501.

Leun, G. C. van der, Beerens, E. G. J. and Lowe, L. B. (1974a) Repair of dermal-epidermal adherence. J. Invest. Derm. 63, 397–401.

Leun, G. C. van der, Lowe, L. B. and Beerens, E. G. J. (1974b) The influence of skin temperature on dermal-epidermal adherence. J. Invest. Derm. 62, 42–46.

MacDonald, R. A. (1961) Lifespan of liver cells. Arch. Internal Med. 107, 335–343.

MacKenzie, I. C. (1970) Relationship between mitosis and the ordered structure of the stratum corneum in mouse epidermis. Nature 226, 653–655.

McLoughlin, C. B. (1961) Importance of mesenchymal factors in differentiation of chick epidermis. II. Modification of epidermal differentiation by contact with different types of mesenchyme. J. Embr. Exp. Morph. 9, 385–409.

Osgood, E. E. (1957) A unifying concept of the etiology of the leukemias, lymphomas, and cancers. J. Natl. Cancer Inst., 18, 155–166.

Palade, G. E. and Farquhar, M. G. (1965) A special fibril of the dermis. J. Cell Biol. 27, 215–224.

Rytömaa, T. and Kiviniemi, K. (1964) In vitro experiments for demonstration of specific feedback factors in rat serum. Proc. XIV Scand. Congr. Pathol. Microbiol., 169. Universitetsforlaget, Oslo.

Rytömaa, T. and Kiviniemi, K. (1968a) Control of granulocyte production. Cell Tiss. Kin. 1, 329–340; 341–350.

Rytömaa, T. and Kiviniemi, K. (1968b) Control of DNA duplication in rat chloroleukaemia by means of the granulocyte chalone. Europ. J. Cancer 4, 595–606.

Schmidt, W., Richter, J. and Geissler, R. (1974) The dermo–epidermal junction of the human skin. Zeitschr. Anat. Entwicklungsgesch. 145, 283–298.

Scott, E. J. van and Ekel, T. M. (1963) Kinetics of hyperplasia in psoriasis. Arch. Derm. 88, 373–381.

Smith, J. A. and Martin, L. (1973) Do cells cycle? Proc. Natl. Acad. Sci. USA 70, 1263–1267.

Smith, J. A. and Martin, L. (1974) Regulation of cell proliferation. In: Cell Cycle Controls (eds. G. M. Padilla, I. L. Cameron and A. Zimmerman), pp. 43–60. New York: Academic Press.

Sumrall, A. J. and Johnson, W. C. (1973) The origin of dermal fibrocytes in wound repair. Dermatologia 146, 107–114.

Weiss, P. and Kavanau, J. L. (1957) A model of growth and growth control in mathematical terms. J. Gen. Physiol. 41, 1–47.

Winter, G. D. (1972) Epidermal regeneration in the domestic pig. In: Epidermal Wound Healing (eds. H. I. Maibach and D. T. Rovee), pp. 71–112. Chicago: Year Book Medical Publishers.

Winter, G. D. (1973) Studies, using sponge implants, on the mechanism of osteogenesis. In: Biology of the Fibroblast (eds. E. Kulonen and J. Pikkarainen), pp. 103–125. London: Academic Press.

Yaoi, Y. and Kanaseki, T. (1972) Role of microexudate carpet in cell division. Nature 237, 283–285.

CHAPTER 3

The history of chalones

OLAV HILMAR IVERSEN

Institute of Pathology, University of Oslo, Rikshospitalet, Oslo 1, Norway

3.1 The name

> What's in a name? That which we call a rose
> By any other name would smell as sweet;
> (*Romeo and Juliet*, Act II, Sc. ii)

The term 'chalone' is surrounded by a good deal of controversy. I have met several research workers who said they believed in growth-inhibitory substances, but not in chalones. The word seems to be emotionally laden with positive values for the congregation of chalone-believers, and with rather strong negative values for many sceptics, especially those of British extraction. There is nothing new in fighting about words ('Mit Wörter lässt sich trefflich streiten', *Faust*, 1790), however, what we choose to call a substance is in the long run of little importance, since reality will either give a specific meaning to the name, or – the name will soon be forgotten.

The word chalone was probably first used at the Seventeenth International Congress of Medicine, the minutes of which were printed in the British Medical Journal of August 16, 1913 (fig. 3.1). In 1906 E. H. Starling had proposed the term 'hormone' as a name for stimulatory signal substances. At the above meeting, Sir E. A. Schäfer suggested that a special name was needed for those substances which were inhibitory in action, and suggested the word 'chalone', from the Greek *chalao*, meaning to loosen or to lower. It is often used in the New Testament, e.g. when the ship with St. Paul as a prisoner on board (The Acts, 27, 17) was caught in a heavy storm off the coast of Crete, the crew had to 'chalone' to reduce the speed of the ship. This has been translated in various English Bible versions as 'shorten the

𝕭𝖗𝖎𝖙𝖎𝖘𝖍 𝕸𝖊𝖉𝖎𝖈𝖆𝖑 𝕵𝖔𝖚𝖗𝖓𝖆𝖑.

AUGUST 16ᴛʜ, 1913.

London, August 6th to 12th.

CONTENTS.

Seventeenth International Congress of Medicine.

Sir E. A. Schäfer dealt with the classification of hormones, and contended that the word "hormone," derived by Professor Starling from ὁρμάω, to stir up or excite, suggested merely an exciting agent, but that nowadays it was applied in too broad a fashion to all internal secretions, whether excitant or inhibitory in nature. He suggested that a special name was needed for those substances which were inhibitory in action, and offered the word "chalone" (from χαλάω, to loosen), leaving the term "hormone" for the excitants. This would necessitate the coining of a comprehensive word to include both hormones and chalones, and for this Professor W. R. Wardle had suggested "autacoid" (ἄκος, a remedy). Thus the expression "autocoid substance" would denote any drug-like principle which was produced in, or can be extracted from, the internally secreting organs. A very active discussion followed.

Fig. 3.1. Collage from the British Medical Journal, August 16, 1913, containing the minutes of the meeting of the Seventeenth International Congress of Medicine in London August 6–12, 1913. An extract of the text is presented. This was probably the first time the word 'chalone' was used for this purpose.

sail', 'lower the gear' or 'float out the sea-anchor'. Schäfer's proposal was not accepted, and today the word 'hormone' signifies either an inhibitor or a stimulant. In 1962, Bullough adopted the word 'chalone' to describe the type of tissue-specific anti-mitotic substances which were at that time being extracted from the epidermis. In a relatively recent paper (1973), he comments on the 'curious coincidence that the first chalone preparation was made in London in a laboratory neighbouring that in which, exactly 60 years earlier, the first hormone preparation had been made' by Bayliss and Starling (1902).

'"When I use a word", Humpty Dumpty said in rather a scornful tone, "it means just what I choose it to mean – neither more nor less". "The question is", said Alice, "whether you *can* make words mean so many different things". "The question is", said Humpty Dumpty, "which is to be Master – that's all".' (Lewis Carroll: *Alice through the Looking-glass*, 1871). In the case of the name 'chalone', let nature be Master, and let future research give a true meaning to the word.

3.2 The present

The organs and tissues of the adult body are constantly kept at a normal size. After cell injury and/or cell loss, regenerative reactions are set in motion. These involve increased cell proliferation with production of new cells, cell migration, and cell differentiation. Some of these reactions are local, like those in the epidermis after a superficial scratch, others are obviously general, like those in the bone marrow after a haemorrhage. Regeneration is seen in its purest form in labile cell populations. In stable and permanent cell families, areas of cell loss are to a varying extent repaired by scar tissue.

It is an accepted hypothesis that cells belonging to the same type have developed a system to keep each other informed about their total number in the body or the area and their degree of differentiation, and that this system consists of certain specific signal molecules produced by the cells for the regulation of growth and differentiation.

During recent years evidence indicating or confirming the presence of many chemical signal molecules with an inhibitory action on cell proliferation has come to light. A few have been concentrated and purified to a certain extent.

Although it is still too early to formulate a definition of chalones, the following ideas are accepted by most of the workers in the field:

1) Chalones are produced in and present in the tissues on which they selectively act.

2) Chalones may act locally by diffusion in the tissue, or generally through the circulation.

3) Chalones are water-soluble molecules.

4) Chalones are tissue-specific, but species-non-specific.

5) Chalones act mainly in the late G_1 phase by delaying the entry of cells into DNA synthesis and/or in the late G_2 phase by controlling mitotic activity.

6) Chalone action is reversible, and chalones do not injure cells or cell membranes.

7) Chalone action is short-lived. This may be due to the presence of chalone antagonists, sometimes called 'anti-chalones'.

8) The mechanism of chalone action is not yet known; it is not even known whether they act within the cells or via the cell membranes.

9) Chalone action is in some way related to stress hormone action and probably also to cyclic AMP (what isn't?), but the exact mechanism of these interactions is not known.

10) Chalones are not the only growth-regulatory factors in the tissues on which they act, but they are possibly the most important. The total system of growth regulation is probably very complex, with different degrees of complexity in different tissue systems.

11) It is tempting to speculate about the possible role of chalones in the treatment of many pathological conditions such as cancer and psoriasis, and to discuss their possible role in preventing rejection reactions after transplantation, etc. Several workers, including myself, have not been able to withstand this temptation. So far, however, there is no direct, convincing evidence for the role of chalones in any type of therapy.

12) Chalones have now been shown, to a greater or lesser extent, to exist in the epidermis proper, sebaceous glands, eccrine sweat glands, hair follicles, melanocytes, granulocytes, erythrocytes, lymphocytes, fibroblasts, liver, kidney, intestinal epithelium, lung alveolar epithelium, endometrium (?), testicular spermatogenic cells, smooth muscle, lens of the eye, ascites tumour cells, leukaemic cells, melanomata, and squamous cell carcinomata.

The fact that it has been impossible to purify and clearly define such an important substance in the course of over 10 years' work is partly due to the instability of the effective signal substances in the tissue extracts (because chalone-degrading enzymes are also present?), but mainly to the fact that up to now all the assay systems available for testing chalone activity involve laborious handiwork. The counting of labelled cells and mitoses is an enormously tedious and time-consuming procedure.

The present situation in chalone research closely resembles that in hormone research 30–40 years ago, as described by Lasnitsky (1965): '. . . the fact that the hormones were not properly quantitated and often contained impurities, makes it hardly surprising that the results were often inconsistent or contradictory . . .'.

3.3 The past

It is not easy to trace the historical origins of the line of reasoning that finally resulted in the concept of chalones, since the first experiments were accompanied by rather vague ideas about tissue-specific growth inhibition. When I tried to look up the history of chalones, I was reminded of an old Danish joke: 'The strangest things happen in history. I once had an old coat, which I gave to my father; he used it for gardening, and when it was worn out he gave it to his father, who gave it to his father again, and so on, until it was lost at the Battle of Stamford Bridge'. I lost the track of such ideas back in the eighteen sixties, apart from those implicit in such classical medical generalizations as *similia similibus curantur* (like cures like), which implies that for example extracts of healthy tissue can favourably influence unhealthy tissue.

3.3.1 The theoretical concept

3.3.1.1 Cybernetics

A cybernetic system is a dynamic system in which an equilibrium is maintained by means of negative feedback. The cybernetic idea in mechanical physics was discussed in detail by J. D. Maxwell in 1868. One of the earliest technical constructions utilizing this principle was the governor constructed by James Watt in 1788 to control the velocity and the effect of the steam engine. At the output side of his engine Watt arranged two spinning flyballs so that they would be impelled outwards from the governor shaft by centrifugal force. The arm at the top of the spinning flyballs regulated the valve that controlled the supply of steam to the engine. In this way the velocity and the effect of the machine could be automatically regulated.

In 1926, Vito Volterra used cybernetic principles in ecology to explain the mutual interaction between two or more species associated together. If one of the species could find sufficient food in its environment, it would multiply indefinitely if left to itself, while the other would perish for lack of nourishment if left alone; but the second feeds upon the first, and so the two species can co-exist together. Volterra states: 'Having determined the laws of this increase and diminution it is possible to establish two differential equations of the first order, non-linear, which can be integrated. The integrals revealed the fact that the number of individuals of the two species are periodic functions of the time, with equal periods, but different phases...'. The Volterra model has some limitations, among them the fact that it cannot be used for small numbers. However, this limitation, which seems to be common to many growth models, does not apply to chalones, since all tissues consist of millions of cells. It is very easy to see the isomorphism between the components in the Volterra model, the eaten and the eating species, and the components in the Weiss–Kavanau model (1957, see below), the generative and the differentiated mass, respectively.

During and after the last world war, the rapid development of automatic control equipment both in industry and in armaments manufacture (gunfire control, guided missiles, etc.) promoted a comprehensive study of the theory of negative feedback systems, with a strong emphasis on the quantitative measurements of the information in the feedback cycles. There is thus a close connection between the theories of feedback systems proper and the communication theory.

In 1948 the mathematician Norbert Wiener published his book *Cybernetics*, in which he coined this term to describe the whole field of control and communication in the machine, in the various biological systems, and even in human sociology. This book inspired a large number of studies using cybernetic models to interpret physiological regulation mechanisms. Thus, Wiener bridged the gap between mathematics and physics on one side and biology on the other. Growth regulation by inhibitors of proliferation is only a special case of general cybernetics.

3.3.1.2 The biological idea

One of the first physiologists to formulate the idea of cybernetic control systems in biology was Claude Bernard (1878). He stressed the importance of a constant 'milieu intérieur' as a necessary condition for the independent life of an organism. To maintain such a constant environment, regulatory forces must be operating: 'La fixité du milieu suppose un perfectionnement de l'organisme tel que les variations externes soient à chaque instant compensées et equilibrées'.

In 1939 W. B. Cannon coined the term *homeostasis* to describe this phenomenon.

From the time of Bizozerro (1894) the different cells in the organism have been classified according to cell kinetics into three categories, viz. labile, stable and permanent cell populations. In the labile cell populations, e.g.

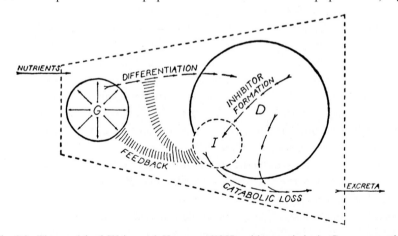

Fig. 3.2. The model of Weiss and Kavanau (1957, with permission). G = generative mass, D = differentiated mass, I = inhibiting principle. For further explanation, see text.
(Reproduced by permission of The Rockefeller University and Dr. Paul Weiss.)

the epidermis or the bone marrow, new cells are continuously being formed to compensate for the cell loss. This has been called physiological or 'orthic' regeneration. Following pathological cell loss, this type of regeneration shifts to a 'pathic' regeneration.

In 1957 Weiss and Kavanau formulated the general idea of growth regulation based on cybernetic principles (fig. 3.2). The essential features of this model are the basis for all later work on chalones. According to Weiss and Kavanau: 'Each specific cell type reproduces its protoplasm by a mechanism in which key compounds ('templates') characteristic of the particular cell type acts as catalysts. Each cell also produces specific freely diffusable compounds antagonistic to the former ('anti-templates') which can block and thus inhibit the reproductive activity of the corresponding 'templates'. The 'anti-template' system acts as a growth regulator by a negative 'feedback' mechanism in which increasing populations of 'anti-templates' render an increasing proportion of the homologous 'templates' ineffective, resulting in a corresponding decline of the growth rate. The attainment of terminal size is an expression of a stationary equilibrium between the incremental and decremental growth components and of the equilibration of the intracellular and extracellular 'anti-template' concentration.'

Weiss and Kavanau used their model to explain the overall growth curves of chickens and it could also be used to explain the well-known phenomenon of 'over-shooting', i.e. the hyperplasia seen when loss of substance is followed by regeneration. The anti-templates described by Weiss and Kavanau correspond directly to chalones.

The main body of this chapter on the history of chalones will be devoted to the history of the epidermal chalones, since this has for a long time been the 'leading edge' of chalone research.

3.3.2 Practical application

3.3.2.1 The epidermal chalone
By the early nineteen sixties the time was ripe for the adoption of the cybernetic theory to explain the growth regulation of the epidermis. In 1960 Bullough and Laurence published their study on wound healing in terms of changes in the epidermal mitotic activity based on a study of the effects of inflicting different sorts of wounds on the mouse ear skin. They concluded: 'The evidence shows that, while the mitotic rate of a tissue may be influenced by hormones, it is not controlled by them. The ultimate control of the mitotic rate evidently resides within the tissues themselves. It is obvious that, in appropriate circumstances, the cells of most tissues are

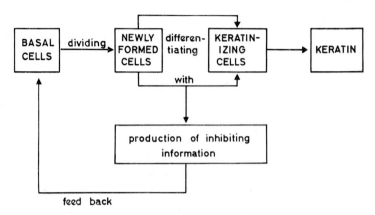

Fig. 3.3. Simple schematic representation of the model suggested by Iversen (1960). The production of inhibiting information is thought to be dependent upon the process of differentiation.

capable of indefinite growth and mitosis, and that each tissue specific control mechanism must be anti-mitotic.' I proposed a similar theory of epidermal growth regulation in March 1960, and elaborated it at the First International Congress of Cybernetic Medicine in Naples in October 1960, as shown in fig. 3.3.

On the basis of a study of the changes induced in the dehydrogenase activity in epidermis following a single application of a carcinogen, I concluded that the 'biphasic, oscillating character of the disturbance in the dehydrogenase activity is interpreted as pointing to a homeostatic control mechanism . . .' (Iversen, 1960b).

The epidermis is a tissue in dynamic equilibrium, whose growth is influenced by many factors: hormones, nerves, condition of vessels, immunological mechanisms, and external wear and tear. To balance the cell proliferation against the cell loss a control system must be operating. Theories explaining regeneration and wound healing in the epidermis fall into two large groups: those involving possible growth-stimulatory factors, the so-called 'wound hormones'; and those involving growth-inhibiting factors, the so-called 'chalones'. A series of observations and theoretical considerations formed the basis for the epidermal chalone theory:

i) The tendency to hyperplasia. It is well known that any superficial injury to the epidermis leads to hyperplasia. If one simply increases the external wear and tear, the number of cells in the epidermis increases (Iversen and Bjerknes, 1963). Careful removal of surface cells by stripping with adhesive tape (Pinkus, 1952; Christophers and Braun-Falco, 1967;

Hennings and Elgjo, 1970) or destroying the upper cell layer with silver nitrate (Oehlert and Block, 1962), leads to an increased proliferation in the basal layer followed by a transient period of hyperplasia. Being an active member of a rowing club results in thickening of the skin of the hands and thinning of the material of the back of the trousers. This is because living tissue, with its growth-regulatory systems, is thickened by wear and tear, whereas dead tissue becomes thinner.

ii) The local type of reaction. If a child falls and scratches his left knee, the healing process starts only in that area. There is no hyperplasia and no rise in mitotic activity in the right knee. The effect of such superficial cell loss, as measured by the proliferative reaction in the basal cells, extends

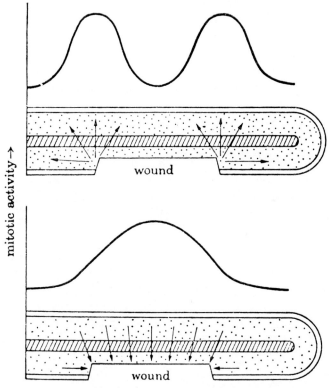

Fig. 3.4. Diagrams from the classical experiments of Bullough and Laurence (1960, with permission) to show the regions of high epidermal mitotic activity expected in uninjured ear epidermis opposite a 3 mm² area from which the epidermis and superficial dermis have been removed, on the assumption (upper diagram) that a 'stimulating wound hormone' is produced by the injured epidermis, and (lower diagram) that the concentration of epidermal inhibitor (chalone) is reduced in the neighbourhood of a wound. (Reproduced by permission of the Royal Society, London, and Dr. William Bullough.)

only about 1 mm beyond the injury (Bullough, 1962). This strongly supports the theory that the regulating signal in the epidermis is a locally acting and probably short-lived chemical substance. This signal substance probably also circulates in the blood, but a small reduction caused by minor local cell loss is not registered by epidermal cells far away from the area of cell loss.

iii) The London Chalone Group (Bullough and Laurence) came to a positive conclusion about the existence of epidermal growth-inhibitory substances by studying *the healing of wounds* on the skin of the mouse ear. The mouse ear is so thin that it might be assumed that a mitotic inhibitor which is freely diffusible would affect even the epidermis on the opposite side of the ear. Fig. 3.4 is a schematic illustration of the situation that would develop after a wound on one side of the mouse ear if (a) a stimulating wound hormone is produced by the damaged epidermis (upper diagram), or if (b) the concentration of an epidermal mitotic inhibitor is reduced in the neighbourhood of a wound (lower diagram). Bullough and Laurence's experiments demonstrated that the situation shown in the lower diagram corresponded best with the facts. From the results of these and other similar

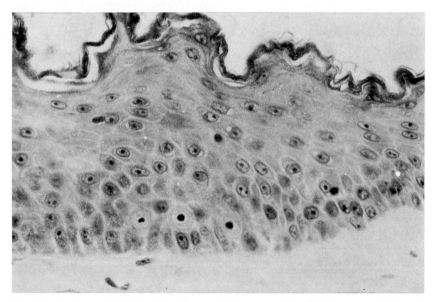

Fig. 3.5. On the ventral side of the African fruit bat web 12 × 50 mm areas of epidermis were removed by adhesive tape stripping. The regenerative reaction close to the wound was studied on both sides of the web. This picture shows a histological section of the hyperplasia seen on the dorsal side in the central area opposite the wound at 120 h. The normal epidermal thickness on the fruit bat web is only two cell layers. Note the heavily increased number of cells and the many mitotic figures.

experiments the authors proposed the existence of a mitotic inhibitory substance in the epidermis. This conclusion was vigourously opposed by some workers, on the grounds that the differences in mitotic activity observed between the areas located opposite the centre and the periphery of the wound were not sufficiently significant.

Finegold's results (1965), however, supported the findings of Bullough and Laurence, and showed that the increase in mitotic activity on the other side of the ear could be prevented by retransplantation of skin to the wounded area. Recently, the Oslo Chalone Group (Iversen et al., 1974) have repeated this type of experiment on the African fruit bat web. This latter study fully confirmed the findings of Bullough and Laurence. The

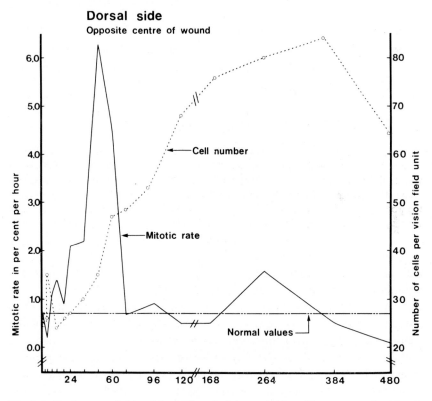

Fig. 3.6. On the ventral side of the African fruit bat web 12 × 50 mm areas of epidermis were removed by adhesive tape stripping. The regenerative reaction close to the wound was studied on both sides of the web by the Colcemid method and by counting cells. This diagram shows the alterations in mitotic rate and cell number at the dorsal side opposite the center of the wound. Following a wave of increased mitotic rate, the cell number increased to about 3–4 times the normal value.

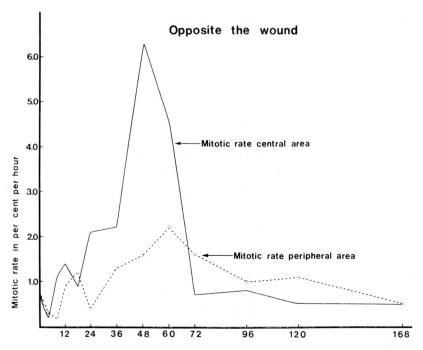

Fig. 3.7. On the ventral side of the African fruit bat web 12 × 50 mm areas of epidermis were removed by adhesive tape stripping. The regenerative reaction close to the wound was studied on both sides of the web by the Colcemid method and by counting cells. This graph shows a comparison of the alterations in mitotic rate on the dorsal side opposite the wound in the central and peripheral area respectively, at different time intervals after the stripping. It is clearly shown how the mitotic rate rose to higher levels in the central than in the peripheral areas.

fruit bat web membrane is very thin and has no central layer of cartilage as in the mouse ear. On the ventral side of the African fruit bat web 12 × 50 mm areas of epidermis were removed by adhesive tape stripping. The regenerative reaction close to the wound was studied on both sides of the web by the Colcemid method and by counting cells. Waves of increased proliferation occurred, followed by an increase in cell number. An example is shown in fig. 3.5. The reaction was local and limited. It was definitely strongest on the dorsal side opposite the centre of the wound (figs. 3.6, 3.7, 3.8 and 3.9).

Retransplantation of epidermis to the wound and four-hourly treatment with aqueous skin extracts prepared from fruit bat webs prevented the development of hyperplasia and an increase in cell proliferation. The authors concluded that the theory which most easily explained the time course,

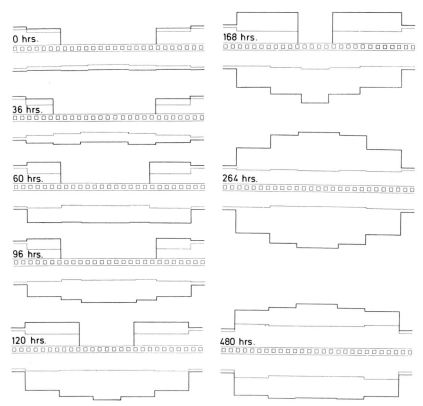

Fig. 3.8. On the ventral side of the African fruit bat web areas of epidermis were removed by adhesive tape stripping. The regenerative reaction on both sides of the web was studied by counting cells. This shows a schematic drawing of the wound and its surroundings at different times after the stripping. The number of basal cells and the number of differentiated cells on both sides of the web are shown. The size of the wound is also indicated. It is seen how hyperplasia develops on the uninjured side of the web and at the edges of the wound and how this hyperplasia started at about 36 h and reached its maximum 168 h after the stripping. The hyperplasia was most pronounced opposite the centre of the wound.

degree and localization of the changes in cell proliferation and cell number, and the prevention of these reactions by administration of chalone powder and retransplantation, was the chalone theory of growth control.

iv) The Oslo Chalone Group (Iversen and Elgjo) became interested in epidermal chalones because of certain observations concerning the *early stages of carcinogenesis*. Experiments in Oslo (Iversen and Evensen, 1962), showed that after a single application of 0.005 ml of a 1% solution of 3-methylcholanthrene (a carcinogen) in benzene to a circumscribed area of the skin of hairless mice (fig. 3.10) the following primary reactions occurred:

O. H. Iversen

72 hours after stripping

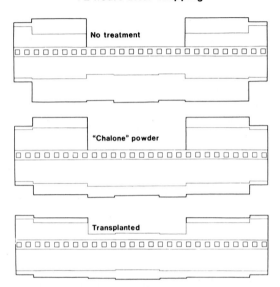

Fig. 3.9. This diagram shows how treatment with chalone powder and retransplantation of epidermis could prevent development of hyperplasia opposite the wound 72 h after stripping. The top diagram shows the situation without any additional treatment, the middle one shows the chalone powder treated animals, and the bottom one shows the situation after transplantation of epidermis.

a) DNA synthesis and mitosis were almost completely blocked for some hours (fig. 3.10, rate of cell renewal), and b) the mitochondria of many cells became seriously injured (fig. 3.10, cell damage). The secondary effects were as follows: a) The rate of cell proliferation increased 24 h after application to about three times the normal. It remained high during the next few days, and thereafter returned to normal (fig. 3.10, rate of cell renewal). b) Many cells destroyed by the carcinogen died and were shed during the first, second and third days after application (fig. 3.10, rate of cell death). This was deduced from calculations based on the experimental findings. c) A transient hyperplasia developed after the second day, reaching its peak on the fifth day, after which it slowly dwindled (fig. 3.10, cell count). When the rate of cell renewal alters as shown in the figure, and the cell loss remains normal and constant, the hyperplasia should have developed as shown in the dotted line labelled m_1. The real hyperplasia, however, followed the curve $m(t)$. This means that the area between these two curves is a measure of increased cell loss. The rate of cell loss can be calculated as shown in the bottom curve, and it was assumed that the cell loss alone led to decrease

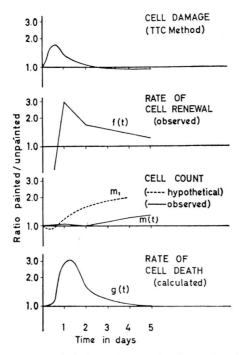

Fig. 3.10. Observations and calculations of the early effects of a single application of 3-methylcholanthrene to hairless mouse skin. For explanation, see text.

in the chalone concentration and thereby triggered the proliferative response. Simulation on an analogue computer showed good isomorphism between the results obtained using a cybernetic model and the findings from the mouse epidermis (Iversen and Bjerknes, 1963). Thus, a biological and cybernetic study confirmed and strengthened the theory that the main growth regulation principle in the epidermis is of a cybernetic nature.

The next problem was then to extract and find this negative feedback signal substance.

3.3.2.2 The extraction of chalone-like substances

As early as 1931 Murphy and Sturm from the Rockefeller Institute for Medical Research in New York reported some preliminary observations of a growth-inhibiting factor extracted from a fowl tumour. They found that this factor, when properly concentrated, could retard the growth of a transplantable mouse sarcoma. On the basis of these observations, Murphy suggested as a working hypothesis that the growth and differentiation of cells are controlled by a balanced system comprising a stimulating force and a retarding force, a suggestion which he regarded as being in line with other known physiological processes. Murphy and Sturm also demonstrated that a substance extracted from placenta and embryo skin retarded the growth of both transplanted and natural cancers in mice.

Today it is difficult to see from their experiments whether the demonstrated effects are of a chalone nature or due to immunological mechanisms or non-specific toxicity, but Murphy clearly expressed the idea of inhibitory and stimulatory growth-regulatory signal substances.

In 1936/1937 Simms and Stillman from the Department of Pathology, College of Physicians and Surgeons, Columbia University, New York, described a growth inhibitor in adult tissue. They stated: 'We believe that the tissue inhibitor described in this paper plays a large role in restraining growth in the adult animal body, thereby keeping the cells in their normal dormant state. It is suggested that the cells elaborate the inhibitor and deposit it in the surrounding intercellular space where it remains because of its insolubility'. This tissue inhibitor was obtained from chicken, dog and sheep aortas. It could be precipitated by an equal volume of alcohol, and further precipitated by calcium chloride. It was destroyed by high temperatures but withstood trypsin.

No further reports on such substances appeared in the literature for many years, and this research probably also suffered from the effects of the Second World War. Fresh interest arose, however, in the nineteen sixties.

Going back to the theoretical concept of cybernetics as applied to epidermal growth regulation described above (the biological idea), the next obvious step was to homogenize epidermis, make extracts and test the effects of these extracts on the mitotic activity of squamous cell epithelium and other cell types. Bullough and Laurence published the first results from testing such extracts in 1964. Simple aqueous extracts of homogenized epidermis turned out to contain a mitosis-inhibiting principle. The first extraction was made with mouse epidermis homogenized with an MSE glass homogenizer.

In 1965, Iversen, Aandal and Elgjo in Oslo published a confirmation of these findings. Their extracts were made from hairless mouse skin. They used the Colcemid technique and an in vivo system for determining the mitotic rate. The mitotic rate was depressed about 50% during the four-hour period measured. The chalone solution was injected intraperitoneally (fig. 3.11).

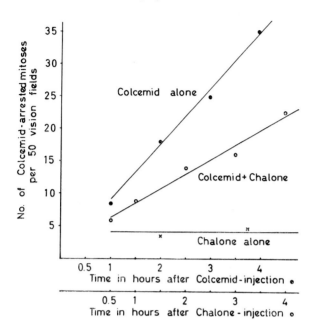

Fig. 3.11. Diagram from the first paper by Iversen, Aandal and Elgjo on the effect of intraperitoneal skin extract injections. The diagram shows the mitotic count at different time intervals after injection with Colcemid alone (upper curve), and chalone alone (lower curve). It is seen that the rate of cell proliferation, symbolized by the angle between the line of accumulation of mitosis and the abscissa, is reduced to about 50% of the normal by chalone injection (middle curve).

Extraction of chalones has since been performed in different ways in different laboratories with different basic materials.

Laurence and W. Hondius Boldingh (1968) prepared chalone-containing crude extracts from pig and cod skin. The slaughtered pigs were immersed in a water bath at 60°C for about 15 min, the hairs were burned off the skin, and the rind (i.e. the epidermis together with some collagenous dermis) was separated. This material was then ground into a fibrous powder after being lyophilized. With this method they found the same effect on mitotic activity as when they initially used freshly prepared rind. Cod skin powder was prepared from frozen cod skin which was processed in a meat-cutter, lyophilized and ground as finely as possible, resulting in a coarse-grained powder. From these powders the crude extracts were made by water extraction at 4°C.

The Oslo Group prepared chalone from hairless mouse skin, mechanically homogenized in a mill cooled with liquid nitrogen. The resulting skin powder was extracted in distilled water at 4°C. After centrifugation, all the foreign parts were spun down and the clear supernatant contained the mitosis-inhibiting principle. This was lyophilized and used as crude chalone. Later, it was partly purified by dialysis before use.

Further purification procedures for the epidermal G_2 chalone were first published by Hondius Boldingh and Laurence in 1968, and Marks in Heidelberg has been working mainly on the purification of the epidermal G_1 chalone (Marks, 1973). As regards other chalones, see below.

3.3.3 Some of the properties of chalones

3.3.3.1 Cell cycle specificity

The first epidermal chalone concept was concentrated on chalone as a mitotic inhibitor. The inhibition was measured by the Colcemid method in short-term organ cultures of mouse ear or in vivo. In 1968 Baden and Sviokla reported that a watery extract of the skin had no effect on epidermal DNA synthesis. Later it turned out that this result was due to the fact that too short a time had been allowed to elapse between the injection and the measurement of the result.

Almost all chalone systems investigated seem to contain both chalones inhibiting cell entrance into the S phase and chalones inhibiting cell entrance into mitosis. The first type of chalone has been called the G_1 factor or the S chalone, and the second type the G_2 factor or the M chalone.

The first indications of the presence of two growth-inhibiting factors in the skin came from Elgjo and Hennings (1971b), who made a study of the epidermal mitotic rate and DNA synthesis after injection of water-extracts made from mouse skin treated with Actinomycin D. Hennings, Elgjo and Iversen (1969) had showed that 9–12 h must elapse between the injection of aqueous skin extract before a significant inhibition of DNA synthesis can be observed.

Through an ingenious method described by Laerum (1970), whereby it was possible to separate basal and differentiating cells of the hairless mouse epidermis, it was shown by Elgjo, Laerum and Edgehill in 1971 and in 1972 that the G_2 inhibitor of epidermis was mainly present in the basal cells and the G_1 inhibitor in the differentiating cell layer.

In 1971 Marks also showed that crude pig skin extract contained two factors that could be separated from each other by various fractionation procedures. In 1971, Bichel also showed that Ehrlich ascites tumour cells produced two different inhibitors, one acting on cells in G_2 and one on cells in late G_1. Thus, chalones appear to have cell cycle specificity both in the late G_1 phase and in the G_2 phase, inhibiting the entrance of cells into mitosis and into DNA synthesis, respectively.

3.3.3.2 Tissue specificity and species nonspecificity

Tissue specificity is said to be characteristic of chalones, but in the early years of chalone research this of all chalone properties was the least founded on experimental evidence.

As regards the epidermal chalone, the concept of tissue specificity has been interpreted in different ways. The proliferation-inhibiting effect of the epidermal chalones may be (i) specific to epidermal tissues, (ii) specific to all ectodermal tissues, or (iii) specific to all ectodermal surface epithelial cells. Tissue specificity may also mean that epidermal chalones (iv) act specifically on keratinizing epithelia, regardless of their ectodermal or endodermal origin.

Laerum and Maurer (1973) proposed certain criteria for the acceptance of a specific chalone action. Ideally a control extract should not show growth-inhibiting action on the type of cells studied, but should preferably contain another chalone with specific action on another cell type. Only by such controls can non-specific growth inhibition be definitely excluded (cf. Houck's Law: 'Dead cells don't divide and dying cells divide damn slowly!') This presupposes, however, that the chalone source is pure. Up to now, these strict criteria can only be used for blood cells such as granulocytes and lymphocytes, and for pure suspension of separated basal and differentiated cells in the epidermis. Most of the chalone preparations used are made from a mixture of tissues.

In 1970(a) Bullough and Laurence, and later Bullough and Deol (1972) indicated that the epidermal appendages, sebaceous glands and eccrine sweat glands, seem to produce chalones which are not identical to the epidermal chalones, because skin extracts from areas not containing these glands had no inhibiting effect on their mitotic rate, whereas skin extracts containing such glands did affect the mitotic rate.

The most thorough study on tissue specificity of the epidermal chalone is that of Nome (1975). He tested many extracts of mouse tissues for growth-inhibitory effect on the epidermis, forestomach, small intestinal epithelium and epithelium from colon. He concluded that the epidermal chalones had tissue specificity in the sense that they were produced by and acted on keratinizing epithelia alone.

Laerum and Maurer (1973) have shown that crude skin extract had no effect on the DNA synthesis of the myelopoietic cells growing in diffusion chambers, whereas extracts of granulocytes did produce an effect.

Saetren (1956) demonstrated that liver and kidney extracts selectively inhibited the mitotic wave found in the rest of the organ after partial hepatectomy cr nephrectomy. Liver extracts had no effect on DNA synthesis of the epidermal cells (Hennings et al., 1969). Bullough et al. (1967) showed that liver extract had only a small effect on the mitotic rate of the epidermis. Verly (1973) reported results indicating the existence of a tissue-specific liver chalone. The literature on growth regulation of the liver is voluminous and difficult to interpret, but a good review was given by Grundmann and Seidel (1969), who tended to accept the theory of a tissue-specific liver chalone.

The finding of Saetren (1956), Simnett and Chopra (1969) and Chopra and Simnett (1970) indicate a tissue-specific kidney chalone. Rytömaa and Kiviniemi (1968a, b) demonstrated tissue-specific granulocyte and erythrocyte chalones, which has since been confirmed by other investigators (Paukovits, 1971; Laerum and Maurer, 1973). Tissue-specific lymphocyte chalones have been demonstrated by several authors (see 'Other chalones', below) and even tumour cells seem to produce tumour-specific inhibitory signal substances. As shown by Bichel (1970, 1971, 1972), simultaneous inoculation of JB-1 and Ehrlich ascites tumour in the same animals is followed by independent growth of both tumours. Cell-free ascites from one of these ascites tumours has an inhibiting effect on the cells in the G_1 and G_2 phases when injected into mice bearing the same tumour type. Foreign cell-free ascites, however, has no effect.

Thus, there is growing evidence in the literature supporting the hypothesis of the tissue specificity of chalones.

Epidermal G_2 chalone has been shown to be species–nonspecific. Extracts of human, pig, mouse and cod skin have been tested both in vivo in Oslo and in vitro in London (Bullough et al., 1967). We observed that epidermal G_2-chalone is not species-specific, nor even class-specific, but is common to man, pig, mouse and cod.

3.3.3.3 Relation to stress hormones and cyclic AMP
Adrenaline played an important role in the early years of chalone research. Initially, it was stated that it acted as a cofactor, forming an adrenaline—chalone complex (Bullough and Laurence, 1964). This was the basis for the so-called discriminative test, the 'adrenaline-wash' technique (Bullough et al., 1964).

Later it was shown that hydrocortisone may be equally important (Bullough and Laurence, 1968).

During recent years, works by Laurence et al. (1972) showed that the stress hormones are only indirectly related to the chalones, and that the phenomena observed may be mediated through chalone-binding or chalone-degrading systems, the 'anti-chalones' (see below).

As suggested by F. Seelich (Vienna) (see Iversen, 1969), the chalones may act via the cyclic AMP (and perhaps also the GMP) system. This idea has been further elaborated by Vorhees et al. (1973). Since stress hormones and cyclic AMP are known to be related, this may enable us to understand the role of these hormones in the mechanism of chalone action.

Quite recently (Elgjo, 1975; Young et al., 1975) it has been shown that both adrenaline and cyclic AMP mainly affect the G_2 phase and are thus probably connected with the M chalone, whereas cyclic AMP has a slight inhibitory effect on the cell transit from G_1 to S.

3.3.4 Other chalones

Other chalones that have recently been described are: chalones in sebaceous glands, eccrine sweat glands and hair follicles by Bullough and Laurence (1970) and Bullough and Deol (1972); melanocyte chalones by Bullough and Laurence (1968) and Dewey (1973); granulocyte chalones by Rytömaa and Kiviniemi (1968) and Paukovits (1971); erythrocyte chalones by Rytömaa and Kiviniemi (1968a) and Kivilaakso (1970); lymphocyte chalones by Moorhead et al. (1969), Lasalvia et al. (1970), Bullough and Laurence (1970a), Houck et al. (1971) and Kiger et al. (1973). As regards the liver and the kidney, the situation is complicated. Saetren (1956) found evidence for the presence of chalone-like substances in these organs, and the question of their presence in the liver has been discussed by e.g. Verly (1973), and in the kidney by Chopra and Simnett (1969). Fibroblast chalones have been reported by Houck et al. (1973), lung alveolar epithelial chalones by Simnett et al. (1969), and chalones in the lens of the eye by Voaden (1968). Chalone-like substances have been found in ascites tumour cells (Bichel, 1970, 1971), granulocytic leukaemic cells (Rytömaa and Kiviniemi, 1968c), melanomata (Bullough and Laurence, 1968a), and squamous cell carcinomata (Bullough and Laurence, 1968b; Elgjo and Hennings, 1971a; Laurence and Elgjo, 1971). Quite recently, evidence has been found for chalones in the testis (Chermont and Mauger, 1974) and in the small intestinal epithelium (Galjaard et al., 1972).

3.3.5 Anti-chalones

The evidence shows that chalones are short-lived. This may be due to their being very unstable, to their quick removal by the bloodstream, to rapid inactivation by degrading enzymes, or to binding to specific sites in the cell membranes. Chalone-like substances have been found in the blood, and even in urine, but this does not exclude the possibility that rapid binding to cell constituents or rapid degradation by enzymes is the main cause of the short-lived nature of the chalones.

The concept of 'anti-chalones' has been evolved to explain this short-livedness, the chalone-antagonistic effect of some extracts, and the different effects on the epidermal cells at different body sites to an injection of the same epidermal chalone (Argyris, 1972; Rytömaa and Kiviniemi, 1968a, b; Laurence et al., 1972; Elgjo and Edgehill, 1973). Recently, Houck et al. (1973) have claimed that his purified serum sialoprotein, which is the mitotic 'trigger' for diploid human fibroblasts in vitro may function as an anti-chalone by displacing the pre-existing fibroblast chalone.

Recently, a theoretical treatment of the concept of anti-chalones was published by Bjerknes and Iversen (1974), showing that 'anti-chalones' need be neither tissue-specific nor directly antagonistic to chalones. For example, the epidermal growth factor extracted from the salivary gland of rodents (Cohen, 1972) may be an anti-chalone.

3.3.6 Chalones, carcinogenesis and cancer treatment

The role of chalones in carcinogenesis and in the treatment of cancer has been much discussed. There seems to be general agreement that malignant tumours can produce the chalone of the tissue of origin, and that the proliferation rate of tumours can be influenced by the specific chalone. It has been suggested that tumours may be less sensitive than normal tissues to chalone inhibition of cell division.

Repeated attempts at using tissue extracts to cure cancer in humans have been made, so far without any proven effect. As already mentioned, in 1931, 1932 and in 1933 Murphy and Sturm and later Macfayden and Sturm (1936) reported on the presence of inhibiting factors which could retard the growth of transplanted and natural cancers in mice. The most interesting experiment was that of Murphy and Sturm in 1933, in which they injected mice intraperitoneally with embryo skin extract and placenta extract. The mice had mammary carcinomas, and after weekly injections with embryonic skin extract, 28% of the tumours were stationary, 12% showed marked regression, and 27% complete absorption. After placental extract injection, 24% were stationary, 25% showed marked regression and 19% complete absorption. No control groups are reported, but the authors conclude:

'There seems to be little doubt that the extracts of the two tissues which have previously been shown to reduce the takes of transplanted cancer have an influence on natural or spontaneous cancer.' The authors, however, make the following reservation: 'We do not consider that the results stated necessarily establish the hypothesis on which the experiment was based, for the complexity of the materials makes it quite possible that this explanation is not the correct one. The general relations between the factors which influence the origin and growth of spontaneous tumours, the balance in mechanism of normal tissues, and the inhibitor which has been isolated from the chicken sarcomas cannot be seriously discussed until further knowledge is available'. (This is good advice, which is still appropriate today.)

In 1965 Parshley reported the inhibiting effects on the growth of a series of tumours in vitro of extracts from adult connective tissue, which seemed to be particularly effective against sarcomas.

In a series of papers in 1968 and 1969 (for a review, see Bullough, 1969), the mitosis-inhibiting and necrotizing effect of certain tissue extracts on four malignant transplantable tumours (the VX2 epithelial tumour, a chloro-leukaemia and two melanomas) were published. These results were interpreted as being due to a chalone effect. The papers also drew attention to the possibility of using chalones in the treatment of cancer, in phrases such as the following: 'The question now obviously arises whether such chalones may be of practical value in cancer chemotherapy to arrest or even reverse tumour growth'. 'Again it is possible that tumour growth in vivo may be prevented or even reversed by repeated injections of either normal or tumour tissue extracts'. 'This suggests the possibility of suppressing neoplastic growth by repeated chalone injections'. 'This fact may be proven to have considerable value in that it may provide a basis for the treatment of malignant tumours by chalone-containing extracts . . .'. It was also stated that a disruption of the normal homeostatic balance between cell gain and cell loss in tumours is 'the basic event in carcinogenesis', and that 'this must depend on some change in the control mechanism of which the chalone forms a part'.

In 1970, I published a critical paper on such statements, in which I objected to attributing the acute necrosis of the melanomata to chalone effects, and stated: 'It seems more likely that the extensive necrosis in the tumour is not due to growth inhibition, but is mediated through the vascular bed, possibly as a local Schwartzman's reaction. The preparing phase might be brought about by the inflammatory reaction around the 'foreign' transplanted tumour. It is well known that widely diverse agents can be active as the provoking factor for Schwartzman's reaction. Contaminating bacterial toxins might, for instance, be present in the tissue extracts, especially from tumours. A secondary immunological mechanism related to the Arthus type reaction must also be ruled out, at least in the cases in which tumour extracts were used'. In 1972 (a, b) Mohr et al. in fact reported that the acute necrosis in the melanomas was not due to chalones, but to toxins from *Clostridium* spores present in the extracts.

The apparent cure of mice with a transplanted chloroleukaemia after repeated injections of granulocyte extracts reported by Rytömaa and Kiviniemi (1969), is a very interesting finding and a great inspiration for further work on this aspect of the chalones.

In a recent systematic investigation of the presence of growth-inhibitory substances in animal tissues, Bardos et al. (1968) tested over 1000 fractions of extracts from 28 different bovine and porcine tissues. Anti-tumour activity was found in 14 fractions from different tissues and cell culture cyto-toxicity was found in 8 fractions from the liver, 1 from the lung and 2 from the pineal gland.

Since we do not yet know the biochemistry and physiology or the chemical constitution of the chalones, it is too early to make any statements about the relationship between chalones and carcinogenesis or chalones and the treatment of cancer. I fully agree with Bullough in his statement in 1969: 'It still remains to be established that the tissue chalones ... have a role to play in the treatment of cancer'. Today it seems to be well documented, and it is also biologically reasonable to accept, that differentiated malignant tumours produce the specific chalone of the tissue of origin, and that the rate of proliferation in such tumours can be influenced by the chalones. However, this does not automatically imply that chalones can be used in cancer therapy.

All scientific experiments have hitherto been performed with transplanted tumours. The tumour–host relationship in such instances is very different from the tumour–host relationship in tumours primarily occurring spontane-ously in an animal or human being, or induced by viruses, irradiation or chemical carcinogens. The rate of cell division, for instance, is generally much higher in transplanted tumours than in spontaneous tumours.

It may be correct to say that up to now we have not solved the problem of the role of chalone in cancer treatment. I am very sceptical of the idea that chalones as such can be directly instrumental in cancer treatment. On the other hand, there is a possibility that chalones may play a role as an adjuvant in cancer treatment, by modulating the cell cycle. If cells are most sensitive to cytostatic drugs and irradiation in DNA synthesis, in the G_2 or the M phase, it might be possible to use chalones to stop all cell division in a certain family of cells. If malignant cells are less responsive than normal cells to a given chalone concentration, it might be possible to regulate the dose and thus have the cancer cells go into cycle in a more or less synchronized manner, while the normal cells are still blocked by chalones in G_1. This would then be the right moment for cytostatic treatment or irradiation.

3.3.7 Organized co-operation on chalones

Cooperation between the European workers interested in chalones began in 1963–64. Chalones were first publicly mentioned at an International Conference on the Control of Cellular Growth in Adult Organisms in Helsinki 1965 (published by Academic Press Inc., 1967). The idea of chalones was received with great scepticism and disbelief, and virtually passed over during the discussion. The first European Chalone Club meeting was held in Oslo in July 1968 (see fig. 3.12), arranged by myself and K. Elgjo. Among the participants were the London Group, the Oslo Group, U. Mohr from West Germany, and T. Rytömaa from Helsinki, the only one working with granulocytic chalones. The meeting lasted for three days, and we discussed mainly the concept of chalones and the biological properties of epidermal and granulocytic chalones as far as they were known at that time. The

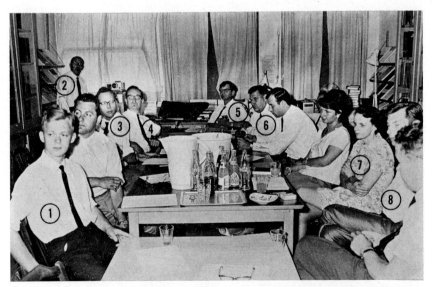

Fig. 3.12. The participants at the first European Chalone Club Meeting in Oslo July 1968. 1) Ole Nome, Oslo; 2) W. S. Bullough, London; 3) Kjell Elgjo, Oslo; 4) W. Hondius Boldingh, Organon, Holland; 5) O. H. Iversen, Oslo; 6) O. Mohr, Hannover; 7) Edna B. Laurence, London; 8) T. Rytömaa, Helsinki.

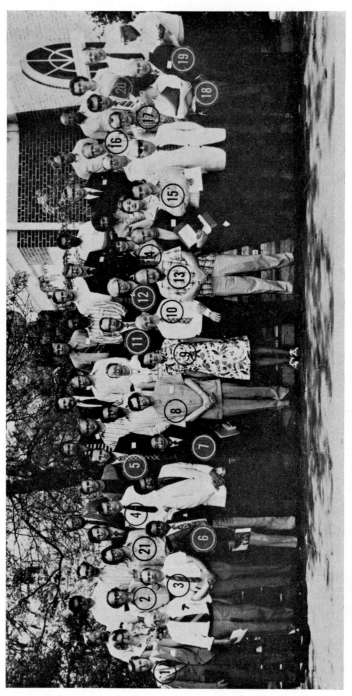

Fig. 3.13. The participants at the first symposium of the International Chalone Conference held at Brook Lodge, Augusta, Michigan, June 1972. 1) T. Rytömaa, Helsinki; 2) J. J. Vorhees, Ann Arbour; 3) D. L. Dewey, London; 4) L. G. Lajtha, Manchester; 5) H. Hennings, Bethesda; 6) D. P. Chopra, Philadelphia; 7) A. C. Chung, Washington; 8) O. H. Iversen, Oslo; 9) Edna B. Laurence, London; 10) W. S. Bullough, London; 11) K. Elgjo, Oslo; 12) Dame Honor Fell, Cambridge; 13) J. C. Houck, Washington; 14) Nicole Kiger, Villejuif; 15) F. Marks, Heidelberg; 16) P. Bichel, Aarhus; 17) W. R. Paukovits, Vienna; 18) W. G. Verly, Montreal; 19) G. Mueller, Madison; 20) M. Rajewsky, Tübingen; 21) D. J. Simnett, Newcastle. The names of all the participants are printed in National Cancer Institute Monograph 38, 1973.

The future of chalone research is still buried under the sand, as shown in fig. 3.14, and with this in mind, it may be appropriate to end this chapter on the history of chalones with what is said to be the last words of Louis Pasteur: 'Il faut travailler!'

References

Argyris, T. S. (1972) Chalones and the control of normal regenerative and neoplastic growth of the skin. Am. Zool. 12, 137–149.

Baden, H. P. and Sviokla, S. (1968) Effect of chalone on epidermal DNA synthesis. Exp. Cell Res. 50, 644–646.

Bardos, T. J., Gordon, H. L., Chmielewicz, Z. F., Kutz, R. L. and Nadkarni, M. V. (1968) A systematic investigation of the presence of growth-inhibitory substances in animal tissues. Cancer Res. 28, 1620–1630.

Bayliss, W. M. and Starling, E. H. (1902) The mechanism of pancreatic secretion. J. Physiol. 28, 325–353.

Bernard, C. (1878) Sur les Phénomènes de la Vie. Paris.

Bichel, P. (1970) Tumour growth inhibiting effect of JB-1 ascitic fluid-I. Europ. J. Cancer 6, 291–296.

Bichel, P. (1972) Specific growth regulation in three ascites tumours. Europ. J. Cancer 8, 167–173.

Bizzozerro, G. (1894) Wachstum und Regeneration im Organismus. Wien Med. Wschr. 16, 699, and 17, 744.

Bjerknes, R. and Iversen, O. H. (1974) Antichalone. A theoretical treatment of the possible role of antichalone in the growth control system. Acta Pathol. Microbiol. Scand. A, Suppl. 248.

Bullough, W. S. (1962) The control of mitotic activity in adult mammalian tissues. Biol. Rev. 37, 307–342.

Bullough, W. S. (1969) The use of tissue extract in the treatment of cancer. In: Fortschritte der Krebsforschung. Molekularbiologie, Wachstum, Klinik (eds.: C. G. Schmidt & O. Wetter) F. K. Schattauer Verlag: New York, pp. 315–319.

Bullough, W. S. (1973) The chalones: A review. In: Chalones: Concepts and current researches (eds.: B. K. Forscher and J. C. Houck) Nat. Cancer Inst. Monogr. 38, 5–15.

Bullough, W. S. and Deol, J. U. R. (1972) Chalone control of mitotic activity in eccrine sweat glands. Brit. J. Dermatol. 86, 586–592.

Bullough, W. S., Hewett, C. L. and Laurence, E. B. (1964) The epidermal chalone. A preliminary attempt at isolation. Exp. Cell. Res. 36, 192–200.

Bullough, W. S. and Laurence, E. B. (1960) The control of epidermal mitotic activity in the mouse. Proc. Roy. Soc. B 151, 517–536.

Bullough, W. S. and Laurence, E. B. (1964) Mitotic control by internal secretion: The role of the chalone-adrenalin complex. Exp. Cell. Res. 33, 176–194.

Bullough, W. S. and Laurence, E. B. (1968a) Control of mitosis in mouse and hamster melanomata by means of the melanocyte chalone. Europ. J. Cancer 4, 607–614.

Bullough, W. S. and Laurence, E. B. (1968b) Control of mitosis in rabbit Vx2 epidermal tumours by means of the epidermal chalone. Europ. J. Cancer 4, 587–594.

Bullough, W. S. and Laurence, E. B. (1968c) The role of glucocorticoid hormones in the control of epidermal mitosis. Cell Tissue Kinet. 1, 5–10.

Bullough, W. S. and Laurence, E. B. (1970a) The lymphocytic chalone and its antimitotic action on a mouse lymphoma in vitro. Europ. J. Cancer 6, 525–531.

Bullough, W. S. and Laurence, E. B. (1970b) Chalone control of mitotic activity in sebaceous glands. Cell Tissue Kinet. 3, 291–300.

Bullough, W. S., Laurence, E. B., Iversen, O. H. and Elgjo, K. (1967) The vertebrate epidermal chalone. Nature (Lond.) 214, 578–580.

Cannon, W. B. (1939) The wisdom of the body. Norton Publ., New York.

Chopra, D. P. and Simnett, J. D. (1970) Stimulation of mitosis in amphibian kidney by organ specific antiserum. Nature (Lond.) 225, 657–658.

Christophers, E. and Braun-Falco, O. (1967) Epidermale Regeneration am Meerschwein-chenohr nach Hornschichtabriss. Arch. Klin. Exp. Dermatol. 231, 85–96.

Clermont, Y. and Mauger, A. (1972) Existence of a spermatogonial chalone in the rat testis. Cell Tissue Kinet. 7, 165–172.

Cohen, S. (1972) Epidermal growth factor. J. Invest. Dermatol. 59, 13–16.

Dewey, D. L. (1973) The melanocyte chalone. In: Chalones: Concepts and current researches (eds.: B. K. Forscher and J. C. Houck) Nat. Cancer Inst. Monogr. 38, 213–216.

Elgjo, K. (1975) Epidermal chalone and cyclic AMP: An in vivo study. J. Invest. Dermatol. 64, 14–18.

Elgjo, K. and Edgehill, W. (1973) Epidermal growth inhibitors (chalones) in dermis and serum. Virch. Arch. B 13, 14–23.

Elgjo, K. and Hennings, H. (1971a) Epidermal chalone and cell proliferation in a trans-plantable squamous cell carcinoma in hamsters. I. In vivo results. Virch. Arch. B 7, 1–7.

Elgjo, K. and Hennings, H. (1971b) Epidermal mitotic rate and DNA synthesis after injection of water extracts made from mouse skin treated with Actinomycin D: Two or more growth-regulating substances? Virch. Arch. B 7, 342–347.

Elgjo, K., Laerum, O. D. and Edgehill, W. (1971) Growth regulation in mouse epidermis. I. G_2-inhibitor present in the basal cell layer. Virch. Arch. B 8, 277–283.

Elgjo, K., Laerum, O. D. and Edgehill, W. (1972) Growth regulation in mouse epidermis. II. G_1-inhibitor present in the differentiating cell layer. Virch. Arch. B 10, 229–236.

Finegold, M. J. (1965) Control of cell multiplication in epidermis. Proc. Soc. Exp. Biol. Med. 119, 96–100.

Galjaard, H., Meer-Fieggen, W. van der and Giesen, J. (1972) Feedback control by functional villus cells on cell proliferation and maturation in intestinal epithelium. Exp. Cell Res. 73, 197–207.

Grundmann, E. and Seidel, H. J. (1969) Die reparative Parenchymregeneration am Bei-spiel der Leber nach Teilhepatektomie. F. Büchner (ed.) Handbuch der allgemeinen Pathologie. Entwicklung. Wachstum II. Springer Verlag, Berlin, 129–243.

Hennings, H. and Elgjo, K. (1970) Epidermal regeneration after cellophane tape stripping of hairless mouse skin. Cell Tissue Kinet. 3, 243–252.

Hennings, H., Elgjo, K. and Iversen, O. H. (1969) Delayed inhibition of epidermal DNA synthesis after injection of an aqueous skin extract (chalone). Virch. Arch. B 4, 45–53.

Hondius Boldingh, W. and Laurence, E. B. (1968) Extraction, purification and preliminary characterization of the epidermal chalone: A tissue specific mitotic inhibitor obtained from vertebrate skin. Europ. J. Biochem. 5, 191–198.

Houck, J. C., Cheng, R. F. and Sharma, V. K. (1973) Control of fibroblast proliferation.

In: Chalones; concepts and current researches. (eds.: B. K. Forcher and J. C. Houck) Nat. Cancer Inst. Monogr. 38, 161–170.

Houck, J. C., Hiltje Irausquin and Sanford Leikin (1971) Lymphocyte DNA synthesis inhibition. Science 173, 1139–1141.

Houck, J. C., Sharma, V. K. and Cheng, R. (1973) Fibroblast chalone and serum mitogen (anti-chalone). Nature New Biol. 246, 111–113.

Iversen, O. H. (1960a) A homeostatic mechanism regulating the cell number in epidermis. Its relation to experimental skin carcinogenesis Proc. 1st Congr. Int. Cybernetic Med., Gianno, Naples.

Iversen, O. H. (1960b) Cell metabolism in experimental skin carcinogenesis. Acta Pathol. Microbiol. Scand. 50, 17–24.

Iversen, O. H. (1969) Chalones of the skin. In: Ciba Foundation Symposium on Homeostatic Regulators (eds.: G. E. W. Wolstenholme and Julie Knight) J. & A. Churchill Ltd., London, pp. 29–53.

Iversen, O. H. (1973) The chalones. Acta Pathol. Microbiol. Scand. A, Suppl. 236, 71–76.

Iversen, O. H., Bhangoo, K. S. and Hansen, K. (1974) Control of epidermal cell renewal in the bat web. Virch. Arch. B 16, 157–179.

Iversen, O. H. and Bjerknes, R. (1963) Kinetics of epidermal reaction to carcinogens. Acta Pathol. Microbiol. Scand. Suppl. 165.

Iversen, O. H. and Evensen, A. (1962) Experimental skin carcinogenesis in mice. Acta Pathol. Microbiol. Scand. Suppl. 156.

Iversen, O. H., Aandahl, E. and Elgjo, K. (1965) The effect of an epidermis specific mitotic inhibitor (chalone) extracted from epidermal cells. Acta Pathol. Microbiol. Scand. 64, 506–510.

Kiger, N., Florentin, I. and Mathé, G. (1973) A lymphocyte-inhibiting factor (chalone?) extracted from thymus: Immunosuppressive effects. In: Chalones: Concepts and current researches (eds.: B. K. Forscher and J. C. Houck) Nat. Cancer Inst. Monogr. 38, 135–142.

Kivilaakso, E. (1970) The response of RNA synthesis to mitotic regulation in the erythron. Acta Physiol. Scand. 80, 436–442.

Laerum, O. D. (1970) The separation and cultivation of basal and differentiating cells from hairless mouse epidermis. J. Invest. Dermatol. 54, 279–287.

Laerum, O. D. and Maurer, H. R. (1973) Proliferation kinetics of myelopoietic cells and macrophages in diffusion chambers after treatment with granulocyte extracts (chalone). Virch. Arch. B 14, 293–305.

Lasalvia, E., Garcia-Giralt, E. and Macieira-Coelho, A. (1970) Extraction of an inhibitor of DNA synthesis from human peripheral blood lymphocytes and bovine spleen. Rev. Europ. Etudes Clin. Biol. 15, 789–792.

Lasnitzki, I. (1965) The action of hormones on cell and organ cultures. E. N. Wilmer (ed.) Cell and tissue in culture. London: Academic Press, 1, 591–658.

Laurence, E. B. and Elgjo, K. (1971) Epidermal chalone and cell proliferation in a transplantable squamous cell carcinoma in hamsters. II. In vitro results. Virch. Arch. B 7, 8–15.

Laurence, E. B., Randers-Hansen, E., Christophers, E. and Rytömaa, T. (1972) Systemic factors influencing epidermal mitosis. Rev. Eur. Etud. Clin. Biol. 17, 133–139.

Macfayden, D. A. and Sturm, E. (1936) Further observations on factors from normal tissues influencing the growth of transplanted cancer. Science 84, 67–68.

Marks, F. (1971) Direct evidence of two tissue-specific chalone-like factor regulating mitosis and DNA synthesis in mouse epidermis. Hoppe-Seylers Z. Physiol. Chem. 352, 1273–1274.

Marks, F. (1973) A tissue-specific factor inhibiting DNA synthesis in mouse epidermis. In: Chalones: Concepts and current researches (eds.: B. K. Forscher and J. C. Houck) Nat. Cancer Inst. Monogr. 38, 79–80.

Maxwell, J. C. (1868) On governors. Proc. Roy. Soc. Lond. 16, 270–283.

Mohr, U., Hondius Boldingh, W. and Althoff, J. (1972) Identification of contaminating Clostridium spores as the oncolytic agent in some chalone preparations. Cancer Res. 32, 1117–1121.

Mohr, U., Hondius Boldingh, W., Emminger, A. and Behagel, H. S. (1972) Oncolysis by a new strain of Clostridium. Cancer Res. 32, 1122–1128.

Moorhead, J. F., Paraskova-Techernozenska, E., Pirrie, A. J. and Hayse, C. (1969) Lymphoid inhibitor of human lymphocyte DNA synthesis and mitosis in vitro. Nature 224, 1207–1208.

Murphy, J. B. (1931) Discussion of some properties of the causative agent of a chicken tumor. Trans. Assoc. Amer. Phys. 46, 182–187.

Murphy, J. B. and Sturm, E. (1931) Further observations on an inhibitor principle associated with the causative agent of a chicken tumour. Science 74, 180–181.

Murphy, J. B. and Sturm, E. (1932) Normal tissues as a possible source of inhibitor for tumors. Science 75, 540–541.

Murphy, J. B. and Sturm, E. (1933) Effect of inhibiting factor from normal tissues on spontaneous tumors of mice. Science 77, 631–633.

Nome, O. (1975) Tissue specificity of the epidermal chalones. Oslo. Virch. Arch. B 19, 1–25.

Oehlert, W. and Block, P. (1962) Der Mechanismus und zeitliche Ablauf der reparativen Regeneration in Geweben mit post- und intermitotischen Zellbestand. Verh. dtsch. Ges. Path. 46, 333–340.

Parshley, M. S. (1965) Effect of inhibitors from adult connective tissue on growth of a series of human tumours in vitro. Cancer Res. 25, 387–401.

Paukovits, W. R. (1971) Control of granulocyte production: separation and chemical identification of a specific inhibitor (chalone). Cell Tissue Kinet. 4, 539–547.

Pinkus, H. (1952) Examination of the epidermis by the strip method. II. Biometric data on regeneration of the human epidermis. J. Invest. Dermatol. 19, 431–447.

Rytömaa, T. and Kiviniemi, K. (1968a) Control of granulocytic production. I. Chalone and antichalone, two specific humoral regulators. Cell Tissue Kinet. 1, 329–340.

Rytömaa, T. and Kiviniemi, K. (1968b) Control of granulocyte production. II. Mode of action of chalone and antichalone. Cell Tissue Kinet. 1, 341–350.

Rytömaa, T. and Kiviniemi, K. (1968c) Control of DNA duplication in rat chloroleukaemia by means of the granulocytic chalone. Europ. J. Cancer 4, 595–606.

Rytömaa, T. and Kiviniemi, K. (1969) Chloroma regression induced by the granulocytic chalone. Nature 222, 995–996.

Saetren, H. (1956) A principle of auto-regulation of growth. Exp. Cell Res. 11, 229–232.

Simms, H. S. and Stillman, N. P. (1937) Substances affecting adult tissue in vitro. II. A growth inhibitor in adult tissue. J. Gen. Physiol. 20, 621–629.

Simnett, J. D. and Chopra, D. P. (1969) Organ specific inhibitor of mitosis in the amphibian kidney. Nature (Lond.) 222, 1189–1190.

Simnett, J. D., Fisher, J. M. and Heppleston, A. G. (1969) Tissue-specific inhibition of lung alveolar cell mitosis in organ culture. Nature 233, 944–946.

Verly, W. G. (1973) The hepatic chalone. In: Chalones: Concepts and current researches (eds.: B. K. Forscher and J. C. Houck) Nat. Cancer Inst. Monogr. 38, 175–184.

Voaden, M. J. (1968) A chalone in the rabbit lens? Exp. Eyes Res. 7, 326–331.

Volterra, V. (1926) Fluctuations in the abundance of a species considered mathematically. Nature 118, 558–560.

Vorhees, J. J., Duell, E. A., Bass, L. J. and Harrell, E. R. (1973) Role of cyclic AMP in the control of epidermal cell growth and differentiation. In: Chalones: Concepts and current researches (eds.: B. K. Forscher and J. C. Houck) Nat. Cancer Inst. Monogr. 38, 47–59.

Weiss, P. and Kavanau, J. L. (1957) A model of growth and growth control in mathematical terms. J. Gen. Physiol. 41, 1–47.

Wiener, N. (1948) Cybernetics. John Wiley & Sons Inc., New York.

Young, J. M., Lawrence, H. S. and Cordell, S. L. (1975) In vitro epidermal cell proliferation in rat skin plugs. J. Invest. Dermatol. 64, 23–29.

CHAPTER 4

Control of cell division during the cell cycle: nuclear protein modifications and new specific phase inhibitors

MARK E. SMULSON

with assistance of Patricia Stark

Department of Biochemistry, Schools of Medicine and Dentistry, Georgetown University, Washington, D. C. 20007, U.S.A.

The understanding of the mechanisms by which cells control their DNA replication and their timing of cell division holds great interest to those investigators concerned with growth regulation and with those compounds, both natural and synthetic, which affect the various synthetic phases of the cell cycle. This review will concentrate on three major areas of the eukaryotic cell cycle: 1) selected aspects of cell synchrony and cell, 2) population kinetics, and 3) chromosomal protein modifications and their relationship to current knowledge on the regulation of cell staging. One particular nuclear protein modification, produced by the chromosomal enzyme poly(ADP-ribose) polymerase, will be utilized as an example of the approach that the authors have taken to study the regulation of cells progressing through the cell cycle. Finally, selected chemotherapeutic agents which inhibit specific stages of the cell cycle will be reviewed.

4.1 Cell cycle phases

The eukaryotic cell cycle is subdivided experimentally into four major stages:

1) Mitosis is characterized by the segregation of chromosomes leading to cell division. Large morphological changes occur in mitotic cells allowing for 'selective detachment' of such cells for further study.

2) G_1 phase occurs after cell division, and its length of time, when studied in vitro and in vivo, has been shown to be the most variable for cells of different origin. Chromatin is still very condensed in early G_1 phase, and cells are extremely active in both transcription and translation. Many studies have indicated fluctuations in key enzyme synthesis during this period.

Those enzymes required for DNA replication are expressed in late G_1 phase in preparation for semi-conservative DNA replication. A certain percentage of a given cell population is, in addition, induced after mitosis into a non-proliferating stage of the cycle which has been termed G_0. Differentiated cellular synthetic and metabolic activity of a cell type might occur in G_0. Under the correct external stimulus, which is not as yet well understood, cells reversibly may re-enter the cell cycle into G_1 phase after having spent various periods of time in G_0 phase.

3) S phase is the unique period in a cell's propagation cycle when semi-conservative scheduled DNA replication occurs. In addition, histone proteins are only replicated in a coupled fashion with DNA during this phase. For many cell types the length of time of S phase, when studied either in vitro or in vivo is approximately 7 to 10 h. The rate of DNA polymerase primed replication of DNA in vivo has been estimated to be approximately one micron of DNA replicated per minute. Multiple sites of initiation on DNA of chromosomes exist during S phase to insure complete replication of DNA during its allotted short period of replicative activity. Each site of initiation in chromosomal DNA has been termed a replicon or a replicating unit; an average chromosome might contain as many as 2000 of such individual replicating units for DNA synthesis (Huberman and Riggs, 1968). Subtle regulations of chromatin replication occur during S phase such that not all types of chromatin are replicated at the same time. For example, heterochromatin, the highly condensed, nonactive transcriptional chromatin, is replicated during the latter part of S phase, whereas euchromatin, which is most active in transcription and the physical form of chromatin least restricted by various nuclear proteins, is in general replicated early during the S phase of the cell cycle. The discussions below will center on the function of various nuclear protein modifications which occur during S phase and how they participate in control mechanisms for this type of selective DNA replication.

4) G_2 phase follows S phase and is a period of time prior to mitosis when cells participate in the induction of those enzymes and proteins required for chromosomal condensations and for mitosis. Recently, as discussed below, new drugs have been studied which specifically block cells in this stage of the cell cycle. In order to obtain an in vitro model of the cell cycle it is desirable to synchronize a population of in vitro cells such that most cells are in approximately the same position of the cell cycle.

4.2 Cell synchrony

Methods of cell synchrony are essentially grouped into three major categories: physical, chemical and nutritional. Each of these has certain advantages depending upon the area of the cycle one wishes to study. During mitosis, cells are morphologically quite unique and tend to loosen from their attachment to their growth substratum. The method of selective detachment has been utilized very successfully to isolate pure populations of mitotic cells which have the advantage of not having been exposed to any type of chemical mediators. In addition, the use of the alkaloid colchicine to arrest cells in metaphase has also been used to collect cells in mitosis for further study.

Arresting cells at the G_1/S boundary has been utilized by many investigators to synchronize cells such that S phase can be initiated in a synchronous fashion. Thymidine, hydroxyurea, methotrexate, cytosine arabinoside, have all been utilized to arrest cells at this boundary.

As an example of this technique, the data described in fig. 4.1, obtained in the laboratory of the author, will be used to illustrate the use of the drug methotrexate to produce a synchronous population of HeLa cells in culture (Roberts et al., 1975; Smulson et al., 1975). Methotrexate is an inhibitor of folic acid requiring enzymes and specifically binds tightly to the enzyme dihydrofolic acid reductase. With the proper supplementation of purines and amino acids, cells are thus induced into a thymineless state by incubation with this drug. Upon the addition of thymidine at zero time in the experiment in fig. 4.1, cells are thus induced into a synchronous wave of semi-conservative DNA replication, as demonstrated by the pulse labeled measurements of thymidine incorporation into DNA. S phase lasts approximately 8 h in HeLa cells, with a peak of DNA replication at approximately 5 h. The data also shows the quantity of DNA per nuclei which also indicates a quantitative increase during S phase. The cell number remains relatively constant until semi-conservative DNA replication has been completed and then during G_2-M phases a doubling of cell number occurs. This population number remains constant during the ensuing 9- or 10-h period of G_1 phase. After 24 h, the experiment illustrated in fig. 4.1 demonstrates that a second wave of DNA synthesis progresses. In cell culture work, such an experiment allows the sampling of cells at various stages of the cell cycle for further analysis, or to investigate the effects of various compounds, such as drugs or natural components on biochemical and biological intracellular events. Clearly, by the appropriate control experiments, one should be able to detect whether a particular inhibitor, for example, is specific for G_1 phase or any other phase of the cell cycle.

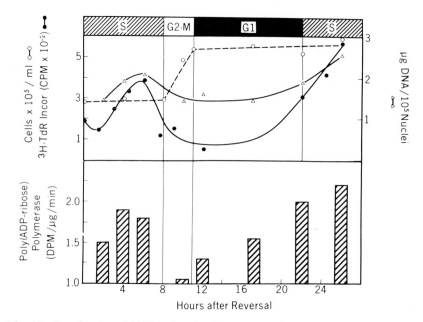

Fig. 4.1. Cytoplasmic poly (ADP-ribose) polymerase and the HeLa cell cycle. A 1500 ml culture of HeLa cells was synchronized at the G_1-S boarder with methotrexate. At zero time the block was released with 10^{-5} M thymidine, and samples were collected at various times. The incorporation of [³H]thymidine into DNA (●—●), the cell number (○—○) and DNA content per 10^5 nuclei (△—△) are shown in the top panel of the figure. Post-mitochondrial extracts were prepared and aliquots containing 140 to 180 μg protein were assayed for poly (ADP-ribose) polymerase activity in the standard 0.5 ml assay mixture. The rate of poly (ADP-ribose) formation (dpm per minute per μg protein) was used to obtain the data shown in the lower panel. Data taken from Roberts et al., 1975.

4.3 In vivo cell population kinetics

One method which has been exploited with great success for in vivo measurements of cell cycle parameters has been the percent labeled mitoses (PLM) method. In this procedure, (³H)thymidine is administered to an animal or an area of tissue or cavity of the body where study of cell kinetics is desired. Because of the rapid degradation of thymidine in mammalian tissues, such a labeling period of thymidine is essentially a pulse measurement of DNA synthesis. After the pulse label, biopsies are obtained in a serial fashion from the organism. Subsequently, each of these tissues is examined microscopically for both total number of mitotic cells and the percentage of labeled mitotic cells. The only cells that will be labeled during the pulse labeling period will be those cells which were in some area of S phase during the pulse labeling period; the first mitoses which will appear as labeled mitoses will thus be the cells which were in the late stages of S phase when labeled thymidine was administered. The period of time required for such cells to appear as labeled mitoses is a measurement of T_{G_2} and a portion of T_M. The last cells to appear as labeled mitoses will be those cells which were just entering S phase upon administration of the label. The period of time in which *all* mitoses examined microscopically are labeled is thus a measurement of T_S. As the cells progress through G_1 (unlabeled) and reach a second cycle, as indicated by a new increase in labeled mitoses, one is capable of calculating the total generation time of the cell (T_C). Thus from such measurements one can in vivo conveniently calculate T_C, T_{G_2}, T_M, T_S, and by difference T_{G_1}. Using such techniques, some typical T_C for man in vivo have been calculated and the results are quite revealing (Lala, 1971). The T_C's vary from 25–50 h (normal intestinal epithelial cells), 2–6 days (human multiple myeloma cells), 1.5 months (normal epidermal cells), to as long as 3 months for cancer of the breast. All of the studies have indicated a rather surprising result; the T_C for cancer cells seems at least as long, and many times even longer, than the generation time for a nearby normal cell in man. The fascinating question is how can this paradox be rationalized with the common view of malignancy as being a rapidly dividing cell? One answer to this question has been established through measurements of the growth fraction (GF) of cell populations; that is, the percentage of the total cell population which actually participates in the cell cycle. The GF is equivalent to one minus the number of cells in G_0 for a population and can be calculated in vivo and in vitro by making use of a measurement of the labeling index (LI). Thus,

$$LI = GF \times \frac{T_S}{T_C}$$

With the exception of the T_S, all other parameters of this equation are conveniently measured by techniques already described. Therefore,

$$GF = \frac{LI}{T_S/T_C}$$

The growth fraction of many normal tissues in man are low; that is, many cells in the population are differentiated and are not displayed throughout the cell cycle. However, the GF for different types of human tumors shows considerable variability and quite high values (100% in the case of Burkett's Lymphoma) have been obtained. With so many cells participating in the cell cycle, especially in the case of malignant cells, after one generation the cell population should increase by:

$$\frac{N}{N_0} = 1 + GF$$

If the *GF* were equal to one, the population would double with each T_C theoretically, but in vivo this does not occur. The malignant cell is found to have a high rate of cell death in comparison with normal cells. Tumor cells die during the cell cycle for a variety of reasons including defective mitoses, outstripping of vascular supply and hence nutrient requirements, and exfoliation of cells into body cavities. Thus the growth rate of a tumor (increase in volume or weight) is generally less than predicted by the *GF* and T_C measurements.

One interesting question concerning the cell cycle kinetics of malignant cells concerns whether such cells can leave the cell cycle, enter into G_0 phase for various periods of time, and then reversibly re-enter the cell cycle. It seems that in the case of malignant cells this is a reversible event and thus it poses an obvious problem for chemotherapy of cancer cells, since G_0 cells would be highly resistant to most chemotherapeutic agents, especially those that are either S phase inhibitors or mitosis inhibitors. It has been observed that, as tumor cells which are participating in the cell cycle age in the body, the T_C increases with time. Thus when a tumor cell population is reduced by chemotherapeutic agents, those cells which have entered G_0 are capable of being called back into the cell cycle, sometimes in even greater numbers than before, and these cells possibly even divide with greater rapidity due to their younger cell cycle age and possibly lower T_C rate.

Clearly, considering the many unknowns pointed out in this brief review of selected aspects of the eukaryotic cell cycle, much work must be accomplished in many areas of cell cycle biochemistry in order to understand the organization of cells during the developmental program. One such area of research is that of the analysis of the structure and function of the chromosomal proteins which presumably control not only the structure of chromosomal subunits in cells but also the expression of genes during the scheduled events of the cell cycle.

4.4 Nuclear proteins during stages of the cell cycle

Nuclear proteins are divided into two classes of molecules, the small molecular weight basic histones, and the larger molecular weight and rather complicated acidic, non-histone proteins (NHP). The histones range in molecular weight from 20,000 (histone F_1) to 10,000 daltons and are divided into five classes, the so called lysine rich histones and arginine rich histones. The composition and structure of these histones are remarkably similar in different organisms or cells as well as in the same organism in various stages of the cell cycle and cell development. For these reasons, histones are considered by most investigators to be very general repressors of DNA functions in the chromosomal control organization. In contrast, the NHP vary considerably in content and apparent species in many different organisms; their rate of synthesis and content in the cell is quite different during various stages of cell activity and the cell cycle. For these reasons the NHP are considered to be involved with subtle control mechanisms involving gene expression during cell differentiation and cell growth. Recent experiments by the group at Glascow, consisting of Stewart Gilmour and John Paul and colleagues (Gilmour and Paul, 1970), as well as experiments by Gary Stein and his colleagues (Stein et al., 1974), have indicated very clearly that reconstitution of chromatin components in vitro can be performed with NHP isolated from cells which synthesize a specific protein. When probed in vitro with RNA polymerase, such reconstituted chromatin is capable of expressing specifically the genes from which the NHP were derived. Since histones are capable of a firm and tight binding to DNA, it is felt that the NHP, due to unique specificity, are capable of binding to histones in specific regions of DNA. Possibly, when such NHP are modified, for example by addition of negative charges due to phosphorylation, such complexes of NHP and histones expose areas of DNA, and hence allow RNA polymerase to express specific genes for ultimate protein synthesis (Stein et al., 1974). Below will be outlined some aspects of nuclear protein modifications, specifically those modifications which possibly influence scheduled cell replication, either at the DNA level or at mitosis.

4.5 Nuclear protein modifications and the cell cycle

It appears, that in order for DNA to be active for transcription, histones and perhaps other nuclear proteins must be altered so that they can be displaced from specific transcribable regions of the genome. A number of histone modifications are directly associated with this mechanism of gene control and these will be only briefly mentioned, in view of the large body of review literature already available in this area (Stein et al., 1974; Hnilica, 1972). The addition of histones to native DNA in vitro drastically inhibits the ability of RNA polymerase to transcribe this template. AcetylCoA serves as a substrate for a series of enzymes which are capable of acetylating the ε-amino group of lysine. It has been demonstrated that when histones are thus modified, their repression of transcription is markedly reduced, presumably by virtue of the loss of positive charges on the histone repressors. This modification has been extensively studied during the synchronized chinese hamster cell cycle and it has been found that histones F_{2A}, F_{2B}, and F_3 reach the highest levels of acetylation by late S phase, in contrast to histone F_1, which reaches its peak of modification in mid-S phase (Shepherd et al., 1971). In PHA stimulated lymphocytes, regenerating liver, and also cortisol induced differentiation in rats, acetylation of histones has been noted as being an early event just prior to stimulation of specific transcriptional effects in such systems.

Another histone modification where cell cycle specificity of function seems suggested is the methylation of the ε-amino group of lysine in histones. Histones F_1 and F_{2A} seem to be the only histones methylated by this modification. The methylation modification tends to make histones more positively charged and hence more firmly attached to DNA. This has been experimentally tested and proven by using the binding of histones to DNA affinity columns. In recent studies, it has been shown that this activity starts at the end of S phase and the beginning of G_2 phase (Bijvoet, 1972). It is thus possible that its function might be related to the condensation of chromosomes and that methylation might stabilize positions of histones in chromatin after S phase.

Phosphorylation of histones and non-histone proteins has received considerable attention as to its relationship to events in the cell cycle and to its role in expression of gene transcription. The phosphorylation of histones falls into two classes, those affected by hormones and mediated by adenyl cyclase and cyclic AMP that are thought to be associated with specific transcriptional gene expression events, and those phosphorylation reactions with histones which are not hormone dependent and are associated with S phase events and cell replication. This latter type of histone modification is probably the best example of a nuclear protein modification which seems directly involved with DNA replication and cell proliferation (Langan, 1973). Histone F_1 has specific amino acid residues (mainly serine and threonine) which are modified by these two control regulations, one concerning hormone reactions relating to transcription and the other relating to cell growth and replication. Since histones are thought to be mainly structural elements involved in repressing functions of DNA, it seems reasonable that during certain periods of the cell cycle, for example during S phase and during mitosis, the phosphorylation of histones, and specifically F_1, might be related to a relaxation of the subunit structure of chromatin required for either replication or mitosis. Alternatively, condensation of chromatin could be achieved by specific phosphorylation of histone F_1, relaxation of its position in DNA, followed by cross-linking of various F_1 histone molecules along the length of chromatin structure.

Another nuclear protein modification that seems directly related to cell proliferation and DNA replication is the ADP-ribosylation of nuclear proteins. The experimental approach to the study of the regulation of DNA replication in our laboratory will be discussed in some detail to illustrate the techniques available for cell cycle analysis in cultured cells.

4.6 Poly-ADP-ribosylation of nuclear proteins as a model of studies probing changes in nuclear proteins as a cellular mechanism of control of cell replication

Poly(ADP-ribose) polymerase is an enzyme tightly bound to the chromatin of eukaryotic organisms. It catalyzes the successive transfer of ADP-ribose from NAD^+ to various nuclear proteins. Chains of 15 to 20 ADP-ribose groups can be isolated from chromatin or nuclei; covalent attachment of this chain is through an alkali labile bond to various nuclear proteins, although histones in vitro serve very favorably as acceptors in assays. The polymer is rapidly turning over in intact cells, since there are a number of enzymes, including a specific glycohydrolase, which cleave the polymer (Miwa, N. and Sugimura, T., 1971). DNA is required for elongation of the polymer and the enzyme is inhibited by not only nicotinamide (the end product of the reaction) but also by thymidine, suggesting a relationship to DNA functional replication. Burzio and Kolde (1973a, b) have shown that in rat liver nuclei or chromatin this modification leads to drastic inhibition of DNA replication. The mechanism underlying their observation seems to involve the poly-ADP-ribosylation of a specific rat liver chromatin endonuclease which normally under in vitro conditions tends to activate DNA into primer sites which serve as initiators for DNA polymerase. This observation stimulated our own interest in the modification and our subsequent studies to relate a function of this nuclear protein modification to events specifically in the S phase of the cell cycle. Peaks of accumulation of polymer in intact cells have been demonstrated by Kidwell and coworkers (Kidwell and Burdette, 1974) to occur in mid-S phase and G_2 phase of the cell cycle. Activity measurements on the enzyme as assayed in either nuclei or chromatin have proved quite complicated because of the complexity of the in vitro assay. The chromatin-enzyme system not only contains active

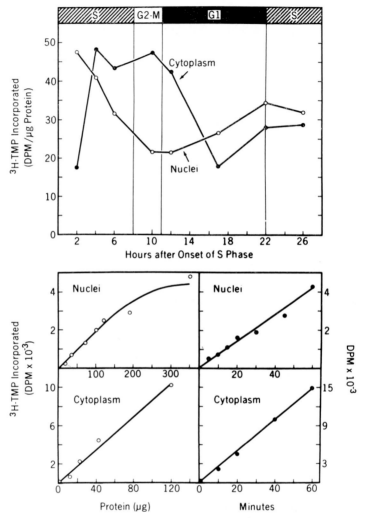

Fig. 4.2. Abscissa: (A) time after onset of S phase (h); (B) (left) μg protein; (right) time (min); ordinate: (A) spec. act. (dpm/μg protein); (B) radioact. (dpm × 10⁻³). Nuclear and cytoplasmic DNA polymerase activity during the cell cycle. (A) Conditions for nuclear DNA polymerases (○—○) and post-mitochondrial cytosol polymerases (●—●) were described; (B) controls for proportionality of protein (○—○) were incubated for 30 min. Controls for linearity of time (●—●) contained constant amounts of nuclei (70 μg protein/assay) and cytosol fraction (50 μg protein). Data taken from Smulson et al., 1975.

enzyme but also species of DNA required for activity as well as various nuclear protein acceptors which may well contain various amounts of endogenous polymer already existing from in vivo cell conditions.

Recently, we have attempted to determine when during the cell cycle this enzyme first appears during biosynthesis on polyribosomes (Roberts et al., 1975). This cytoplasmic assay of the nuclear enzyme was designed in order to allow us experimentally to control the assay by strict input of both histones (as acceptors) and DNA. The assay should thus reflect the period during the cell cycle when the enzyme is of importance to the cell. Although our chromatin and nuclear assays indicated low activity of the enzyme in S phase relative to other stages of the cell cycle (Smulson et al., 1971, 1975), the data in fig. 4.1, where cytoplasmic activity of the enzyme is assayed under optimal conditions of input histones and DNA, shows that the enzyme is synthesized at a high level during mid-S phase of the cell cycle. Synthesis or appearance of the enzyme in the cytoplasm is quite low subsequent to S

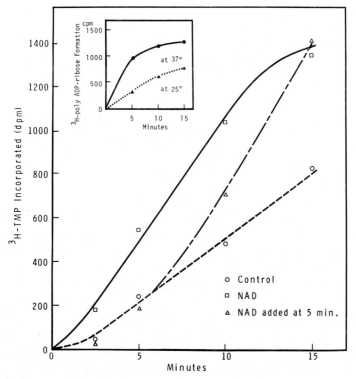

Fig. 4.3. Kinetics of [³H]dTMP incorporation during poly (ADP-ribose) formation. The normal mixture for DNA synthesis was increased by a factor of five. The reaction was started by addition of 2×10^7 nuclei and incubation was done at 37 °C. The inset shows the amount of poly (ADP-ribose) formed at 37 °C in the DNA synthesis assay and at 25 °C in the normal poly (ADP-ribose) polymerase assay. Data taken from Roberts et al., 1974.

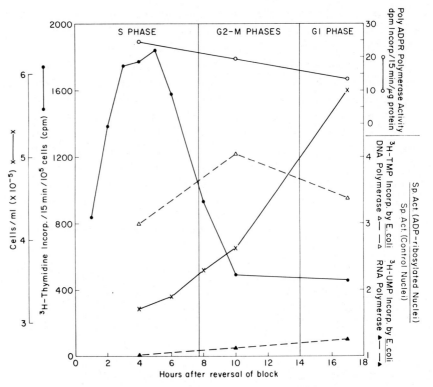

Fig. 4.4. Extent of ADP-ribosylation of nuclear proteins during the cell cycle and effect on RNA and DNA synthesis. Data taken from Roberts et al., 1973.

phase and during G_1 and G_2 phase, but again shows high activity in cytoplasm during a second round of S phase promoted by this method of cell synchrony. In this regard, the enzyme reflects the specific activity of nuclear DNA polymerase (fig. 4.2) also assayed in the cell cycle. Eukaryote DNA polymerase α has a molecular weight of about 100,000 and exists in both the cytoplasm and the nucleus, while DNA polymerase β (40,000 to 50,000 daltons) is found primarily in the nucleus.

As mentioned above, this nuclear protein modification appears to lead to inhibition of DNA polymerase in rat liver nuclei; however, based on the data shown in fig. 4.1, we were prompted to assess the effect of the modification on HeLa cell nuclei and chromatin under conditions of exogeneous DNA polymerase addition. In contrast to the results with rat liver chromatin or nuclei, the data (fig. 4.3) indicates that in HeLa nuclei, formation of poly(ADP-ribose) on nuclear proteins leads to *increased* activity for DNA polymerase (Roberts et al., 1973, 1974). Since a high proportion of liver cells are not included in the GF of the liver cell population, and hence not in one of the phases of the cell cycle, it was felt that perhaps the differences between liver and HeLa systems could be resolved by analysis of the effect of this modification on DNA synthesis during different phases of the HeLa cell cycle. However, the data (fig. 4.4) indicate that enhancement of DNA polymerase activity was evident throughout the cell cycle of the HeLa cell system and inhibition was never found (Roberts et al., 1974). The data also indicate that, when chromatin is probed with RNA polymerase, in contrast

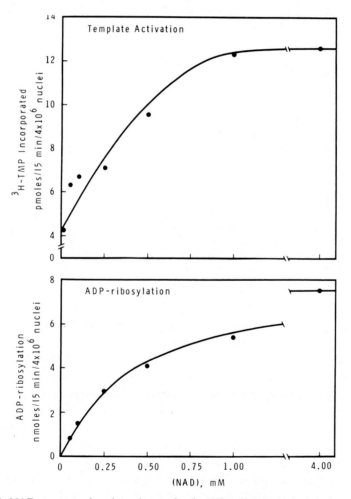

Fig. 4.5. NAD concentration dependence of poly (ADP-ribose) synthesis and template activation of HeLa nuclei for DNA synthesis mediated by *E. coli* DNA polymerase I. Data taken from Roberts et al., 1974.

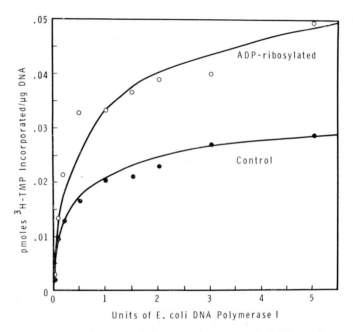

Fig. 4.6. Incorporation of a single deoxynucleotide as a function of increasing concentration of *E. coli* DNA polymerase I. Aliquots containing 8×10^6 nuclei were added to the poly (ADP-ribose) polymerase mixture (1.0 ml final volume) containing either no NAD or 4 mM NAD. After 15 min at room temperature, the solutions were diluted with 5 ml of 0.25 M sucrose containing 2 mM $MgCl_2$ and 40 mM nicotinamide. The nuclei were collected by centrifugation and resuspended in twice-concentrated DNA polymerase mixture containing various amounts of DNA polymerase I and [^{3}H]dTMP but no other deoxynucleoside triphosphates. Data taken from Roberts et al., 1974.

to DNA polymerase, no effect appears to be evident on transcription as promoted by the poly(ADP-ribose) modification.

We were further able to show that the stimulation by NAD$^+$ noted in nuclei could also be obtained in either sonicated nuclei or chromatin, indicating that permeability of substrate or exogeneous DNA polymerase was not being influenced by NAD$^+$ (Roberts et al., 1974). In addition, there was essentially no effect on activity of *E. coli* DNA polymerase I by NAD$^+$ or free poly(ADP-ribose) directly; the phenomenon is directly related to the covalent attachment of chains of poly(ADP-ribose) to various nuclear proteins in either chromatin or nuclei. The experiment described in fig. 4.5 further demonstrates that there is a direct proportionality between the extent of ADP-ribosylation of nuclear proteins and the template activation for DNA polymerase promoted by this system in HeLa nuclei.

One might anticipate that a covalent attachment of a long polyanion polymer to histones bound to DNA in chromatin would tend to release these modified proteins from their tight binding to DNA and expose regions for binding of DNA polymerase. We tested this hypothesis by the experiment shown in fig. 4.6, where the number of primer sites accessible to binding by exogeneous bacterial DNA polymerase was measured directly. The experimental model consists of the measurement of the incorporation into phosphodiester bond of only one *single* deoxynucleoside triphosphate in the presence of increasing concentrations of DNA polymerase until enzyme saturation is reached. At saturation the amount of deoxynucleotide incorporated can be interpreted as a *measurement of the degree of complexity of nuclear protein binding to DNA*. For example, this absolute value should be low when chromatin is isolated from stages of the cell cycle where DNA and nuclear proteins are highly condensed, such as the G_2 phase. It should be noted that in this measurement the formation of poly ADP-ribosylated proteins significantly stimulated the number of primer sites that were accessible for DNA polymerase (upper curve, fig. 4.6). It is not yet clear whether the nuclear proteins are selectively released from areas of DNA, exposing already existing primer sites for DNA polymerase, or whether protein release during modification allows nicks in DNA to be generated by endogenous endonucleases.

4.7 Effect of ADP-ribosylation during the cell cycle

Since the modification catalyzed by poly (ADP-ribose) polymerase in HeLa cells seems to change the ultrastructure of regions of chromatin and we wished to finally attempt to answer two major questions: 1) would this measurement suggest an important physiological function for poly (ADP-ribose) polymerase, and 2) whether a particular phase in the cell cycle is particularly sensitive to the change of DNA polymerase binding promoted by this enzyme.

Cells were synchronized by the methotrexate method and eight samples throughout the cell cycle were obtained, nuclei prepared, and analysis similar to that described in fig. 4.6 performed (fig. 4.7). The extent of natural protein condensation in chromatin is shown in fig. 4.7B (this is essentially the bottom curve of an experiment such as performed in fig. 4.6). Chromatin is especially condensed at the end of S phase and in the beginning of early G_1 phase, as assessed by this method. Template availability for DNA polymerase as promoted by poly(ADP-ribose) polymerase is shown in fig. 4.7D and 4.7E. Late S and early G_1 phases seem to be the most sensitive areas of the

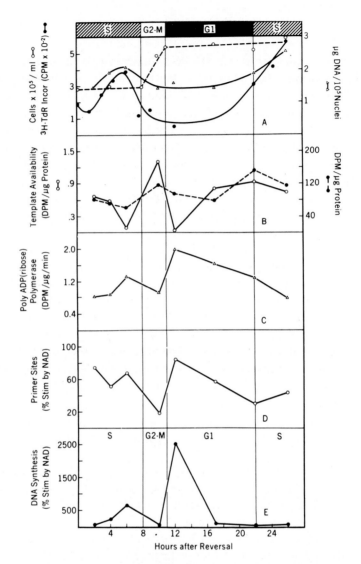

Fig. 4.7. Abscissa: time after initiation of S phase (h); ordinate: see below. ADP-ribosyla-tion and its effect on template-primer of HeLa cell nuclei during the cell cycle. (A) Cell synchrony. Pulse measurements of thymidine (cpm × 10^{-2}) into DNA/10^5 cells (●—●), cell density × 10^3/ml (○—○) (both left of ordinate) and DNA (µg) content/10^5 nuclei (△—△); (B) template availability in intact nuclei to single deoxynucleotide (^{3}H-TTP) incorporation by excess *E. coli* DNA polymerase I (●—●) (dpm/µg protein, right). Template accessibility to DNA polymerase under total DNA synthesis conditions (dpm/µg protein, left) is shown (○—○). (C) Poly (ADP-ribose) polymerase assay (dpm/µg/min); (D) enhancement of primer site accessibility by ADP-ribosylation. Primer site analysis was performed in presence and absence of NAD (1 mM) results expressed as % stim by NAD; (E) total DNA synthesis with *E. coli* DNA polymerase. Per cent stimulation is the result of incubation with NAD (1 mM). Data taken from Smulson et al., 1975.

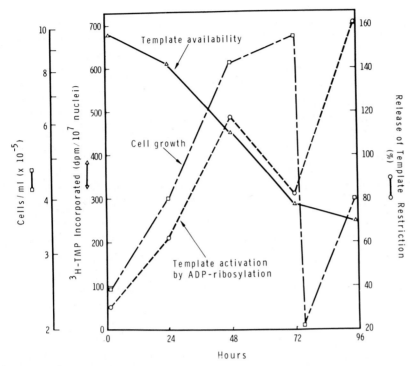

Fig. 4.8. Relationship of nuclear template activity and release of template restriction by poly (ADP-ribose) formation as a function of the asynchronous growth cycle of HeLa cells. HeLa cells were grown and cell samples were collected at the indicated times. At 72 h, the culture was diluted with fresh medium to restore growth. The template availability ($\triangle$) of isolated nuclei was determined by measurement of [³H]dTMP incorporation with *E. coli* DNA polymerase I. Release of template restriction ($\bigcirc$) is defined as the amount of [³H]dTMP incorporated by *E. coli* DNA polymerase I in the presence of 4 mM NAD divided by the amount of [³H]dTMP incorporated in the absence of NAD multiplied by 100. Data taken from Roberts et al., 1974.

cell cycle affected by this reaction. A similar experiment during asynchronous growth of HeLa cells is shown by the data in fig. 4.8, where both normal template availability is measured as well as enhancement of this template availability due to poly(ADP-ribose) polymerase. One major comment can be made about the results of both these experiments. It would seem that there exists an inverse correlation biologically between the extent of natural restriction of DNA polymerase binding to DNA due to histones and other nuclear proteins and the ability of this nuclear protein modification to release this response. That is, wherever, physiologically, chromatin is highly condensed, poly(ADP-ribose) polymerase is able to relax this condensation and expose regions which can be probed by binding of DNA polymerase. However, it is clearly too early to conclude that poly(ADP-ribose) polymerase has a function either in control of S phase events evolving replicon recognition sites for DNA polymerase or, alternatively, a role in the condensation and decondensation of chromatin components. However, these experiments indicates one approach for the study of the roles of nuclear protein modifications and their effects during the cell cycle.

4.8 Cell cycle specific inhibitors

One very important biochemical tool allowing investigators to probe various phenomena of the cell cycle involves selective inhibitors, either natural or synthetic, which are capable of selective arrestment of cells in specific stages of the cell cycle. In the concluding portions of this review we would like to categorize and describe a number of new and promising drugs and agents which seem to be specific for arresting specific areas of the cell cycle.

The knowledge of cell cycle specificity of antineoplastic drugs has proved to be of great importance in the timing of chemotherapeutic regimens. The cycle phase where maximum inhibition of macromolecular synthesis occurs may or may not correspond to the period of maximum cell death which may occur many hours following the drug effect, if at all. Even without cell death, the failure to divide can be important in chemotherapy.

An equally important reason for which drugs inhibitory to specific phases of the cell cycle are sought is that they can be essential aids in the elucidation of the basic biochemical processes of cell growth. The timing and site of action of the drug indicates what processes are essential for division and when they occur in relation to other cell cycle events. The development of understanding of the action of hydroxyurea (HU) is an example. This drug inhibits ribonucleotide reductase, the enzyme responsible for the conversion of ribonucleotides to deoxyribonucleotides (Sinclair, 1965). HU inhibits cells entering S phase presumably because dNTP pools are insufficient for the onset of DNA replication.

Table 4.1 indicates some of the better known cell synchrony agents (S and M phase inhibitors) and their actions on the eukaryote cell.

Several methods have been presented in the recent literature for testing anti-cancer drugs to determine their cell cycle specificity. It is desirable to have a quick and reliable means to screen the ever growing number of drugs for their site of action, the knowledge of which is preliminary to more probing biochemical studies of the drug.

Tobey and his colleagues at Los Alamos have developed two valuable

Table 4.1

Cell synchrony agents affecting S phase and mitosis.

Phase affected	Drug	Drug type	Action
S	Methotrexate	Folic acid analog	Inhibits dihydrofolate reductase
	5-FUdR	Nucleoside	Converted to 5F-dUMP; inhibits thymidylate synthetase
	Hydroxyurea	Hydroxylamine analog	Inhibits ribonucleotide reductase
	Cytosine arabinoside	Pyrimidine analog	Blocks deoxycytidine formation
	Thymidine (high conc.)	Nucleoside	Blocks initiation of DNA synthesis; dTTP inhibits TdR kinase, UdR kinase, dCMP deaminase, CDP and UDP reduction
M	Vinblastine	Plant alkaloid	Inhibits assembly of microtubules; precipitates tubulin
	Colchicine	Plant alkaloid	Inhibits assembly of microtubules; binds to tubulin
	Colcemid	Plant alkaloid derivative	Inhibits assembly of microtubules

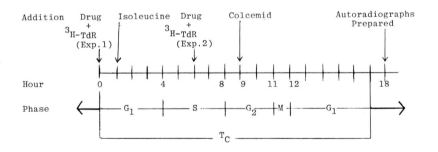

CHO cells starved of isoleucine to G_1 block are given drug and ^3H–TdR at either t = 0 (Exp. 1) or t = 6 (Exp. 2). Cells are enriched with isoleucine at t = 1 and colcemid added at t = 9 to block cells in mitosis. Autoradiographs are prepared at t = 18 to determine mitotic and labeled fractions. See test for interpretations.

* Ref. 26

Fig. 4.9. Experimental protocol for testing cell cycle specific drugs (Nagatsu et al., 1972).

methods for analysis of cell cycle specificity (Tobey, 1972a; Tobey and Crissman, 1972). Both methods utilize Chinese hamster ovary (CHO) cells blocked in G_1 arrest with isoleucine deficiency. By this procedure cells are accumulated four hours before the G_1/S boundary (see fig. 4.9). CHO cells have a Tc of approximately 17 h with $G_1 = 9$, $S = 4$, $G_2 = 3$ and $M = 1$. The drug and low levels of ^{3}H-TdR are added at either $t = 0$ (Exp. 1) or $t = 6$ (Exp. 2). The block is reversed by the addition of isoleucine at $t = 1$. Cells progress into S phase at approximately $t = 4$. Colcemid is added to the culture at $t = 9$ and autoradiographs are prepared at $t = 18$ to determine the labeled and mitotic fractions (fig. 4.9). In Experiment 1, if the resultant culture is devoid of labeled and mitotic cells, then the drug blocks G_1 or G_1-S; if the labeled fraction of cells is equal to the control but the mitotic cells are much fewer, the drug blocks G_2. In Experiment 2, if the labeled and mitotic cells are much fewer than the control culture, the drug blocks cells already in S phase; and again, if the fraction of labeled cells is equal to that of the control but the mitotic index lower, then the drug inhibits G_2 phase. If the labeled and mitotic fractions of the drug treated culture are equal to the control in Experiment 1 and Experiment 2, then the agent is without effect on the cell cycle.

Another method proposed by Tobey utilizes flow microfluorometry analysis of the population distribution of DNA content, and autoradiography (Tobey and Crissman, 1972). Using this method one can accurately determine the total number of cells in G_1, S and G_2 by their respective DNA content. CHO cells in isoleucine mediated G_1 arrest are supplemented with isoleucine and the drug. Ten hours later a portion of the cells are fixed with formalin and stained with fluorescent-Feulgen and acriflavine. A flow microfluorometry pattern is obtained that shows the DNA distribution pattern. A second portion of the same culture is washed free of the drug (at least partial reversibility is assumed) and resuspended in warm medium containing ^{3}H-TdR. Each hour following resuspension an aliquot is removed for determination of labeled fraction and cell number. Three major responses are possible: 1) The agent blocks G_1 so that FMF analysis yields G_1 DNA content, and the cells require at least four hours to enter S after removal of the drug; 2) The agent blocks G_1–S with a similar FMF pattern to I, but after drug removal the cells immediately begin DNA synthesis; 3) The agent prevents neither G_1 or initiation of S so that FMF yields cells with a greater DNA content than G_1 cells, and after removal of the drug they divide within a short period. Noting minor variations and rates of change can yield even more information on the drug action.

Many of the new drugs currently being investigated block cells in G_2

Table 4.2

Specific inhibitors of G₂ phase of the cell cycle.

Drug	Drug type	Proposed action
Macramomycin	Antibiotic	Binds to cell surface
Daunomycin	Anthracycline antibiotic	Intercalates into DNA, causing breaks and chromosomal damage
Adriamycin	Anthracycline antibiotic	Intercalates into DNA, causing breaks and chromosomal damage
Mithramycin	Antibiotic	Binds to DNA, inhibits RNA polymerase
Neocarzinostatin	Acidic protein	Induces degradation of DNA
Bleomycin	Glycopeptide antibiotic	Causes DNA damage

phase (see table 4.2) enabling us to learn much about cell requirements immediately prior to cell division. One of the most interesting is macramomycin. This is a weakly basic polypeptide antibiotic, molecular weight 15,000, isolated from cultures of *Streptomyces macromomyceticus* (Chimura et al., 1968) and has been shown to inhibit growth of mouse leukemia 1210 and mouse sarcoma 180. Kunimoto et al. show that with HeLa and Yoshida sarcoma cells macramomycin binds to the cell membrane (Kunimoto et al., 1972). It inhibits DNA synthesis but not drastically, and has no effect on RNA synthesis or protein synthesis during the cell cycle. The lethal effect of macramomycin on cell growth occurs after S phase and this effect is reversible by brief treatment with trypsin. Kunimoto has ruled out the possibilities that the drug interferes with uptake of precursors, or induces degradation of DNA. He concludes that the cell surface is functional in replication and that macramomycin interferes by its interaction with the surface. Lippman (1974), using 1210 leukemia cells and TA3Ha mouse ascites tumor cells has shown that macramomycin is cytostatic, that is, cell division is inhibited but the cell remains viable. At low cytostatic concentrations, DNA synthesis is not inhibited. The macramomycin treated cell is greatly enlarged so that the DNA content is 2 to 40 times greater than that of a normal cell. This endoreduplication suggests a G₂ block. Reversal of the cytostatic effect can be accomplished with trypsin.

Daunomycin and adriamycin are two additional antitumor antibiotics, closely related in structure, which seem to be G₂ inhibitors. Daunomycin is a glycosidic anthracycline compounds isolated from *Streptomyces peuceticus*

(Acamone, 1964). Adriamycin is isolated from a mutant of the same strain and differs from daunomycin by a single hydroxyl group (Chirigos and Papas, 1975). Both compounds prevent cells from reaching mitosis at low concentrations. DNA and RNA synthesis is affected although the cells progress smoothly from G_1–S. Tobey suggests that in the presence of the drugs the genome that is replicated is abnormal such that the cells are unable to complete G_2 (Tobey, 1972b). There is evidence suggesting that these antibiotics form complexes with DNA. Sawada et al. have shown that the two antibiotics increase the T_m of calf thymus DNA indicating a marked change in chromosome stability (Sawada, et al., 1974). However, Dalgleish et al. (1974) on the basis of circular dichroism studies finds that the complex of daunomycin-DNA does not behave as a typical intercalating drug–DNA complex. Various investigators (Kim and Kim, 1972; Bhuyan and Fraser, 1974) have shown that adriamycin is most cytotoxic during S phase, so that one might assume that the major drug effect occurs during the DNA synthetic processes. This supports Tobey's suggestion that the observed G_2-M block is a consequence of S phase abnormalities.

Mithramycin is another antibiotic known to bind to DNA. It is isolated from *Streptomyces plicatus* (Chirigos and Papas, 1975) and has been used, clinically to treat embryonic cell carcinoma of the testes, hypernephroma, and glioblastoma multiforme (Tobey, 1972). Although a G_2-M inhibitor, mithramycin differs from adriamycin and daunomycin in that its primary inhibitory effect is on transcription (Bhuyan and Fraser, 1974). The compound has very little effect on DNA synthesis, and does not effect cell entry into S phase. Mithramycin bridges complementary strands of the DNA duplex in the presence of Mg^{2+} to form a stable intermediate that is unable to be transcribed by RNA polymerase. Cells accumulate in G_2 and the inhibitory mechanism of this compound illustrates the importance of an RNA process associated with G_2 phase (Tobey, 1972).

Yet another G_2-M inhibitory drug is neocarzinostatin (NCS) an acidic polypeptide of molecular weight 10,000 isolated from *Streptomyces carzinostaticus*. It has significant growth inhibitory effect on mouse ascites tumor (Sawada et al., 1974). Bhuyan has shown with synchronized DON cells that the most sensitive phases of the cell cycle in terms of plating efficiency reduction are M and G_1 (Bhuyan et al., 1972). Exposure during S phase did not appear to inhibit DNA synthesis. Sawada, however, observes that with L1210 cells NCS inhibits ^{3}H-TdR incorporation in a rapid and striking manner (Sawada et al., 1974). Uridine incorporation was less affected. This drug does not affect uptake of the precursors into the cell nor does it affect DNA polymerase (crude L1210) in a cell free system. It does, however, interact with the DNA template, causing a slight decrease in the T_m of calf thymus DNA. When L1210 cells were incubated with NCS and subsequently the DNA analyzed on alkaline sucrose gradients, the size of the DNA was shown to be reduced considerably in comparison to the control. The decrease in T_m caused by incubation with NCS is probably the result of DNA strand scission (Sawada et al., 1974). This could explain Tobey's observation that cells are blocked at the G_2-M border, since the genome is considerably damaged and unable to undergo mitosis. An additional observation with this compound has been that the mitotic index is higher in the cells treated at $t = 0$ and than at $t = 6$, suggesting that the inhibitory effect is reversible perhaps by repair (Tobey, 1972).

Bleomycin is a complex glycopeptide isolated from *Streptomyces verticullus* and is active against a variety of human neoplasms including squamous cell carcinoma, melanomas, and lymphomas (Tobey, 1972), and has been used by Barranco (Barranco et al., 1973) as a successful in vivo synchronizing agent for human malignant melanomas. Belomycin has been found to induce a G_2-M block with CHO cells, and to allow initiation and synthesis of the total DNA at a normal rate (Tobey, 1972). Krishnan and Paika observed a G_2 block with HeLa, mouse fibroblasts, and human lymphoblasts in a system where asynchronous cells exposed to the drug and ^{3}H-TdR are then exposed to colcemid for four hours; no mitotic cells are seen to have been synthesizing DNA (Paika and Krishnan, 1973). Nagatsu reports a bleomycin induced G_2 block with Ehrlich ascites tumor cells, noting that a portion of the cells continue on to a second DNA synthetic phase without having divided (Nagatsu et al., 1972). These results are explained by the fact that bleomycin causes damage to the chromosome in the form of chromatid breaks, translocations, and cross-overs. Hittelman and Rao (1974) also found bleomycin to cause a G_2 block in CHO cells. In their studies they utilized the technique of fusing interphase cells with mitotic cells by incubation with UV inactivated Sendai virus. This procedure causes premature condensation of the interphase chromosome (PCC) such that the immediate effect of the drug can be assessed and the drug effect can be measured at any time throughout the cell cycle. Utilizing this technique they found a 5–9-fold increase in chromosome aberrations in the treated PCC than when it was allowed to reach mitosis. Within one hour 36% of the DNA gaps and breaks were shown to be repaired; 44% of the cells delayed in G_2 were unable to reach M. This suggests that there is a maximum amount of chromosome damage which a cell can sustain and repair.

Thus macramomycin, daunomycin, adriamycin, mithramycin, NCS, and bleomycin all tend to act to inhibit cells in G_2 phase of the cell cycle. Four of the compounds also alter the state of the genome to the extent that the cell is unable to undergo division and thus pose interesting questions as to the controls affecting initiation of mitosis. Further work with these drugs seems imperative, as does further biochemical studies on the effects upon cell cycle of the antineoplastic drugs presently being developed in laboratories throughout the world.

Acknowledgments

Parts of this work have been supported by U.S. Public Health Service Grants CA13195 and CA11950.

References

Arcamone, F., et al. (1964) Daunomycin. I. The structure of daunomycinone. J. Am. Chem. Soc. 86, 5334–5335.

Barranco, S. C., Luce, J. K., Romsdahl, M. M. and Humphrey, R. M. (1973) Bleomycin as a possible synchronizing agent for human tumor cells in vivo. Cancer Res. 33, 882–887.

Bhuyan, B. K. and Fraser, T. J. (1974) Cytotoxicity of antitumor agents in a synchronous mammalian cell system. Cancer Chem. Rep. 58, 149–155.

Bhuyan, B. K., Scheidt, L. G. and Fraser, T. J. (1972) Cell cycle phase specificity of antitumor agents. Cancer Res. 32, 398–407.

Burzio, L. and Koide, S. S. (1970) A functional role of polyapdr in DNA synthesis. Biochem. Biophys. Res. Commun. 40, 1013–1026.

Burzio, L. and Kiode, S. S. (1973) Activation of the template activity of isolated rat liver nuclei for DNA synthesis and its inhibition by NAD. Biochem. Biophys. Res. Commun. 53, 572–579.

Byvoet, P. (1972) In vivo turnover and distribution of radio-N-methylin arginine-rich histones from rat tissues. Arch. Biochem. Biophys. 152, 887–888.

Chimura, H., Ishizuka, M. and Hamada, M. (1968) A new antibiotic macramomycin, exhibiting antitumor and antimicrobial activity. J. Antibiotics 21, 44–49.

Chirigos, M. and Papas, T. S. (1975) Immunological and chemotherapeutic prevention and control of oncogenic viruses. Adv. in Pharm. and Chemotherapy, Vol 12 (eds. S. Garattini et al.) Academic Press, New York, pp. 111–113.

Chu, M. Y. and Fischer, G. A. (1962) A proposed mechanism of action of 1-B-D-Arabinolfuraadsyl-sytosine ASAN. Biochem. Pharmacol. 11, 423–430.

Dalen, H., Oftebro, R. and Engeset, A. (1965) The effect of methotrexate and leucovorin on cell division in chang cells. Cancer 18, 41–48.

Dalgleish, D. G., Fey, G. and Kersten, W. (1974) Circular dichroism studies of complexes of the antibiotics caunomycin, nogalamycin, chromomycin and mithramycin with DNA. Biopolymers 13, 1757–1766.

Gilmour, R. S. and Paul, J. (1970) Role of non-histone components in determining organ specificity of rabbit chromatins. FEBS Letters 9, 242.

Hittleman, W. and Rao, P. (1974) Bleomycin-induced damage in prematurely condensed chromosomes and its relationship to cell cycle progression in CHO cells. Cancer Res. 34, 3433–3439.

Hnilica, L. S. (1972) The Structure and Biological Functions of Histones. CRC Press, Cleveland, Ohio.

Huberman, J. A. and Riggs, A. P. (1968) On the mechanism of DNA replication in mammalian chromosomes. J. Mol. Biol. 32, 327–341.

Kidwell, W. R. and Burdette, K. E. (1974) Poly (ADP-ribose) synthesis and cell division. Biochem. Biophys. Res. Commun. 61, 766–773.

Kim, S. H. and Kim, J. H. (1972) Lethal effect of adriamycin on the division cycle of HeLa cells. Cancer Res. 32, 323–325.

Kunimoto, T., Hori, M. and Umezawa, H. (1972) Macramomycin, an inhibitor of the membrane function of tumor cells. Cancer Res. 32, 1251–1256.

Lala, P. K. (1971) Studies on tumor cell population kinetics. Methods Cancer Res. 6, 3–95.

Lambert, W. S. and Studzinski, G. P. (1969) Thymidine as a synchronizing agent. II. Partial recovery of HeLa cells from unbalanced growth. J. Cell Physiol. 73, 261–266.

Langan, T. A. (1973) Protein kinase and protein kinase substrates. In: Advances in Cyclic Nucleotide Research, Vol 3 (eds.: P. Greengard and G. A. Robison) Raven Press, New York, pp. 99–153.

Lippman, M. M. (1974) In vitro studies on macromycin (NCS-170105): effects on cultured TA3Ha and L-1210 cells. Can. Chem. Rep. 58, 181–187.

Maranz, R. and Shelanski, M. L. (1970) Structure of microtubular crystals induced by vin blastine in vitro. J. Cell Biol. 44, 234–238.

Miwa, M. and Sugimura, T. (1971) Splitting of the ribose-ribose linkage of poly(adenosine diphosphate-ribose) by a calf thymus extract. J. Cell Biol. 44, 234–238.

Nagatsu, M., Richart, R. and Lambert, A. (1972) Effects of bleomycin on the cell cycle of Ehrlich ascites carcinoma. Cancer Res. 32, 1966–1970.

Paika, K. D. and Krishan, A. (1973) Bleomycin-induced chromosomal aberrations in cultured mammalian cells. Cancer Res. 33, 961–965.

Puck, T. T. and Sheffer, J. (1963) Life cycle analysis of mammalian cells. I. A method for localizing metabolic events within the life cycle and its application to the action of colcemide and sublethal doses of X-irradiation. Biophys. J. 3, 379–397.

Roberts, J. H., Stark, P. and Smulson, M. (1973) Stimulation of DNA synthesis by adenosine diphosphoribosylation of HeLa nuclear proteins during the cell cycle. Biochem. Biophys. Res. Commun. 52, 43–50.

Roberts, J. H., Stark, P. and Smulson, M. (1974) Poly (ADP-ribose): Release of template restriction in HeLa cells. Proc. Natl. Acad. Sci. U.S. 71, 3212–3216.

Roberts, J., Stark, P., Giri, C. and Smulson, M. (1975) Cytoplasmic poly (ADP-ribose) polymerase during the HeLa cell cycle. Arch. Biochem. Biophys. (in press).

Sawada, H., Tatsumi, K., Sasada, M., Shirakawa, S., Nakamura, T. and Watisaka, G. (1974) Effect of neocarzinostatin on DNA synthesis in L1210 cells. Cancer Res. 34, 3341–3346.

Shepherd, G. R., Noland, B. J. and Hardin, J. M. (1971) Histone acetylation in synchronized mammalian cell cultures. Biochem. Biophys. Acta 228, 544–549.

Sinclair, W. K. (1965) Hydroxyurea: differential lethal effects on cultured mammalian cells during the cell cycle. Science 150, 1729–1731.

Smulson, M., Henriksen, O. and Rideau, C. (1971) Activity of polyadenosine diphosphoribose polymerase during the human cell cycle. Biochem. Biophys. Res. Commun. 43, 1266–1273.

Smulson, M., Stark, P., Gazzoli, M. and Roberts, J. (1975) Release of template restriction for DNA synthesis by poly DAP (ribose) polymerase during the HeLa cell cycle. Exp. Cell Res. 90, 175–182.

Stein, G. S., Spelsberg, T. C. and Kleinsmith, L. J. (1974) Non-histone chromosomal proteins and gene regulation. Science 183, 817–824.

Taylor, E. W. (1965) The mechanism of colchicine inhibition of mitosis; kinetics of inhibition and the binding of ^{3}H colchicine. J. Cell Biol. 25, 145–160.

Taylor, J. H., Haut, W. F. and Tung, J. (1962) Effects of fluororodeoxyudine on DNA replication, chromosome breakage, and reunion. Proc. Natl. Acad. Sci. 48, 190–198.

Tobey, R. A. (1972a) A simple, rapid technique for determination of the effects of chemotherapeutic agents on mammalian cell cycle traverse. Cancer Res. 32, 309–316.

Tobey, R. A. (1972b) Effects of cytosine arabinoside daunomycin, mithramycin, adriamycin, and camptothecin on mammalian cell cycle traverse. Cancer Res. 32, 2720–2725.

Tobey, R. A. and Crissman, H. A. (1972) Use of flow microfluorometry in detailed analysis of effects of chemical agents on cell cycle progression. Cancer Res. 32, 2726–2732.

CHAPTER 5

The assay of cell proliferation inhibitors

B. I. LORD

Paterson Laboratories, Christie Hospital and Holt Radium Institute,
Manchester M20 9BX, U.K.

The assessment of substances which increase the proliferation rate of cell populations presents many problems. When attempting to assess proliferation inhibitors the problems are considerably greater. The basis of this statement lies in the fact that cell proliferation processes are so readily inhibited by a wide variety of materials and conditions. The problem is magnified when one has to rely on in vitro techniques which, without the protective effects of a reticulo–endothelial or macrophage system, is at best a compromise which keeps the cells in a relatively 'happy' condition. For example, simple short term suspension and monolayer cultures of haemopoietic tissues are invariably running down and their successful use depends on the lack of a disturbance which merely increases the 'unhappiness' of the system. Where measurements have to be extended over several hours, as will be shown to be necessary, a culture system may be totally inadequate to demonstrate the true effect of an inhibitor. Thus, a culture system must be sufficiently stable and preferably growing, rather than simply maintained, to be capable even of demonstrating inhibitory effects on cell proliferation.

Since such systems are subject to so many artefactual parameters, it is necessary to demonstrate adequately that an effect is not simply non-specific. No 'chalone' preparation can as yet be considered even reasonably pure. At best, they are cocktails of many cellular constituents. Thus, the definition of cell line specificity for a potential 'chalone' represents a very acute problem and consequently it is necessary either that a culture contains a variety of cell lines which can be separately identified or that a series of directly comparable cultures of different cell types is available. In this way, the control cell populations can be treated with an extract in an identical manner to the test cell populations. Conversely, in order to determine whether a particular cell extract is unique, it is necessary to prepare extracts of very closely related cell populations and to test them against equally closely related cell types. Thus, for example, cell line specificity is not adequately indicated if granulocyte extracts affect granulocytic cells whilst brain extracts do not, because the two extracts are so different in their origin. Neither is it indicated if granulocyte extracts affect granulocytic cells but do not affect a cultured malignant cell line like HeLa cells; in this case because the two test systems are so dissimilar. Assay systems must, therefore, be capable of demonstrating, unequivocally, the cell line specificity of inhibitory cell extracts.

A further requirement for any assay system is that the errors of measurement shall be smaller than the changes to be measured. While this factor may seem very obvious, in biological systems variations in measurable parameters are often very large and, as will be demonstrated below, may be comparable with the magnitude of the probable change expected.

The assay techniques available cover a wide spectrum of end points ranging from those where 'improvement was obvious to the naked eye' (Rytömaa and Kiviniemi, 1970) to the sophistication of a definition of molecular organisation due to the intramolecular biophysical forces within a cell (Cercek and Cercek, 1972). Many of these techniques are based on the definition of the subdivisions in the cell cycle and involve the measurement of the mitotic interval and/or the incorporation of tritium labelled thymidine into cells synthesising DNA. This latter method is the one most universally applied throughout the field of 'chalone' research.

Measurement of the structuredness of the cytoplasmic matrix (SCM) of cells affords a unique way of making some very precise observations about the behaviour of cells which may well be related to their proliferative status.

Since one is interested in studying the population growth controlling properties of 'chalones', one of the more realistic end points should be to investigate whether or not cell production is affected. The diffusion chamber technique in which a cell population is isolated within a physiological environment and yet can be studied quantitatively is an obvious candidate for such a measurement. Similarly, colony techniques, both in vitro and in vivo afford the opportunity to study the development of a single population of cells.

Biologically orientated end points may serve to demonstrate the effectiveness of cell extracts in limiting cell production or function. For example, it should be possible to measure the survival of animals bearing tumours after encountering the appropriate extract; the change in the rate of wound healing after treatment with epidermal extracts; changes in lymphocyte proliferation and the graft versus host reaction following the application of lymphocyte extracts.

Clearly, a variety of techniques is available for the assay of cell extracts containing proliferation inhibitory or 'chalone-like' compounds and each of these will be examined in the light of the criteria discussed above and for the information they may afford. Ultimately, however, if the 'chalone' hypothesis is to hold as a physiological control process over cell proliferation then it is necessary to demonstrate the effects under physiological conditions. The use of artificially produced cell extracts, applied in grossly supraphysiological dose, is no test of homeostatic control. Experiments to assess 'chalone-like' activity in such situations are, however, notoriously difficult to design and are therefore somewhat limited.

It is not the purpose of this chapter, however, to present a series of detailed recipes for the various techniques used by 'chalone' workers. Since most of them are standard methods, it is intended to discuss only the principles of the techniques. I shall then attempt to analyse the information that can be obtained and to examine their advantages, pitfalls and short-comings.

5.1   The cell cycle

The key to direct measurements of effects of any agent on cell proliferation lies in a knowledge of the phases of the cell generation cycle. Howard and Pelc (1951, 1953) subdivided the cycle into four well defined phases related to DNA content as shown in fig. 5.1. Following through the cycle, the DNA content remains constant at the $2N$ level for the G_1 period during which the cell is preparing itself for DNA synthesis. During DNA synthesis (S phase), the DNA content rises to the $4N$ level (not necessarily in a linear manner as illustrated in the figure). The DNA content then remains constant again (G_2 phase) while the cell prepares for mitosis (M phase). If, as in all normal in vivo situations, the cell population is in a steady state of cell proliferation, it is highly probable that the population is largely, if not completely, asynchronous. The lower part of the diagram represents, therefore, an asynchronous cell population where the cells are distributed throughout the phases of the cycle in proportion to the duration of those phases. If all the cells are in the proliferation cycle, i.e. the growth fraction is unity, then a measurement of the proportion of cells in any one phase compared to the total population is a measure of the relative times spent in each phase (t_G, t_s, t_{G_2}, t_m), the duration of the complete cycle being shown as t_c. The

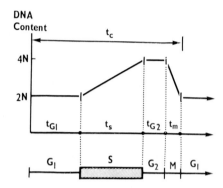

Fig. 5.1. Change in DNA content of a cell nucleus as it progresses through the cell cycle. The lower part of the diagram represents an asynchronous cell population illustrating that the relative number of cells in each phase of the cycle is proportional to the duration of that phase.

exception to this may lie in a tissue which exhibits a high degree of diurnal rhythm in its proliferative activity, skin tissues, for example, when it is important that experiments always be carried out at the same time of day, and preferably, since one is investigating inhibitors, at the time when the proliferation rate is highest. This aspect of methodology has been stressed for example by Laurence (1973). Under these conditions it is possible that there may be some degree of synchronous proliferation in the population which may affect the observations.

In cell culture conditions, a different set of rules applies. If the cell population is growing then the proportion of cells in, say, the DNA S phase of the cycle bears a logarithmic relationship to the size of the population. These functions are well worked out and are explained fully in text books relating to cell proliferation kinetics (e.g. Cleaver). For example, the proportion of cells in DNA synthesis is given by the equation

$$[\exp(t_s/t_c \times \ln 2) - 1] \times \exp(t_{G_2}/t_c \times \ln 2)$$

(Cleaver, 1967).

As far as the measurement of the phases of the cell cycle is concerned, the two G intervals cannot at present be observed because there is no sufficiently well recognised marker for these phases. Mitosis is clearly recognisable as a cell with changed morphology and has therefore been the traditional method of observing changes in the cell cycle. It is, however, a phase of short duration relative to the total cycle time and therefore few mitotic cells are to be found. The situation can be improved using metaphase arrest agents as described below and, as such, measurement of the proportion of cells in mitosis is a valuable technique in studying the effects of inhibitors. Since the synthesis of tritiated thymidine in 1957/8 (Hughes, 1957, and Verly, Firket and Hunebelle, 1958), however, the study of cell kinetics has been revolutionised. On average, over a wide range of tissues, the ratio of cells in DNA-S to mitosis is between 8:1 and 15:1 (Schultze and Oehlert, 1960) and consequently the accuracy of measuring cells in the S phase is considerably higher than for those in mitosis. As a result, detailed analyses of the cell parameters for a wide variety of tissues have been made and can serve as a basis for investigating changes in the cell cycle.

5.2 *Measurement of the stathmokinetic index*

As mentioned above, the mitotic phase of the cell cycle is relatively short and in most cases is measured in minutes rather than hours. By the use of spindle poisons or stathmokinetic agents (agents which prevent spindle formation and block mitosis at the metaphase stage) cells entering metaphase are accumulated. Thus, an increasing number of mitotic figures is seen in the preparation. The proportion of metaphase figures at a predetermined time is known as the stathmokinetic index. The phases of mitosis are illustrated in fig. 5.2, the stathmokinetic agent acting to prevent movement into the anaphase stage. For most practical purposes, prophase is not so readily definable as is metaphase and consequently only metaphase figures are counted. The rate of accumulation of metaphase figures should represent the rate of flow of cells through mitosis provided that the agent used has no effect on any other phase of the cell cycle and that the time scale of observation is too short for the system to recognize a disturbance due to

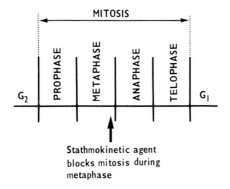

Fig. 5.2. The mitotic phase of the cell cycle and its subdivisions. Stathmokinetic agents block mitosis during the metaphase stage.

the loss of arrested cells. Thus, a test agent applied at, say, time zero followed by a stathmokinetic agent at half or one hour later should reflect any inhibition (or stimulation) taking place at the $G_2 \rightarrow M$ boundary, by a reduction (or increase) in the rate of accumulation of arrested metaphase figures.

Lack of an effect on the mitotic process under these conditions, however, does not necessarily mean there is no effect on cell proliferation. A block at the $G_1 \rightarrow S$ boundary would not, for example, be seen until all the cells in the S and G_2 phase had passed through mitosis. Consequently, if the normal cell cycle analysis is known, it is possible to start the mitosis arrest at a time when the unaffected S and G_2 cells have passed through mitosis and hence check on the possible $G_1 \rightarrow S$ blockage. Used to its fullest capacity, the mitotic arrest rate should be measured at a series of times after application of the extract (e.g. Elgjo, 1973). In this way, it is theoretically possible to fix the timing of the effect of an extract with respect to the cell cycle.

Colchicine was the earliest of the agents used for blocking mitosis (Dustin, 1936). Colcemid, a synthetic drug closely related to colchicine was found in many cases to be superior. More recently, the vinca alkaloids, vinblastine and vincristine have become available as stathmokinetic drugs. An assessment of colchicine for the measurement of mitotic rate was made by Hooper (1961) and an excellent comparison of the relative efficiencies of these four agents has been presented by Tannock (1966). He suggested that an effective stathmokinetic agent should possess the following characteristics:

i) There must be an optimum dose at which it arrests all metaphases in the tissue of interest over a certain period of time;

ii) The arrested metaphases should not degenerate into an unrecognisable state before the tissues are fixed and examined;

iii) The mitotic arrest properties should not be highly sensitive to dose;

iv) There should be no effect on interphase cells.

Tannock showed that for each of these agents there was an optimum dose level and that to exceed it, the loss through pyknotic degeneration may already be important before the peak of mitoses has been achieved. He concluded that colchicine, vinblastine and vincristine all come near to meeting these requirements and that their optimum doses are in the region of 0.5 to 2 μg/g body weight used in vivo for the two tissues tested. Colcemid was less satisfactory, requiring a dose of greater than 5 μg/g body weight. In fact, it showed relatively poor metaphase arrest properties and gave no peak of mitoses over the dose range tested. It was subsequently abandoned. To use less than the optimum dose means that a number of cells may escape the block, thereby underestimating the rate of entry into mitosis and consequently underestimating the proliferation rate.

When working on sectioned material, an important and previously overlooked, geometrical factor must be taken into account. For example, mitoses in the crypt cells of the small intestine are invariably out of line with the interphase nuclei resulting in an overestimate of the stathmokinetic index (Tannock, 1966).

It has normally been assumed that, when the optimum dose is used, the accumulation of metaphase figures is linear and that satisfactory results are obtained as long as one works on the linear part of the curve i.e. before cells are beginning to escape from the block and before pyknotic degeneration occurs. Tannock, however, demonstrated that the accumulation curve is rarely linear and that to assume linearity resulted in large systematic errors which tend to overestimate cell cycle and turnover times. In recognising all these sources of error, it is perhaps not surprising that colchicine and colcemid, applied to a tumour tissue, overestimated the doubling time by a factor of two while vinblastine and vincristine, though better, still gave overestimates of about 40%. This observation has been borne out in recent studies using vinblastine on haemopoietic cell populations (Lord, unpublished results) where the rate of accumulation of mitotic figures has been found to be considerably slower than would be predicted by thymidine labelling studies (see below). Tannock applied these stathmokinetic agents to only two tissues but his results were sufficient to show that their conditions of use will depend on the tissue to be investigated. It is clearly important, therefore, in using this technique to determine the optimum conditions of use for a particular spindle poison on the cell population investigated.

In spite of the precautions which must be taken in using this technique it represents a very valuable tool in assessing some aspects of changes in cell proliferation and as such has been widely used. The initial demonstrations of the epidermal 'chalone' for example were made from the reduced numbers of mitotic figures in colcemid-arrested cultures consisting of small pieces of mouse ear incubated in standard buffered saline containing glucose (Bullough and Laurence, 1960, 1961). With regard to this latter point, Bullough and Laurence (1961, 1964) laid down stringent requirements for the demonstration of a 'chalone' effect. They found that the 'chalone' effect for skin tissues exhibits an adrenalin dependency and accordingly defined the presence of a 'chalone' only when the mitotic rate of the epidermis was reduced in the first 4 h with colcemid, was normal after 9 h but was reduced again after an adrenalin wash. More recently studies were made in vivo

using a dose of 4 μg colcemid/g body weight (Hondius Boldingh and Laurence, 1968; Laurence and Randers-Hansen, 1971) for studies on epidermal
and epithelial cell mitotic rates. In both cases the number of mitoses/cm
was determined on sections of epidermis. Bullough and Laurence (1970)
used a similar dose of colcemid (4 μg/ml) on a mouse lymphoma in culture.
This dose may possibly be a little on the low side in view of the information
processed by Tannock. In fact a careful survey by Nome (1974) on dose and
time responses showed that the optimum dose of colcemid for a variety of
skin tissues was about 6 μg/g, a dose also chosen by Elgjo (1973). At the
extremes, Chopra (1973) used 25 μg/ml in cultures of embryonic kidney
cells while Simnet and Fisher (1973) used as little as 0.4 μg/ml in cultures
of various organs, principally rat lungs.

From the practical point of view, stathmokinetic agents can be used
both in vivo and, providing the culture conditions are satisfactory for the
continued proliferation of the cells, in vitro. The method has the advantage
that the cells are directly and individually assessed under the microscope so
that cell extracts can be tested for specificity of effect. This is particularly
useful in preparations of haemopoietic tissue where several cell types may
be present. In this case, however, the loss of some of the identifying characteristics of the cells during the mitotic phase can introduce confusion. By
suitable manipulations (see below) haemopoietic population test systems can
be prepared in which this problem is minimised. It appears that the errors
involved in measuring the accumulation rate of mitoses are rather high, but
providing that optimum doses of the chosen stathmokinetic agents are used
and that measurements are all relative then the technique can be used satisfactorily.

5.3 Methods involving the incorporation of tritiated thymidine (^{3}HTdR)

For nearly two decades, [^{3}H]thymidine incorporation into proliferating cell
populations has been used as a measure of cell proliferation. Although
thymidine is not a naturally occurring DNA precursor in mammalian systems
it can enter the DNA synthetic pathway specifically and if labelled in some
way it will be recognised in the newly-synthesised DNA. The labelling of
thymidine with tritium (Hughes, 1957; Verly et al., 1958) opened the way
for extensive studies of DNA synthesis and cell proliferation kinetics.

In using tritiated thymidine as a label for DNA it is assumed that (i) DNA
turnover is due solely to cell division, (ii) DNA synthesis, in general, destines

a cell to divide again, (iii) re-utilisation of labelled materials is insignificant, (iv) there is no perturbation of the normal cell generative cycle by radiation injury from the tritium incorporated into DNA or from the formation of labelled degradation products.

The specificity of tritiated thymidine for labelling cells in pre-mitotic DNA synthesis has been questioned by Pelc (1962, 1964) and Pelc and Gahan (1959) who described the labelling of metabolic DNA synthesis in some tissues. In slowly dividing tissues they found an excess of labelling over cell division. In the seminal vesicle, for example, only 13% of the labelled cells were found to divide. The labelled cells which did not divide, however, took up the label at only 2% of the rate of the other group. In tissues with high proliferation rates, the degree of labelling is highly compatible with the division rate and while a certain level of non-pre-mitotic DNA synthesis may be taking place it must be very low by comparison with that in preparation for mitosis. Premises (i) and (ii), are, therefore, effectively valid for the rapidly turning over tissues though for the more slowly proliferating tissues, they are less tenable.

The breakdown of labelled DNA and the re-utilization of the products represents a more serious problem. DNA catabolites, including thymidine, its nucleotides or nucleotide chains, may be re-utilized by direct intercellular exchange. In the bone marrow for example extruded normoblast nuclei are largely phagocytosed in the marrow making labelled materials directly available for re-utilization. Feinendegen et al. (1966) measured the regression rate of tritium activity in the bone marrow of rats and compared it with the regression rate of [131]iodine incorporated from 5-iododeoxyuridine, another specific label of DNA synthesis. Over a period of ten days, they found that ^{131}I disappeared from the marrow almost twice as quickly as tritium. As a result, they calculated that 35–40% of the thymidine or its nucleotides released from DNA by catabolism is physiologically re-utilized.

Radiation damage from intranuclear tritium is another factor which is a problem only in extended experiments. It has been found, for example, that a dose of 1 μCi ^{3}HTdR/g body weight gave deleterious effects on mouse spermatogonia four days later i.e. cells were failing to pass through two divisions (Johnson and Cronkite, 1959). Grisham (1960) found that a dose of 1–2 μCi/g had an inhibitory effect on the regeneration of rat liver. Two μCi/g also had a delaying effect on the second generation cycle in small intestinal crypt cells. Consequently, if cells are to remain unaffected for any length of time 1–2 μCi/g appears to be about the maximum dose permissible for in vivo studies. In vitro, a dose of 0.25 μCi/ml ^{3}HTdR for 3 h has recently been shown to produce a substantial level of chromosomal aberrations in three successive cell cycles of PHA stimulated lymphocytes (Geard, 1975). Dosages in vitro therefore must be kept considerably lower than for in vivo work. In particular, since tritium has a long half life, its continued presence in a culture effectively constitutes a continuous labelling process.

The problem of cell killing by intranuclear irradiation also arises in relation to the specific activity of the tritiated thymidine. It appears that, provided adequate thymidine is available, a constant amount will be incorporated. With specific activities of ^{3}HTdR up to about 60 Ci/mmole now commercially available, large quantities of tritium may be incorporated. For example, in a repeated labelling experiment, injecting 0.5 μCi ^{3}HTdR every 6 h for 7 days (provided premise (ii) holds, no cell will receive more than twice the dose of a single injection) and then measuring haemopoietic stem cells (i.e. CFU$_s$, see below) it was found that ^{3}HTdR at 5 Ci/mmole had no effect on the total number of CFU$_s$ (table 5.1) but at 23 Ci/mmole there was a 50% reduction in the number of CFU$_s$ (Lord and Murphy, unpublished results).

A similar observation was made when measuring the proportion of haemopoietic stem cells in DNA-synthesis. It appeared that there is some uptake of ^{3}HTdR into non-S cells if the specific activity is greater than about 20 Ci/mmole. This extra thymidine was not bound in DNA, could easily be removed by washing but could apparently become incorporated into the DNA of haemopoietic stem cells when further synthesis started (Lord et al., 1974). Additionally, Peterson and his co-workers also observed an unusually high toxicity in P388 lymphoma cells when using high specific activity ^{3}HTdR (Peterson et al., 1971, 1973). This does, however, have a compensatory advantage because some workers have warned that certain unpurified cell extracts can contain significant quantities of *cold* thymidine which may dilute the activity of the *hot* thymidine and result in an apparently

Table 5.1

Effect of specific activity of ^{3}HTdR on the killing of CFU$_s$ by repeated injections of 0.5 μCi^{3}HTdR/g body weight.

	CFU$_s$/femur
Saline injected control	6100
^{3}HTdR 23 Ci/mmole injected every 6 h for 7 days	3200
^{3}HTdR 5 Ci/mmole injected every 6 h for 7 days	6120

reduced ³HTdR incorporation. Lenfant et al. (1973), for example, showed that one of the fractions of liver extracts inhibitory to ³HTdR incorporation in regenerating liver was due primarily to the presence of cold thymidine in the extract. The use of a lower specific activity ³HTdR is therefore advisable.

Most of these points present possible problems in extended experiments only and even these can be eliminated or at least minimised. A single 'flash' labelling of an asynchronous cell population gives thymidine incorporation in proportion to the amount of DNA synthesis taking place provided that the interval between injection and sacrifice is shorter than the G_2 phase but longer than the time required for complete incorporation of the thymidine. This latter time appears to be of the order of 15 min (Rubini et al., 1960). Cronkite et al. (1959) reported intense labelling in cells within minutes of injecting the thymidine and Appleton (1964) using the technique of water soluble autoradiography showed that the thymidine was irreversibly bound in the cell nucleus within 15 min.

It thus seems that tritiated thymidine should be a convenient and suitable marker for DNA synthesis and since, in most tissues, there are about ten times as many cells in S as in mitosis (Schultze and Oehlert, 1960) greater accuracy can be obtained by measuring labelled cells. There are two basic ways of doing this (i) direct counting of incorporated radioactivity and (ii) autoradiography, which is more reliable and more informative in that cells are individually scored.

5.3.1 Direct measurement of incorporated tritium

Tritium is normally measured as that bound to DNA in the acid insoluble fraction of the cells and counted in a liquid scintillation counter. Since the tritium is in this form it is assumed that the total counts recorded give a relative measure of the degree of DNA synthesis in the population. However, such measurements have been made in a very generalized manner with little allowance for variations in experimental design. In the same way that the correct choice of timing is important in investigating inhibition at the $G_2 \rightarrow M$ boundary, so it is important in studying inhibition at the $G_1 \rightarrow S$ boundary and in the S phase. A short interval of ³HTdR incorporation indicates the amount of DNA synthesis at the time of injection. A longer period of incorporation illustrates, in addition, the amount of new DNA synthesis started during the incorporation time. Thus the wide variations in incorporation times used by various workers e.g. Elgjo, 30 min; Marks, 45 min; Rothberg et al., 4 h; Houck et al., 6 h; Garcia-Giralt et al., 24 h; Kiger et al., 6 h; Verly, 1 and 2 h (all reported in Chalones: Concepts and

Current Researches 1973) are in fact all measuring different aspects of the cell cycle and no comparison of the results is possible. In addition, as with the stathmokinetic techniques, when testing cell extracts, the amount of ^{3}HTdR incorporated will also depend on its time of application relative to the application of the extract.

The following sections give an analysis of some of the cell systems in which ^{3}HTdR incorporation has been used and of the information that may be obtained from the measurements.

5.3.1.1 Bone marrow cell populations

Incorporation of ^{3}HTdR into bone marrow cell populations can be carried out either in vivo or in vitro but the latter method has found most common use. Rytömaa (1968), Rytömaa and Kiviniemi (1968), Paukovits (1971) have used short term coverslip cultures of bone marrow and the general principle of the method is to add the test extract at the start of the culture and then add ^{3}HTdR at some chosen time later. The cultures are then killed, the DNA extracted and counted in a scintillation counter.

As discussed in the introduction, the important factor in using a cell culture is that proliferation should at least be maintained. Rytömaa (1968), however, found that these coverslip cultures do in fact run down in their cellularity and unless one can show that ^{3}HTdR uptake will be as good in the later stages of the culture as at the beginning, one ends up with a system in which an extract may simply be contributing as an 'unhappiness' factor. Consequently, unless the method is restricted to very short term observations the use of such a culture is rather limited. In addition, it is well known that in bone marrow populations, some cell types will attach to the glass while others will not and this itself is likely to upset the balance of the cell populations. It may be better, therefore, for these short term measurements to use suspension cultures in siliconised glassware.

Simnett and Fisher (1973) were able to underline the inadequacy of extended cultures in that thymidine incorporation in neonatal rat lung cultures bore no relationship to the rate of cell proliferation. By contrast, there was a good relationship for adult rat lung cultures. They concluded that the usefulness of ^{3}HTdR incorporation measurements as a method of measuring cell proliferation rate may vary according to the age and possibly the type of the organ under investigation.

However, it is worthwhile considering what is known of the proliferation characteristics of the bone marrow cell populations and to estimate how much inhibition of thymidine incorporation might be expected. Several cell lines are present in the same culture and it is not practicable to separate

Table 5.2

Simplified myelogram of rodent bone marrow showing the distribution of the major cell groups and the proportions of these groups in DNA-synthesis.

	% Total cells	% in DNA-S	No. of cells in S
Erythroid cells	30	33	10
Granulocytic cells	45	22	10
Lymphoid cells	25	20	5
Total cells	100	25	25

Table 5.3

Calculated reduction in DNA-synthesising cells based on the specific inhibition of synthesis in any one cell type.

	Cells in DNA synthesis			
	Normal	Treat with RCE	Treat with GCE	Treat with LNE
Erythroid cells	10	0	10	10
Granulocytic cells	10	10	0	10
Lymphoid cells	5	5	5	0
Net cells in S	25	15	15	20
% reduction in DNA synthesising cells	0	40	40	20

them for tritium counting. Consequently, it is not possible to demonstrate the specificity of an extract for a particular cell type. Table 5.2 represents an approximate myelogram of rat or mouse bone marrow illustrating that three major cell series constitute virtually 100% of the cells: about 30% erythroid, 25% lymphoid and 45% granulocytic. Of this latter group, about half are relatively mature and beyond the proliferative phase. From autoradiographic studies, about 25% of the total cells are labelled, 10 being erythroid, 10 granulocytic and 5 lymphoid. The elimination of DNA synthesis from any one series will result in a relatively small fall in thymidine incorporation as illustrated in table 5.3 by the percentage reduction in DNA synthesising cells. This reduction is calculated on the assumption that the extracts are completely cell line specific in their effect; that all existing DNA synthesis is stopped in a specific cell line and that there is a complete block to further DNA synthesis at the $G_1 \rightarrow S$ boundary. It is clear from this table that the maximum depression obtainable is around 40% and this means that any reduction in incorporation greater than about 40% cannot be inhibition which is specific to one cell line. Rather its effects must spread to other cell lines, indicating that the extract tested is more probably demonstrating non-specific toxicity.

In fact, several studies have shown that it is often difficult to get greater than about 50% inhibition in the apparent proliferation rates (e.g. Chopra, 1973; Elgjo, 1973; Laurence, 1974). It is quite possible, therefore, that the maximum inhibition of ^{3}HTdR incorporation in a bone marrow system may be as small as about 20%. Equally, if the effect is restricted to a block at the $G_1 \rightarrow S$ boundary, even incubating the marrow with ^{3}HTdR for 4–5 h then a depression of more than about 20% would not be expected.

5.3.1.2 Sensitivity of the measurement of ^{3}HTdR incorporation
The fact that one is now interested in measuring a difference in incorporation of the order of 20% raises the question of whether the technique is sufficiently sensitive to measure this difference.

It is currently the practice in our laboratories, having made a Sephadex fractionation of an extract, to assay all of 100 fractions for an effect on

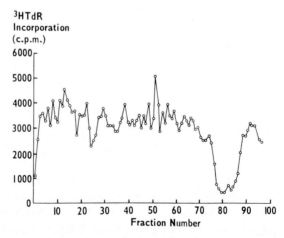

Fig. 5.3. Tritiated thymidine incorporation by bone marrow following treatment by 100 consecutive Sephadex G-15 fractions of physiological saline. The marked depression of ^{3}HTdR incorporation between fractions 76–89 represents all the salt coming out in supra-hypertonic concentrations. Over the rest of the fractions, a two-fold variation in counts is seen between tubes 24 and 51. (Diagram kindly supplied by Dr. D. J. Pillinger.)

Table 5.4

Errors of observation of thymidine incorporation by rat bone marrow cells. Errors for the 15 replicate measurements were made from data kindly supplied by Dr. D. J. Pillinger.

System	Standard deviation	Standard error
15 replicate measurements		
Non-siliconised tubes	20%	5%
Siliconised tubes	10%	3%
3 replicate measurements*		
Non-siliconised tubes	27%	16%
Siliconised tubes	15%	9%

* Calculated values from the 15 replicate measurement experiments, using the same range of values.

thymidine incorporation. Fig. 5.3 kindly supplied by Dr. D. J. Pillinger illustrates the type of result obtained from a G-15 fractionation of physiological saline. Clearly, there are very marked fluctuations from one tube to the next though in such a system, any sequence of at least three tubes should give effectively the same result.

Using a preparative system whereby losses of DNA and, therefore, tritium are minimised, Dr. Pillinger (personal communication) made 15 replicate measurements on bone marrow cultured in non-siliconised tubes and 15 in siliconised tubes. Table 5.4 shows the standard deviations and errors which bearing in mind that 15 replicate measurements were made, are high. In practice, perhaps as few as 3 replicate measurements only can be made. In that case, these deviations and errors are of the same order as the maximum effect that can be expected for bone marrow. For example, using non siliconized glassware with a 5% standard error on 15 replicate counts would, for a 20% inhibition, read $20 \pm 6\%$. If the measurements were reduced to 3 replicate counts this would become $20 \pm 18\%$ and, therefore, barely significant. In other words, under conditions as ideal as possible one requires a large inhibition to be significant and, in the base of bone marrow cells, this may be difficult.

5.3.1.3 Phytohaemagglutinin stimulated lymphocyte cultures
The phytohaemagglutinin (PHA) stimulated lymphocyte culture system is now a highly standardised proliferating cell culture in which normal non-proliferating circulating lymphocytes are separated from blood and stimu-

lated by PHA to undergo blast transformation and eventual cell proliferation. Only one proliferating cell type is present in the population thus giving the investigator a far greater chance to quantitate changes in proliferation by the simple expedient of measuring ^{3}HTdR incorporation. The actual accuracy of measurement is of course no greater than for the bone marrow populations but in this case, a reduction of 50% in the number of lymphocytes in DNA synthesis now represents a reduction of 50% of the ^{3}HTdR incorporation into the culture, a difference which can be measured with confidence.

The possibility of unknown quantities of cold thymidine being present in the test extracts still exists and again it has been found advantageous in our laboratories to use the relatively low specific activity ^{3}HTdR ($\sim$ 5 Ci/mmole) in making such measurements. Under these conditions, the variations between replicate measurements are minimised.

In practice, investigators have added the test extract at the start of the culture and then waited until the time at which cells would normally be going through DNA-synthesis before adding ^{3}HTdR. This procedure introduces two limitations on the system. At the start of the culture, the cells are not stimulated for proliferation; certainly not yet in cell cycle. Any inhibitory effect exercised by the extract at that point would be outside the concept of a proliferation inhibitor. However, it is not clear from the literature whether PHA and the test extract are added simultaneously or slightly separated in time. Certainly, PHA initiates the stimulation within minutes (Cercek and Cercek, 1974) but changes in the structuredness of the cytoplasmic matrix (see below) of the lymphocytes demonstrate that PHA is ineffective if an inhibitory lymphoid extract is already present (Lord et al., 1974b). If the PHA and the inhibitor are added together, therefore, it would not be surprising to obtain virtually 100% elimination of the thymidine incorporation. This limitation, however, can be overcome quite simply by allowing the stimulation process to be completed before adding the test extract.

The second limitation is more severe though not insuperable. In the situation where the culture is allowed to proceed for 66 h before adding thymidine, an extract with a long half life in culture may be affecting the lymphocytes at any stage of its pre-proliferative phase, of the G_1 phase, at the $G_1 \rightarrow S$ boundary or during the S phase. Conversely, if the extract has a short half life, then any effect seen must reflect an effect on the early stages of the culture and as such be quite different from the effects normally ascribed to a 'chalone'. It is not possible, from this type of experiment, to estimate the effective half life of an extract nor, consequently, its point of action. Thus it can illustrate that a particular extract is capable of inhibiting thymidine incorporation but can give no information as to the stage of the process which is inhibited. Recent experiments carried out in these laboratories (Shah and Lord, unpublished results) in which cultures were treated at different times following PHA stimulation, followed by removal of the extract from the culture after 2 h, indicate that lymphoid tissue extracts will inhibit subsequent ³HTdR incorporation from any point in the entire process. Using this type of procedure, the unknown half life of the extract is effectively controlled and its effects in time can be located.

Since the culture carries only one type of proliferating cell, specificity determinations for lymphoid cell extracts are straightforward. Comparable extracts from other blood cells should not produce any inhibition of the ³HTdR incorporation.

5.3.1.4 *Other systems*

³HTdR incorporation has also been used routinely both in vivo and in vitro for other tissues; in particular to study epidermal and liver 'chalones' (Elgjo, 1973; Marks, 1973; Rothberg and Arp, 1973; Verly, 1973). For epidermal tissues, if hair follicles are involved, it is essential that animals of the correct stage of follicular development be used i.e. the second telogen phase (Silver et al., 1969) which occurs for example in *male* mice aged 7–8 weeks. In female mice, disturbances caused by the oestrous cycle make the appearance of this phase erratic. In this way it is possible to obtain a reasonably unique proliferating cell population which, although apparently difficult to inhibit to less than 50% of the normal level of ³HTdR incorporation can be expected to give significantly-measurable degrees of inhibition.

With respect to liver studies, effects on liver regeneration have been studied both in vivo by injecting 'purified chalone' and ³HTdR (1 μCi/g) and in vitro by means of a simple culture of 0.5-mm thick slices of regenerating liver in Hanks' balanced salt solution containing 'purified chalone' and ³HTdR (4 μCi/ml) (Simard et al., 1974). Lenfant and his colleagues (1973), however, have demonstrated that crude liver extracts do contain thymidine which produces a non-specific inhibition of ³HTdR incorporation. Thus, thymidine contamination constitutes a very real problem which must always be considered and if present must be removed before assays can have any validity.

5.3.2 *Autoradiographic measurements of incorporated* ³*HTdR*

The measurement and analysis of the cell cycle by means of high resolution autoradiography with tritiated thymidine have been developed into an extensive field of research and have wide applications. In the field of 'chalone' research therefore, it should take a prime role and it does have the advantage that the cells involved are assessed individually under the microscope. In a mixed cell population for example, it should, therefore, be possible to observe directly whether a test extract is cell line specific. Observation of the DNA-S phase has two advantages over observation of mitosis: firstly there are many more cells in S and secondly, the morphology of the cells is not disturbed so that in mixed cell populations there is less risk of wrongly identifying a cell.

In principle and timing, the technique is the same as for simple thymidine incorporation. Extract and ^{3}HTdR are applied to the tissue under investigation at the appropriate times. The culture or animal is killed, histological preparations (smears or section) of the tissue made, covered with a photographic emulsion and allowed to expose for sufficient time to permit the incorporated tritium to produce a latent image. The image is developed, the preparation stained and labelled cells counted under the microscope. Tritium is a weak β-particle emitter with a maximum energy of 18 KeV and a mean energy of 5.7 KeV. This means that 99% of the emitted β-particles are absorbed in a photographic emulsion within one micron from its origin. Thus tritium is an ideal isotope for autoradiographic purposes giving such high resolution that autoradiographic grains are located precisely over the nuclei of the labelled cells; there is no spillage of grains into the cytoplasmic regions.

As shown above, a simple measurement of the proportion of cells labelled (labelling index, I_L) in an asynchronous steady state cell population, following a 30-min exposure to ^{3}HTdR, gives the ratio t_s/t_c where t_s is the time spent in DNA-synthesis and t_c is the duration of the cell cycle. A reduction in this ratio following shortly after the application of a test extract would appear primarily to be the result of a direct inhibitory effect on DNA synthesis. The exact nature of the effect does, however, depend to a large extent on the duration of DNA synthesis. For example, with $t_s = 4$ h and ^{3}HTdR injected 1 h after the test extract (fig. 5.4a), one would expect a reduction of 25% in the labelling index if the effect were to block the $G_1 \rightarrow S$ boundary only and have no effect on S itself. For longer duration t_s ($\geqslant$ 10 h say) the drop in labelling index in the first hour would become insignificant (fig. 5.4.b). If a significant effect is seen under these conditions then it would have to be related to a direct effect on cells in S (fig. 5.5). In this case, one should expect an immediate drop in the labelling index; to zero if the blockage is complete.

When longer intervals are allowed between applying the test extract and

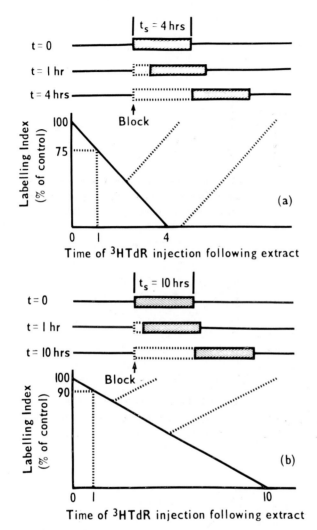

Fig. 5.4. Loss of cells in DNA-synthesis following a blockage at the $G_1 \rightarrow S$ boundary. The duration of DNA-synthesis is 4 h in (a) and 10 h in (b).

carrying out the flash labelling experiment, the effect seen will depend on the biological life time of the extract. Since a 'chalone' is considered to have a reversible effect one would expect the effect to last at least as long as the concentration of the inhibitor remains above some critical threshold value. During the time for which the inhibitor remains effective, a continuous reduction of the labelling index would indicate a continued block at the $G_1 \rightarrow S$ boundary (fig. 5.4). In this case, the rate of fall of the labelling index

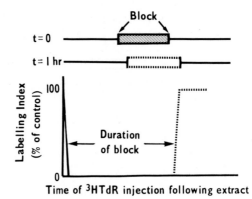

Fig. 5.5. Loss of cells in DNA-synthesis following a total block on DNA-synthesis.

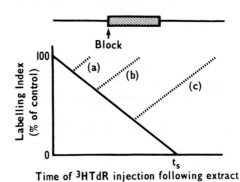

Fig. 5.6. Recovery of DNA-synthesising cells following release from a blockage at the $G_1 \to S$ boundary: The duration of the blockage is approximately (a) $1/6 \times t_s$, (b) $1/3 \times t_s$, (c) $2/3 \times t_s$.

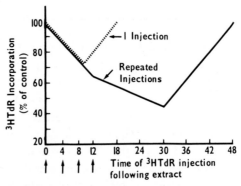

Fig. 5.7. Diagramatic representation of epidermal DNA-synthesis following injection of single (-----) or repeated (——) doses of a skin extract. The arrows indicate the injection times for mice receiving 4 doses of the extract. (Adapted from Elgjo, 1973.)

will represent the rate of flow of cells out of DNA synthesis which is, initially at least, the normal rate of flow of cells through the cycle. Thus, if the duration of the normal cell cycle is known it will be possible to determine whether the reduced labelling index is due solely to a $G_1 \rightarrow S$ block or due partly to a block in DNA synthesis itself.

Subsequent recovery of the labelling index depends on how soon the inhibitor ceases to be effective. When this happens, if the block has been at the $G_1 \rightarrow S$ boundary one would expect the flow of cells into S to restart and recovery of the labelling index to correspond to the renewed rate of flow of cells (fig. 5.4 dotted lines). Alternatively, release from an S block may result in a return to the normal labelling index in a very short space of time (fig. 5.5).

If a $G_1 \rightarrow S$ block is of short duration by comparison with the cell flow rate (fig. 5.6) as may occur in some of the more slowly proliferating tissues then recovery will take place before the labelling index has fallen very significantly. In this case, even repeated injections of the inhibitors may not be very effective. An example of this effect may be seen in work published by Elgjo (1973) and diagrammatically illustrated in fig. 5.7. Following a single injection of an epidermal extract, thymidine incorporation fell to about 70% of control in about 9 h. By 18 h it had returned to normal. Four repeated injections over a period of 12 h reduced the incorporation only to 45% of control. The small reduction in ^{3}HTdR incorporation after a single injection followed by a return to normal indicates a DNA synthesis of long duration (cf. fig. 5.4b) and both the rate of fall of thymidine incorporation and the subsequent rates of recovery suggest the long cell cycle time characteristic of epidermal cells.

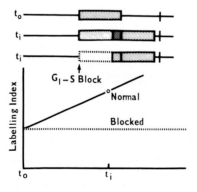

Fig. 5.8. Proportion of labelled cells following repeated doses of tritiated thymidine in a normal cell population and in a cell population blocked at the $G_1 \rightarrow S$ boundary.

Complementary information can be obtained by allowing continuous incorporation of ³HTdR in an in vitro system or by giving repeated injections in an in vivo system (fig. 5.8). Providing that the interval between injections is shorter than the duration of DNA synthesis and that labelled cells are not lost from the tissue immediately following the last division in their proliferation sequence, determination of the rate of increase of labelling index measures the rate of flow of cells into DNA synthesis, a reduced rate of increase probably reflecting a block at the $G_1 \to S$ boundary.

These arguments, of course, presuppose that the effect of an extract is not one of blocking the entry of thymidine into the cell. Such an effect could be checked directly by the use of the water soluble autoradiography technique (Appleton, 1964) though a subsequent reduction in the mitotic index could be accepted as evidence that the rate of flow of cells through S had been reduced.

A brief example of the use of autoradiography in such studies can be made with reference to the effect of an erythrocyte extract in vivo on proliferating erythroid cells (Lord, unpublished results). Normal bone marrow cells are often proliferating at below their maximum capacity (Lord, 1964, 1965) and since potentially inhibitory materials are under investigation it is advantageous to start with cells proliferating at their maximum rate. This was achieved by lethally-irradiating mice and then grafting 5.10^5 normal bone marrow cells to promote recovery. Along the lines of the spleen colony forming technique (Till and McCulloch, 1961), haemopoietic stem cells derived from the bone marrow graft proliferate in the spleens of the recipient mice to produce the various kinds of haemopoietic cells. Erythroid cells,

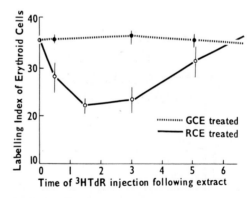

Fig. 5.9. Variation in the labelling index of erythroid cells in regenerating mouse spleens following a single injection of a partially purified red blood cell extract. The controls were treated with a similarly prepared granulocyte extract.

however, develop rather faster than granulocytic cells and if one selects the mice at 7 to 8 days after grafting, the spleens consist of about 40% rapidly proliferating erythroid cells, 55% lymphoid cells and only 5% granulocytic cells. (Alternatively, before grafting, the recipient animals can be hyper-transfused with red blood cells to suppress subsequent erythropoiesis. On waiting for 10 to 11 days after grafting, a large degree of granulopoiesis has developed and the spleens are now 50% granulocytic and 50% lymphoid). In this way, it is possible to select for a high proportion of the cells in which one is interested and, in addition, they are in a state of rapid proliferation. Fig. 5.9 shows the ^{3}HTdR labelling indices of erythroid cells in such preparations, labelled for 0.5 h at up to 5 h after an injection of a partially purified red blood cell extract (RCE) or granulocyte extract (GCE). The GCE has not affected the labelling index but following RCE, the index falls for 1.5 h from 36% to 22%. If this is produced by a total block at the $G_1 \rightarrow S$ boundary, it represents a flow rate of 14% in 1.5 h or an average cell cycle time of 10.5 h. During the first half hour only there is a fall of 8% which represents a fastest cycle time of around 6 h and this agrees well with that calculated by Lajtha et al. (1971) for the development of an erythroid colony.

Autoradiography is thus a very versatile technique, well-suited to a study of factors which might change the nature of the cell cycle. There is a variety of techniques available for complete measurement of the cycle: the percent labelled mitosis curve method (Quastler, 1959; Quastler and Sherman, 1959) is capable of giving the duration of all the cycle's phases though since this requires extended observations it would be necessary to maintain the concentration of the inhibitor throughout the experiment. Repeated labelling measurements, again over an extended time period, can also be used to measure the cell cycle and the duration of DNA-synthesis (Lord, 1965, 1968). Double labelling with tritium labelled and carbon-14 labelled thymidine is potentially the most powerful technique for analysing the cell cycle, requiring only three or four measurements over a relatively short time period (Wimber and Quastler, 1963). To date, however, no real attempts have been made to use these techniques, which are particularly useful for in vivo measurements, in the study of cell proliferation inhibitors.

5.4 Measurement of the structuredness of the cell cyptoplasmic matrix SCM

Measurement of the structuredness of the cytoplasmic matrix (SCM) of cells is potentially a very powerful technique for the basic assay of the inhibitory activity of cell extracts. The cytoplasmic matrix is an organisation of the molecules within the cytoplasm which is the result of physical interactions between macromolecules such as proteins, water molecules and solutes (Ling, 1972). Measurement of changes in the structure of cytoplasm were originally developed from observations of the gravitational sedimentation of statoliths in root-cap cells of barley (Cercek, 1969; Cercek and Cercek, 1971). Very few other cells, certainly none of them mammalian, were known which could be used for this type of study. Cercek and Cercek, however, combined the technique of fluorescence polarization (Perrin, 1929) with the phenomenon of fluorochromasia (Rotman and Papermaster, 1966) to develop a highly precise and reproducible measurement of this structuring which they used initially for studies on logarithmically-growing yeast cells (Cercek and Cercek, 1972) and then for mammalian cells (Cercek et al., 1973). Chen and Bowman (1965) had demonstrated that the use of ultraviolet polarizing filters with large apertures allow corrections to be made for diffraction grating induced polarization anomalies. In addition, the good transmission properties of these filters permit the entrance of sufficient light so that small slits and dilute solutions can be used. As a result, they showed that under optimum conditions, polarization can be measured with a precision of $\pm$ 0.002. More recently Cercek and Cercek (1974) have measured the fluorescence polarization value of lymphocytes from 72 different healthy human donors and have obtained a value of $P = 0.206$ with a standard error of $\pm$ 0.002. Clearly, therefore, this is a technique that is capable of giving extremely precise measurements, changes of 10% for any sample being highly significant, and, as shown below, has been able to demonstrate unequivocally specific and reversible effects of extracts from mature blood cells on their own precursor cells.

In practice, although individual measurements are complete within a short period of time, the SCM of a population of cells does not change over a period of several hours, a control measurement made about 4 h after the start of an experiment being less than 5% higher than at the start. It is practicable, therefore, to make a series of measurements on aliquots of a given cell suspension extending over several hours.

5.4.1 Principle of the measurement of SCM

The basis of SCM measurements lies in the fact that living cells exhibit fluorochromasia, a phenomenon first described by Rotman and Papermaster in 1966 and used then as a viability test for cells. This phenomenon is illustrated in fig. 5.10. A non-fluorescing substrate of fluorescein, in this case fluorescein diacetate (FDA), is introduced to a cell, the cytoplasm of which it enters. Once inside the cell, it is broken down by enzymatic hydrolysis to liberate free fluorescein molecules which do, of course, fluoresce. These fluorescein molecules are free to move within the cytoplasm of the cell but in a manner dependent on the molecular organisation of the cytoplasm. They are also free to leave the cell. Fluorescein molecules outside the cell, however, cannot pass the cell membrane back into the cytoplasm. Thus, provided that the cell is in a medium completely free of hydrolytic enzymes, any fluorescein observed must have been produced within that cell's cytoplasm.

Fig. 5.11 shows the principle on which the fluorescence is measured using a polarizing fluorescence spectrophotometer. Incident monochromatic light of wavelength 473 nanometers is polarized before entering the cuvette containing cells suspended in a solution of fluorescein diacetate. Molecules of

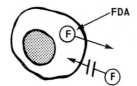

Fig. 5.10. The phenomenon of fluorochromasia. Fluorescein diacetate (FDA) may enter the cell and liberate fluorescein (F) which can leave the cell. (F), however, can not enter the cell.

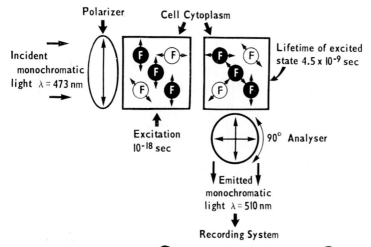

Fig. 5.11. Fluorescence polarization. (F) excited fluorescein molecules: (F) non-excited fluorescein molecules. The arrow heads on the fluorescein molecules denote the direction of the electric vector of the dipole oscillator responsible for light absorption and emission.

fluorescein, whose electric vector of the dipole oscillator responsible for light absorption and emission is parallel with the plane of polarization, will be excited by that light and will fluoresce. This excitation process takes only 10^{-18} sec and so effectively selects a specific group of fluorescein molecules. The lifetime of the excited state, however, is considerably longer, 4.5×10^{-9} sec. Rotational relaxation of the fluorescein molecule between absorption and emission depolarizes the fluorescence. Since the ease of rotation of a molecule is inversely related to the viscosity of its medium (Einstein, 1906), changes in the viscosity of the cytoplasm, i.e. the molecular organisation of the cytoplasmic matrix, will affect the rotation of the fluorescein molecules and consequently the degree of fluorescence polarization. In effect, the polarization will increase if the ease of rotation of the fluorescein molecules in the cytoplasm decreases, and vice versa. In essence, the technique, there-fore, gives a measure of the average relative microviscosity of the cytoplasm. In this context, however, the term viscosity is misleading since the cytoplasm of a cell is not a homogeneous liquid but a structured heterogeneous and polyphasic system. Accordingly, the term 'Structuredness' has been used to describe the state of organisation of the cytoplasm (Cercek and Cercek, 1972).

In practice, the fluorescence is measured as a continuous process. The build up of fluorescein molecules is recorded by observing the light emission through the emission monochromator set at 510 nm with the emission

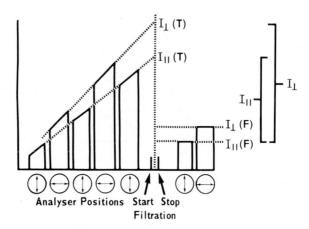

Fig. 5.12. Diagramatic representation of the chart recording from the fluorescence spectrophotometer. I(T), fluorescence components in the cell suspension: I(F), fluorescence components in the cell free filtrate: $I_|$ and $I_{||}$ are the corrected fluorescence intensities in the parallel and perpendicular phases.

polarizer set alternately parallel and perpendicular to the plane of polarization of the incident light.

A diagrammatic representation of the type of recording obtained is shown in fig. 5.12. Depending upon the ease of rotation of the fluorescein molecules, the parallel and perpendicular components diverge. Since fluorescein is also leaving the cells however, each component contains a contribution from the fluorescein in the medium and this must be removed. To do this, the cells are filtered from the suspension on Millipore paper (pore size 0.22 μm), the start and finish of the filtration process being recorded on the chart. Finally, fluorescence in the medium is recorded in both the parallel and perpendicular planes. Since the hydrolytic enzymes are not present in the medium, no further fluorescein production will take place and the traces will be horizontal. Subtraction of these values, $I_1(F)$ and $I_{11}(F)$, from the values obtained with the cells present (projected to the mid point of the filtration times, $I_1(T)$ and $I_{11}(T)$, give the intensities, I_1 and I_{11}, of the two components of the fluorescence polarization in the cells. The polarization value, P, or SCM of the cells is then calculated from the formula

$$P = \frac{I_1 - GI_{11}}{I_1 + GI_{11}} \quad \text{(Chen and Bowman, 1965)}$$

where I_1 is the emission intensity with the polarizors parallel; I_{11} is the emission intensity with the polarizers perpendicular; G is a grating factor which corrects for the small degree of polarisation produced by the diffraction grating. It is a function of the instrument and must be determined under conditions of use. This is carried out using the method of Azumi and McGlynn (1962). Since the gratings are normally ruled vertically, it is usual for normal use to have the excitation polarizing filter vertical. To measure G, the sample is excited with horizontally polarized light and the emission analysed in the vertical (I_{HV}) and horizontal (I_{HH}) planes. The ratio $I_{HV}:I_{HH}$ ($= G$) should be unity since the fluorescence is observed along the direction of the electric vector of the activating light. In practice it is generally less than one and must therefore be determined.

5.4.2 *Relationship of SCM to the cell generation cycle*

Since this technique is not one directly related to measuring cell proliferation kinetics, it is necessary to consider the relationship between SCM and cell proliferation. In a series of experiments carried out by Cercek et al. (1973), chinese hamster ovary cells were synchronised at mitosis and the fluorescence polarization values (SCM) of the cells measured at various times up to 12 h later. The cell cycle of these cells can be divided into the following phases, $G_1 = 2$ h, $S = 7.5$ h, $G_2 = 2$ h, $M = 0.5$ h (Williams and Ockey, 1970) and measurements during these phases show that polarization is highest during mitosis ($P = 0.158$). It decreases slightly during the G_1 phase ($P = 0.153$), falls rapidly in early S ($P = 0.115$) and continues to fall throughout S ($P = 0.092$ in late S). In G_2, however, the SCM rapidly increases again ($P = 0.149$) to reach a value close to its former level.

It is clear, therefore, that changes in the pattern of cell proliferation will be reflected by changes in the structuredness of cytoplasm. A rapidly proliferating population of cells will contain a small proportion of cells in G_1 and G_2 and will therefore have a low polarization value. Conversely, a slowly proliferating population of cells will contain a large proportion of cells in G_1 and G_2 and will therefore have a high polarization value. It, therefore, follows that any treatment which causes an increase in structuredness is at least compatible with a reduction in the rate of proliferation of the cells.

There are, however, examples of the use of this technique in which changes in structuredness cannot be related directly to changes in the cell cycle. Changes in the structuredness of normal human lymphocytes for example are observed within one minute of the application of the mitogen, phytohaemagglutinin. Neither before nor immediately after PHA stimulation can lymphocytes be considered to be in cell cycle. Lymphoid cell extracts can, however, increase the structuredness of such PHA stimulated lymphocytes back to their pre-stimulated level (Lord et al., 1974a). In this situation, the lymphoid cell extract cannot be considered as an inhibitor of cell proliferation though used on proliferating lymphocytes it may well have such an effect (Lord et al., 1974a).

In spite of this problem, it will be shown below that the technique can show the specificity and reversibility of changes in the structuredness of the cytoplasmic matrix of cells. In a simple incubation mixture of cells in Medium 199, it is unlikely that the original proportion of cells in the S phase will be maintained. As mentioned above, however, the SCM of these cells remains constant over a period of several hours but since the measurement of structuredness is, strictly speaking, related to the cytoplasmic processes the constancy of the measurement perhaps indicates that these are maintained during incubation much better than nuclear processes.

5.4.3 Practical application of the test

Measurement of the SCM of cells has been made in several haemopoietic cell populations. Lymphocytes from normal human blood, proliferating granulocytic cells grown in a liquid suspension culture (Dexter et al., 1973) and proliferating normoblasts from mouse foetal livers were thoroughly washed and resuspended at a concentration of 5×10^6 cells/ml in medium TC199. Aliquots of each of these cell suspensions were treated with fractionated extracts of lymphocytes, granulocytes or erythrocytes at a final concentration of 33 μg/ml for 30 min. Aliquots of the incubated samples were then suspended at a concentration of about 10^5 cells/ml in 2.5 μmol/l fluorescein diacetate solution in phosphate buffered saline. This suspension was rapidly transferred to a 1-cm cuvette and put into the thermostatically controlled cuvette holder of the spectrophotometer which was maintained at 27 °C. An example of the type of recording obtained is shown in fig. 5.13.

As a result of these experiments, it was possible to demonstrate a complete

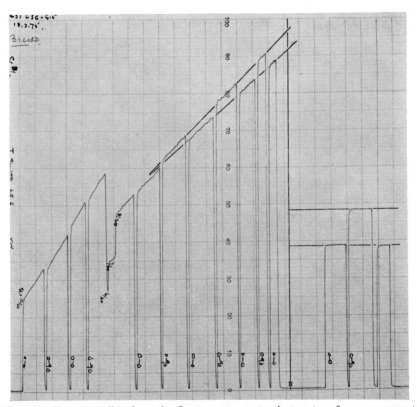

Fig. 5.13. Chart recording from the fluorescence spectrophotometer of a measurement made on mouse bone marrow cells. (The amplification change part way through was made by changing the emission slit width.)

Table 5.5

Percentage change in SCM of haemopoietic cells when treated with mature blood cell extracts.

Test extract		Cell type tested		
Extract	Molecular weight range	Normal lymphocytes	Cultured granulocytic cells	Foetal liver normoblasts
Lymph node	500–1000	+2	+4	+2
extract (LNE)	1000–10000	+7	−2	+5
	30000–50000	*+44*	+2	+2
Granulocyte	*500–1000*	+1	*+42*	−3
extract (GCE)	*1000–10000*	+1	*+13*	+4
	30000–50000	0	+4	+4
Erythrocyte	*500–1000*	−1	−2	*+51*
extract (RCE)	*1000–10000*	−1	−2	*+48*
	30000–50000	−1	−4	*+46*

Molecular weight ranges shown in italics are the ranges containing active inhibitory material according to the reported data. Highly significant changes in the SCM of the test cells are also shown in italics. (Reprinted from the British Journal of Cancer 29 (1974) 173.)

pattern of specificity of effect of the cell extracts for proliferating cells of their own lineage. The SCM's of the untreated controls were (i) PHA stimulated lymphocytes, $P = 0.191$, (ii) cultured granulocytes, $P = 0.176$ and (iii) foetal liver normoblasts, $P = 0.147$. Table 5.5 (reprinted from the Br. J. Cancer 29 (1974) 173) illustrates this specificity and, in fact, for the most part limits the effect to the molecular regions where 'chalones' have been suggested. The changes shown in this table as percentage change compared to the control values are all highly significant increases in structuredness and therefore compatible with an effect of proliferation inhibition. In view of the fact that cytoplasmic processes are being measured, it seems likely, therefore, that the effect is occurring in the G_1 phase, probably at the $G_1 \rightarrow S$ boundary.

In a further publication (Lord et al., 1974b) it was possible to demonstrate the complete reversibility of these increases by the simple expedient of washing out the extracts. In addition these were all xenogeneic experiments and so it would appear that, used in this way, such measurements were able to demonstrate that extracts of mature blood cells may fulfil three of the basic requirements for specific 'chalone-like' proliferation inhibitors.

One of the principal advantages of this technique is that all tests can be carried out under identical conditions. This means that direct comparisons of very closely related cell types and cell extracts can be used to determine in an unequivocal manner the specificity of an effect.

An additional feature of these measurements is their sensitivity to the effects of the extracts. Preliminary dose response studies of the effect of erythrocyte extracts on regenerating erythroid spleens for example have shown that maximal increases in SCM are obtained with doses of about 10^{-1} μg/ml. Significant measurable changes, i.e. greater than 10% increase, were obtained with a dose as low as 2×10^{-5} μg/ml (Lord, unpublished results). Assuming a uniform molecular weight for the contents of the extract, this represents a molar concentration of less than 10^{-11} M and since the extract is very much a cocktail, it indicates that the active constituent is effective at extremely low concentrations.

5.5 *Measurements involving the assessment of cell growth*

Since a 'chalone' is required ultimately to modify cell production one should ideally be able to measure the effect by a reduction in cell growth. A number of techniques is available for this purpose though apart from a small number of specialised cell systems, definitive growth techniques are largely confined to the haemopoietic system. These include the diffusion chamber technique, the spleen colony forming technique and the agar colony forming technique in which primitive granulocyte precursors develop through all the stages of granulocytosis. Many basic data are available for these techniques and in addition the extensive information they afford is well understood. A technique comparable to that for primitive granulocytic precursors but for early erythrocyte precursors has recently been developed (Stephenson et al., 1971). Its understanding, however, is still elementary and consequently not ready for consideration as assay method for growth modifying factors.

Other colony producing methods such as HeLa cell cultures or P388 lymphoma cultures have a limited applicability, perhaps as crude specificity or toxicity tests but since they are so far removed even from their own original characteristics, their usefulness is questionable. Cell growth in other established cell lines can be used similarly but these are clearly subject to the same limitations. Houck et al. (1972) have used cultures of human fibroblasts and have been able to demonstrate that medium conditioned by fibroblasts grown to the confluent stationary phase will inhibit cell growth in further log phase growing cultures. Measurement of the rate of growth of cells is sufficient here to demonstrate growth inhibitory activity of the conditioned media.

5.5.1 The diffusion chamber method

The diffusion chamber method of studying the effects of substances on cell proliferation was developed by Benestad (1970, 1972) and represents a compromise between a culture technique and an in vivo test system. As such, it represents a superior cell culture using the animal host as the incubator and culture medium. Such an arrangement has several advantages, not the least of which is the fact that the medium is more physiological although somewhat anoxic. This medium is continuously buffered and balanced and allows for the effective removal of any toxic products as they are produced. As far as can be determined, for granulocytic cells, the parameters of proliferation are comparable to those measured in granulo-poietically stimulated in vivo systems (Benestad, 1972; Bøyum and Breivik, 1973). At the same time, the cells under investigation are isolated and the problems associated with mixed cell populations can be effectively avoided. Quantitation of cell numbers in the chambers is somewhat limited, however, since a fibrin clot forms over the membranes and must be dissolved using a proteolytic enzyme in order to release the cells.

The chamber is constructed by sealing two Millipore membranes (pore size 0.22 μm) on to either side of a 14-mm perspex ring. The ring contains a small hole through which the chamber can be filled with cell suspension. After sterilizing, filling and sealing the chamber, it is implanted in the peritoneal cavity of a host mouse.

So far, this technique has been used only for stem cells and for studying granulocyte (and macrophage) proliferation. Benestad, for example, has employed cell fractionation techniques such as those described by Bøyum (1968). In this way, it is possible to fill the chamber with specific cell population types and thus control, to a large extent, the type of cell which will grow in the chamber. Potentially however, a number of other cell types could be grown in the chambers.

Application of potential inhibitors to test cells can be applied in a variety of ways. They may be injected into the host animal and allowed to come into contact with the chamber cells by diffusion through the Millipore membranes. Alternatively, potential inhibitor producing cells (e.g. granulocytes) can be added directly into the chamber with the test cells. A newer adaptation of this method of application is to make a double chamber containing the test cells on one side of the central membrane and the potential inhibitor producing cells on the other side. An alternative way of using the chamber is to measure the effects on the chamber cell population on implantation into animals bearing tumours or for example a transplantable leukaemia which may be expected to produce high endogenous levels of inhibitor.

The end point for assessments using this technique can also take several forms. Much basic work has been carried out by Benestad (1972) characterising the growth of granulocytic and mononuclear cell populations. Consequently, changes in the growth patterns of the cells can be measured. Thymidine incorporation and/or mitotic index studies may also be carried out but these are subject to the limitations discussed above.

Chamber cell populations may also be assayed for the growth of stem cells (in the case of haemopoietic tissue, stem cell assays are discussed in the next section). For such measurements, the timing and the manner in which the cells are exposed to the potential 'chalone' are critical if one is to distinguish between direct cytotoxicity and reversible inhibition. An experiment of this kind, however, can be used to give vital information on the specificity of action and the location of an effect in a cell's developmental sequence.

5.5.2 Colony formation methods

5.5.2.1 Spleen colony technique

The spleen colony technique was developed in 1961 by Till and McCulloch and has since been used extensively for the assay of haemopoietic stem cells. Mice are lethally irradiated (800–850 rads X-rays) and then injected intravenously with a suspension of syngeneic bone marrow cells (or any syngeneic haemopoietic tissue) containing the stem cells to be assayed. Seven to eleven days (normally nine days) later, the mice are killed, their spleens removed and fixed in Bouin's solution. When fixed, the spleen surface is seen to contain whitish nodules which can readily be counted under a dissecting microscope. It was found that the number of colonies produced is directly proportional to the number of cells initially injected (Till and McCulloch, 1961; McCulloch and Till, 1962). For normal bone marrow, on average about 20 colonies are produced for every hundred thousand cells injected, varying slightly with the strain of mouse used. In addition, it was found from chromosomal aberration studies that each colony had developed from a single donor cell (Becker et al., 1963). Since the colonies contain developing and mature blood cells and since they themselves can colonize further irradiated mouse spleens, the cells initiating the colonies satisfy the definition of a stem cell and are known by their functional definition as spleen colony forming units, CFUs.

In itself, a study of inhibitory effects on the CFUs has little application at present except as a test for toxicity. A treatment of the donor cells prior to injection can, unless toxic to CFUs, only be expected to induce a delay of a few hours in the cells which are not going to start proliferating significantly for about 72 h anyway.

Growing colonies, however, contain proliferating haemopoietic cells and effects on the growth of the cells can be measured in vivo. By establishing regenerating spleens as described in the section on autoradiography it is possible to treat the animal repeatedly during colony development and study the effect on colony size and number. A suitable experimental regime would be to inject 5×10^4 normal bone marrow cells into lethally irradiated mice and wait until day 5 of colony development when the spleens will be rich with all stages of erythroid development. From days 5 to 8 inclusive, the test extract is injected every eight hours in an attempt to arrest the erythropoiesis. A parallel set of mice, irradiated but not injected with cells, must be included in order to obtain the background cellularity. At 9 days, some of the mice are killed and their spleens fixed for colony counting. From the rest, the spleens are removed and their cellularity measured. The non-injected mice are similarly treated so that the average cellularity per colony can be calculated.

An illustration of the use of this technique is given in a preliminary series of experiments (Shah and Lord, unpublished data), in which 1 mg of a partially purified extract from rat red blood cells (molecular weight range 500–1000 daltons) was injected according to the above regime. One mg of a comparable extract from rat granulocytes or an equal volume of saline was injected into the controls. At 9 days, after subtracting the background spleen cellularity, the mean colony cellularity in the red cell extract treated mice was about 30% lower than in the granulocyte extract and saline treated controls; 1.51×10^6 cells per colony for RCE treated mice compared to 2.32×10^6 cells per colony and 1.97×10^6 cells/colony for the GCE and saline treated mice respectively (table 5.6). The number of colonies produced is also reduced by about 23% but this almost certainly relates to the reduced colony cellularity which makes some colonies too small to count. The error on a colony count can be up to about 10% so the reduction of colonies in the GCE-treated mice is barely significant although a small reduction might be expected due to effects on the granulocytic part of the spleen regeneration.

If indeed this is a 'chalone' type of inhibition, then colony growth should rapidly be resumed after stopping the routine treatments. Thus a comple-

Table 5.6

Repeated treatment of developing erythroid spleen colonies with cell extracts. One mg of extract injected every 8 h on days 5 to 8 inclusive following bone marrow graft to an irradiated mouse. The mice were killed on day 9 or 12.

	Cols/spleen	Corrected spleen cellularity ($\times 10^{-6}$)	Cells/colony ($\times 10^{-6}$)
9 days			
Saline treated	12.2	24.0	1.97
GCE treated	11.1	25.8	2.32
RCE treated	9.0	13.6	1.51
12 days			
Saline treated	13.3	37.3	2.80
GCE treated	13.9	40.2	2.89
RCE treated	12.8	28.8	2.25

mentary experiment in which the treatments were stopped at day 8 but the animals allowed to live up to 12 days is also shown in table 5.6. A feature of the colony experiment is that the total number of colonies does not increase between day 5 and 13 (Lewis and Trobough, 1964; McCulloch, 1963) and as seen in the table, colony numbers in the saline treated controls are not significantly different at 9 and 12 days but in the RCE treated animals both the colony counts and the colony cellularity are showing a marked recovery. The GCE treated mice are not significantly different from the controls.

5.5.2.2 The agar colony technique
In the agar colony technique developed by Pluznik and Sachs (1965) and by Bradley and Metcalf (1966), colonies are grown in a medium of agar and a colony stimulating factor. It is now generally accepted that the cells from which the colonies develop are primitive cells committed primarily to granulocyte development. As such, it should be a system favourable for the assay of potential granulocyte inhibitors. As with the spleen colony technique, however, a short treatment of the cells before plating could not reasonably be expected to have a noticeable effect unless the treatment is toxic to the colony forming cells.

Treatment of the developing colonies should be possible as for the spleen colonies. However, this is an in vitro culture system with the attendant difficulties of interfering with the culture conditions. In order for the colonies

B. I. Lord

to grow in agar, a conditioned medium containing colony stimulating factor (CSF), itself a cell extract, is necessary and any potential inhibitor is therefore in competition with the CSF. In addition, the cells are growing in a semi-solid medium which may hinder diffusion of the test materials to the cells. On the other hand, this may be countered by the test materials having a relatively long half life in a culture system. The kinetics of growth of the colony cells have been measured and shown to compare well with granulocytic cells grown in diffusion chambers. In addition, the cell cycle is closely comparable to in vivo myelopoiesis under a high degree of demand (Testa and Lord, 1973). Since it is possible to measure colony size distributions for the cultures the technique is potentially a useful and valid way of assessing inhibitors of granulocytopoiesis and the specificity of other inhibitors.

5.6 Measurement of tumour regression

A number of tumour systems may also be used to test out potential inhibitors. Some of these are based on tumour cell lines grown in vitro. For example, melanoma cells can be grown in plastic tissue culture dishes and the amount of growth can be assessed by removing the cells from the dish with trypsin, putting them into suspension and counting the cells (Dewey, 1973). Assessment of melanoma cell extracts can be made in this culture by the change in cell numbers produced. The method affords little opportunity of assessing definitive specificity but can be useful, as in the case of modifying fibroblast growth, as a closed system for studies on melanocytes and melanoma cells.

In vivo, Rytömaa and Kiviniemi have used chloroma tumours growing in rats (Rytömaa and Kiviniemi, 1969). This is the shay granulocytic chloro-leukaemia, which is transplantable as a localized tumour whose gross dimensions can be measured with calipers. This was not initially seen as an assay technique but since tumour regression was observed it could potentially be developed as a rough activity test for the granulocyte extracts though in order to produce significant changes in tumour size a repeated dosage schedule would appear to be essential.

5.7 Miscellaneous test systems

Other systems exist in which inhibitory effects have been demonstrated and which could conceivably be developed as 'chalone' assay techniques. Rytömaa extended his studies of the modification of chloroma growth by testing granulocyte extracts against the same chloro-leukaemia grown as a generalized leukaemia (Rytömaa and Kiviniemi, 1970). The end point in this case was extended survival but, as with the tumour, this is a rather crude end point and a repeated dose schedule is necessary to produce any significant change.

Any true 'chalone' with a relatively short, reversible, inhibitory action however can, from a single treatment, produce only a minimal delay in cell production and therefore cannot produce any significant prolongation of survival. Consequently, the end point of survival is relatively insensitive and its use is therefore limited.

A similar end point has, however, been used in assessing the value of lymphoid cell extracts (Garcia-Giralt et al., 1973) by virtue of their ability to allow an allogeneic graft to protect an irradiated animal. In this type of experiment, the test extracts are injected into the donor animals prior to transplanting lymphoid cells into irradiated recipient mice. An active lymphoid extract produced a change in the 30 day survival from about 25% to about 80%. Similarly, Kiger et al. (1973a) assessed inhibitory activity of thymic extracts by their ability to prevent the normal graft versus host reaction as measured by lymph node enlargement, splenomegaly or mortality when donor parental lymphoid cells were incubated with the extract. They further demonstrated this activity in vivo by measuring the survival of allogeneic skin grafts (Kiger et al., 1972). The thymic extract, injected 3 days per week, increased the graft survival from 18.5 days to 22.0 days. Similarly, Houck et al. (1973) also increased the survival of allogeneic skin grafts from 10.5 days to 29 days by injecting a spleen extract 3 times per week.

It appears therefore that any in vivo test based on long term (> 24 h say) endpoints invariably requires a repeated dosage schedule which may limit its value as an assay technique for showing the presence of some degree of inhibition.

Two further immunologically based techniques followed up by Houck et al. (1973) illustrate what may represent excellent quantitative assays of lymphocyte extracts. These are the inhibition of proliferation in mixed lymphocyte cultures and inhibition of the macrophage migration inhibitory factor (MIF). The mixed lymphocyte culture system is simply an extension of the phytohaemagglutinin stimulated lymphocyte culture with the same advantages and disadvantages (p. 111). The MIF test as applied by Houck and Chang (1973) is quick and sensitive and it was found that the release of MIF activity into the supernatant medium of cultures treated with extracts was inversely proportional to the dose of extract used. The lower limit of its sensitivity is of the order of 5 μg/ml and as such does not compare with measurement detecting 50 pg/ml by the SCM test. It is, however, a technique which may successfully be exploited in assaying inhibitory activity obtained from lymphoid tissues. It is clearly useful for confirming the activity of an extract and since the measurement is based on a homogeneous population of cells, it should be ideal for checking and confirming cell line specificity.

5.8 Conclusion

An attempt has been made to analyse some of the assay techniques most commonly used in the 'chalone' field of research. This aspect of the subject has probably been the major reason for the slow development of the 'chalone' hypothesis of cell proliferation control by feedback inhibition processes. All of these techniques are subject to quite serious experimental pitfalls which have made interpretation of the results rather hazardous. Consequently an attempt has been made to assess what information may be obtained from them without giving details of their actual use. Of the newer techniques, such as that which measures cytoplasmic structuredness, more details are presented. Similarly extended applications of the more standard methods, such as autoradiography, are also discussed in more detail together with examples of their use.

In vitro methods in particular require a very careful understanding and it would be hoped that the future of culture techniques might be developed along the lines of the perfusion culture systems of Kruse (1972). The advantages of such systems are very obvious since they were primarily designed for working with cells in vitro under environments approaching steady state conditions. One obtains a relatively constant pH, constant levels of nutrient input and constant levels of metabolic product concentrations. Closed culture systems may control the pH fairly well but cannot control the other two factors. Since all living systems are open systems, Kruse expresses surprise that almost all in vitro work with mammalian cells, including the assay of 'chalones', has been carried out in closed culture systems whose environments are in a constant state of flux (Kruse, 1973). Such an approach is at present simulated only by the diffusion chamber method among the culture techniques available for measuring cell growth and proliferation. Continuous perfusion techniques for other cell systems would contribute greatly to bridging the gap produced by the simplicity but artificiality of in vitro culture compared with the complexity, reality and often indeterminacy of in vivo studies.

The ultimate definition of any physiological control process, however, depends on its unequivocal demonstration in an in vivo situation and one can do no better than to conclude by reiterating the warning of Joseph

Barcroft: '. . . but I claim for those who are prepared to study "life as a whole" than man places an undue limitation on his intellect if he is not prepared to look at living things as they are, but will merely study artefacts about which he can obtain more precise information'.

References

Appleton, T. C. (1964) Autoradiography of soluble labelled compounds. J. R. Microscop. Soc. 83, 277.

Azumi, T. and McGlynn, S. P. (1962) Chem. Phys. 37, 2413.

Becker, A. J., McCulloch, E. A. and Till, J. E. (1963) Cytological demonstration of the clonal nature of spleen colonies derived from transplanted mouse marrow cells. Nature 197, 452.

Benestad, H. B. (1970) Formation of granulocytes and macrophages in diffusion chamber cultures of mouse blood leukocytes. Scand. J. Haematol. 7, 279.

Benestad, H. B. (1972) Cell kinetics in diffusion chambers: survival, resumption of proliferation, and maturation rate of murine haemopoietic cells. Cell Tissue Kinet. 6, 147.

Hondius Boldingh, W. and Laurence, E. B. (1968) Extraction, purification and preliminary characterisation of the epidermal chalone: A tissue specific mitotic inhibitor obtained from vertebrate skins. Europ. J. Biochem. 5, 191.

Bradley, T. R. and Metcalf, D. (1966) The growth of mouse bone marrow cells in vitro. Aust. J. Exp. Biol. Med. Sci. 44, 287.

Bullough, W. S. and Laurence, E. B. (1960) The control of epidermal mitotic activity in the mouse. Proc. R. Soc. Lond. (Biol) 151, 517.

Bullough, W. S. and Laurence, E. B. (1961) The control of mitotic activity in mouse skin. Dermis and hypodermis. Exp. Cell Res. 21, 394.

Bullough, W. S. and Laurence, E. B. (1970) The lymphocytic chalone and its antimitotic action on a mouse lymphoma in vitro. Europ. J. Cancer 6, 525.

Bøyum, A. (1968) Separation of leukocytes from blood and bone marrow. Scand. J. Clin. Lab. Invest. 21, Suppl. 97.

Bøyum, A. and Breivik, H. (1973) Kinetics of murine haemopoietic cell proliferation in diffusion chambers. Cell Tissue Kinet. 6, 101.

Cercek, L. (1969) Effects of ^{14}MeV neutrons and 300 kVp X-rays on geotrophic response and sedimentation velocity of statoliths in barley roots. Int. J. Radiat. Biol. 16, 419.

Cercek, L. and Cercek, B. (1971) Effects of O_2-concentration, dose rate, LET and cysteamine on the radiation induced changes in viscosity of the cytoplasm in the statocytes of barley roots. Int. J. Radiat. Biol. 19, 361.

Cercek, L. and Cercek, B. (1972) Studies on the structuredness of cytoplasm and rates of enzymatic hydrolysis in growing yeast cells. I. Changes induced by ionizing radiation. Int. J. Radiat. Biol. 21, 445.

Cercek, L. and Cercek, B. (1974) Involvement of cyclic-AMP in changes of structuredness of cytoplasmic matrix (SCM) Rad. Environm. Biophys. 11, 209.

Cercek, L., Cercek, B. and Ockey, C. H. (1973) Structuredness of the cytoplasmic matrix and Michaelis–Menten constants for the hydrolysis of FDA during the cell cycle in chinese hamster ovary cells. Biophysik. 10, 187.

Chen, R. F. and Bowman, R. C. (1965) Fluorescence polarization measurement with ultraviolet-polarizing filters in a spectrophotometer. Science 147, 729.

Chopra, D. P. (1973) Regulation of mitosis in the embryonic kidney *(Xenopus laevis)* by kidney growth inhibitor (chalone). In: Chalones: concepts and current researches (eds.: B. K. Forscher and J. C. Houck) Natl. Cancer Inst. Monogr. 38, p. 189.

Cleaver, J. E. (1967) In: Thymidine metabolism and cell kinetics (eds.: A. Neuberger and E. L. Tatum) North-Holland, Amsterdam. p. 104.

Cronkite, E. P., Fliedner, T. M., Bond, V. P., Rubini, J. R., Brecher, G. and Quastler, H. (1959) Dynamics of haemopoietic proliferation in man and mice studied by ^{3}H-thymidine incorporation into DNA. Progr. Nucl. Energy Series VI 2, 92.

Dewey, D. L. (1973) The melanocyte chalone. In: Chalones: concepts and current researches (Eds.: B. K. Forscher and J. C. Houck) Natl. Cancer Inst. Monogr. 38, p. 213.

Dexter, T. M., Allen, T. D., Lajtha, L. G., Schofield, R. and Lord, B. I. (1973) Stimulation of proliferation and differentiation of haemopoietic cells in vitro. J. Cell Physiol. 82, 461.

Dustin, A. P. (1936) La colchine réactif de l'imminence caryocinétique. Arch. Portug. Sc. Biol. 5, 38.

Einstein, A. (1906) Ann. Physics 19, 37.

Elgjo, K. (1973) Epidermal chalone: cell cycle specificity of two epidermal growth inhibitors. In: Chalones: concepts and current researches (eds.: B. K. Forscher and J. C. Houck) Natl. Cancer Inst. Monogr. 38, p. 71.

Feinendegen, L. E., Bond, V. P. and Hughes, W. L. (1966) Physiological thymidine reutilization in rat bone marrow. Proc. Soc. Exp. Biol. Med. 122, 448.

Garcia-Giralt, E., Rella, W., Morales, V. H., Diaz-Rubio, E. and Richaud, E. (1973) Extraction from bovine spleen of immunosuppressant with no activity on haemopoietic spleen colony formation. In: Chalones: concepts and current researches (eds.: B. K. Forscher and J. C. Houck) Natl. Cancer Inst. Monogr. 38, 125.

Geard, C. R. (1975) Chromosomal aberrations in three successive cell cycles of *Wallabia bicolor* leukocytes after tritiated thymidine incorporation. Radiat. Res. 61, 18.

Grisham, J. W. (1960) Inhibitory effect of tritiated thymidine on regeneration of the liver in the young rat. Proc. Soc. Exp. Biol. Med. 105, 555.

Houck, J. C. and Irausquin, H. (1973) Some properties of the lymphocyte chalone. In: Chalones: concepts and current researches (eds.: B. K. Forscher and J. C. Houck) Natl. Cancer Inst. Monogr. 38, 117.

Houck, J. C., Attallah, A. M. and Lilly, J. R. (1973) Immunosuppressive properties of the lymphocyte chalone. Nature 245, 148.

Houck, J. C. and Chang, C. M. (1973) A new sensitive assay for macrophage inhibitory factor. Proc. Soc. Expl. Biol. Med. 142, 800.

Houck, J. C., Weil, R. L. and Sharma, V. K. (1972) Evidence for a fibroblast chalone. Nature New Biol. 240, 210.

Hooper, C. E. S. (1961) Use of colchicine for the measurement of mitotic rate in the intestinal epithelium. Am. J. Anat. 108, 231.

Howard, A. and Pelc, S. R. (1951) Nuclear incorporation of ^{32}P as demonstrated by autoradiographs. J. Exp. Cell Res. 2, 178.

Howard, A. and Pelc, S. R. (1953) Synthesis of deoxyribonucleic acid in normal and irradiated cells and its relation to chromosome breakage. Heredity 6, 261 (Suppl.)

Hughes, W. L. (1957) Brookhaven National Laboratory Progress Reports 473 (S-38) p. 35.

Johnson, H. A. and Cronkite, E. P. (1959) The effect of tritiated thymidine on mouse spermatogonia. Radiat. Res. 11, 825.

Kiger, N., Florentin, I. and Mathé, G. (1972) Some effects of a partially purified lymphocyte-inhibiting factor from calf thymus. Transplantation 14, 448.

Kiger, N., Florentin, I. and Mathé, G. (1973) A lymphocyte-inhibiting factor (chalone?) extracted from thymus: immunosuppressive effects. In: Chalones: concepts and current researches (eds.: B. K. Forscher and J. C. Houck) Natl. Cancer Inst. Monogr. 38, 135.

Kiger, N., Florentin, I. and Mathé, G. (1973) Inhibition of graft-versus-host reaction by preincubation of the graft with a thymic extract (lymphocyte chalone). Transplantation 16, 393.

Kruse, P. F. Jr. (1972) Use of perfusion systems for growth of cell and tissue cultures. In: Nutrition and metabolism of cells in culture (eds.: G. A. Rothblat and V. J. Cristofalo). Vol. 2, Academic Press Inc., New York, p. 11.

Kruse, P. F. Jr. (1973) Commentary on 'Control of Fibroblast proliferation' by J. C. Houck, R. F. Cheng and V. K. Sharma. In: Chalones: concepts and current researches (eds.: B. K. Forscher and J. C. Houck) Natl. Cancer Inst. Monogr. 38, p. 171.

Lajtha, L. G., Gilbert, C. W. and Guzman, E. (1971) Kinetics of haemopoietic colony growth. Brit. J. Haematol. 20, 343.

Laurence, E. B. (1973) The epidermal chalone and keratinizing epithelia. In: Chalones: concepts and current researches (eds.: B. K. Forscher and J. C. Houck) Natl. Cancer Inst. Monogr. 38, p. 61.

Laurence, E. B. and Randers-Hansen, E. (1971) An in vivo study of epidermal chalone and stress hormones on mitosis in tongue epithelium and ear epidermis of the mouse. Virchows Arch. Abt. B. Zellpath. 9, 271.

Lenfant, M., Kren-Proschek, L. and Verly, W. G. (1973) Thymidine as one of the factors in a beef liver extract decreasing tritiated thymidine incorporation into DNA. Can. J. Biochem. 51, 654.

Lewis, J. P. and Trobough, F. E. Jr. (1964) Haematopoietic stem cells. Nature 204, 589.

Ling, G. N. (1972) Hydration of macromolecules. In: Water and aqueous solutions: structure thermodynamics and transfer processes (ed.: R. A. Horne) Wiley Interscience, New York, London, p. 692.

Lord, B. I. (1964) The effects of continuous irradiation on cell proliferation in rat bone marrow. Brit. J. Haematol. 10, 496.

Lord, B. I. (1965) Cellular proliferation in normal and continuously irradiated rat bone marrow studied by repeated labelling with tritiated thymidine. Brit. J. Haematol. 11, 130.

Lord, B. I. (1968) Distribution of cell cycle times of normoblasts in the bone marrow of normal and continuously irradiated rats. In: Effects of radiation on cellular proliferation and differentiation I.A.E.A. Symposium, Vienna p. 247.

Lord, B. I., Cercek, L., Cercek, B., Shah, G. P., Dexter, T. M. and Lajtha, L. G. (1974a) Inhibitors of haemopoietic cell proliferation?: Specificity of action within the haemopoietic system. Brit. J. Cancer 29, 168.

Lord, B. I., Cercek, L., Cercek, B., Shah, G. P. and Lajtha, L. G. (1974b) Inhibitors of haemopoietic cell proliferation: Reversibility of action. Brit. J. Cancer 29, 407.

Lord, B. I., Lajtha, L. G. and Gidali, J. G. (1974c) Measurement of the kinetic status of bone marrow precursor cells: Three cautionary tales. Cell Tissue Kinet. 7, 507.

Marks, F. (1973) A tissue specific factor inhibiting DNA synthesis in mouse epidermis. In: Chalones, concepts and current researches (eds.: B. K. Forscher and J. C. Houck) Natl. Cancer Inst. Monogr. 38, p. 79.

McCulloch, E. A. (1963) Les Clones de cellules hématopoiétiques in vivo. Rev. Fr. Etud. Clin. Biol. 8, 15.

McCulloch, E. A. and Till, J. E. (1962) The sensitivity of cells from normal mouse bone marrow to γ-radiation in vitro and in vivo. Radiat. Res. 16, 822.

Nome, O. (1974) Tissue specificity of the epidermal chalones. Thesis for medical doctorate at the University of Oslo.

Paukovits, W. (1971) Control of granulocyte production: separation and chemical identification of a specific inhibitor (chalone). Cell Tissue Kinet. 4, 539.

Pelc, S. R. (1962) Incorporation of tritiated thymidine in various organs of the mouse. Nature 193, 793.

Pelc, S. R. (1964) Labelling of DNA and cell division in so called non-dividing tissues. J. Cell Biol. 22, 21.

Pelc, S. R. and Gahan, P. B. (1959) Incorporation of labelled thymidine in the seminal vesicle of the mouse. Nature 183, 335.

Perrin, F. (1929) La fluorescence des solutions. Ann. Physics 10, 169.

Peterson, A. R., Fox, B. W. and Fox, M. (1971) Toxicity of tritiated thymidine in P388F lymphoma cells. I. Incorporation into DNA and cell survival. Int. J. Radiat. Biol. 19, 123.

Peterson, A. R., Fox, B. W. and Fox, M. (1973) Alkaline sucrose sedimentation studies of DNA from P388F lymphoma cells treated with difunctional alkylating agents. Biochim. Biophys. Acta. 299, 385.

Pluznik, D. H. and Sachs, L. (1965) The cloning of normal 'mast' cells in tissue culture. J. Cell Comp. Physiol. 66, 319.

Quastler, H. (1959) Some aspects of cell population kinetics. In: Kinetics of cellular proliferation (ed.: F. Stohlman Jr.) Grune and Stratton, New York, N.Y., p. 218.

Quastler, H. and Sherman, F. G. (1959) Cell population kinetics in the intestinal epithelium of the mouse. Exp. Cell Res. 17, 420.

Rothberg, S. and Arp, B. C. (1973) Epidermal chalone and inhibition of DNA synthesis. In: Chalones, concepts and current researches (eds.: B. K. Forscher and J. C. Houck) Natl. Cancer Inst. Monogr. 38, 93.

Rotman, B. and Papermaster, B. W. (1966) Membrane properties of living mammalian cells as studied by enzymatic hydrolysis of fluorogenic esters. Proc. Natl. Acad. Sci. U.S. 55, 134.

Rubini, J. R., Cronkite, E. P., Bond, V. P. and Fliedner, T. M. (1960) The metabolism and fate of tritiated thymidine in man. J. Clin. Invest. 39, 909.

Rytömaa, T. (1968) Granulocytic chalone and antichalone, in Hemic cells in vitro (ed.: P. Farnes) A symposium of the Tissue Culture Association 4, 47.

Rytömaa, T. and Kiviniemi, K. (1968) Control of granulocyte production. I. Chalone and antichalone, two specific humoral regulators. Cell Tissue Kinet. 1, 329.

Rytömaa, T. and Kiviniemi, K. (1969) Chloroma regression induced by the granulocytic chalone. Nature 222, 995.

Rytömaa, T. and Kiviniemi, K. (1970) Regression of generalised leukaemia in rat induced by the granulocytic chalone. Europ. J. Cancer 6, 401.

Schultze, B. and Oehlert, W. (1960) Autoradiographic investigation of incorporation of [³H]thymidine into the cells of the rat and mouse. Science 131, 737.

Silver, A. F., Chase, H. B. and Arsenault, C. T. (1969) Early anagen initiated by plucking compared with early spontaneous anagen. In: Advances in Biology of Skin (ed.: W. Montagna) Pergamon Press, New York. Vol. IX, p. 265.

Simnett, J. D. and Fisher, J. M. (1973) An assay system for humoral growth factors. In: Chalones: concepts and current researches (eds.: B. K. Forscher and J. C. Houck) Natl. Cancer Inst. Monogr. 38, p. 19.

Stephenson, J. R., Axelrad, A. A., McLeod, D. L. and Shreeve, M. M. (1971) Induction of colonies of hemoglobin-synthesising cells by erythropoietin in vitro. Proc. Natl. Acad. Sci. U.S. 68, 1542.

Simard, A., Corneille, L., Deschamps, Y. and Verly, W. G. (1974) Inhibition of cell proliferation in the livers of hepatectomized rats by a rabbit hepatic chalone. Proc. Natl. Acad. Sci. U.S. 71, 1763.

Tannock, I. F. (1967) A comparison of the relative efficiencies of various metaphase arrest agents. Exp. Cell Res. 47, 345.

Testa, N. G. and Lord, B. I. (1973) Kinetics of growth of haemopoietic colony cells in agar. Cell Tissue Kinet. 6, 425.

Till, J. E. and McCulloch, A. E. (1961) A direct measurement of the radiation sensitivity of normal mouse bone marrow cells. Radiat. Res. 14, 213.

Verly, W. G. (1973) The hepatic chalone. In: Chalones: concepts and current researches (eds.: B. K. Forscher and J. C. Houck) Natl. Cancer Inst. Monogr. 38, 175.

Verly, W. G., Firket, H. and Hunebelle, G. (1958) Preparation of tritium labelled thymidine and its use for the study by the autoradiographic method of the synthesis of DNA in culture cells. Proc. 2nd Int. Conf. on Peaceful Uses of Atomic Energy 25, 181.

Williams, C. A. and Ockey, C. H. (1970) Distribution of DNA replicator sites in mammalian nuclei after different methods of cell synchronization. Exp. Cell Res. 63, 365.

Wimber, D. E. and Quastler, H. (1963) A ^{14}C and ^{3}H-thymidine double labelling technique in the study of cell proliferation in tradescantia root tips. Exp. Cell Res. 30, 8.

CHAPTER 6

Regulation of cell growth in vitro and in vivo: point/counterpoint

ABDELFATTAH M. ATTALLAH

Biochemical Research Laboratory, Research Foundation of Children's Hospital, Washington, D. C. 20009, U.S.A.

6.1 Introduction

For this review, I have chosen to summarize and compare the existing growth regulation theories with the chalone concept. It has long been evident that in any typical adult mammalian tissue the dynamic equilibrium between cell gain and cell loss must be controlled by some precise homeostatic mechanism (see Bullough Review, 1965). There are numerous theories concerning the regulation of growth and cell division. Some propose the operation of inhibitors; others propose stimulators. One group would have each organ and tissue control its own growth; others claim a central control of all growth. I shall first give a brief history of several of these theories and then consider in detail a theory of growth regulation controlled by a feedback inhibition.

6.2 Growth stimulators

In 1892, Wiesner first proposed that injured cells might liberate substances capable of stimulating growth. In a theory about possible growth-stimulating factors or the so-called 'wound hormone', Abercrombie much later (1957) proposed a 'wound hormone' released locally in response to local injury. He suggested that the mitotic activity of tissue around the wound was due to the stimulating action of this hormone, which was produced by the damage to cells and which acted generally on all local tissues. 'The stimulus mechanisms that we may regard as in a broad sense hormonal can be classified according to two criteria: 1) the degree of dispersion in the body of the 'hormone': either the stimulant is systematically distributed by the blood stream, the response being localized only because the sensitive cells are localized; or the stimulant is predominantly local, the responding cells being not so much those sensitive to as those exposed to stimulation . . .' (Abercrombie, 1957).

Bucher et al. (1951) reported that, when partial hepatectomy was performed on one member of a parabiotic pair or two of parabiotic triplet rats, the number of mitoses in the intact liver of the parabiotic partner (that had not undergone partial hepatectomy) was increased. Serum from hepatectomized rats was injected into rats that had intact livers and also produced an increase of the mitotic rate of the intact liver (Friedrich-Freksa and Zaki, 1954).

Recently, Demetriou et al. (1974) reported that serum from unilateral nephrectomized normal rats or human patients had no effect on liver cells grown in vitro. In contrast, the effect of serum from rats or patients who underwent hepatectomy alone was not different from serum of rats or patients subjected to (unilateral) hepatectomy and nephrectomy, suggesting to them that the stimulating effect of serum on cell growth in vitro was a result of hepatectomy alone. These authors reported that the molecular weight of this stimulating factor for liver cells was less than 12,000 daltons.

6.3 Growth inhibitors

Adult tissue is characterized by a lag period of several days preceding the onset of growth in vitro. Before planting fresh adult tissue in culture medium, the tissues are usually treated with trypsin (Simms and Stillman, 1936). This use of trypsin was originally intended to stimulate growth by virtue of the protein split products released by the digestion of the proteins (Baker and Carel, 1928). Simms and Stillman (1936) confirmed that treatment of chicken aorta tissue with trypsin before planting in culture flasks stimulated the tissues to grow sooner and more rapidly. Washing these tissues after trypsin treatment resulted in even better growth stimulation. They were confronted with a new question: Why should the enzymatic digestion of tissue protein stimulate growth? These workers suggested that the enzyme digested away an inhibitory protein material and thus removed it from the environment of the cells. In support of their idea, they found a growth inhibitor in the fluid after adult aorta tissue has been digested with trypsin. The unheated digestion fluid itself when mixed with serum was seen to inhibit the growth of fresh tissue as compared with the serum control. This tissue inhibitor had been obtained from chicken, dog, and sheep aorta. It was precipitated by an equal volume of alcohol and it was non-dialyzable. Simms and Stillman also believed that the inhibitor was produced by the cells of the adult animal to regulate the growth of the adult animal body. 'We believe that the tissue inhibitor described in this paper plays a large role in restraining growth in the adult animal body, thereby keeping the cells in their normal dormant state. It is suggested that the cells elaborate the inhibitor and deposit it in the surrounding intercellular space where it remains because of its insolubility' (Simms and Stillman, 1936).

Working in vivo, Saetren (1956) has studied the effects of the introduction of kidney macerate on the mitotic rate of rat kidney after partial nephrectomy. A strong mitotic depression was obtained, particularly when the amount of kidney macerate introduced equalled the amount of kidney removed. If the rats suffered partial hepatectomy as well as partial nephrectomy, the kidney macerate acted selectively on the kidneys and left the liver unaffected. The mitotic rate of the kidney was similarly unaffected by macerates of liver, spleen, testis, or brain. Saetren indicated that the inhibitory substances produced by the kidney and the liver were relatively unstable, thermolabile, and non-dialyzable.

Rose (1952) made a proposal along similar lines in which he conceived of growth limitation as a mass action phenomenon. He suggested that during development, each tissue might inhibit its own growth when an appropriate mass had been attained. In support of this proposal, he offered some data on the effect of amphibian differentiation when the embryos are reared in a medium to which specific extracts of adult organs have been added. Under such conditions, he reported inhibition of brain growth by brain extract and heart and circulatory differentiation by heart extract. Shave (1954) also submitted data showing the inhibition of nervous tissue development in the frog by tissue fractions of the appropriate adult organ.

A high mitotic activity during regeneration following partial hepatectomy had been demonstrated (see Abercrombie, 1957; Swann, 1958). Similarly, when one kidney is removed, the other hypertrophies until the remaining organ reaches a size comparable to the size of both organs before the operation (Eigsti and Dustin, 1955). It has been suggested (see Swann, 1958) that each tissue secretes into the general body space a specific mitotic inhibitor and when part of the tissue is removed, this results in a decrease of the existing inhibitor concentration. Thus, a high mitotic activity will start and continue in the tissue until the normal size of the tissue is reestablished, consequently building up enough inhibitor to prevent further cell division.

Glinos and Gey (1952) found that mere dilution of plasma caused mitosis in the liver of normal rats, and Glinos (1956) has shown that regeneration can be inhibited by increasing the plasma concentration and that the active fraction is in the plasma albumin. In Glinos' words (1960), 'These findings were considered to indicate an inverse relationship between the concentration of certain serum constituents and the rate of cell division in the liver.' Stich and Florian (1958) have also shown that serum from normal adults inhibits liver regeneration, whereas serum from hepatectomized animals did not. This circulating inhibitor of liver growth has been shown to be active on a parabiotic partner. When a partially hepatectomized rat was joined parabiotically to a normal rat, the liver of the normal rat also developed an increased mitotic rate (Wehneker and Sussman, 1951).

Kamrin's report (1959) initiated the search for immunosuppressive α-globulins. From mammalian plasma, immunosuppressive α-globulins were isolated by Mowbray (1963). Cooperband et al. (1968) used a similar technique to isolate immunoregulatory α-globulin (IRA) from human plasma. IRA inhibited several immune responses including the rejection of renal allografts in vitro (1974).

6.4 Growth inhibitors and tumors

Murphy and Sturm (1931) extracted a material from 'chicken tumor I' that inhibited the transplantation of this tumor into the appropriate host. This inhibitor reduced the acceptance and growth of the tumor by 86%, while all the control animals had actively growing tumors. This inhibitor was stable after heating at 55°C for 30 min but was destroyed by heating to 65°C. This inhibitor had no effect upon transplantable mouse carcinoma. However, extracts of 'chicken tumor I' definitely inhibited the growth of a mouse sarcoma in 83 mice out of 94 (88%). The untreated control mice, however, showed no tumor development in only 21% of the animals. Tumor growth was not different from the control when mice were treated with extracts of chicken serum or with chicken tumor extract heated to over 65°C.

The effect of homologous embryo skin extracts and placenta extract on the spontaneous mammary tumors of mice was also studied by Murphy and Sturm (1934). The tumor was removed and the wound was treated with the extracts. It was found that tumor recurrences in the control (untreated mice) was 50.9%, in the embryo skin extract-treated mice 25.9% demonstrated recurrence, and only 6% of the mice treated with placenta extract contained tumors. In another experiment, Murphy and Sturm surgically removed the tumor from the animal and incubated it with tissue extracts for short periods. They then transplanted the tumor back into the same mice. These autografts either failed to grow, or their subsequent growth was significantly retarded. Cessation of growth of more than 2/3 of the mice with established mammary tumors was found when these animals were injected intraperitoneally with placental extracts.

There are other reports of homologous growth inhibition in solid tumor systems. Goodman (1957) found that at death, the total mass of tumor tissue was the same in mice with two tumors as it was in mice with a single tumor. If two tumors were present and one was surgically removed, the growth rate of the remaining tumor was accelerated. Laird, in 1964, states that 'exponential growth of tumors has been observed only rarely and then for relatively brief periods'. The slowing of growth was demonstrated in almost all tumors studied as the tumor increased in size (Laird, 1964), eventually reaching a maximum.

6.5 Growth stimulators versus growth inhibitors

Another hypothesis explained overall body growth in terms of both inhibitors and stimulators. Tanner (1963) suggested that, since in the course

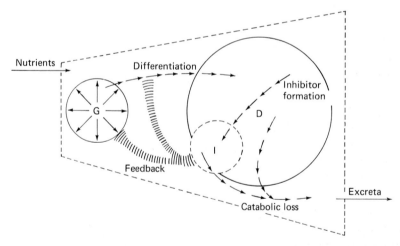

Model 6.1. Shows the main features of the Weiss–Kavanau model of growth control (1957). G, generative compartment; D, differentiating compartment; I, inhibiting principle. In this model cells from the generative compartment are transferred to the differentiated compartment, and from there lost by catabolism. The differentiated compartment produces an inhibitor substance which diffuses back and probably regulates both the cell proliferative activity of the generative compartment as well as the rate of cell differentiation. This model can be used to explain the experimental finding concerning the regulation of cell proliferation in the cell populations of the mammalian body. (Reproduced by courtesy of the authors and J. Gen. Physiol.)

of normal ontogeny the brain develops earlier than any other part of the body, it might be a likely site of growth regulation. According to Tanner's hypothesis, the body produces inhibitors that are monitored by the control center (brain). Thus, the brain may constantly compare the actual size of the body with the size it should be at any given age and produce growth stimulators in proportion to the discrepancy detected.

A somewhat similar hypothesis, this one advanced by Burwell (1963), Burch and Burwell (1965), and Burch (1969), likewise contends that one kind of tissue regulates the growth of all others. In this case, it is suggested that the lymphatic system kept track of how big each organ was and produced regulatory growth substances accordingly. The mass of each target organ is supposedly monitored by the lymphocyte system via tissue coding factors (TCF), which are tissue-specific substances produced by each organ in the body. Should the size of any such organ fall below normal, the number of specific TCF's produced would decline, and the lymphatic tissues would secrete growth stimulators called mitotic control protein (MCP). Thus, the output of growth stimulators would be inversely proportional to the concentration of target organ products. According to this idea, growth is initiated by stimulants and turned off in their absence.

A much more elaborate model of growth has been proposed by Weiss (1947) and Weiss and Kavanau (1957). The basic assumptions of this model are:

1) 'Living mass' has the ability to reproduce and, in the absence of restraining factors, will reproduce exponentially.

2) A living system consists of two components: 'generative mass' which remains in reproductive activity, and 'differentiated mass', derived from the former and consisting of terminal products and other secondary derivatives that do not possess the ability to reproduce. In development, there is a gradual transition from 'generative' to 'differentiated' mass and progressive differentiation is one factor checking unlimited growth.

3) Protoplasmic reproduction or growth is essentially based upon cell-specific catalysts, 'templates' which reproduce the living mass of the same cell type. In addition, each cell also produces freely diffusable compounds antagonistic to the former ('antitemplates') which can block and thus inhibit the reproductive activity of the corresponding 'templates'.

4) Hence, a second growth-regulating and limiting factor provides a negative feedback control in the way that an increasing population of 'antitemplates' checks a corresponding proportion of 'templates', so leading to a decline of growth rate.

5) Attainment of a terminal size is an expression of the steady state

between incremental and decremental growth components and between self-reproducing, intracellular 'templates' and inhibiting, freely diffusable 'antitemplates'.

6) Both 'generative' and 'differentiated' mass (including 'antitemplates') undergo continual metabolic degradation and replacement by catabolic loss of generative mass is in the first approximation negligible in comparison with other growth-inhibiting components.

Weiss (1952) supports this idea by an in vitro experiment in which embryonic chick heart and kidney were cultured in extracts of whole chick embryo or of whole embryos minus the homologous organ, and the results were obvious. Kidney growth was more active when the kidney component was missing from the embryo extract.

Murgita and Tomasi Jr. (1975a, b) have demonstrated the existence of non-dialyzable, non-cytotoxic immunosuppressive α fetoprotein (AFP) in mouse amniotic fluid (MAF). It inhibited both primary and secondary antibody production and also inhibited the stimulation of lymphocytes in vitro by either mitogen or antigen. They also reported that MAF was composed of approximately 14% transferrin, 36% albumin, and 50% AFP. In these studies, transferrin acted as a lymphocyte stimulator, whereas AFP acted as an inhibitor. These workers speculate that AFP could be the factor responsible for depressing the maternal immune response during pregnancy which, in turn, could contribute to the delayed rejection of the developing histoincompatible fetus.

6.6 Chalones as the preexisting endogenous specific inhibitor of growth

From studies of the changes in the cell metabolism during experimental skin carcinogenesis of epidermal cells, Iversen (1960) proposed a theory for epidermal growth regulation which he discussed at the First International Congress of Cybernetic Medicine in Naples in October 1960. He proposed that the differentiating cells produced an inhibitor which acted on the basal epidermal cells to prevent them from multiplying too rapidly.

In the same year, Bullough and Laurence (1960) demonstrated a high mitotic activity of mouse ear epidermis after wounding. If a piece of skin was actually removed, the highest mitotic activity was found on the unwounded portion opposite the damage. Injury to the dermis produced no effect on the epidermis. Furthermore, the zone of activity was restricted to an area 1 mm away from the wound edge, regardless of wound size. Maximum

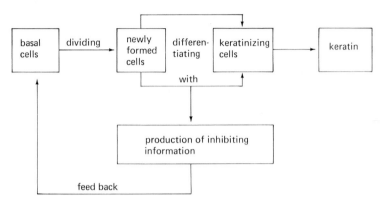

Fig. 6.1. Schematic representation of Iversen's model of epidermal growth control by negative feedback (from Iversen, 1969).

mitotic activity occurred after 36–42 h. Three possible explanations suggested themselves: (i) a 'wound hormone' released by damaged tissue stimulated mitosis; (ii) increased blood supply encouraged mitosis; or (iii) the wound resulted in a loss of inhibitory substance which was normally present. The first idea was unlikely because the maximum growth was nowhere near the damaged tissue. Rather, it was in the center on the opposite side, and the zone of mitotic activity remained the same width, regardless of wound size. The second was disproved by doing an experiment in tissue culture where all of the samples had equal access to nutrients and oxygen and still the maximum growth was nowhere near the damaged tissue. There remained the third explanation, namely a loss of a preexisting mitotic inhibitor.

The word hormone was first used by Starling in 1906 in reference to the substance secretin discovered by Bayliss and Starling in 1902. Starling Later (1914) defined a hormone as 'any substance normally produced in the cells of some part of the body and carried by the blood stream to distant parts which it affects for the good of the body as a whole'.

Huxley (1935) indicated that Schafer introduced the word autocoid to denote substances of this sort which were produced in specific tissues and wished to use the word hormone to include other substances (parahormones) with non-specific sites and effects. This terminology, however, has not passed into general use. 'Schafer's subdivision of his class of autocoids into "harmazones" and "chalones" according to whether their action is stimulative or inhibitory, has also not met with favour, chiefly because it is unworkable in practice' (see Huxley, 1935). The word chalone refers to the slacking off of the main-sheet on a sailing vessel, thereby slowing down its rate of speed through the water. Bullough adopted the word chalone in 1962 to denote the type of tissue-specific antimitotic substance he claimed to be endogenous to epidermal cells.

Finegold (1965) extended the ideas of Bullough and Laurence to show that the replacement of the removed tissue with a graft of intact epidermis suppressed the proliferation opposite the wound, thereby providing further supporting evidence for the existence of epidermal chalone. It was soon noticed that hormones had a marked influence on the activity of the epidermal inhibitory substance which had been crudely prepared from an aqueous extraction of epidermal homogenates. Many experiments, too numerous to be mentioned singly, were done to determine what effects were due to the time of day of the experiment, the state of excitement of the subjects, the endogenous hormone level, and the interaction of various hormones. The most important fact arising from all of these studies was the necessity for adrenalin, either endogenous or supplied in the medium, for chalone activity (Bullough and Laurence, 1962). If the endogenous adrenalin was allowed to exhaust itself, no further addition of chalone would have any inhibitory effect until more catecholamines were supplied. However, lymphocyte chalone activity is independent of both hydrocortisone phosphate and adrenalin (Houck et al., 1971; Attallah et al., 1975).

In the course of all these experiments, the concept of the chalone as a tissue-specific, but not species-specific, endogenous mitotic inhibitor emerged (Bullough, 1965). Chalone from the epidermis of mouse, pig, or dogfish would affect the skin from any of these species regardless of origin, whereas liver tissue or some other organ extract had no effect upon epidermal mitoses. Further, the epidermal 'chalone' did not affect mitoses in any other tissues (see Bullough, 1965).

Attempts to purify the inhibitor substances met with little success. The simplest method was merely to grind frozen cells, extract with water and NaCl, centrifuge at 25,000 g for 15 min, and use this crude material as the 'chalone' on the assumption that any material in this extract would have no significant effect upon the assay system.

In 1967, Bullough and coworkers said that epidermal chalone was a non-dialyzable glycoprotein of mol.wt. 25,000 and unstable unless lyophilized. The most thorough report of purification was that of Hondius Boldingh and Laurence (1968). These investigators performed almost every possible identification procedure on water extracts of pig skin which had been further purified by ethanol extraction. The chalone was found to be stable at pH 3.0 and 6.0 but unstable at pH 9.0. The isoelectric point was 5.2–6.0.

In the last decade there has been active research into the extraction and

Table 6.1

Negative feedback inhibitors (chalones).

	*Cell cycle stage at which inhibition has been shown	Active material mol. wt. (daltons)	Source appropriate tissues from several species	Assay system in vitro	in vivo	Cell specificity	Species specificity
Colon	G_1	30,000–50,000	T	T	NT	yes	none
Epidermis	G_1	ca. 100,000	T	T	T	yes	none
Erythrocyte	G_1	2,000–4,000	T	T	NT	yes	none
Fibroblast	G_1	30,000–50,000	T	T	NT	yes	NT
Granulocyte	G_1	4,000	T	T	T	yes	none
Kidney	G_2	NT	T	T	T	yes	none
Lens	G_2	20,000–30,000	T	T	NT	NT	NT
Liver	G_1	1,000	T	T	T	yes	none
Lymphocyte	G_1	30,000–50,000	T	T	T	yes	none

*Cell cycle events: G_1 = Gap_1 (diploid DNA content); S = period of DNA synthesis; G_2 = Gap_2 (tetraploid DNA content); M = mitosis
T = tested; NT = not tested.

purification of chalone from different tissues (see table 6.1) which led to the First International Chalone Conference (see NCI Monograph #38, 1973) and this volume.

Elgjo et al. (1971, 1972) and Elgjo (1973) introduced the idea that there might be two epidermal chalones acting at different stages of the cell cycle. They separated cells from the basal layer and cells from the differentiating layers. Extracts of each cell type were prepared in order to determine their chalone activity. Basal cells were found to contain primarily G_2 chalone activity by counting mitotic figures, while the differentiating cells contained mostly a chalone active in the G_1 by measuring labeled thymidine uptake phase of the cell cycle. Marks (1971) called Bullough's original adrenalin-requiring chalone the M factor and claimed that it was a glycoprotein of mol.wt. 30,000–40,000 which was destroyed by heat and trypsin. The other factor he called an S factor, which was larger and had more carbohydrate residues. This factor inhibited the transition to S phase. With an estimated 50,000-fold purification, it was still heterogeneous. In contrast to M factor, the activity of the S factor was not affected by boiling at neutral pH or by exhaustive digestion with trypsin or pronase, and it was tissue-specific. Marks (1973) suggested that the G_1-inhibitor was a glycoprotein with an apparent mol.wt. of 100,000–300,000 daltons and consisting of a large protein 'coat' which could be removed by proteolytic digestion, and a small active 'core', probably a glycopeptide, with a mol.wt. of 10,000–20,000 daltons.

Houck and Hennings (1973) suggested that factors acting in G_1 should properly be designated 'chalones' for clarity in the literature and chalones should be referred to as 'G_1 chalone', 'G_2 chalone', 'maturation chalone', etc., depending on the assay used for estimating chalone activity, whether by measuring the inhibition of the incorporation of labeled thymidine or by estimating the mitotic index. Further, there seems to exist two lymphocyte chalones, one specific for T lymphocytes and one for B lymphocytes (Florentin et al., 1973; Attallah et al., 1975; Attallah and Houck in this book).

6.7 Chalones and tumors

6.7.1 Ascites tumors

Burns (1968) has produced recurrent growth of Ehrlich ascites tumor (EAT) cells previously not engaged in DNA synthesis by removal of a small portion of the cells from the tumor when it was at maximal size. Burns also demonstrated that EAT cell growth seemed to be limited by the attainment of a

Table 6.2

Chalones and cancer.

Chalone source	Cell cycle stage at which inhibition has been shown	Liability to treatment by proteases	Mol. wt. (daltons)	Assay system		Tumor inhibition
				in vitro	in vivo	
Ascites	G_1	yes	10,000–50,000	NT	T	JB-1 ascites tumor (mice)
	G_2	yes	1,000–10,000	NT	T	JB-1 ascites tumor (mice)
Colon	G_1	yes	30,000–50,000	T	NT	SW-48 colon carcinoma cells
Epidermis	G_1	no	100,000	T	T	Hamster carcinoma
	G_2	yes	30,000–40,000	T	T	Mitotic depressions of V × 2 epidermal tumor
Fibroblast	G_1	yes	30,000–50,000	T	NT	Human osteosarcoma
Granulocyte	G_1	yes	4,000	T	T	Chloroleukemia (rat) chronic myeloid leukemia (man)
Melanocyte	G_1	yes	2,000	T	T	Melanoma
Lymphocyte	G_1	yes	30,000–50,000	T	T	Leukemia cell in mouse and man

G_1 = Gap before DNA synthesis; G_2 = gap before mitosis; T = tested; NT = not tested.

critical number or mass of viable tumor cells but not by the metabolic inability of the host to support tumor growth. Brown (1970) and later Bichel (1972) showed that after simultaneously inoculating two quite different ascites tumors intraperitoneally into the same mouse, the tumor cells reached twice the number as that found following the inoculation of one tumor. This phenomenon could result from two cell-specific and endogenous negative feedback inhibitors: each tumor inhibiting its own growth but having little effect on the other (Bichel, 1973a). The presence of two inhibitors in cell-free ascites fluid has been demonstrated (Bichel, 1973b). One inhibitor was found for the G_1 phase of the cell cycle with a mol.wt. between 10,000 and 50,000 daltons and the other for the G_2 phase with a mol.wt. between 1,000 and 10,000 daltons (table 6.2).

6.7.2 *Epidermal chalone*

Bullough and Laurence (1968a) extracted the rabbit V × 2 epidermal tumor (a poorly differentiated, fast-growing, metastatic squamous cell carcinoma) derived from the Shope papilloma and were able to demonstrate epidermal chalone activity in these extracts (see table 6.2 for biological characteristics), using mouse cell cultures.

This tumor also responded to the addition of pig skin-derived epidermal chalone extracts with a decreased mitotic index in vivo. Further, the presence of a large V × 2 tumor was found to depress the epidermal mitotic rate in the host animal. This suggested that epidermal chalone activity was systemically released into the circulation by the tumor.

The Hewitt epidermal keratinizing squamous carcinoma is fast-growing in WHT/Ht albino mice and typically shows central keratinizing and peripheral mitosis. Its cells apparently synthesize a tissue-specific epidermal chalone that is released into the blood (Bullough and Deol, 1971). Mice carrying this carcinoma have epidermal mitotic rates which are depressed by about 50%, although the mitotic rates of their sebaceous glands are unaffected. Thus, the fall in mitotic rate apparently was epidermal-specific and not due to a general metabolic deterioration or to stress.

The Hewitt epidermal carcinoma was also found to contain appreciable quantities of the tissue-specific epidermal chalone which was active in the first 4 h but not in the second 4 h of incubation in vitro, unless the epidermis was washed in a dilute adrenalin solution (Bullough and Deol, 1971). There was no significant mitotic depression in the tumor cell with bigger levels of chalone concentrate, and thus, this effect presumably was due either to some intrinsic inadequacy in the chalone control mechanism of the tumor

A. M. Attallah

Table 6.3

The presence of epidermal chalone in both normal and epidermal carcinoma cells and its effect on these tissues in vitro and in vivo.

Epidermal chalone source	Bullough and Laurence, 1968a				Elgjo and Hennings, 1971; Laurence and Elgjo, 1971			
	Inhibition of in vitro growth		Inhibition of in vivo growth (rabbit)		Inhibition of in vitro growth		Inhibition of in vivo growth (hamster)	
	Epidermal carcinoma cells	Normal epidermis	Epidermal carcinoma	Normal epidermis	Squamous carcinoma	Normal epidermis	Squamous carcinoma	Normal epidermis
Normal skin	+	+	+	+	−	+	+	+
Epidermal carcinoma	NT	+	NT	+	NT	+	NT	+

+ = Inhibition; − = no inhibition; NT = not tested.

cell or to preexisting abnormally low chalone concentration within the tumor cells.

Elgjo and Hennings (1971) chose a transplantable keratinizing hamster epithelioma to see if the rates of mitosis and DNA synthesis of this tumor were influenced by the addition of exogenous epidermal chalone. After injection of epidermal chalone, DNA synthesis and the mitotic rate of the tumor in the epithelium, ear epidermis, and the cheek pouch were depressed. The cells were sensitive to the chalone action in both G_1 and G_2 phase but not in S phase. However, in the groups of hamsters treated with repeated injections of chalone, there was no decrease in tumor size or change in histology after treatment.

In an in vitro study of the same tumor, Laurence and Elgjo (1971) found that the tumor tissue contained a mitotic inhibitor biologically identical to epidermal chalone. However, epidermal chalone had no effect on the mitotic rate of the tumor cells in vitro. Their explanation for these results was that there may be a difference in the dose of colcemid needed for different tissues to arrest cells in metaphase to study the mitotic rate of these cells. The results of both groups of investigators are summarized in table 6.3.

6.7.3 Melanocyte chalone

Since skin contains a large population of melanocytes, extracts of skin presumably contain melanocyte chalone (Bullough and Laurence, 1968b; Mohr et al., 1968). This has been studied with Harding-Passey melanomata transplanted into mice and hamsters. Bullough and Laurence (1968b) injected mice subcutaneously with partially purified extracts of pig skin and found that 4 h later the mitotic activity of the outermost growing zone of the melanomata decreased by about 50%. They also cut pieces from the outermost mitotically active zone of hamster tumor and incubated them in vitro with chalone extract and found that melanocyte chalone activity required adrenalin and hydrocortisone. Mohr et al. (1968) found that after daily injections of melanocyte chalone into tumor-bearing animals for 5 days, the tumors became soft and necrotic, the amelanotic melanomata darkened, regressed, then ulcerated, and finally healed. In contrast, highly purified skin extracts which were very active against epidermal mitosis, showed no inhibition of melanomata either in vivo or in vitro (Bullough and Laurence, 1968b; Mohr et al., 1968).

Recent studies (Dewey 1973; Seji et al., 1974), using melanoma cells in vitro, show a reduction in cell numbers directly related to the concentration of melanocyte chalone added to the cultures. This chalone is heat-labile, consists of protein and RNA, has a mol.wt. less than 5000 daltons, and its growth-inhibiting action is cell-specific but not species-specific. Its biological activity seems to depend on both protein and RNA moieties (Seiji et al., 1974). Biological characteristics of melanocyte chalone are shown in tables 6.1 and 6.2.

6.7.4 Granulocyte chalone

Chloroleukemia cells are a malignant derivative of the granulocytic cell system which, when transplanted subcutaneously, cause a local tumor that has a relatively slow growth rate; when injected intraperitoneally, they cause a typical generalized leukemia.

Studies were performed, using chloroleukemic rats, in which regression of local tumors and survival were used as criteria for chalone activity subsequent to the intraperitoneal injection of chalone extract (Rytömaa and Kiviniemi, 1970; Rytömaa, 1973).

Granulocyte chalone has been found in normal and leukemic blood of several species, including man and rat (Rytömaa and Kiviniemi, 1968a, b, 1970; Rytömaa, 1973). The amount of chalone in tumor cells, however, is only 1/40 to 1/10 that found in normal cells, while the amount in the serum of leukemic animals is in great excess of that found in normal serum (Rytömaa and Kiviniemi, 1968a, b). Thus, tumor cells may be producing a normal amount of chalone which is escaping into the serum (table 6.4).

While both normal and tumor cells respond to the addition of granulocyte chalone to the culture medium, normal cells are significantly more sensitive to the chalone (Rytömaa and Kiviniemi, 1968b). Thus, there may be at least two reasons for the rapid proliferation of tumor cells: (i) escape of chalone from the cell, and (ii) decreased sensitivity of the cells to the chalone (Rytömaa and Kiviniemi, 1968b).

Table 6.4

Characteristics of granulocyte chalone and its presence in both normal and granulocytic leukemia cells.

	Granulocytic leukemia	Normal granulocyte
Amount of chalone in the cell	small	large
Amount of chalone in the serum	large	small
Cell response to granulocyte chalone	weak	strong
Cell-specific, not species-specific	yes	yes

In rats with generalized leukemia, no spontaneous remissions were observed and all control animals died within 24 days of tumor induction; a significant number of the treated animals showed permanent regression of their chloroleukemia (Rytömaa and Kiviniemi, 1970; Rytömaa, 1973).

Several experiments show the effect of long-term chalone treatment of the growth rate of baby rats (Rytömaa and Kiviniemi, 1970). Because the treatment did not retard whole growth, the granulocyte chalone was considered to have had no generalized inhibitory effect upon the proliferation of the cells primarily involved in whole body growth. Also, when a crude preparation effective in vitro was tested on the mitotic activity of epidermal cells in vitro, no effect could be seen (Rytömaa, 1973). Lord et al. (1974) found that extracts of lymph node or red blood cell did not have activity but that granulocytes did when tested against granulocytes.

Finally, recent studies (Benestad et al., 1973) using a diffusion chamber implanted intraperitoneally indicated that only the proliferation of the granulocytic portion of the bone marrow cells was inhibited by the administration of granulocyte chalone concentrates in vivo. These latter studies provide the strongest evidence for the cell specificity of the granulocyte chalone. Therefore, it appears that granulocyte chalone has been shown to be cell-specific.

Paukovits (1973) isolated a highly purified polypeptide granulopoiesis-inhibiting factor (GIF) from medium which had contained bone marrow cells. The action of GIF was strongly cell type-specific and was not species-specific. Paukovits thinks that GIF may be identical with granulocyte chalone (Paukovits, 1973). See table 6.1 for biological characteristics.

Recently Lozio et al. (1973) reported the isolation of a small inhibitory peptide or glycoprotein with mol.wt. less than 10,000 daltons from human and bovine spleen. This spleen inhibitor (SI) has been found to be very cytotoxic to a human chronic myelocytic leukemia (CML) established cell line containing the Philadelphia chromosome as a marker. SI was highly cytotoxic to CML cells after incubation for 24 h; by 48 h all the cells were dead. Marked inhibition of RNA synthesis started to be seen after 15 h incubation, while no change in DNA synthesis was seen before 24 h incubation.

There are differences between the Rytömaa and Kiviniemi and the Paukovits assay procedure and that used by Lozio et al., namely: (a) Rytömaa and Kiviniemi and Paukovits used a short-term tissue culture incubation (about 5 h); (b) Lozio and co-workers used longer periods of incubation (more than 24 h); and (c) only Lozio and co-workers always used an established CML cell line.

It could be that these three groups of investigators are dealing with the same factor; however, the cytotoxicity could be demonstrated only against leukemic cells incubated with the factor for a large portion of the cell cycle. This may explain the in vivo chloroleukemia regression after prolonged treatment of rats carrying this tumor with granulocyte chalone (Rytömaa and Kiviniemi, 1968, 1969, 1970). We have found that lymphocyte chalone was uniquely cytotoxic for lymphocytic leukemia cells in vitro after 24 h incubation (Attallah and Houck, 1974, 1975).

6.7.5 Leukemic specific cytotoxic effect of lymphocyte chalone

The 30,000–50,000-dalton range of extracts of spleen or thymus has been shown to contain a specific inhibitor of the mitotic activity of normal stimulated lymphocytes (Houck et al., 1971; Houck et al., 1973a; Attallah et al., 1975). This specific endogenous mitotic inhibitor, or chalone, was not cytotoxic for normal lymphocytes but appeared to be cytotoxic for leukemic lymphocytes from established cell lines of either mouse or human cells after 24 h incubation in vitro. This lymphotoxic effect could also be demonstrated on fresh primary cultures of leukemic lymphocytes. Lymphocyte chalone was more cytotoxic to L-1210 cultures under crowded conditions (cell in G_0–G_1), in contrast to cytosine arabinoside, which showed more inhibition toward cells in uncrowded cultures (cell in S phase) (table 6.5). This lympho-cytotoxicity of chalone on L-1210 cells was directly correlated with the incubation time and was maximal after almost one complete cycle. The inhibition of DNA synthesis and the cytotoxic effect upon leukemic cells

Table 6.5

Comparison of lymphocyte chalone cytotoxicity by (S phase-specific) chemotherapy drugs upon normal and leukemic cells.

Drug	Leukemic lymphocyte cells		Normal cells
	Uncrowded cells in S phase of growth	Crowded cells mostly in G_0–G_1 phase	
Lymphocyte chalone	+	+++	―――
Cytosine arabinoside	+++	+	+++
Methotrexate	+++	+	+++

S phase = cells in DNA synthesis; G_0–G_1 = cells in dormant state; ――― = no cytotoxic effect; + = very weak cytotoxic effect; +++ = strong cytotoxic effect.

was irreversible, however, while the chalone-produced inhibition of both DNA synthesis and proliferation of normal lymphocytes was reversible. Kinetic studies have shown that protein synthesis was inhibited first, followed by inhibition of RNA and DNA synthesis by these leukemic cells. Finally, thymus chalone did not effect DNA synthesis or alter the viability of lymphoblasts with B cell characteristics; it was cytotoxic toward lymphoblasts with T cell characteristics, however, suggesting the presence of two inhibitors, one specific for B cell lymphocytes and the other for T cell lymphocytes (see Attallah and Houck in this volume for details).

6.7.6 Plasmacytomas

It has been shown that various plasmacytoma cells (PC) significantly depress the primary immune response of their host. The degree of suppression was proportional to the size of the tumor. It has been shown that this immuno-suppression was not due to nutritional competition between tumor and normal cells or to the feedback inhibition by the myeloma protein on antibody-producing cells or by the takeover of the immune system of the host animals by neoplastic plasma cells (Zolla et al., 1974). Normal spleen cells have been enclosed in Millipore chambers and implanted in either normal mice or mice carrying PC, or thymic lymphoma, or melanoma. The ability of these normal spleen cells to mount primary immune response to sheep red blood cells has been investigated. Tanapatchaiyapong and Zolla (1974) have shown that PC release a humoral chalone-like material that inhibited the response of normal spleen cells to produce antibody to sheep red blood cells, and this inhibition was not shown in mice carrying other tumors. This inhibitory factor seems to be specific for B lymphocytes.

6.8 Chalones and antichalones

In rats, the entry of large numbers of mature granulocytes into the blood from the bone marrow is followed by a reduction in the amount of granulo-cyte chalone and the concomitant appearance of a specific stimulator, the granulocyte 'antichalone', in the serum (Rytömaa and Kiviniemi, 1968b). Thus, a balance between chalone (mol.wt. 4000) and antichalone (mol.wt. 35,000) may be required for granulocytopoiesis. Chalone prevents and anti-chalone promotes the entry of granulocytic precursor cells into the DNA synthesis phase of the cell cycle. Under normal conditions, the chalone prevents the excessive proliferation of granulocyte precursors, while under conditions of acute functional demand, 'antichalone', a tissue-specific

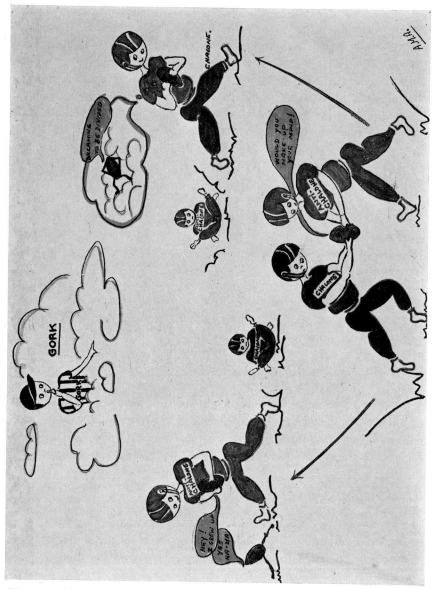

The competitive action of chalone and antichalone. Regulation of cell growth. GORK, God only really knows.

stimulator, replaces chalone in the serum (Rytömaa and Kiviniemi, 1968b).

Colony-stimulating factor (CSF) (antichalone?) is a glycoprotein factor specifically required for granulocyte and macrophage colony growth in vitro. The mol.wt. of mouse lung CSF is 15,000 while the mol.wt. of CSF obtained from human urine is 45,000 (Metcalf, 1974). Metcalf (1971) reported the finding of dialyzable CSF inhibitor (chalone?) from normal and neoplastic hemopoietic cells. Metcalf's group has found an imbalance in the CSF–CSF inhibitor regulatory system of chronic and acute myeloid leukemia. The CSF level in the serum of patients with leukemia was elevated above normal; in contrast, the CSF inhibitor in the serum of these patients was very low (Metcalf, 1974). It will be of great interest to find out the resemblance between CSF–CSF inhibitor and granulocyte chalone–anti-chalone by using the same assay to evaluate the two regulatory systems.

Houck et al. (1972) have shown that extracts of fibroblasts in culture and of a similar mol.wt. portion of their used medium after cultivation in vitro contained a mitotic inhibitor which is not cytotoxic to fibroblasts and which apparently is specific for these cells in vitro. Houck and Cheng (1973) have isolated and purified completely a sialoprotein from mammalian serum which is stringently required for diploid human fibroblasts in vitro prolifera-tion. Houck showed that, during the wound repair in vivo, the normally mitotically arrested fibroblasts begin to proliferate at a considerable rate in that portion of the tissue adjacent to the injury. Thus, it is probable that the fibroblast mitogen derived from the serum flooding into the injured tissue area around the site of the wound would displace chalone from the fibroblast contained within this marginal area and therefore permit the entrance of these cells into the mitotic cycle (Houck et al., 1973; Houck and Attallah, in press; Houck in this volume).

6.9 A hypothetical mechanism for growth control by chalone

6.9.1 Contact inhibition and cell transformation

Normal cell populations appear to be inherently able to regulate their own growth; this ability is manifested in vitro as post-confluence inhibition or contact inhibition of cell division (see Martz and Steinberg, 1971). Some normal cells, when infected by an oncogenic virus, undergo a characteristic change called transformation. A similar 'spontaneous' transformation supposedly occurs in the absence of a virus infection, in cell cultures kept growing in vitro for long periods. However, we have shown (Merril et al. 1972) that tissue culture medium contains serum which is often contaminated with viruses. This observation raises questions concerning the origin of 'spontaneously' transformed cells in vitro.

An understanding of the nature of the changes involved in the transformation can be gained from comparative in vitro studies of normal cells and of cells which have reached an advanced stage of transformation (Sheppard, 1971).

Contact inhibition has two aspects: inhibition of cell division and inhibition of cell locomotion. With loss of the first characteristic, cells continue to divide, even after confluence is achieved, forming multiple cell layers and giving a marked increase in the cell saturation density (the number of cells per unit area). Loss of inhibition of cell movement leads to a loss of orientation of the cells (Todaro and Green, 1966). The loss of these growth restraints represents an early morphologic manifestation of viral transformation; the degree to which each is altered affects the morphology of the transformed colony.

There appears to be a complete failure of mutual growth inhibition between all virus-transformed cells so that they grow to saturation densities 10–25 times greater than do non-transformed cells (Todaro et al., 1967). This lack of contact inhibition between cells of a transformed line may be attributed to either (i) alteration of the cell surface so as to render cell-to-cell contact no longer effective in suppressing macromolecular synthesis, or (ii) destruction of the system in the nucleus that responds to the cell-to-cell interaction. Cells transformed by polyoma virus (PV) (Stoker, 1963), carcinogenic hydrocarbons, or 'spontaneously' (Borek and Sachs, 1966), can be contact-inhibited by normal cells; also lethally X-irradiated cells from PV-transformed cell lines can contact-inhibit unirradiated cells from the same cell line.

6.9.2 'Second messenger' hypothesis

Adenosine 3',5'-cyclic monophosphate (cyclic AMP) has a clearly defined role as a 'second messenger' in the action of many hormones (Robison et al., 1968). Also the intracellular level of cyclic AMP in transformed and rapidly growing normal cells is lower than in slowly dividing or stationary normal cells (Sheppared, 1972). Addition of dibutyryl cyclic AMP to the medium of cultured cells changes their morphology temporarily and restores controlled growth to transformed cells (Inbar and Sachs, 1969). It has been proposed (Hadden et al., 1972; Rudland et al., 1974) that cell growth is regulated by the balance of cyclic AMP and cyclic GMP in the cell, high cyclic AMP:cyclic GMP ratios being associated with the proliferative state. Cyclic GMP could act as a positive signal, while cyclic AMP acts as a negative intracellular signal for controlling the growth of the cell (Hadden et al., 1972; Rudland et al., 1974).

Pharmacological agents which raise the endogenous level of cyclic AMP markedly inhibit the stimulation of lymphocytes (Smith et al., 1971). Insulin causes a decrease in the concentration of intracellular cyclic AMP and inhibits membrane-bound adenylate cyclase (Jimenet et al., 1973). Cyclic AMP inhibits the mitotic activity of mouse epidermis in vitro (Voorhees et al., 1972) and prevents lymphocytes from differentiating into antibody-producing cells when it is present during a critical period of immune induction in vitro (Bosing-Schneider and Kolb, 1973).

Cyclic AMP is capable of significantly inhibiting the uptake of [^{3}H]TdR into DNA from hamster ovary (CHO) fibroblast-like cells (Hauschka et al., 1972) and this cyclic AMP inhibition of thymidine uptake is mediated through the inhibition of nucleoside kinase activity. Iversen (1969) was the first to propose that cyclic AMP may play a role in epidermal differentiation.

6.9.3 Chalone action possibly involving the cyclic AMP system

Although chalones have been found in all tissues in which they have been sought and a number of chalone systems have been identified (Attallah, 1974b), the mechanism of action at the cellular level is not yet understood.

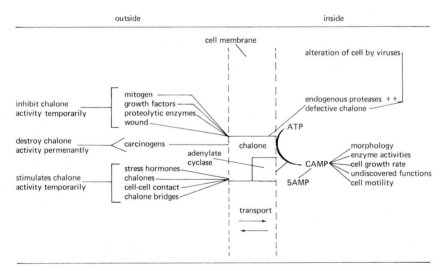

Fig. 6.2. An overview of the hypothesized chalone-cyclic AMP system. An increase of chalone activity would elevate cyclic AMP intracellularly, and lower cyclic AMP would result from a decrease of chalone activity. cAMP, adenosine 3′, 5′-cyclic monophosphate; ATP, adenosine triphosphate; 5AMP, 5′-monophosphate.

However, if we postulate that chalone is a part of the cell membrane which regulates the cyclic AMP system, we can construct a simple model (fig. 6.2) of growth regulation which is consistent with various experimental observations which follow.

6.9.3.1 *Factors which stimulate chalone activity temporarily*

Strains of normal cells attain relatively low population densities and inhibit each other in mixed culture (Eagle and Levine, 1967). This interstrain inhibition is not species-specific. Contact inhibition through temporary chalone bridges between adjacent cell membranes has recently been proposed (Attallah, 1972, 1974; Houck et al., 1973b). Supporting the observation, normal fibroblasts from different species inhibit the growth of transformed cells but only if the cells are in contact (Stoker and Shearer, 1966; Eagle and Levine, 1967). Also, at the time cultures become confluent and rates of cell division decrease, human skin fibroblasts show greater adenyl cyclase activity prior to confluence (Zacchello et al., 1972).

6.9.3.2 *Factors which inhibit chalone activity temporarily*

A transient reduction of the cellular cyclic AMP level occurs after confluent monolayers of normal mouse fibroblast (3T3) cells have been exposed to serum, trypsin, or insulin (Sheppard, 1972). The mitogenic factor from serum which apparently acts as an antichalone has been purified (Houck and Cheng, 1973). It apparently displaces preexisting chalone from the surface of the fibroblast and permits the cell to enter the mitotic phase (Houck et al., 1973b). Proteolytic enzymes very likely could have the same effect either by destroying the existing chalone on the cell membrane or the sites to which it is bound. This would allow the cell to escape from mitotic control until the necessary amount of new chalone is synthesized; then the chalone shared by these cells would again be sufficient to control mitosis. Other compounds acting on the cell surface to stimulate growth include proteases bound to sepharose beads (Burger, 1971) and neuraminidase (Vaheri et al., 1972). Their effects are transitory and generally permit only one round of cell division after the agent is removed. Wound healing in vitro is initiated when a small patch of cells is scraped away from a stationary phase monolayer (Raff and Houck, 1969). This could lower the amount of chalone that regulates the cyclic AMP system, subsequently lowering cyclic AMP in cells which, in turn, start dividing, repair the wound, and accumulate enough chalone to become contact inhibited through chalone bridges (Attallah, 1972, 1974a).

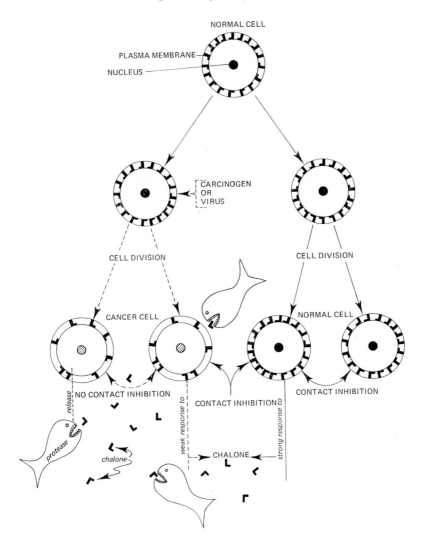

Fig. 6.3. The possible relationships between chalone, normal cells, and cancer cells. One of the manifestations of cell transformation is the alteration of the plasma membrane after treatment with oncogenic viruses or carcinogens. Cancer cells apparently have lower chalone (Bullough and Laurence, 1968; Rytömaa and Kiviniemi, 1968) and adenyl cyclase activity (Peery et al., 1971), but increased proteolytic enzymes (Schnebli, 1972). The cancer cell does not respond as well as normal cells to the mitotic inhibition of chalones (Bullough and Laurence, 1968; Rytömaa and Kiviniemi, 1968). Note: inhibition of growth by contact between normal cell and normal cell, between normal and transformed cells, but not between transformed and transformed cells.

6.9.3.3 Factors which destroy chalone activity permanently
Volm et al. (1969) have shown that the supernatant of rat liver treated with the carcinogen diethylnitrosamine has no inhibitory activity to DNA synthesis of liver explant, in contrast to liver chalone in the supernatant of normal liver. A difference in the chemical nature of the plasma membranes of normal as compared with transformed cells has been found (Hakomori et al., 1968; Wu et al., 1968). This alteration could be the cause of decreased activity of chalone and/or adenylate cyclase. Also, the activity of adenyl cyclase is permanently lower in transformed cells than in untransformed cells (Peery et al., 1971). A decreased response of adenyl cyclase in psoriatic skin to epinephrine and lower amounts of chalone activity in psoriatic skin has been found (Wright et al., 1973).

Several transformed cell lines produce a protease that depends on serum for its activation (Ossowski et al., 1973). Also, an increase in such protease-like activity has been reported in DNA virus-transformed cells (Schnebli, 1972). A number of protease inhibitors selectively inhibited the growth of transformed cells (Schnebli and Burger, 1972).

Cancer cells do not contain as much chalone and will not respond to chalone as effectively as normal cells do (Bullough and Laurence, 1968; Rytömaa and Kiviniemi, 1968). Furthermore, chalones apparently escape from cancer cells into the blood stream of tumor-bearing animals (Bullough and Laurence, 1968; Rytömaa and Kiviniemi, 1968).

The difference between neoplastic and normal cells might be attributed to the large amount of proteolytic enzymes produced by these cancer cells, consequently altering either the chalone or its binding site. Another possibility would be the modification of all or part of the genome to produce a possibly defective chalone (see fig. 6.2).

6.9.4 The putative mechanism of chalone action

A unifying explanation for all of the above results would be that the chalone glycoprotein contains two active sites: one site specific for the cell membrane, and the other site non-specifically stimulating the adenyl cyclase activity on the membrane. As a consequence of the action of this cell-specific stimulator of adenyl cyclase activity, the intracellular concentration of cyclic AMP would be maintained at a relatively high level. The cell would then be unable to enter the mitotic cycle because of a decrease in nucleoside kinase activity and hence a lack of DNA and RNA precursors. Since DNA synthesis requires the continuous recruitment of nucleoside precursors, it is tempting to speculate that chalone shuts off the supply of precursors for macromolecular synthesis at some stage before the incorporation of deoxy-nucleoside triphosphates into DNA, but allows the completion of DNA synthesis from those triphosphates formed prior to chalone addition (Attallah and Houck, in this volume). The possibility that chalone involves the cyclic AMP system clearly deserves further investigation; a necessary proof of this proposed mechanism for chalone activity would be the demonstration of an increased adenyl cyclase activity in broken membrane preparations after the addition of an appropriate chalone.

References

Abercrombie, M. (1957) Localized formation of new tissue in an adult mammal. Symposium Soc. Exp. Biol. 11, 235.

Attallah, A. M. (1972) Mechanism of chalone action involving the cyclic AMP system: a new hypothesis. Unpublished paper presented to the Genetics Committee, George Washington University.

Attallah, A. M. (1974) Partial purification and characterization of lymphocyte chalone. Ph.D. thesis in Genetics, George Washington University.

Attallah, A. M. and Houck, J. C. (1974) Specific cytotoxic effects of lymphocyte chalone upon leukemic lymphocytes in vitro. Ninth Leucocyte Conference (Abstract).

Attallah, A. M. and Houck, J. C. (1975) Lymphocyte chalone concentrates and their effects upon leukemic cells in vitro. Proceedings of International Symposium of Haematology, Milan, Italy, September, 1975. Boll. 1st. Sieroter-Milanese 54, 3.

Attallah, A. M., Sunshine, G., Hunt, C. V. and Houck, J. C. (1975) The specific and endogenous mitotic inhibitor of lymphocytes (chalone). Exp. Cell Res. 93, 283.

Bayliss, W. M. and Starling, E. H. (1902) The mechanism of pancreatic secretion. J. Physiol. 28, 325

Benestad, H , Rytömaa, T. and Kiviniemi, K. (1973) The cell-specific effect of the granulocytic chalone demonstrated with the diffusion chamber technique. Cell Tissue Kinetics 6, 147.

Bichel, P. (1972) Specific growth regulation in three ascitic tumors. Europ. J. Cancer 8, 167.

Bichel, P. (1973a) Self-limitation of ascites tumor growth: a possible chalone regulation. NCI Monogr. 38, 197.

Bichel, P. (1973b) Further studies on the self-limitation of growth of JB-1 ascites tumors. Europ. J. Cancer 9, 133.

Borek, C. and Sachs, L. (1966) The difference in contact inhibition of cell replication between normal cells and cells transformed by different carcinogens. Proc. Natl. Acad. Sci. U.S. 56, 1705.

Bosing-Schneider, R. and Kolb, H. (1973) Influence of cyclic AMP on early events of immune induction. Nature 244, 224.

Brown, H. R. (1970) The growth of Ehrlich carcinoma and Crocker sarcoma ascitic cells in the same host. Anat. Rec. 166, 283.

Bucher, N. L. R., Scott, J. F. and Aub, J. C. (1951) Regeneration of the liver in parabiotic rats. Cancer Res. 11, 457.

Bullough, W. S. (1965) Mitotic and functional homeostasis: a speculative review. Cancer Res. 25, 1683.

Bullough, W. S. and Deol, J. U. (1971) Chalone-induced mitotic inhibition in the Hewitt keratinizing epidermal carcinoma of the mouse. Europ. J. Cancer 7, 425.

Bullough, W. S. and Laurence, E. B. (1960) The control of epidermal mitotic activity in the mouse. Proc. R. Soc. B. 151, 517.

Bullough, W. S. and Laurence, E. B. (1964) Mitotic control by internal secretion: the role of the chalone-adrenalin complex. Exp. Cell Res. 33, 176.

Bullough, W. S. and Laurence, E. B. (1968a) Control of mitosis in rabbit V × 2 epidermal tumors by means of the epidermal chalone. Europ. J. Cancer 4, 587.

Bullough, W. S. and Laurence, E. B. (1968b) Melanocyte chalone and mitotic control in melanomata. Nature 270, 137.

Burch, P. R. J. (1969) An Inquiry Concerning Growth, Disease and Ageing. University of Toronto Press, Buffalo.

Burch, P. R. J. and Burwell, R. G. (1965) Self and not-self. A clonal induction approach to immunology. Quart. Rev. Biol. 40, 252.

Burger, M. M. (1971) Current Topics in Cellular Regulation. Academic Press, New York, Vol. 3, p. 135.

Burns, E. R. (1968) Initiation of DNA synthesis in Ehrlich ascites tumor cells in their plateau phase of growth. Cancer Res. 28, 1191.

Burwell, R. G. (1963) The role of lymphoid tissue in morphostasis. Lancet 2, 69.

Cooperband, S., Bondevik, H., Schmid, K. and Mannick, J. A. (1968) Transformation of human lymphocytes: inhibition by homologous alpha globulin. Science 159, 1243.

Demetriou, A., Seifter, E. and Levenson, S. (1974) Effect of sera obtained from normal and partially hepatectomized rats and patients on the growth of cells in tissue culture. Surgery 76, 779.

Dewey, D. L. (1973) The melanocyte chalone. NCI Monogr. 38, 213.

Eagle, H. and Levine, E. (1967) Growth regulatory effects of cellular interaction. Nature 213, 1102.

Eagle, H., Levine, E. and Koprowski, H. (1968) Species specificity in growth regulatory effects of cellular interaction. Nature 220, 266.

Eigisti, O. and Dustin, P. (1955) Colchicine in Agriculture, Medicine, Biology, and Chemistry. Iowa: Iowa State College Press.

Elgjo, K. (1973) Epidermal chalone: cell cycle specificity of two epidermal growth inhibitors. NCI Monogr. 38, 71.

Elgjo, K. and Hennings, H. (1971) Epidermal chalone and cell proliferation in a transplantable squamous cell carcinoma in hamsters. I. In vivo results. Virchows Arch. Zellpathol. 7, 1.

Elgjo, K., Laerum, O. and Edgehill, W. (1971) Growth regulation in mouse epidermis. I. G_1 inhibitor present in the basal cell layer. Virchows Arch. Zellpathol. 8, 277.

Elgjo, K., Laerum, O. and Edgehill, W. (1972) Growth regulation in mouse epidermis. II. G_1 inhibitor present in the differentiating cell layer. Virchows Arch. Zellpathol. 10, 229.

Finegold, M. M. (1965) Control of cell multiplication in epidermis. Proc. Soc. Exp. Biol. Med. 119, 96.

Florentin, I., Kiger, N. and Mathe, G. (1973) T lymphocyte specificity of a lymphocyte inhibiting factor (chalone) extracted from the thymus. Europ. J. Immunol. 3, 135.

Friedrich-Freksa, H. and Zaki, F. (1954) Spezifische Mitose-Auslösung in normaler Rattenleber durch Serum von partiell hepatektomierten Ratten. Z. Naturforsch. 98, 394.

Glinos, A. D. (1958) The mechanism of liver growth and regeneration, in The Chemical

Basis of Development (eds.: W. D. McElroy and B. Glass). Johns Hopkins Press, Baltimore.

Glinos, A. D. (1960) Environmental feedback control of cell division. Ann. N. Y. Acad. Sci. 90, 592.

Glinos, A. D. and Gey, G. O. (1952) Humoral factors involved in the induction of liver regeneration in the rat. Proc. Soc. Exp. Biol. Med. 80, 421.

Goodman, G. J. (1957) Effects of one tumor upon the growth of another. Proc. Am. Assoc. Cancer Rec. 2, 207.

Hadden, J. W., Hadden, E. M., Haddox, M. K. and Goldberg, N. D. (1972) Guanosine 3'; 5'-cyclic monophosphate: a possible intracellular mediator of mitogenic influences in lymphocytes. Proc. Nat. Acad. Sci. U.S. 69, 3024.

Hakomori, S., Teather, C. and Andrews, H. (1968) Organizational differences of cell surface 'hematoside' in normal and virally transformed cells. Biochem. Biophys. Res. Commun. 33, 563.

Hauschka, P. V., Everhart, L. P. and Rubin, R. W. (1972) Alteration of nucleoside transport of Chinese hamster cells by dibutyryl adenosine 3'; 5'-cyclic monophosphate. Proc. Nat. Acad. Sci. U.S. 69, 3542.

Hondius Boldingh, W. H. and Laurence, E. B. (1968) Extraction, purification, and preliminary characterization of the epidermal chalone: a tissue-specific mitotic inhibitor obtained from vertebrate skin. Europ. J. Biochem. 5, 191.

Houck, J. C. and Attallah, A. M. (1975, in press) Tumor Biology (ed.: F. Becker) Plenum Press, New York, Vol. 3.

Houck, J. C. and Cheng, R. F. (1973) Isolation, purification, and chemical characterization of the serum mitogen for diploid human fibroblasts. J. Cell. Physiol. 81, 257.

Houck, J. C. and Hennings, H. (1973) Chalones: specific endogenous mitotic inhibitors. FEBS Letters 32, 1.

Houck, J. C., Irausquin, H. and Leikin, S. (1971) Lymphocyte DNA synthesis inhibition. Science 173, 1139.

Houck, J. C., Attallah, A. M. and Lilly, J. R. (1973a) Some immunosuppressive properties of lymphocyte chalone. Nature 245, 148.

Houck, J. C., Cheng, R. F. and Sharma, V. K. (1973b) Control of fibroblast proliferation. NCI Monogr. 38, 161.

Huxley, J. (1935) Chemical regulation and the hormone concept. Biol. Rev. 10, 427.

Inbar, M. and Sachs, L. (1969) Structural differences in sites on the surface membrane of normal and transformed cells. Nature 223, 710.

Iversen, O. H. (1960) A homeostatic mechanism regulating the cell number in epidermis. Its relation to experimental skin carcinogenesis. Proc. First Int. Congr. Med., Naples. 420.

Iversen, O. H. (1969) Homeostatic Regulators (eds.: E. Wolstenholme and J. Knight). J. and A. Churchill, Ltd., London, pp. 29–56.

Jimenez, L., Surian, E., Flawia, M. and Torres, H. (1973) Effect of insulin on the growth pattern and adenylate cyclase activity of BHK fibroblasts. Proc. Natl. Acad. Sci. U.S. 70, 1388.

Kamrin, B. B. (1960) Studies on the healing of successful skin homeografts in albino rats. Ann. N. Y. Acad. Sci. 87, 323.

Laird, A. K. (1964) Dynamics of tumor growth. Brit. J. Cancer 18, 490.

Laurence, E. B. and Elgjo, K. (1971) Epidermal chalone and cell proliferation in a transplantable squamous cell carcinoma in hamsters. II. In vitro results. Virchows Arch Zellpathol. 7, 8.

Lord, B., Cercek, L., Cercek, B., Shah, G., Dexter, T. and Lajtha, L. (1974) Inhibitors of hemopoietic cell proliferation?: specificity of action within the hemopoietic system. Brit. J. Cancer 29, 168.

Lozzio, B. B., Lozzio, C. B. and Banberger, E. G. (1973) Human spleen inhibitor of leukemic cell growth. Experientia 15, 87.

Marks, F. (1971) Direct evidence of two tissue-specific chalone-like factors regulating mitosis and DNA synthesis in mouse epidermis. Hoppe-Seylers Z. Physiol. Chem. Bd. 552, 1273.

Marks, F. (1973) A tissue-specific factor inhibiting DNA synthesis in mouse epidermis. NCI Monogr. 38, 79.

Martz, E. and Steinberg, M. S. (1971) The role of cell-cell contact inhibition of cell division: a review and new evidence. J. Cell. Physiol. 79, 189.

Merril, C., Friedman, T., Attallah, A., Geier, M., Krell, K. and Yarkin, R. (1972) Isolation of bacteriophage from commercial sera. In Vitro 8, 91.

Metcalf, D. (1971) Inhibition of bone marrow colony formation in vitro by dialyzable products of normal and neoplastic hemopoietic cells. Aust. J. Exp. Biol. Med. Sci. 49, 351.

Metcalf, D. (1974) Regulation by colony-stimulating factor of granulocyte and macrophage colony formation in vitro by normal and leukemic cells, In: Control of Proliferation in Animal Cells (eds.: B. Clarkson and R. Baserga). Cold Spring Harbor Laboratory, New York, pp. 887–907.

Mohr, U., Althoff, J., Kinzel, V., Suss, R. and Volm, M. (1968) Melanoma regression induced by chalone: a new tumor-inhibiting principle acting in vivo. Nature 220, 138.

Mowbay, J. F. (1963) Ability of large doses of an alpha-2 plasma protein fraction to inhibit antibody production. Immunology 6, 217.

Murgita, R. A. and Tomasi Jr., T. B. (1975a) Suppression of the immune response by alpha-fetoprotein. I. The effect of mouse alpha-fetoprotein on the primary and secondary antibody response. J. Exp. Med. 141, 269.

Murgita, R. A. and Tomasi Jr., T. B. (1975b) Suppression of the immune response by alpha-fetoprotein. II. The effect of mouse alpha-fetoprotein on mixed lymphocyte reactivity and mitogen-induced lymphocyte transformation. J. Exp. Med. 141, 440.

Murphy, J. B. and Sturm, E. (1931) Further observations on an inhibitor principle associated with the causative agent of a chicken tumor. Science 74, 180.

Murphy, J. B. and Sturm, E. (1934) The effect of a growth-retarding factor from normal tissues on spontaneous cancer of mice. J. Exp. Med. 60, 305.

Ossowski, L., Unkeless, J., Tobia, A., Quigley, J., Rifkin, D. and Reich, E. (1973) An enzymatic function associated with transformation of fibroblasts by oncogenic viruses. J. Exp. Med. 137, 112.

Paukovits, W. R. (1973) Granulopoiesis-inhibiting factor: demonstration and preliminary chemical and biological characterization of a specific polypeptide (chalone). NCI Monogr. 38, 147.

Peery, C. V., Johnson, G. S. and Pastan, I. (1971) Adenyl cyclase in normal and transformed fibroblasts in tissue culture. J. Biol. Chem. 246, 5785.

Raff, E. C. and Houck, J. C. (1969) Migration and proliferation of diploid human fibroblasts following 'wounding' of confluent monolayers. J. Cell. Physiol. 74, 235.

Robison, G. A., Butcher, R. W. and Sutherland, E. W. (1968) Cyclic AMP. Ann. Rev. Biochem. 37, 147.

Rose, S. M. (1952) A hierarchy of self-limiting reactions as the basis of cellular differentiation and growth control. Am. Naturalist 86, 337.

Rudland, P. S., Seeley, M. and Seifert, W. (1974) Cyclic GMP and cyclic AMP levels in normal and transformed fibroblasts. Nature 251, 417.

Rytömaa, T. (1973) Chalone of the granulocyte system. NCI Monogr. 38, 143.

Rytömaa, T. and Kiviniemi, K. (1968a) Control of DNA duplication in rat chloroleukemia by means of the granulocytic chalone. Europ. J. Cancer 4, 595.

Rytömaa, T. and Kiviniemi, K. (1968b) Control of granulocyte production. I. Chalone and antichalone, two specific regulators. Cell Tissue Kinetics 1, 329.

Rytömaa, T. and Kiviniemi, K. (1970) Regression of generalized leukemia in rat induced by the granulocytic chalone. Europ. J. Cancer 6, 401.

Saetren, H. (1956) A principle of autoregulation of growth. Production of organ-specific mitotic inhibitors in kidney and liver. Exp. Cell Res. 11, 229.

Schnebli, H. P. (1972) A protease-like activity associated with malignant cells. Schweiz Med. Wschr. 102, 1194.

Schnebli, H. P. and Burger, M. (1972) Selective inhibition of growth of transformed cells by protease inhibitors. Proc. Natl. Acad. Sci. U.S. 69, 3825.

Seiji, M., Nakano, H., Akiba, H. and Kato, T. (1974) Inhibition of DNA and protein synthesis in melanocytes by a melanoma extract. J. Invest. Dermatol. 62, 11.

Shaver, J. (1954) Inhibition of nervous system development in the frog produced by tissue fractions of adult homologous organ. Anat. Rec. 118, 646.

Sheppard, J. R. (1971) Restoration of contact-inhibited growth to transformed cells by dibutyryl adenosine 3′, 5′-cyclic monophosphate. Proc. Natl. Acad. Sci. U.S. 68, 1316.

Sheppard, J. R. (1972) Difference in the cyclic adenosine 3′, 5′-monophosphate levels in normal and transformed cells. Nature New Biol. 236, 14.

Simms, H. S. and Stillman, N. P. (1936) Substances affecting adult tissue in vitro. II. A growth inhibitor on adult tissue. J. Gen. Physiol. 20, 621.

Smith, J. W., Steiner, A. L. and Parker, C. W. (1971) Human lymphocyte metabolism. Effects of cyclic and non-cyclic nucleotides on stimulation by phytohemagglutinin. J. Clin. Invest. 50, 442.

Starling, E. H. (1906) Die chemische Koordination der Körpertätigkeiten. Verh. Ges. Naturforsch. Arzte (Stuttgart), Pt. 1, 246.

Starling, E. H. (1914) Discussion on the therapeutic value of hormones. Proc. Royal Soc. Med. (London), vii, Therap. and Pharmacol. Sect., 29–31.

Stich, H. F. J. and Florian, M. L. (1958) The presence of a mitosis inhibitor in the serum and liver of adult rats. Canad. J. Biochem. 36, 855.

Stoker, M. (1964) Regulation of growth and orientation in hamster cells transformed by polyoma virus. Virology 24, 164.

Stoker, M. and Shearer, O. C. (1966) Growth inhibition of polyoma-transformed cells by contact with static normal fibroblasts. J. Cell Science 1, 297.

Swann, M. M. (1958) The control of cell division: a review. II. Special mechanisms. Cancer Res. 18, 1118.

Tanapatchaiyapong, P. and Zolla, S. (1974) Humoral immunosuppressive substance in mice bearing plasmacytomas. Science 186, 748.

Tanner, J. M. (1963) Regulation of growth in size in mammals. Nature 199, 845.

Todaro, G. J. and Green, H. (1966) Cell growth and the initiation of transformation by SV$_{40}$. Proc. Natl. Acad. Sci. U.S. 55, 302.

Todaro, G. J., Matsuya, Y., Bloom, S., Robbins, A. and Green, H. (1967) Stimulation of RNA synthesis and cell division in resting cells by a factor present in serum. In: Growth Regulating Substances for Animal Cells in Culture (eds.: V. Defendi and M. Stoker). Wistar Institute Press, Philadelphia, Wistar Inst. Symposium, Monogr. 7, 87–98.

Vaheri, A., Ruoslahti, E. and Nordling, S. (1972) Neurominidase stimulates division and sugar uptake in density-inhibited cell cultures. Nature New Biol. 238, 211.

Volm, M., Kinzel, V., Mohr, U. and Suss, R. (1969) Inactivation of tissue-specific inhibitors by a carcinogen (Diethylnitrosamine). Specialia 16, 68.

Voorhees, J. J., Duell, E. A. and Kelsey, W. H. (1972) Dibutyryl cyclic AMP inhibition of epidermal cell division. Arch. Dermatol. 105, 384.

Weiss, P. (1952) Self-regulation of organ growth by its own products. Science 115, 487.

Weiss, P. and Kavanau, J. L. (1957) A model of growth and growth control in mathematical terms. J. Gen. Physiol. 41, 1.

Wenneker, A. and Sussmann, N. (1951) Regeneration of liver tissue following partial hepatectomy in parabiotic rats. Proc. Soc. Exp. Biol. Med. 76, 683.

Wright, R. K., Mandy, S. H., Haprin, K. M. and Hsia, S. L. (1973) Defects and deficiency of adenyl cyclase in psoriatic skin. Arch. Dermatol. 107, 47.

Wu, H., Meezan, E., Black, P. and Robbins, P. (1969) Comparative studies on the carbohydrate-containing membrane components of normal and transformed fibroblasts. I. Glucosamine-labeling patterns in 3T3, spontaneously transformed 3T3, and SV$_{40}$-transformed 3T3 cells. Biochem. 8, 2509.

Zacchello, F., Benson, P. F. and Giannelli, F. et al. (1972) Induction of adenylate cyclase activity in cultured human fibroblasts during increasing cell population density. Biochem. J. 126, 27.

Zolla, S., Naor, D. and Tanapatchaiyapong, P. (1974) Cellular basis of immunodepression in mice with plasmacytomas. J. Immunol. 112, 2068.

CHAPTER 7

The epidermal chalones

FRIEDRICH MARKS

Deutsches Krebsforschungszentrum (German Cancer Research Center), Institute of Biochemistry, D-6900 Heidelberg, Federal Republic of Germany

7.1 Introduction

The main function of epidermis is to protect the body from harmful external influences and from water loss. This is accomplished in two ways:

1) by the biosynthesis of keratin, which is one of the most resistant biological materials known, and

2) by the ability to repair physical and chemical damage by means of cell migration and cell proliferation which frequently goes along with transient dedifferentiation and reversible development of hyperplasia.

The biosynthesis of keratin is a suicide maturation pathway in that the epidermal cells acquire their optimal and final stage of functionalization only as dead horny scales. The latter are continuously being shed from the skin surface. To compensate for this permanent cell loss, a permanent production of new cells is required which is restricted to the undermost cell layer (basal layer, stratum germinativum). Usually the mitosis is horizontally orientated (Bullough, 1964; Iversen et al., 1968); both daughter cells remain in the basal layer and an adjacent cell is pushed out. This cell matures (keratinizes) and finally dies when moving upwards to the skin surface. Since basal cells – at least in mouse epidermis – are already engaged in a slow production of keratin precursors (Christophers, 1971), it is assumed that the extruded cell is a cell which is at the given moment most advanced in keratinization and has, therefore, the weakest grip on the underlying connective tissue (Bullough, 1964, 1973; Iversen et al., 1968).

Mammalian epidermis is not only built up by horizontally orientated strata but is also vertically organized by stacking of the flattened keratinized cells to form columns of polygonal cross-section (Mackenzie, 1969; Christophers, 1971; Karatschai et al., 1971). Beneath each column several (8–10 in mice) basal and suprabasal cells are aligned forming a helical pattern. Since each column is produced by its underlying basal cells, the whole structure has been called an epidermal proliferative unit (EPU) (Potten, 1974). Obviously mitotic activity seems to occur more frequently in those cells lying beneath the periphery of the column, whereas the central basal cells are proliferating more slowly (Mackenzie, 1972; Potten, 1974).

In order to maintain tissue homeostasis, or the constancy of tissue mass and function, the rate of cell loss and the rate of cell gain and cell maturation have necessarily to be interconnected within a regulatory circuit. This feedback requires the exchange of information between differentiated cells and proliferative cells. As far as we know, any intercellular transport of information is brought about by chemical messengers. Since in cybernetic systems of this kind stability is guaranteed only by negative feedback, it is reasonable to assume that these messengers are inhibitory molecules, which are produced either by the proliferating cells to inhibit cell maturation or by the differentiating cells to control cell proliferation and the onset of maturation. In the case of epidermis the second possibility is backed by considerably more evidence than the first one.

It seems to be almost unnecessary to emphasize that mechanisms controlling tissue homeostasis must have the ability of rapid adaption since otherwise repair and regeneration processes would not work in the proper manner.

7.2 Evidences for feedback regulation of epidermal cell proliferation

Feedback control of epidermal cell proliferation is suggested by simple evidence. For example, under stress conditions the tissue never disappears although the mitotic activity is considerably depressed. Vice versa, psoriatic epidermis showing an abnormally high proliferative activity does not become thicker and thicker but reaches a homeostatic equilibrium.

If keratinized or keratinizing cells are removed, for example by means of stripping with adhesive tape (Pinkus, 1952) or by friction, the underlying basal cells respond by a burst of mitotic activity so that the cell loss is rapidly and locally compensated. As in the case of a deeper wound, the enhanced cell proliferation is – apart from a period of overshooting – automatically reduced to its normal value when the repair has been finished.

From this it is obvious that experiments on wound healing and tissue repair can provide insight into the regulatory mechanisms governing epidermal cell proliferation, although the repair of skin lesions is a highly complex process including primarily epithelial cell migration as well as division of epidermal cells and a response of the underlying connective tissue. By focussing their interest on the proliferative response, Bullough and Laurence (1960a) in London came to most important and conclusive results. Since their investigations must be considered to be true pioneer work, they will be described here in more detail.

In order to provoke the repair process, a cut 1 cm long was made in the dorsal skin of mice which extended down through the panniculus carnosus. This resulted in a stimulation of mitotic activity which reached a peak after 36–48 h. This enhanced proliferative response was almost completely restricted to a zone with a width of 1 mm from the cut edge. Within this zone a gradient of mitotic activity with the highest activity proximal to the wound edge could be observed.

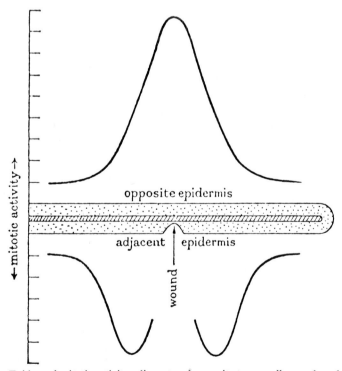

Fig. 7.1. Epidermal mitotic activity adjacent and opposite to a small wound made on one side of a mouse ear 2 days previously. From Bullough and Laurence (1960a). (With permission of the authors and of the Royal Society, London.)

In a second series of experiments the authors investigated the influence
of a small cut made through the epidermis on one side of a mouse ear on
the mitotic activity of the epidermis on the opposite side of the ear. A mouse
ear is only about 0.15 mm thick and its two epidermal layers are separated
by a very thin layer of connective tissue. It could be expected, therefore,
that the zone of high mitotic activity adjacent to the wound would extent
to the uninjured opposite side of the ear. Indeed, it was observed that the
opposite undamaged epidermis showed a mitotic response which was as
powerful as that adjacent to the wound (fig. 7.1). With proper control
experiments, this effect was shown not to be due to the greatly enriched blood
supply around the damaged area. The authors were thus left with the conclusion that the enhanced mitotic activity in the vicinity of the wound as
well as on the opposite side of the ear was the consequence of either the
production of a mitogenic agent (wound hormone, see Abercrombie, 1957;
Teir et al., 1967) or the loss of an endogeneous inhibitor which is synthesized
within the skin.

By means of an ingenious technique Bullough and Laurence (1960a) made
a wound in the subcutaneous tissue including hairroots without damaging
the overlying epidermis (fig. 7.2). Under these conditions no significant
mitotic response of the epidermis was observed (though the wounded area
developed a rich blood supply and suffered a heavy invasion of leucocytes).
The whole effect turned thus out to be obviously tissue-specific (see also
Bullough and Laurence, 1960b). If the wound was not only a simple cut but a
more extended lesion, the highest mitotic activity on the undamaged opposite
side was found opposite to the *center* of the lesion (fig. 7.3). The authors

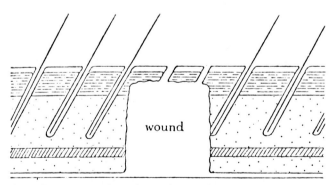

Fig. 7.2. Schematic representation of a subcutaneous and dermal wound made by
Bullough and Laurence in order to investigate the specificity of the epidermal mitotic
response to wounding. From Bullough and Laurence (1960a). (With permission of the
authors and of the Royal Society, London.)

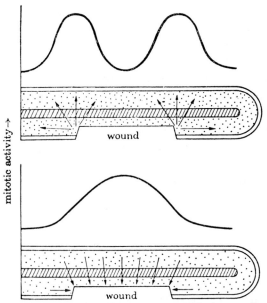

Fig. 7.3. Distribution of mitotic activity in mouse epidermis opposite to an extended epidermal wound. The upper diagram shows the pattern which is expected on the assumption that a stimulating 'wound hormone' is released from the damaged epidermis at the wound edges. The lower diagram represents the observed distribution. From Bullough and Laurence (1960a). (With permission of the authors and of the Royal Society, London.)

considered this observation not to be consistent with the assumption of a wound hormone thought to be released from the *wound edges* but took it as strong evidence for the loss of a pre-existing mitotic inhibitor:

'The present results suggest that normally an inhibitory substance is in constant production, and that it may be lost partly with the cornified cells which are shed from the surface and partly by diffusion into the dermis. It may also be unstable. In the neighbourhood of a wound there appears to be both a reduced inhibitor production and a drainage away of inhibitor into the wound' (Bullough and Laurence, 1960a).

Two years later Bullough (1962) proposed to call the inhibitor a chalone referring to a term which was created in 1916 by E. A. Schäfer in order to define 'an endocrine product which inhibits or diminishes activity, as distinguished from a hormone, which excites to increased activity' (Schäfer, 1916) but which never was accepted by endocrinologists. This adoption of chalone by Bullough for the negative feedback inhibitor of epidermal proliferation was connected with a new definition:

'A chalone may be defined as an internal secretion product produced by a tissue for the purpose of controlling by inhibition the mitotic activity of that same tissue' (Bullough, 1962). In this formulation the word chalone is practically synonymous with the antitemplate of Weiss and Kavanau (1957). In a famous theory, which is based on a large body of experimental evidence, these authors suggested that tissue growth is controlled by an interplay between stimulatory ('templates') and inhibitory ('antitemplates') impulses. The production of antitemplates (which were supposed to be chemical messengers) was thought to be a normal consequence of differentiation; the differentiated tissue mass secretes these freely diffusible inhibitors which control cell proliferation in the generative tissue mass:

'The antitemplate system acts as a growth regulator by a negative feedback mechanism in which increasing populations of antitemplates render an increasing proportion of the homologous templates ineffective resulting in a corresponding decline of the growth rate. The attainment of terminal size is an expression of a stationary equilibrium between the incremental and decremental growth components and of the equilibrium of the intercellular and extracellular antitemplate concentration' (Weiss and Kavanau, 1957).

For many biologists this concept still offers the most concise and conclusive interpretation of tissue homeostasis. In 1960 it was directly adapted by Iversen (1960a, b, 1961) in order to explain growth regulation in epidermis (see below).

Interestingly, almost at the same time when Bullough and Laurence published their results on wound healing, Mazia (1961) postulated that 'the stimulation of cell division in multicellular systems is the removal of a block . . . the stimulus is nor more than the permission of the cell to do what it would have done if it had been left alone in the first place'. In other words: the background of Bullough's concept is the idea that a cell (at least an undifferentiated or stem cell) has an inborn tendency to replicate and that it is this tendency which, for the benefit of the multicellular organism, has to be strictly controlled by means of a tissue-specific inhibitory mechanism.

Bullough's results were strongly confirmed by the experiments of Finegold in 1965. Again it was shown that a wound made on one side of a hamster ear induced a mitotic response not only at the wound margins but also in the undamaged opposite ear epidermis. This reaction could be suppressed by the presence of a skin graft in the wound provided that the graft was metabolically active (as measured by the uptake of labelled thymidine) thus proving that the hyperplastic response was not prevented by toxic substances from dying tissue. The author considered his results as being entirely inconsistent with the concept of a wound hormone: 'Since wounds of equal size were made in each ear, the number of injured host cells at the margins was the same. The addition of a graft to one side provided another group of injured cells, those bordering the inserted tissue. If injured cells were responsible for release of a material that stimulates mitotic activity, the epidermis opposite a graft should have displayed even greater cell labelling than that opposite a wound. Yet, as shown, grafting suppressed the proliferative response' (Finegold, 1965). Since there was no mitotic inhibition adjacent to a skin graft, Finegold concluded that other influences on mitotic activity such as decreased cellular adhesiveness and cell migration must be considered which probably outweigh the potency of available inhibitor.

Recently Iversen et al. (1974) have repeated and extended this type of experiment on wound healing in an impressive study using the web membrane of the African fruit bat. Since this tissue resembles a mouse ear in many aspects (the two epidermal layers are separated by a thin connective tissue sheet with a diameter of 1 mm or less) but is much larger and easier to handle, it was found to be an almost ideal object for the purpose envisaged.

When an area of epidermis was removed from the ventral side of the web by stripping with adhesive tape, several waves of increased mitotic activity and the development of epidermal hyperplasia were observed adjacent to the wound as well as on the undamaged opposite side. Again the *local* character of the response was confirmed excluding a general blood-borne mechanism or a nerve impulse as the cause, but supporting strongly the concept of a diffusible signal substance generated or lost in the direct vicinity of the lesion. As in the study of Bullough and Laurence (1960a), the maximum response was found opposite the *central* area of the wound. This observation again excluded the possibility of a wound hormone produced by the damaged epidermal cells at the *wound edges*. Several other possible explanations of the hyperplasia such as increased nutritional supply to the wounded epidermis (wick effect), shrinking of the basement membrane, prolongation of cell maturation, a critical cell surface/volume ratio, an inflammatory reaction etc. could also be ruled out with a high degree of confidence. Therefore, the authors were again left with the chalone concept as an explanation of their results. This was strongestly supported by the observation that skin grafting as well as local treatment of the wound with freeze-dried skin extract inhibited or prevented the proliferative response on both sides of the web. The authors concluded that 'the results . . . *do not* by themselves *prove* the existence of epidermal chalones, but taken together with other evidence . . . they may be said to give strong evidence for the chalone hypothesis. The final proof has to await the chemical purification and characterization of the chalones' (Iversen et al., 1974).

Other strong evidence for the existence of a self-regulatory mechanism in epidermis has been provided by the elegant studies of Mizuno and Fujii (1969) (Fujii and Mizuno, 1969) which, surprisingly, have often been overlooked in the chalone literature. Employing a technique which was originally developed by Locke (1967), they implanted thin sheets of cellophane, Teflon or Millipore filters into mouse skin through a cut in the back skin. When the material was impermeable (cellophane, teflon or paraffin-impregnated Millipore filter) the epidermis grew around both sides of the implant ultimately forming a pocket (fig. 7.4). However, after implantation of a porous filter the epidermis did not move around the sheet but remained separated by the implant (fig. 7.5). After treatment of the skin with various

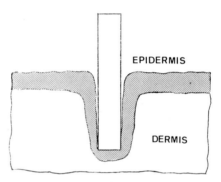

Fig. 7.4. Behaviour of epidermis when a disk of impermeable material was inserted after wounding. The epidermis migrates around both sides of the implant. The same growth pattern was observed when a permeable filter was implanted into carcinogen-treated skin. According to Mizuno and Fujii (1969).

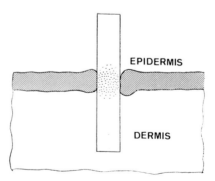

Fig. 7.5. Behaviour of epidermis when a permeable filter was inserted after wounding. The epidermis remains separated on both sides of the implant. According to Mizuno and Fujii (1969).

carcinogens – but not after application of non-carcinogenic hydrocarbons or croton oil – the epidermis grew also around a permeable implant (fig. 7.4). By proper control experiments it could be excluded that the observed growth pattern of epidermis was due to the different surface characteristics of the implanted materials. From their results the authors drew the conclusion that in the normal tissue, control of cell growth and cell migration is brought about by an intercellular exchange of regulatory substances which were able to penetrate the filter; in carcinogen-treated tissue this communication seems to be profoundly disturbed.

By means of proper staining and labelling methods Mizuno and Fujii tried to characterize the material which was penetrating the filter and which they believed to be the carrier of information. Their finding that it was glycoprotein containing a heparin-like mucopolysaccharide seemed to be rather peculiar at that time. However, as will be shown below, it is now highly consistent with recent results on the possible chemical nature of the epidermal G_1 chalone. Therefore, the investigations of the two Japanese authors may turn out to become of crucial importance for the understanding of epidermal growth control.

Studying the response of mouse epidermis to carcinogens Iversen and co-workers (Iversen and Evensen, 1962; Iversen and Bjerknes, 1963) also came to the conclusion that epidermal cell proliferation is controlled according to the negative feedback principle. In those experiments the time course of cell damage and cell renewal caused by a single application of 3-methyl cholanthrene was found to be well matched to model curves, which

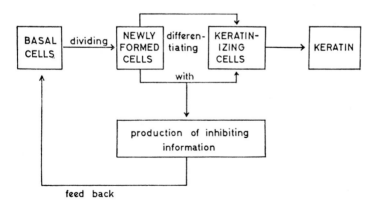

Fig. 7.6. Schematic representation of Iversen's model of epidermal growth control by negative feedback. The production of inhibiting information is dependent upon the process of differentiation. From Iversen (1969). (With permission of the author and of the Ciba Foundation, London.)

had been calculated by means of an analogue computer on the basis of a cybernetic model which was developed by Iversen (1960b, 1961) according to the concept of Weiss and Kavanau (fig. 7.6).

As the author pointed out (Iversen, 1969) 'it is interesting to see how time was ripe in the years 1960 and 1961 for applying such a theory to the epidermis. From studies of the changes in cell metabolism in experimental skin carcinogenesis I proposed such a theory for epidermal growth regulation in March 1960 (Iversen, 1960b) and elaborated it at the First International Congress of Cybernetic Medicine in Naples in October 1960 (Iversen, 1960a) ... In the same year, Bullough and Laurence published their study on wound healing ... In 1961 Mercer proposed a similar theory for epidermis in his book Keratin and Keratinization'.

A similar approach was employed by Tsanev (1963). Having studied originally the response of epidermis to pressure damage and having employed the method of computer simulation he, together with Sendov (Tsanev and Sendov, 1966, 1968), developed a model of growth control which again based on the principle of negative feedback.

7.3 Two or more epidermal chalones?

Despite its unquestionable advantages in explaining theoretically a large number of experimental observations, the chalone concept was afflicted with a serious flaw for a long time: Bullough's hypothesis included, as an essential postulate, that chalones act by switching between cell division and cell maturation (differentiation). As a consequence, Bullough (1965) assumed the cell is prevented from entering the phase of DNA replication so that the point of attack of a chalone must necessarily be somewhere around the G_1–S boundary, i.e. in the late G_1 phase of the mitotic cycle. During this period – called dichophase by Bullough (1965) – the cell has to 'decide' between entering a new mitotic cycle or taking its path toward functionalization. This is consistent with the fact that in normal epidermis as well as in other tissues the great majority of cells are found to be in a diploid state. Nevertheless, for almost ten years the effect of chalone extracts had been measured by means of the colcemid technique. By this method, however, only a block in the G_2 phase could be observed.

To overcome this discrepancy, Bullough (1965) postulated that chalones, beside their proposed effect on the dichophase, are able to slow down the whole mitotic cycle. However, under the conditions of Bullough's in-vitro assay no effect of skin extracts on thymidine incorporation into DNA of epidermal explants could be found (Baden and Sviokla, 1968).

In the meantime, Bullough's hypothetical view cannot be maintained any longer, especially since the most purified preparations of the mitosis-inhibiting chalone so far available do not inhibit epidermal DNA synthesis at all (Thornley and Laurence, 1975).

In order to save the chalone concept in its original formulation, a second factor acting on DNA replication had necessarily to be postulated. Evidence for the existence of such a factor in skin extracts was provided independently in Iversen's laboratory in Oslo and by Marks in Heidelberg. Already in 1969 Hennings et al. demonstrated a reversible inhibitory effect of mouse skin extracts on thymidine incorporation into DNA of mouse epidermis in vivo. The inhibition showed a delay of several hours and reached its maximum 8 h after injection of the extract. Since at that time the authors did not try to characterize the inhibitor, the effect could still be attributed to the antimitotic chalone described by Bullough and Iversen (Elgjo, 1969) thus apparently supporting the idea of a cellcycle unspecific action of the chalones.

Two years later, however, Elgjo et al. (1971) presented evidence that the factor inhibiting DNA synthesis was probably not identical with Bullough's epidermal chalone: after treatment of mouse skin with actinomycin D only the inhibitor of DNA synthesis (now called 'G_1 chalone') could still be demonstrated in extracts made from the skin, whereas the inhibitor of mitosis (now called 'G_2 chalone') obviously had disappeared. The authors concluded that the G_1 chalone was metabolically more stable than the G_2 chalone. Working with the same ethanol precipitates from pig-skin extracts which were used as starting material for an extensive purification of the epidermal G_2 chalone (Hondius Boldingh and Laurence, 1968) Marks (1971, 1973a) at about the same time provided more direct evidence for the existence of two chalone-like inhibitors. After having confirmed the observations of the Oslo group on a delayed and apparently tissue-specific inhibition of thymidine incorporation into mouse epidermis DNA in vivo, he showed that the inhibitor in question differed considerably from the G_2 chalone (Hondius Boldingh and Laurence, 1968): it could not be inactivated by heat, proteolytic digestion or denaturing agents, and was eluted from a sephadex column with an apparent molecular weight of more than 10^5 daltons whereas for the G_2 chalone a value of 3–4 $\times$ 10^4 daltons had been reported (Hondius Boldingh and Laurence, 1968).

The concept of two chalone-like inhibitors in epidermis was strongly supported by experiments on the localization of inhibitory activity within different epidermal cell layers performed by Elgjo et al. Employing a sophisticated technique for separating germinative basal cells from differenti-

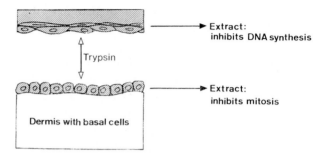

Fig. 7.7. Diagram illustrating the experiment of Elgjo et al. to demonstrate the distinct distribution of the two epidermal chalones within the epidermal cell layers (Elgjo, Laerum and Edgehill, 1972).

ating and keratinized superficial cells they found most of the G_2 chalone in the basal cells (Elgjo et al., 1971) whereas the G_1 chalone was almost entirely restricted to the superficial layers (Elgjo et al., 1972) (fig. 7.7). According to Iversen's feedback hypothesis, a chalone is expected to be produced by differentiating cells; therefore, the authors considered the G_1 chalone to be the epidermal chalone proper whereas the role of the G_2 chalone seems to be somewhat obscure.

In continuation of this study Elgjo et al. (Elgjo 1974a; Elgjo and Edgehill, 1974) recently reported that only the G_2 chalone but not the G_1 chalone seems to diffuse into the dermis. Serum was found to neutralize the anti-mitotic activity of epidermal extracts whereas the inhibitory action on DNA synthesis was only slightly diminished. The serum effect was lost after heating. From these results the authors concluded that the well-known stimulatory effect of connective tissue and serum on epithelial cell growth might have something to do with the ability to bind or to inactivate epithelial growth inhibitors. Another possibility, the production by connective tissue of chalone antagonists (growth factors), will be discussed below.

The existence of two epidermal inhibitors acting either on DNA synthesis or on mitosis is in accordance with observations in Gelfant's laboratory (Gelfant, 1966; Gelfant and Candelas, 1972; Candelas, 1974). Investigating the process of epidermal wound healing by means of the labelled mitosis technique Gelfant and co-workers came to the conclusion that the basal cell layer is built up by at least two different cell populations, a G_2 population and a G_1 population. In mouse ear epidermis, the great majority (90–95%) of basal cells are G_1 cells which move through the cycle in the usual manner. In contrast, the G_2 cells (5–10%) are held up in the G_2 phase for a rather long period of time; Gelfant even believes that G_2 cells are blocked indefinitely in G_2 (Gelfant and Candelas, 1972). Nevertheless, these apparently slow – or non-cycling – cells have retained their capacity to divide and they do so, for example, after wounding.

The G_2-character of the cells triggered into mitosis after wounding was unequivocally confirmed by the following evidence (Candelas, 1974):

1) they entered mitosis as early as one hour after the stimulus;

2) after prelabelling with [^{3}H]thymidine over two days, unlabelled mitoses were still found;

3) the early mitotic activity could not be inhibited by hydroxyurea, a S-phase blocker, or by inhibitors of transcription (actinomycin D and ethidium bromide).

Gelfant postulated that in normal epidermis cell proliferation is controlled by two blocks, a G_1 block regulating the flow of cells into the phase of DNA replication, and a G_2 block controlling the transition from G_2 into mitosis, and that there are two cell populations which are controlled *either* in G_1 *or* in G_2. Furthermore, he suggested, that at least the G_2 block is due to the activity of the epidermal G_2 chalone (at that time the existence of a G_1 chalone was still unknown).

More indirect evidence for the existence in epidermis of G_2-cells has been recently provided also by experiments with mitogens such as vitamin A acid (Zil, 1972) and phorbolesters (Krieg et al., 1974) or after stripping (Bertsch, 1975).

When investigating the distribution of cell proliferation within the epidermal proliferative units (EPU) Potten (1974) came to similar results. He observed that when mice were continuously labelled with [^{3}H]thymidine the labelling index in the basal layer rose with time and reached a plateau at about 90%; 100% levels were not achieved. This result is in accordance with Gelfant's observations. At the time when the plateau was reached, about half of the unlabelled basal cells were located beneath the center of the EPU indicating that the central cells are cycling at a slower rate than the rest and that a few of these cells may even be temporarily out of cycle. Interestingly, the unlabelled basal cells were intensely Feulgen or alum carmine positive, which was taken as an indication that they were perhaps held in the G_2 phase. Those central cells seem to be more responsive to external stimulation than the outer cells, and Potten believes them to be responsible for the triggering of epidermal regeneration after severe wounding. From these and other observations Potten drew the conclusion that the basal cell layer is heterogeneous in the sense of a two-compartment proliferative model similar to that proposed for the haemopoietic system (Lajtha,

1973). In his concept the central basal cell of the EPU is thought to be a clonogenic stem cell similar to the pluripotential stem cells of the haemopoietic system whereas the basal cells in the periphery of the EPU might be considered to be committed stem cells. If G_2 cells are located preferently in the center of the EPU, one could assume that the epidermal G_2 chalone acts primarily on the clonogenic epidermal stem cells. This would be in accordance with the observation that in fetal or neonatal mouse epidermis the G_2 chalone mechanism is obviously already established (Krieg, 1975), whereas no response of the cells to G_1 chalone was found (Bertsch and Marks, 1974; Bertsch, 1975). Independently, the concept of a two-compartment stem cell population in epidermis was proposed also by Krieg et al. (1974); it was emphasized that such a model is most suitable to explain the reaction of hyperplastic skin to epidermal chalones (see below).

7.4 Epidermal G_2 chalone

7.4.1 Extraction

Considering their observations on wound healing, Bullough and Laurence (1960a) were convinced that the epidermal chalone they had postulated had to be a freely diffusible substance. In order to demonstrate the existence of such a factor it was, therefore, only reasonable to prepare an aqueous extract from homogenized epidermis or skin and to check this preparation for tissue-specific antimitotic activity. Experiments of this kind have been done in 1964 by Bullough and Laurence as well as in 1965 by Iversen et al. Whereas Bullough and Laurence extracted epidermis, which had been scraped from depilated mouse-skin, with isotonic saline at 0°C, the Oslo group worked with a whole skin preparation from hairless mice which was homogenized in a mortar or a mill cooled with liquid nitrogen prior to extraction with water or saline at 4°C. After centrifugation of the homogenate the antimitotic factor was found in the clear supernatant. By means of a similar technique extracts were made also from codfish skin and human skin.

   Lateron these extraction methods were – with minor variations – adapted by several authors (Baden and Sviokla, 1968; Frankfurt, 1971; Marrs and Voorhees, 1971a; Chopra et al., 1972; Wiley et al. ,1973).

7.4.2 Assay

The antimitotic activity of epidermal G_2 chalone has been assayed in vivo and in vitro. In each case the decrease of epidermal mitotic activity as measured by means of the 'colcemid technique' is determined. For the in vivo assay nearly identical methods have been employed by several authors working in this field (Iversen et al., 1965; Hondius-Boldingh and Laurence, 1968; Elgjo, 1969). In general, the extract to be tested is intraperitoneally injected into mice together with an appropriate dose of a stathmokinetic agent (colchicin, colcemid or vincristin). Four hours later the animals are killed. Pieces of back or ear skin are fixed, sectioned and properly stained for histological examination (counting of metaphase figures). It has been shown (Elgjo, 1969) that by a single i.p. injection of 5 mg of lyophylized mouse skin extract the mitotic rate in back skin epidermis of mice is depressed for about 4 h with a minimum in the first two h. This inhibition was not followed by a compensatory overshooting in the subsequent 22 h.

The in vitro assay originally designed by Bullough and Johnson (1951) has also widely been used (Bullough and Laurence, 1961a; Hondius-Boldingh and Laurence, 1968; Marrs and Voorhees, 1971). For this purpose small pieces of mouse ear are incubated in phosphate-buffered saline containing 0.02 M glucose and the test sample in an oxygen atmosphere. In order to permit those mitoses already present when the skin was dissected to pass the metaphase, one hour is allowed to pass before colcemid (4 μg/ml) is added. After 4 h incubation with colcemid at 37 °C the ear fragments are fixed, sectioned and stained for histological examination.

A variation of this assay was described by Chopra et al. (1972); here 7-day old epidermal outgrowths which appeared around explants of human skin grown in tissue culture were used.

To ascertain that the inhibition found in the in vitro assay is not due to a non-specific (toxic?) factor, Bullough and Laurence (1964) have introduced a discriminative test which is based on the observation that adrenalin is a necessary cofactor for the epidermal G_2 chalone in vitro (see below). It has been shown that after a 5 h incubation period (normal in vitro assay) the tissue has apparently lost its ability to respond to chalone so that the mitotic rate of the mouse ear epidermis treated with chalone equalled that of the control at the end of a further 4 h period of incubation. The responsiveness can be restored by an adrenalin wash. For this purpose the ear pieces, which have been incubated before for 5 h, are removed from the Warburg flask and immersed for 30 min in another flask containing buffered saline plus glucose and 0.25 μg/ml adrenalin bitartrate. After this treatment the tissue is put back into the original flask and incubated for a further four hours. According to Bullough et al. only an inhibition which is lost after 5 h but is restored by the adrenalin wash is caused by chalone whereas a non-specific inhibitor always shows the same inhibition. The adrenalin-wash test has for example been used to demonstrate a chalone-effect in human skin (Iversen, 1968).

Based on the in vitro assay Bullough and Laurence (1964) have defined a unit of epidermal chalone as the amount, which is required to reduce the epidermal mitotic rate by about 50%; in the early studies this amount turned out to be roughly equivalent to 1 mg dried epidermis.

7.4.3 Attempts on purification and characterization

The first successful attempt to purify and characterize the epidermal G_2 chalone was made by Bullough et al. (1964) in collaboration with the Organon company. It was shown that the factor as extracted with water from back skin epidermis of mice was not dialysable and could be completely inactivated by heating its solution to 100 °C for 10 min. A crude extract was found to loose its activity at 0 °C within a few days and at −20 °C within several weeks but remained active over at least 12 months after freeze-drying. Most of the activity could be precipitated with 60–80% ethanol.

In the late sixties a large scale preparation of G_2-chalone was started (Hondius-Boldingh and Laurence, 1968). The source was mainly commercial rind (epidermis together with dermis). This was obtained from slaughtered

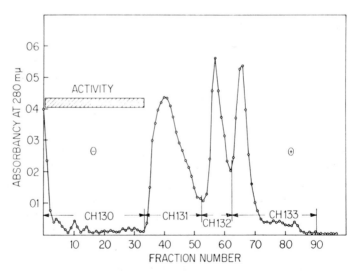

Fig. 7.8. Fractionation of a G_2 chalone-containing ethanol fraction from pig skin by means of preparative electrophoresis (cellulose, 0.1 M acetic acid). From Hondius-Boldingh and Laurence (1968). (With permission of the authors and of the Federation of European Biochemical Societies.)

pigs which had been immersed in a water bath at 60 °C for about 15 min. The hair was then burned off after which the skin was removed and the rind was separated. After lyophilization, the tissue was completely defatted with petroleum ether for 2 h at 45 °C and then ground to a fibrous powder. From this material an aqueous extract was made at 0–4 °C in an atmosphere of nitrogen by means of a high speed mixer. The extract was centrifuged and fractionated by the slow addition of ethanol at 0–4 °C. Usually most of the chalone activity was found in the 71–82% ethanol precipitate; however some activity was also collected with the 55–72% ethanol precipitate as well as with the 81% ethanol supernatant. For further purification, preparative electrophoresis on cellulose columns at pH 3 (0.1 M acetic acid) proved to be superior to other techniques such as gel or ion exchange chromatography. The chalone was found to move towards the cathode faster than the greater

Table 7.1

Amino acid composition of a purified G_2 chalone preparation from pig skin. Tryptophan was not analyzed. (From Hondius-Boldingh and Laurence, 1968.)

Amino acid	Content in sample (corrected for water uptake during hydrolysis)
	% (w/w)
Lysine	3.7
Histidine	1.2
Arginine	4.8
Hydroxyproline	5.4
Aspartic acid	4.5
Threonine	2.0
Serine	2.8
Glutamic acid	7.9
Proline	7.9
Glycine	10.7
Alanine	4.2
Cysteine	0.0
Valine	2.0
Methionine	0.7
Isoleucine	1.1
Leucine	2.3
Tyrosine	0.6
Phenylalanine	1.3
Total amino acid content	63.1

part of the accompanying material (fig. 7.8). A further separation from a large amount of inactive contaminants was achieved by dialysis at 4 °C against water. Finally the authors ended up with a chalone preparation which was purified approximately 2000 times over the crude skin extract.

In the in vivo assay, between 30 and 180 μg of the dialyzed fraction injected per mouse were sufficient to reduce the epidermal mitotic activity to about 50%. Under in vitro conditions the same effect could be achieved with as little as 1.5 μg/ml assay mixture. In the adrenalin wash test the material behaved as expected for a chalone.

The amino acid composition of the purified preparation (table 7.1) shows a remarkably high content of proline and hydroxy-proline. About 63% of the weight of the sample was accounted for by amino acids. Further analysis rendered possible a crude estimate of about 15% carbohydrate.

The chalone was resistant to pepsin but could be destroyed by trypsin; it was stable at pH 3–6 in aqueous solution for at least 3 days but was in-activated at pH 9. The isoelectric point was estimated to be in the range of pH 5.2–6.0. The preparation was found to be almost homogeneous in the ultracentrifuge, and the sedimentation behaviour as well as gel chromatography indicated a molecular weight of $2.5–4 \times 10^4$ dalton.

The authors concluded that their most purified fraction was either a glycoprotein or a mixture of protein and polysaccharides. In the meantime it has become customary in the literature to call the epidermal G_2-chalone a glycoprotein. This is certainly a premature conclusion. Hondius-Boldingh and Laurence (1968) did not claim to have isolated the pure epidermal chalone but refer strictly to the possible heterogeneity of their preparation.

For example, the molecular weight given by the authors should be taken with caution since no precautions have been taken to prevent aggregation of skin proteins. It is well known that these proteins show a strong tendency to aggregate, and polyacrylamide gel electrophoresis of the lyophilized ethanol precipitate used by Hondius-Boldingh and Laurence (1968) demonstrates that it is in fact highly aggregated (Marks, 1973). It should be taken into consideration, therefore, that the G_2 chalone might be a rather small molecule which sticks to a larger protein, perhaps a derivative of collagen as indicated by the amino acid analysis of the highly purified fraction. In this connection Iversen's observation may be recalled that after gel chromatography of epidermal extracts most of the antimitotic activity was found in a fraction with an apparent molecular weight of only 3000 dalton (Iversen, 1969). A similar finding has been mentioned by E. Laurence (1973): during gel chromatography of the active preparation from pig skin on Sephadex G-75 some activity was spread throughout; also with an ion exchange column no definite condensation of activity could be achieved. A behaviour of that kind strongly indicates aggregation.

Although often employed, ethanol precipitation also does not seem to be a reliable method for enriching epidermal chalones. The distribution of the activity over the different fractions seems to depend largely on the particular extract used as source. Thus, Hondius-Boldingh and Laurence (1968) reported that when codfish skin was used as the starting material, the chalone was concentrated in the 81% ethanol supernatant. Working with human skin Chopra et al. (1972) found most of the activity to be precipitated at 81% ethanol and Marrs and Voorhees (1971b) localized the main activity in the 70–80% ethanol precipitate as well as in the 90% ethanol supernatant of rat epidermis extracts. These differences may be also due to aggregation of the chalone with different compounds present in different amounts in the extracts.

Using epidermis of newborn rats as starting material the latter authors (Marrs and Voorhees, 1971b) have greatly confirmed the results of the London group on water solubility, nondialyzability, susceptibility to heat and trypsin and adrenalin requirement in vitro of the chalone.

Recently Chopra et al. (1972) reported on the partial purification of G_2 chalone from human epidermis. After ethanol precipitation the chalone activity was tracked down in a rather strong protein band by means of polyacrylamide gel electrophoresis. However, some doubts may be raised to the conclusion that this band represents the chalone. If one assumes that the concentration of a chalone in a given tissues is on the order of magnitude of that of a hormone, a simple calculation shows that it is highly improbable to stain a chalone on polyacrylamide gels run with a preparation which had been purified only about 200-fold by ethanol precipitation. Again, no precautions against unspecific aggregation had been taken. It must be stated, therefore, that the purification and chemical characterization of the epidermal G_2 chalone is a problem which still awaits its final solution.

7.4.4 Reversibility and tissue-specificity of action

Obviously, for most investigators the reversibility (non-toxicity) and tissue-specificity of chalone action is thought to be a 'conditio sine qua non'.

The adrenalin wash test can be considered to be an evidence for the reversibility of the chalone effect (Bullough and Laurence, 1964). Using this assay and the in vivo test (Bullough et al., 1967) epidermal G_2 chalone activity could be demonstrated in the skin of male and female mice, guinea pigs, pigs, rabbits, man (Chopra et al., 1972), codfish and rats (Marrs and

Voorhees, 1971a; Frankfurt, 1971). Therefore, it is considered to be neither sex- nor species-specific. Beside skin, G_2 chalone was also found in related epithelia such as esophagus (Laurence, 1973b), and lens (Voaden, 1968; Voaden and Leeson, 1970) as well as in palate (Laurence and Randers-Hansen, 1972), gingiva (Laurence and Randers-Hansen, 1972) and urine (Laurence, 1973a). It was furthermore extracted from epidermal (Bullough and Laurence, 1968b; Bullough and Deol, 1971; Laurence and Elgjo, 1971) and lung (Laurence, 1973a) tumors. No epidermal chalone could be detected in other tissues (Laurence, 1973a).

In order to demonstrate tissue-specificity of the action of epidermal G_2 chalone, the inhibitory activity of epidermal extracts was compared with that in extracts of kidney, lung, liver (Iversen, 1969; Elgjo and Hennings, 1971), brain, rectum, as well as of resting and growing hair bulbs. In no case was any inhibition of epidermal mitosis found; therefore, the epidermal extract was considered to be unique in its power of action (Bullough and Laurence, 1964). Vice versa, epidermal extracts did not exhibit any effect on the mitotic activity in growing hair follicles and rectal crypts but inhibited cell division – beside epidermis – in cornea, esophagus, sebaceous glands (Bullough and Laurence, 1964) and eye lens (Voaden, 1968). Moreover, neither epidermis nor liver extracts inhibited the growth of monkey kidney cells in vitro (Chopra et al., 1972).

An important study of the chalone tissue-specificity for epidermis and its appendages has been made by Bullough and Laurence (1970b). It was shown that extracts from skin areas containing sebaceous glands inhibited mitoses in both interfollicular epidermis and sebaceous glands, whereas extracts from epithelia without those glands (oral epithelium, esophagus, codfish skin) did not exhibit any effect on sebaceous glands but still inhibited the mitotic activity in interfollicular epidermis. Moreover, the ethanol precipitate of pig skin extracts inhibited both epidermal and glandular mitotic activity; during further purification, however, the glandular chalone could be separated from the epidermal chalone. In addition, epidermal or glandular extracts did not inhibit eccrine sweat glands, whereas human sweat was shown to contain a chalone-like sweat gland inhibitor which, vice versa, did not act on sebaceous glands or interfollicular epidermis (Bullough and Deol, 1972). Similar differences seem to exist between hair follicles and interfollicular epidermis (Bullough, 1967), between epidermis and skin melanocytes (Bullough and Laurence, 1968b) and between dermis and epidermis (Bullough and Laurence, 1970b; Elgjo, Laerum and Edgehill, 1971).

Another extensive study of tissue-specificity was reported from Iversen's

Table 7.2

Percentage reduction of mitotic activity in different mouse epithelia after injection of 5 mg tissue extract. (From Nome, 1974.)

Tissue in which mitoses were counted	Tissues from which extracts were made								
	Skin	Fore-stom-ach	Glan-dular stom-ach	Lung	Liver	Kidney	Spleen	Stri-ated muscle	Small in-testine
Epidermis	70	59	27	5	14	13	9	8	—
Forestomach	25	44	30	—	10	—	—	3	24
Jejunum	2	12	1	—	—	—	11	—	10
Colon	8	10	2	—	7	3	13	9	21

laboratory. In an experimental *tour de force* using the in vivo assay, O. Nome (1974) has measured the effect of extracts made from different tissues on the mitotic activity in four epithelia: epidermis, forestomach, jejunum and colon. These tissues were chosen because they all have a well defined proliferating pool and are both of ectodermal and endodermal origin. Epidermis is an ectodermal, forestomach an endodermal keratinizing epithelium, whereas the epithelia of the crypts of jejunum and colon have a one-layered columnar structure. A summary of Nome's results is shown in table 7.2: based on a practical minimum of 25% inhibition as an indication of a real chalone effect, a specific inhibitory effect of extracts from squameous cell epithelia on squameous cell epithelia was found, regardless of whether the epithelium was of ectodermal or endodermal origin. As the author pointed out, this may mean that the production of G_2 chalone is related to differentiation (keratinization).

Using the in vivo assay, an inhibitory effect of extracts from rat epidermis on the mitotic activity of forestomach but not of the crypts of the small intestine has also been reported by Frankfurt (1971).

Recently, Laurence and Randers-Hansen (1972) reported that in the in vivo assay extracts from oral epithelium depressed the mitotic rate of tongue epithelium more than did similar extracts from skin and, conversely, skin extracts were more effective in ear epidermis than oral epithelial extracts. A similar observation was made by Nome (1974) when comparing skin and forestomach. These results point to the possibility not only of a epithelia-specific chalone effect but also of structural differences among the epithelial chalones. For a final conclusion on this point we have to await the purification and chemical characterization of the G_2 chalones from different epithelia.

In summary, it may be said that the tissue-specific but species-nonspecific action of epidermal G_2 chalone, which is considered to be one of the most important characteristics of a chalone, is a fairly well documented fact.

Regional differences in epidermal growth control seem to exist when different body sites are compared. Thus, it has been reported that the diurnal variation of epidermal mitotic activity in mouse ear epidermis is somewhat different from that of dorsal epidermis (Pilgrim et al., 1965; Tvermyr, 1969). Rather large differences between the mitotic rates of epithelia from ear, sole of foot, tongue and esophagus have been found and by means of the in vivo assay it was observed that the degree of mitotic inhibition by G_2 chalone was small when the mitotic activity was high and vice versa (Bullough and Laurence, 1966; Christophers and Laurence, 1973; Laurence, 1973b).

Furthermore, when increasing amounts of chalone were injected into mice the degree of inhibition was never 100% but reached a plateau of 50–60% (ear) or 20% (tongue). In contrast, with adrenalin a depression of 75% or more could be achieved in both epithelia (Laurence and Randers-Hansen, 1971, 1972).

This finding may be interpreted in several ways: Laurence et al. (1972; Laurence, 1973b) suggested that the chalone activity is modulated by an antagonist (anti-chalone) and that adrenalin acts by blocking the effectiveness of that factor. Whereas the latter assumption is entirely speculative, the presence in skin of growth factors which may be considered to be anti-chalones, has been repeatedly demonstrated. Beside of the hormone-like Epidermal Growth Factor (EGF) described and purified by Cohen and co-workers (Cohen, 1972), stimulants of epidermal cell proliferation have been found in guinea-pig skin (Hell, 1970; Hell and Cooper, 1973) and in dermis (Karasek, 1972; Melbye and Karasek, 1973). Factors of that kind are considered to be responsible for the well known ability of connective tissue to sustain and modulate epithelial growth and function. Presumed that they do so by neutralizing chalones, it should be expected that their action can be overcome by exogenous administration of rising amounts of chalone so that the mitotic activity finally can be depressed down to zero. Since this is obviously not the case (Laurence and Randers-Hansen, 1971; Laurence, 1973b) some doubts may be raised in the interpretation of Laurence et al. It seems to be more probable that only a distinct proportion of germinative epidermal cells is able to *respond* to G_2 chalone and that the ratio between chalone-susceptible and chalone-unsusceptible cells differs from tissue to tissue (perhaps depending on the functional demands or on the tissue's level of cyclic AMP (see below)).

7.4.5 Hormones and cyclic AMP

It has been known for a rather long time that adrenalin strongly depresses epidermal proliferative activity. Gelfant (1963) has provided evidence that this is due to an inhibition of mitosis rather than DNA synthesis. This was recently confirmed by proper in vitro studies (Young et al., 1975). In several admirable papers Bullough and Laurence (1961b, 1964, 1966, 1968a) have described their investigations on the mechanisms of the antimitotic effect of adrenalin.

It was shown (Bullough and Laurence, 1961b) that the mitotic activity in mouse ear epidermis was low when the animals were active and high when they were resting (diurnal variation) and that it could be artificially decreased by exposing the mice to stress situations such as starvation, exercise or prevention of sleep. Since any decrease of mitotic activity could be counteracted by adrenal-ectomy whereas any increase could be prevented by injections of adrenalin, those effects were attributed to the action of that hormone.

When skin from animals with a decreased mitotic rate (after starvation, exercise or adrenalin injection) was separated and placed in a saline medium in vitro, an abnormally high number of mitoses was seen within the first few hours. This result indicated that under the influence of stress or adrenalin the cells were arrested in the late G_2 phase of the cell cycle and that this inhibition was fully reversible so that it disappeared rapidly under in vitro conditions. Since the release from inhibition could again be counter-acted by small amounts of adrenalin in the incubation medium, it was attributed to washing-out or destroying endogeneous hormone. Interestingly, the high mitotic activity adjacent to a wound turned out to be less sensitive to the inhibitory effect of adrenalin and was shown not to be subject to a diurnal rhythm.

In a painstaking experimental approach the authors subsequently tried to track down the relationships between the adrenalin effect and the chalone mechanism (Bullough and Laurence, 1964). Firstly, they demonstrated that in the in vitro assay identical mitotic depressions of approximately 50% were achieved with either 1 unit of chalone or 0.01 μg adrenalin per 4 ml. However, whereas with the hormone the highest depression was already seen after 1 h, the chalone effect reached its maximum only after 4 h.

Unexpectedly, in both these cases the inhibitory action was only temporary. Epidermis lost its ability to respond to chalone extracts, whether these were fresh or old, within a 5-h incubation period (after exactly 1 h). Adrenalin, on the other hand, lost its inhibitory power within 5 h in vitro, but with fresh adrenalin the previously treated epidermis reacted for a second time. The susceptibility of the tissue to chalone could be easily restored by short term incubation with fresh adrenalin in rather high concentrations (adrenalin wash, see above); but, in the absence of chalone, this treatment did not cause any reduction of the mitotic activity. Later this result was confirmed by Marrs and Voorhees (1971a).

Therefore, the loss of chalone responsiveness was traced back to an inactivation of endogeneous adrenalin under in vitro conditions, whereas the loss of adrenalin responsiveness was probably due to a washing-out of endogeneous chalone. Consequently, the authors concluded 'that epidermal chalone is powerless to cause any mitotic depression in the absence of sufficient adrenalin, just as adrenalin may be powerless in the absence of sufficient chalone, and that, when present together, the chalone and the adrenalin combine to form a complex which is the actual inhibitor' (Bullough and Laurence, 1964). This complex was thought to be extremely unstable breaking down rapidly under in vitro conditions.

In a subsequent paper (Bullough and Laurence, 1966) it was shown that either chalone or adrenalin not only reduce, through G_2-inhibition, the number of mitoses developing in vitro but also that they delay the passage of any mitoses that may develop, thus increasing the mitotic duration. This finding, however, could not be confirmed by Iversen et al. (1965) or by Elgjo (1969).

Since it was known that not only catecholamines but also glucocorticoids can inhibit epidermal mitosis, a further attempt was made to determine the relationship between adrenalin, hydrocortisone and chalone (Bullough and Laurence, 1968a). Whereas, in the in vitro assay chalone and adrenalin inhibited epidermal mitoses equally well, hydrocortisone alone did not show such an effect. When used alone, either chalone or adrenalin had lost its antimitotic power after 5 h; however in the presence of hydrocortisone (0.01 μg) the inhibitory activity of both chalone and adrenalin was greatly preserved. Thus, the glucocorticoid was obviously sustaining the action of chalone and adrenalin.

At first sight, the concept of a chalone–adrenalin complex is, without doubt, the most obvious and elegant interpretation of the phenomena observed by Bullough and Laurence as well as by others. However, all attempts to demonstrate such a complex by means of biochemical methods have completely failed (Laurence, 1973a).

Independent of its theoretical interpretation the results of Bullough and Laurence clearly demonstrate that epidermal cells respond to G_2 chalone only when they are properly 'programmed' by adrenalin and, to a certain sense, by hydrocortisone. This became especially clear when the effect on epidermal tumor cells was studied: here the antimitotic action of chalone in vitro was shown to be *absolutely* dependent on adrenalin and vice versa (Bullough and Laurence, 1968b; Bullough and Deol, 1971; Laurence and Elgjo, 1971).

Surprisingly enough, Laurence and Randers-Hansen (1971, 1972) have recently reported that after administration of G_2 chalone to adrenalectomized mice the same mitotic depression in ear epidermis and in tongue epithelium was observed as in normal animals. From this result the conclusion was drawn that adrenalin has no direct action on the epidermal chalone, for example by forming an adrenalin–chalone complex, but might perhaps react by neutralizing a hypothetical chalone antagonist. As mentioned above, such antichalones might indeed exist in skin or serum; nevertheless, the hypothesis of Laurence and Randers-Hansen (1972) is as yet lacking any experimental evidence.

A new aspect was added to this story since it has become clear that adrenalin obviously never penetrates the membrane of its target cell but is bound by a receptor at the cell surface. In turn, this reaction leads to a stimulation of adenyl cyclase and to the formation of cyclic AMP which is the second messenger of the hormone within the cell. This prompted Iversen (1969) to postulate that in epidermis Bullough's chalone–adrenalin complex rather than adrenalin alone might be the activator of the cyclic AMP system. Subsequently, cyclic AMP, its dibutyryl derivative or theophylline (a specific inhibitor of the cAMP-destroying enzyme phosphodiesterase) were indeed shown to display a pronounced antimitotic effect in the in vitro assay with mouse epidermis, which was quite similar to that observed with adrenalin or chalone (Marks and Rebien, 1972; Voorhees et al., 1972). Furthermore, the complete second messenger system including the enzyme adenyl cyclase (Mier and Urselmann, 1970; Duell et al., 1971; Marks and Rebien, 1972), guanyl cyclase (Marks, 1973b), phosphodiesterase (Mier and Urselmann, 1972; Voorhees et al., 1973; Marks and Raab, 1974) and protein kinase (Kumar et al., 1971, 1972; Mier and Van der Hurk, 1972) could be demonstrated in epidermis and it was found that the epidermal adenyl cyclase was coupled to a β-adrenergic receptor (Duell et al., 1971; Marks and Rebien, 1972) which reacts with adrenalin and corresponding catecholamines. This reaction causes an increase of intraepidermal cyclic AMP in vivo (Marks and Grimm, 1972) as well as in vitro (Brønstad et al., 1971; Duell et al., 1971;

Marks and Rebien, 1972). It seems to be fairly well established now, that the antimitotic effect of catecholamines is mediated by cyclic AMP (for reviews see Voorhees and Mier, 1974; Voorhees et al., 1974). However, as yet any attempt to demonstrate an effect of epidermal G_2 chalone on the epidermal cyclic AMP level, on the β-adrenergic stimulation of adenyl cyclase or on any other component of the second messenger system have failed (Marks and Grimm, 1972; Marks and Rebien, 1972; Marks, 1973b; Marks and Raab, 1974). It has to be concluded, therefore, that chalone does not directly affect the epidermal cyclic AMP system and, thus, the interaction between chalone and adrenalin must be more indirect.

Recent experiments carried out by Elgjo (1975) may throw some light on the possible nature of this interaction. It was found that injections of the β-adrenergic blocker propranolol prevented the inhibition by skin extracts of epidermal mitotic activity in mice. However, when the blocker was administered together with caffeine, an inhibitor of cyclic AMP degradation in the cell, the skin extract showed full inhibitory activity. Therefore, the chalone cannot be considered to be a β-adrenergic agonist, but it seems to be quite probable now that a certain intracellular level of cyclic AMP is necessary for epidermal cells to respond to G_2 chalone. This critical level is maintained and controlled by β-adrenergic agonists.

As already mentioned, the maximal mitotic depression which can be obtained by injections of G_2 chalone is never 100% but levels off at a value which obviously depends on the tissue (Laurence and Randers-Hansen, 1971; Laurence et al., 1972; Christophers and Laurence, 1973). This phenomenon was interpreted by suggesting that the chalone activity was modulated by an antagonist (Laurence et al., 1972). Regarding the observations on the cyclic AMP system another interpretation seems to be more probable, namely that neither chalone nor an antichalone but the cyclic AMP level in a given tissue is the limiting factor of the mitotic depression. This is strongly supported by the observation that in adrenalectomized animals the level of chalone-dependent inhibition is absolutely increased whereas with adrenalin nearly 100% mitotic depression can be achieved (Laurence and Randers-Hansen, 1971).

Regarding the action of hydrocortisone (Bullough and Laurence, 1968a) the mechanism is entirely unknown. Like other steroids this hormone does not act via cyclic AMP as a second messenger. However, there are many examples of a concerted action of steroid hormones together with cyclic AMP, for example in the sense that the steroid induces an enzyme (for instant a protein kinase) which in turn is stimulated or inhibited by cyclic

AMP. Another possibility is the induction of a substrate protein for cyclic AMP-dependent phosphorylation.

Finally, it should be mentioned that epidermal cell proliferation is also influenced by the sex hormones (Hooker and Pfeiffer, 1943; Montagna et al., 1949; Stumpf et al., 1974; Holzmann et al., 1972).

In summary, it may be concluded that in epidermis the flow of cells from the G_2 phase into mitosis is controlled by an endogenous inhibitor called G_2 chalone. This autonomous regulation is modulated by several hormonal influences causing diurnal, stress- and sex-dependent variations of epidermal mitotic activity.

7.4.6 On the mechanism of action of epidermal G_2 chalone

Adapting the theory of Jacob and Monod on gene regulation in bacteria, Bullough (1965) postulated that the epidermal chalone might act as a repressor of a mitosis operon which he thought to code for all activities related to cell division. This concept is of ingenious simplicity but still lacks any experimental evidence.

Another hypothesis which is backed by considerable more facts, had been put forward by Gelfant and Candelas (1972) and Candelas (1974). The data of these authors demonstrate quite unequivocally that the number of mitoses seen after stimulation of G_2-cells by wounding (see above) is decreased by inhibitors of translation (cycloheximide, chloramphenicol, puromycin) but increased by actinomycin D. This paradoxical actinomycin effect is interpreted within the framework of the concept of superinduction (Tomkins et al., 1972). In this theory on translational control of protein synthesis, which is based on rather hard experimental facts, it is proposed that the expression of a given mRNA of some stability is regulated by a post-transcriptional repressor and that the biosynthesis of the mRNA coding for this repressor is inhibited by actinomycin D. Gelfant and Candelas postulate that the epidermal G_2 chalone might be such a post-transcriptional repressor for a mRNA coding for a protein which is essential for a G_2-cell to enter mitosis. Although it seems rather early to speculate about the molecular mechanism of chalone action this idea is nevertheless appealing enough to provoke further experiments. Considering the time course of the paradoxical actinomycin effect as well as the cybernetic standpoint a post-transcriptional repressor has to be rather short-lived. This would be in agreement with the observation of Elgjo et al. (1971) that the epidermal G_2 chalone has disappeared shortly after treatment of skin with actinomycin D.

The presumptive dependency of chalone-dependent G_2 inhibition on cyclic AMP or adrenalin points to the possibility that the post-transcriptional repressor (G_2 chalone) has to be phosphorylated by a cyclic AMP-dependent protein kinase to be fully active. The phosphorylation of enzymes or regulatory molecules which are believed to combine with nucleic acids is a quite common phenomenon (Huijing and Lee, 1973).

Gelfant and Candelas believe that G_2 cells represent a cell population designed to deal with emergency situations such as wounding. On the other hand Elgjo (Elgjo and Edgehill, 1974; Elgjo, 1975) has called attention to the possibility that the G_2 chalone is primarily involved in cell differentiation and that it inhibits mitosis only as a secondary phenomenon.

This assumption is based on evidence that at least some cell types are committed for differentiation in the following G_1 phase while they are still in G_2 phase (Mueller, 1971; Holtzer, 1972). Since cyclic AMP frequently is involved in expression of tissue function, Elgjo (1975) believes the effect of the nucleotide on epidermal G_2 cells to lend additional support to his hypothesis.

7.4.7 G_2 Chalones in other tissues

Specific mitotic inhibitors resembling the epidermal G_2 chalone have been demonstrated in many different tissues. Thus, eye lens does not only respond to epidermal G_2 chalone but produces its own inhibitor which might be identical with the factor from skin (Voaden, 1968; Voaden and Leeson, 1970). The mitotic inhibition in lens exhibits exactly the same dependency on adrenalin as that in epidermis (Voaden, 1968). Recently it could be demonstrated that the catecholamine-induced effect in lens is also mediated by cyclic AMP (Grimes and van Sallmann, 1972); unfortunately, neither the point of attack in the cell cycle nor a possible relationship to the chalone mechanism were investigated. The significance of a G_2 chalone system in lens is stressed by the fact that in this tissue just as in epidermis, a small percentage of cells are inhibited in the G_2-phase (Hanna, 1965).

The existence in sebaceous glands (Bullough and Laurence, 1970b) and in eccrine sweat glands (Bullough and Deol, 1972) of specific G_2 chalones which are not identical to the epidermal G_2 chalone has already been mentioned above. Like the epidermal chalone both these factors are fully active in vitro only in the presence of adrenalin and hydrocortisone; in vivo stress or adrenalin injection inhibits and adrenalectomy enhances mitotic activity in both glandular tissues (Bullough and Laurence, 1970b; Bullough and Deol, 1972).

Specific G_2-inhibition by homologous extracts which was strengthened by adrenalin in vitro has been furthermore demonstrated in lung alveolar cells (Simnett et al., 1969) and in pronephros of *Xenopus laevis* (Simnett and Chopra, 1969; Chopra, 1973). The existence of a G_2 chalone in kidney (see also Saetren, 1956) might be correlated to the occurrence of a distinct population of G_2-cells in this tissue (Gelfant, 1966).

G_2 cells have been demonstrated also in esophagus (Cameron and Cleffman, 1964; Gelfant, 1966) and peripheral leucocytes (Gelfant, 1966). Interestingly, in both these tissues an adrenalin-dependent G_2-inhibition by homologous extracts was also found (Bullough and Laurence, 1970a). In the case of esophagus – not in leucocytes – the factor is obviously similar to if not identical with the epidermal G_2 chalone (Laurence, 1973b).

Mitotic activity, DNA synthesis and protein synthesis of melanocytes and melanoma cells are specifically depressed by melanoma extracts in vivo and in vitro (Bullough and Laurence, 1968c; Seiji et al., 1974). Under in vitro conditions adrenalin and hydrocortisone were essential for the inhibitory effect.

A chalone-like inhibitor was also demonstrated in the 'used' medium of chinese hamster cells which were grown to confluency. Again its effect was increased by adrenalin and at least partially restricted to the G_2 phase (Froese, 1971). Furthermore, the growth of Ehrlich ascites tumor cells is obviously controlled by two chalone-like factors acting either on G_1 or on G_2 phase (DeCosse and Gelfant, 1968; Bichel, 1971, 1973).

A similar observation was made in the case of embryonic intestine (Brugal and Pelmont, 1974). Moreover, extracts from crypt cells of the small intestine of the adult rat contain an intestinal G_2-inhibitor which does not act on epidermis, esophagus or colonic crypts. Like the epidermal chalone it was found to be heat-labile and is apparently produced by the proliferating cells rather than by the differentiated cells of the tissue (Tutton, 1973). Beta-adrenergic agonists such as isoproterenol inhibit mitosis in intestinal crypts, too, but did not augment the chalone effect. Moreover, it was shown that the stress-induced mitotic depression of intestinal mitosis was reduced by sympathectomy rather than by adrenalectomy or beta-adrenergic blockade (Tutton and Helme, 1973, 1974).

Aqueous extracts from chick stomach mucosa were found to suppress selectively mitosis in embryonic chick stomach epithelium in vitro. Epidermis, mesenchyme and intestine were not affected. The inhibitory principle was heat-labile and did not exhibit a requirement for stress hormones (Philpott, 1971). Recently it was demonstrated that injection of aortic tissue extract into swine resulted in a considerable reduction of the rate of entry of arterial smooth muscle cells into mitosis which was obviously due to

G_2 inhibition (Florentin et al., 1973). The extracts could also inhibit the pro-liferative response of arterial smooth muscle cells to injury (Nam et al., 1964).

Plant tissues are known to contain sometimes a rather high percentage of cells arrested in G_2 phase (Evans and Van 't Hof, 1974). Recently a diffusible and heat-stable factor has been demonstrated in the cotyledons of *Pisum* which inhibits root and shoot meristem cells in G_2 (Evans and Van 't Hof, 1974). This 'G_2 factor' resembles the mammalian G_2 chalone in many respects, for instance in its lack of species specificity; it does not seem, however, to be tissue-specific.

Summarizing these results, it has to be concluded that mitotic inhibition by chalone-like factors affecting the G_2-phase of the mitotic cycle is by no means restricted to epidermis but obviously a more general phenomenon. Since G_2 cell populations have been demonstrated in a great variety of tissues (Clarkson et al., 1965; Pederson and Gelfant, 1970) cell cycle control by G_2-chalones might be even more widespread than indicated by the examples cited above. In many – but not all – cases the antimitotic action is augmented by adrenalin and hydrocortisone, probably involving a similar mechanism (including cyclic AMP as a second messenger) as in epidermis. If the elevation of the intracellular level of cyclic AMP is the key event, a strengthening of the chalone effect can be expected to be accomplished not only by catecholamines but also by other hormones or factors acting on the adenyl cyclase system.

7.5 Epidermal G_1 chalone

7.5.1 Extraction

Epidermal G_1 chalone has been extracted from skin and epidermis homo-genates in the same manner as described above for G_2 chalone (Hennings et al., 1969; Elgjo et al., 1971; Marks, 1971, 1973a; Wiley et al., 1973; Bertsch and Marks, 1974).

7.5.2 Assay

The only test for the activity of epidermal G_1 chalone which can be con-sidered to be reasonably reliable, is the in vivo assay. Unless hairless mice are used, only animals in the telogen phase of their hair cycle should be used (Marks, 1971, 1973a) (age 7–8 weeks); otherwise the considerable DNA synthesis in hair follicle cells might overwhelm the determination of the rather low synthetic rate in interfollicular epidermis. Since epidermal DNA synthesis shows pronounced diurnal variations (Tvermyr, 1972), provisions should be made for a constant day–night rhythm in the animal house. Furthermore, all experiments should be done at the same hour of the day (the same is – by the way – recommended for investigations of the G_2 chalone).

The animals are injected intraperitoneally with the test sample. At the time when the inhibitory effect of the chalone has reached its maximum (8–15 h later) (Hennings et al., 1969; Marks 1971, 1973a), the epidermal DNA is pulse-labelled with [^{3}H]thymidine. This has been done either in vitro or in vivo. For the in vivo approach the animals are intraperitoneally injected with thymidine and killed 30–60 min later. Five min prior to sacrifice, the hair of the back is removed by means of a cosmetic depilator. Immediately after killing the depilated skin is dissected and immersed in icecold perchloric acid. The epidermis is scraped off with a scalpel. After homogenization the specific radioactivity of the DNA, which had been isolated by means of the Schmidt–Thannhauser procedure, is measured (Marks, 1973a).

Instead of isolating the DNA one can evaluate the labelling by autoradiography (Elgjo et al., 1972; Elgjo, 1974a; Nome, 1974). Since autoradiography is, of course, much more time consuming it is not suitable for routine testing but should be used as a control of the biochemical method. The pro and con of both methods have been discussed in detail by Hennings and Elgjo (1970) and by Lord in this volume.

If in vitro labelling (Marks, 1971, 1973a) is required, the assay should be done with animals which had been shaved 3–6 days prior to the experiment. Eight to fifteen hours after chalone injection the mice are killed and the back skin is immediately dissected. After scraping off the subcutaneous tissue by means of a scalpel the remaining skin is cut into small pieces and incubated with labelled thymidine in Eagle's medium at 37 °C for 45 min. The medium is then replaced by icecold water containing an excess of unlabelled thymidine and the tissue fragments are homogenized by means of a loosely fitting Potter–Elvejhem homogenizer. After having removed connective tissue by filtration through gauze, the DNA is isolated from the filtrate in the usual manner and checked for specific radioactivity.

The in vitro assay of epidermal G_1 chalone in short-term tissue culture is subject to some severe handicaps. Since the inhibitory effect of chalone is delayed for several hours, skin explants used for the test not only have to be kept alive but also maintained in an active state of DNA synthesis over a rather long period of time. This has not yet been successfully managed. It has been shown (Marks et al., 1971; Dahl and Shuster, 1972; Young et al.,

1975) that epidermis from freshly sacrificed animals rapidly declines in its ability to synthesize DNA in vitro approaching a minimum somewhere between 10 and 24 h. Obviously only those cells, which have already entered the S-phase at the moment of sacrifice, will synthesize DNA in vitro. Only after 40 h does thymidine incorporation reach a new high value, most probably due to an entry of new cells from the G_1 into the S phase. Therefore, short term cultures limit observations to S-phase alone rather than to the G_1-S transition which is most probably the point-of-attack of G_1 chalone. Moreover, explants resemble damaged skin and there is some evidence that wounded epidermis does not respond to G_1 chalone in the proper manner (Bertsch and Marks, 1974; Bertsch, 1975; Bertsch, Csontos, Schweizer and Marks, in press).

In some laboratories long term tissue cultures of skin or epidermis have been used as a test system for G_1 (Delescluse et al., 1971, 1972a, b; Wiley et al., 1973) and G_2 chalone (McGuire and Arensen, 1972) effects. However, the results are rather conflicting and cannot be easily compared with in vivo results. Obviously epidermal DNA synthesis in vitro seems to be very susceptible to many external influences and it is always extremely difficult to decide whether an inhibition observed is due to a chalone or to more nonspecific or cytotoxic effects. Since the living animal acts like a filter, difficulties of that kind are believed to be minimized under in vivo conditions.

Especially dangerous is the use of cultures prepared from fetal or neonatal skin, because it has been shown that they respond only to extremely high doses of skin extract (Bertsch and Marks, 1974; Bertsch, 1975; Fusenig, Raab and Marks, unpublished results). This may have something to do with the fact that – at least in mice – embryonic and neonatal epidermis is obviously not controlled by G_1 chalone but the chalone, responsiveness of the tissue seems to be developed at the earliest one week after birth (Bertsch and Marks, 1974).

7.5.3 Attempts on purification and characterization

Thus far the most extensive attempt on isolation and chemical characterization of the epidermal G_1 chalone has been made by Marks and coworkers in collaboration with the Organon company (Marks, 1971, 1973a, 1974).

Their starting material was the same pig-skin extract which was used for the purification of the epidermal G_2 chalone (Hondius-Boldingh and Laurence, 1968). In the in vivo assay ethanol fractions from this extract exhibited a reversible and dose-dependent depression of thymidine incorporation into epidermal DNA. The effect showed some delay similar to that originally reported by Hennings et al. (1969) for mouse epidermis extract and reached its maximum at about 12 h after injection (Marks, 1971, 1973a). In contrast to the G_2 chalone approximately 5–10 times more activity was found in the 55–72% ethanol precipitate as compared with the 72–81% precipitate whereas the 81% ethanol supernatant was lacking any activity (Marks, 1974, and unpublished results). The inhibitor could neither be destroyed by heating the neutral solution to 100 °C (for 1 h) nor by denaturing agents such as phenol, urea, 1 M formic acid (70 °C), or ionic detergents (100 °C) (Marks, 1971, 1973a). Furthermore, it was completely resistant to trypsin, pronase, ribonuclease, desoxyribonuclease, β-neuraminidase, collagenase and hyaluronidase (Marks, 1971, 1973a and unpublished results) digestion. However, complete inactivation was achieved by brief heating in 0.1 M sodium hydroxide. Despite its extreme stability the factor was not dialysable and was eluted from Sephadex G-200 with the void volume indicating a molecular weight of at least 3×10^5 daltons (Marks, 1973a). This high value, which was retained even after extensive proteolytic digestion, was partially due to non-specific intermolecular interactions (Marks, 1973a). Because of this strong aggregation and its complicating consequences, the starting material had to be disaggregated prior to any purification procedure. This was achieved by incubating the solution of the 55–72% ethanol precipitate with an excess of dithiothreitol and sodium dodecyl sulfate (SDS) and afterwards by blocking free sulphhydryl groups by alkylation with iodoacetamide or iodoacetic acid. The mixture was then digested with pronase over several days (Marks, 1974 and unpublished results). The active material in the digest was retained on DEAE cellulose and could be eluted only with 0.3–0.5 M NaCl (Marks, 1974, and unpublished results); this indicates a rather acidic compound. From Biogel P-100 most of the activity was eluted by 7 M urea/0.5% SDS with the void volume. Therefore the factor has an apparent molecular weight of more than 2×10^4 daltons. This was in accordance with the observation that after proteolytic digestion the chalone was still non-dialyzable even in the presence of 1% SDS or 7 M urea. From the dialyzed pronase digest most of the activity could be separated by precipitation with cetylpyridinium chloride. This quaternary ammonium salt forms insoluble complexes with polyanionic compounds such as nucleic acids or acidic mucopolysaccharides. From the aqueous solution of the precipitated material the chalone-activity could be quantitatively extracted with 80% aqueous phenol. By this procedure it could be separated from the bulk of polyanionic material. Finally, a 2000-fold purification over

the ethanol precipitate or a 400,000-fold enrichment over the crude lyophilized skin extract was achieved (Marks, unpublished results).

According to the preliminary analyses the purified fraction consists
roughly of 35% protein, 16% neutral sugar, 8% polyanionic material,
probably mucopolysaccharide and RNA and 2% hexosamin. Since the
activity cannot be destroyed by RNase, the active principle is most likely
a mucopolysaccharide-containing glycoprotein. As shown by its resistance
to hyaluronidase digestion the chalone activity does not involve hyaluronic
acid (Marks, unpublished results).

A dose of as little as 0.05–0.1 μg of this preparation intraperitoneally injected into an adult mouse turned out to be sufficient for a 50–70% inhibition of epidermal DNA synthesis (Marks, unpublished results). This
dose can probably still be lowered by further purification. Therefore, the
activity of the G_1 chalone is expected to be in the range of that of a hormone.
One can easily calculate that for the isolation of a few milligrams of pure
material one has to start with several kilograms of lyophilized and defatted
skin powder.

A pronase- and heat-resistant G_1 inhibitor of high molecular weight could
also be demonstrated in extracts from pure mouse epidermis which had
been isolated either by scraping or by means of the acetic acid procedure
(Schweizer and Marks, unpublished results). In those extracts another inhibitor with a molecular weight between 10^3 and 10^4 daltons was found.
It is also resistant to heat and proteases. Whether there are any relationships
between the high – and the low – molecular weight fractions is still unknown.

Recently Wiley et al. (1973) demonstrated G_1 inhibitor in the 60% and
the 70–80% ethanol precipitate of pig-skin extract whereas the 80% ethanol
supernatant was shown to enhance thymidine incorporation in an in vitro
test system (cell culture of guinea pig epidermis).

7.5.4 Reversibility and tissue-specificity of action

Since the inhibitory effect of epidermal G_1 chalone was observed only with
adult mice and not with newborn animals (Bertsch and Marks, 1974) in vivo
or in primary cultures of fetal mouse epidermis cells or explants of chick
embryo epidermis (Bertsch, 1975; Fusenig, Raab and Marks, unpublished
results), it must be considered to be non-toxic. This is supported by the
extremely high specific activity of the most purified preparations (Marks,
unpublished results) and by the results of Elgjo (1974a) indicating that the
inhibition is fully reversible.

The first evidence of tissue-specificity was provided by Hennings et al.

(1969) by showing that a liver extract which was prepared in the same way as the epidermis extract did not inhibit epidermal DNA synthesis in vivo. Marks (1971, 1973a) reported similar results: in his experiments neither liver, lung nor kidney extracts depressed thymidine incorporation into epidermal DNA. Conversely, pig-skin extract did not inhibit thymidine incorporation into diaphragm, kidney, lung, spleen and adipose/connective tissues. Recently, Elgjo and Edgehill (1974) failed to demonstrate any epidermal G_1 chalone activity in extracts from dermis or serum.

Again an important demonstration of tissue-specificity comes from Nome (1974) in Oslo. He compared the effect of extracts made from several tissues on the labelling index and the thymidine incorporation in epidermis and the epithelia of forestomach, jejunum and colon. As shown in table 7.3, tissue-specificity of the inhibition of DNA synthesis was of the same nature as shown for the G_2 chalone (see table 7.2): skin extract depressed the DNA synthesis of epidermis and forestomach but not of jejunum and colon. Vice versa, forestomach extract acted only on forestomach and epidermis. Extracts from glandular stomach and small intestine were found to be completely inactive when tested in epidermis. Nome pointed out that 'the results are in agreement with a hypothesis that squamous cell epithelia produce and contain a G_1 chalone which acts specifically on such epithelia, regardless of their ectodermal or endodermal origin' (Nome, 1974). The finding that in mouse epidermis the G_1 chalone seems to be restricted almost entirely to the keratinizing cell layers (Elgjo et al., 1972) is in accordance with the assumption that this factor is produced in the course of keratinization.

An inhibitory effect of epidermal extracts, but not of liver extracts, on

Table 7.3

Percentage reduction in different mouse epithelia of labelling index (LI) and specific incorporation of labelled thymidine into DNA after injection of 10 mg tissue extract (nd means 'not done'). (From Nome, 1974.)

Tissue on which effect was measured		Tissue from which extracts were made			
		Skin	Fore-stomach	Glandular stomach	Small intestine
Epidermis	LI	41	50	—	12
	Incorp.	41	60	nd	nd
Forestomach	LI	36	55	—	9
	Incorp.	nd	nd	nd	nd
Jejunum	LI	11	7	—	3
	Incorp.	—	7	nd	nd
Colon	LI	19	15	—	6
	Incorp.	22	14	nd	nd

DNA synthesis in mouse forestomach in vivo has also been reported by Frankfurt (1971). After four injections over a period of 11 h the percentage of labelled cells was significantly lowered whereas no significant difference in intensity of labelling (grains per cell) could be detected. Measuring the labelling index in mouse epidermis after in vivo treatment with skin extract Elgjo came to the same conclusion (K. Elgjo, personal communication). These results indicate that the effect of epidermal G_1 chalone is due to a true inhibition of the transition of cells from the G_1 to the S phase instead of to more indirect effects such as a delay of the labelling of the intercellular thymidine pool or a direct blockade of the S phase.

Of course, an endogenous regulator such as a chalone has necessarily to be expected to control the flow of cells into the S-phase whereas an inhibition of DNA replication itself would be meaningless from the biological and cybernetic point of view.

Yamaguchi et al. (1974) have measured the effect of extracts from guinea pig epidermis on the labelling index and the mitotic activity in mouse ear epidermis 2 days after wounding in vivo. A rapid decrease in the grain counts 1 h after injection of extract was observed. This effect lasted for about 4 h and may reflect either a direct inhibition of cells in S-phase or a delay of labelling of the intracellular thymidine pool. A significant decrease in the number of labelled cells was not observed before the sixth hour (unfortunately the authors did not follow up their experiment for a longer time). The early effect is in contrast to the observations of Hennings et al. (1969) and Marks (1971, 1973a). This discrepancy may be explained by the different ways of chalone administration: in the study of Yamaguchi et al. the extract was injected subcutaneously instead of intraperitoneally. Moreover, since crude epidermal extract was used, the effect on S-phase (or pool-labelling) and the effect on G_1-S-transition may be due to different factors rather than to one and the same inhibitor, the epidermal G_1 chalone.

As compared with intraperitoneal administration, subcutaneous injection is more closely related to in vitro conditions. Indeed, in in vitro studies with epidermal tissue cultures an early effect of skin extracts on thymidine incorporation (S-phase inhibition?) has been repeatedly observed (Marks et al., 1971; Dahl and Shuster, 1972; Delescluse et al., 1972b). In this connection the important results of Gradwohl have to be mentioned, which have been published only as a short communication (Gradwohl, 1973) but which came to the author's knowledge in more detail by personal contact. While an apparently tissue-specific inhibition by skin extract of DNA synthesis was observed in vivo the results obtained in vitro (explants of mouse ear and P-815 mastocytoma cells) were highly conflicting. Thus, the activity of the extract could not be concentrated in a distinct fraction. Furthermore, the inhibition observed was not tissue-specific and was at least partially due to the strong cytotoxicity of the extract.

Tissue-nonspecificity of epidermal extracts under in vitro conditions has also been reported by Rothberg and Arp (1973, 1975) (and – regarding G_2 inhibition – by McGuire and Arensen (1972)). It has been recently shown that unlabelled thymidine in tissue extracts may simulate the effect of a G_1 chalone (Lenfant et al., 1973). The danger of being misled in this or another way is especially given when the extract is tested in tissue culture or by local (subcutaneous) administration in vivo. In the author's opinion tissue cultures are therefore not suitable for testing specificity unless the fraction to be tested has been rigorously purified.

7.5.5 Hormones

Whereas adrenalin and other catecholamines as well as cyclic AMP are mitotic inhibitors (G_2-phase blocker) in epidermis and apparently enhance the activity of epidermal G_2 chalone in vitro, no such an effect could be observed regarding DNA synthesis and G_1 chalone (Gelfant, 1963; Baden and Sviokla, 1968). Frankfurt (1968, 1971) has even found a stimulation of thymidine incorporation in forestomach cells after injection of adrenalin.

Moreover, no correlation between G_1 chalone and the cyclic AMP system has as yet been detected (Marks and Rebien, 1972; Marks and Grimm, 1972; Marks, 1973b; Marks and Raab, 1974; Elgjo, 1975). This statement seems to be in contrast to the findings of Teel (1972) in which an additive inhibitory effect of dibutyryl cyclic AMP and a homologous extract on hamster cheek pouch epithelium in tissue culture was demonstrated. However, in these experiments the tissue was preincubated together with the cyclic nucleotide and the extract for 6–18 h prior to a 6-h pulse-labelling with thymidine. Therefore, the inhibition of DNA synthesis could well have been the consequence of an early G_2-blockade. The investigation of Teel was based on a study of Hall (1970) demonstrating a complete inhibition of thymidine incorporation when hamster cheek pouch epithelium was cultured for 20 h in the presence of a homologous tissue extract. The inhibitory activity was shown to be thermolabile and could not be found in connective tissue extracts. Since neither cytotoxicity, tissue-nonspecificity nor an effect on the G_2-phase was excluded by the author, some doubts may be raised against his conclusion that the inhibition was due to an epidermal G_1 chalone.

In contrast to catecholamines, glucocorticoids have been proven to inhibit both mitosis and DNA synthesis in squamous epithelia. Frankfurt (1968) reported on a blockade of the transition of forestomach cells into the phase of DNA synthesis when mice were injected with hydrocortisone. His experiments indicate that for the hormone effect there is a critical point in the late G_1 phase when the cells are preparing for DNA synthesis. In accordance with these findings Hennings and Elgjo (1971) have observed a *delayed* response of DNA synthesis in mouse epidermis to local administration of hydrocortisone: after a lag phase of several hours a maximal inhibition of 60% was reached at 12 h. This time course and its dose-dependency as well as the maximal response show a striking similarity to that observed after injection of epidermal G_1 chalone and it may be proposed that both hydrocortisone and chalone act at the same critical point in the late G_1-phase of the cell cycle. However, whereas hydrocortisone also inhibited the increased epidermal DNA synthesis produced by croton oil treatment (Hennings and Elgjo, 1971) no such effect could be achieved with epidermal G_1 chalone (Krieg et al., 1974). Therefore, both agents seem to have different receptor sites.

A delayed inhibition of epidermal DNA synthesis and a blockade of the G_1-S-transition in forestomach cells was also observed after application of actinomycin D (Frankfurt, 1968). It may be assumed, therefore, that at the critical point of the G_1-phase the synthesis of mRNA essential for the cell to enter the S-phase takes place.

The effect of hydrocortisone on the mitotic activity turned out to be biphasic: an early transient inhibition at 6 h – most probably due to G_2 inhibition (see above) – was followed by a late long-lasting depression reaching its maximum between 16 and 24 h (Hennings and Elgjo, 1971). The second inhibition was probably related to the preceding G_1-blockade.

In the light of these results the well known diurnal variation of epidermal DNA synthesis (Tvermyr, 1972) has to be considered to be the consequence of the inhibitory effect of glucocorticoids rather than of adrenalin.

It may be proposed that whereas the flow of cells into the phase of DNA replication is controlled by the endogeneous G_1 chalone mechanism, this autonomous regulation is overwhelmed or modulated by hormonal influences.

7.5.6 On the mechanism of action of epidermal G_1 chalone

The epidermal G_1 chalone seems to fulfil all the requirements of a 'chalone proper': it is apparently produced by the differentiating cells and inhibits the proliferation of the germinative cell population. Like a hormone, it displays its effect in minute amounts; its action is reversible, non-toxic and tissue- but not species-specific. The point-of-attack is in the late G_1-phase of the mitotic cycle, probably when the cell has to 'decide' between proliferation and maturation (dichophase).

Its unique chemical (Marks, 1973a) and metabolic (Elgjo et al., 1971) stability is consistent with the findings of Marks (unpublished) indicating that it is a mucopolysaccharide-containing glycoprotein (although the possibility that it is only firmly aggregated with a mucopolysaccharide has not yet been excluded). These findings are in accordance with the results of Mizuno and Fujii (1969; Fujii and Mizuno, 1969) indicating that the epidermal carrier of growth-controlling information is a glycoprotein containing a heparin-like mucopolysaccharide (see above). In general, mucopolysaccharides seem to be a main component of the 'intercellular cement' of epidermis (see for example Flesch and Esoda, 1964; Kligman, 1964). Recently the occurrence in keratinosomes (Odland bodies) of acidic mucopolysaccharides among other substances has been demonstrated (Ohashi et al., 1973). These lamellar granules enclosed by membranes are formed and extruded by the prickle cells just below the horny layer. They seem to discharge their contents into the intercellular space. However, the function of this material is not been yet fully understood. Beside the assumption that it is an intercellular cement, the possibility should be taken into consideration that it contains growth regulating substances such as the G_1 chalone. A chalone is thought to bring about the feedback between functionalized and germinative cells. Therefore it has to be discharged into the intercellular space. Since keratinized cells are dead, the chalone should be secreted just before this final stage of differentiation is reached. However, at that time the cell membrane might be already so thick that a secretion is possible only by means of an extrusion of granules such as the Odland bodies.

Another interesting site of mucopolysaccharide accumulation is the desmosomes which form intercellular junctions by means of a cement which perhaps stems from the keratinosomes (Orfanos, 1972). It has recently been postulated by the author (Marks, 1973a) that the G_1 chalone might act at the cell membrane, a hypothesis which is based on the assumption that epidermal cell proliferation is controlled by means of a special kind of 'contact inhibition'. The migration of the cell from the basal layer to the skin surface is thought to cause a local loosening of intercellular contacts (desmosomes?); as a consequence, the proliferation of the corresponding basal cell is induced, whereas the injection of G_1 chalone leads to an inhibition by covering the exposed contact sites (fig. 7.9).

Cell contact, cell movement and cell proliferation are closely related

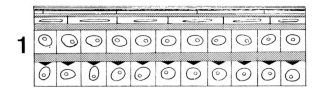

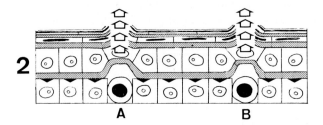

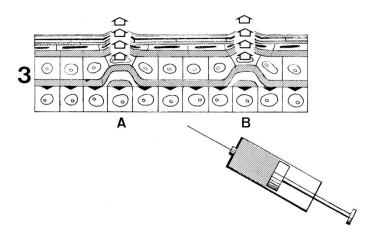

Fig. 7.9. Tentative mechanism of epidermal growth control by membrane-bound G_1 chalone. Diagram 1: schematic representation of a mitotically resting epidermis; specific cell-to-cell contact via G_1 chalone (hatched zones) prevents the G_1-S transition in basal cells. Diagram 2: local loosening of contact due to cell migration (or 'degeneration') in the course of keratinization causes a local release of basal cells (A and B) from chalone inhibition; these cells are going to enter the S phase. Diagram 3: covering of receptor sites on the membranes of the cells A and B after injection of epidermal G_1 chalone; the cells are again inhibited at the G_1-S transition.

processes. For example, it is well known that epidermal wounds are closed primarily by the active migration of epidermal cells with cell proliferation being of secondary importance. Implying that the process of wound repair is only an amplification of the situation occurring normally in epidermis, Winter (1972) has proposed that migration of epidermal cells from the basal layer to the skin surface might be the consequence of active cell movement rather than of direct or indirect mitotic pressure, so that the everyday physiological regeneration of epidermis might be primarily a matter of cell migration. This has been recently supported by results of Potten and Allen (1975) showing that the immediate reaction of epidermis to a removal of the layer of keratinized cells (stripping) is a rapid movement of cells from the underlying basal layer to the superficial layers. This results in a depopulation of the stem cell compartment which is secondarily compensated by enhanced cell proliferation causing transient hyperplasia. The whole process is accompanied by profound alterations of desmosomal structures (Potten and Allen, 1975) and by a temporary loss of the tissue's responsiveness to epidermal G_1 chalone (Bertsch, 1975; Bertsch, Csontos, Schweizer and Marks, in preparation). It should be taken into consideration, therefore that the primary effect of a chalone – especially of the epidermal G_1 chalone – may be the inhibition of cell migration with depression of cell proliferation being the secondary consequence. This idea is again consistent with the results of Mizuno and Fujii (1969; Fujii and Mizuno, 1969) indicating control of epidermal cell proliferation *and* cell movement by means of an exchange of chemical messengers (see above).

7.6 Epidermal chalones and hyperplasia

Despite its great heuristic value, several objections may be raised against the concept of a *simple* negative feedback regulation of epidermal cell proliferation. Bullough (1965, 1973) has emphasized that, if the epidermal tissue mass is controlled only in that way, any increased mitotic activity must lead to increased tissue mass. Actually, however, in undamaged epidermis any change of the mitotic rate is so exactly matched by corresponding changes in the rate of cell maturation that the ratio of both these rates is a constant (Bullough, 1972). Therefore, Bullough postulated that a chalone has three functions, firstly to inhibit cell proliferation, secondly to delay cell maturation and thirdly to 'decide' whether a cell runs through the mitotic cycle once more or enters the ageing pathway. Whereas the first function – inhibition of cell proliferation – is now fairly well established by experimental evidence, direct experimental approaches to confirm the other functions of chalone have not yet been made. In the case of epidermis this was primarily due to the lack of proper biochemical methods to measure the rate of epidermal differentiation as well as to the impurity of chalone preparations.

However, the question may be asked as to whether it is really necessary to postulate a chalone effect on differentiation: if one assumes – according to Weiss and Kavanau as well as to Iversen – that a change of mitotic activity is always the *consequence* of a corresponding change in the rate and degree of cell differentiation (and at present there are no facts which could disprove this) the mitotic rate is necessarily and directly coupled to the rate of cell maturation.

In damaged epidermis, however, the situation seems indeed to be more complicated, because the automatic response of epidermis to any type of injury is not simply compensatory growth but transient hyperplasia. This hyperplasia is not only an overshooting of the regenerative reaction but obviously a rather long lasting transformation of the tissue involving a complete breakdown of the columnar structures and a dearrangement of the epidermal proliferative units (see, for example, Potten and Allen, 1975). Bullough (1972) has tried to explain the hyperplastic response by assuming the existence of epidermis in at least two different phases which he believes to be related to the intraepidermal chalone concentration. 'Phase 1 epidermis', as realized in mice, rats and senile man, is thin, has a flat junction to the underlying dermis and a low mitotic rate. The basal layer exists of mitotic and early post-mitotic cells; the latter are committed to keratinization and are extruded into the superficial layers. As long as the mitotic rate does not exceed a certain limit the thickness of phase 1 epidermis depends solely on the post-mitotic lifespan of the keratinocytes and is independent of the proliferative activity in the basal layer. This limit is thought to be controlled by the chalone level. Beyond it, phase 1 epidermis is transformed into 'phase 2 epidermis', which is realized in guinea pigs, pigs and man and any condition of benign hyperplasia. In phase 2 epidermis the chalone concentration is thought to be so low that all basal cells are in the mitotic cycle so that no post-mitotic cells remain to be driven out. As a consequence the basal layer is folded due to the pressure generated by cell divisions. This, in turn, leads to a thickening of the tissue, because the number of mitotic cells per unit area of skin is increased. Since – according to Bullough's view – the chalone controls both proliferative activity and the rate of cell ageing, the increased mitotic rate in phase 2 epidermis is matched by a decreased post-mitotic life span. This concept offers an elegant explanation of many observations on morphology and cell kinetics. However, its underlying principle – the relation of the phases to the chalone level and the emphasis on cell proliferation as the driving force – is as yet highly speculative. Furthermore, the existence of *two* epidermal chalones has not been taken into consideration.

Recent investigations indicate that the situation might be in fact even more complex. First of all, the metabolic stability of G_1 chalone leads to the assumption that it is the chalone responsiveness of the target cells rather than the absolute level of the inhibitor by which regenerative processes are induced and controlled. This is indeed supported by experiments showing that epidermal hyperplasia is always accompanied by a temporary decrease or even abolition of the tissue's ability to respond to G_1 chalone, regardless whether it is induced by chemical or mechanical means (Krieg et al., 1974; Bertsch, 1975; Bertsch, Csontos, Schweizer and Marks, unpublished results).

Hyperplastic epidermis morphologically resembles (at least in mice) fetal or neonatal tissue. As already mentioned above, it has been shown by Bertsch and Marks (1974) that neonatal mouse epidermis does not respond to G_1 chalone although it is obviously able to synthesize the factor (this is consistent with the concept that chalone production is an automatic consequence of tissue differentiation: neonatal mouse epidermis is a fully keratinized epithelium). However, the responsiveness is established within the first weeks post natum. This clearly indicates that G_1 chalone is not *absolutely* necessary for maintaining growth control in epidermis but that it is essential for the maintenance of the *adult* stage of the tissue. During hyperplastic transformation this configuration breaks down into a 'pseudo-embryonic' state. It has been mentioned already that in hyperplastic epidermis also the ordered structure of the epidermal proliferative units is broken down. This striking coincidence points to the possibility that the G_1 chalone mechanism is closely related to a particular architecture of the tissue, which again is an expression of a highly ordered system of intercellular contacts. It must be emphasized, therefore, that growth regulation cannot be properly understood without regarding morphological facts. This seems to be self-evident; nevertheless, it has been neglected in the chalone literature quite often.

In analogy to the haemopoietic system, where the inhibitory effect of G_1 chalones is restricted to the committed stem cells whereas the pluripotential stem cells do not respond, it was proposed (Krieg et al., 1974; Bertsch and Marks, 1974) that also in epidermis only committed stem cells can be blocked by G_1 chalone. This assumption, which is closely related to Potten's concept of a two-compartment stem cell population in epidermis (Potten, 1974), implies that the physiological regeneration of neonatal mouse epidermis is almost exclusively brought about by G_1 chalone – insensitive pluripotential stem cells which will be replaced by G_1 chalone – sensitive committed stem cells during maturation of the animal. After treatment with hyperplasiogenic agents, wounding or other damage, the state of this cellular commitment is more or less reversed, either by an enhanced proliferation of residual pluripotential stem cells (G_2 cells?, see Gelfant and Candelas, 1972) or by transient dedifferentiation of 'committed' to 'pluripotential' cells or both. Dedifferentiation has indeed been demonstrated after treatment of mouse epidermis with tumor-promoting mitogens (Raick, 1973, 1974) and is thought generally to accompany wound healing. It is most probably the cause of metaplastic processes such as the repair of interfollicular epidermis by cells from hair roots or sebaceous glands as well as, for example, lens regeneration from iris epithelium (Yamada, 1972). Any metaplasia, during which a differentiated cell population 'reverses its commitment and asumes a type of differentiation distinct from the original one' (Yamada, 1972), must necessarily be accompanied by a temporary 'switching-off' of cell-line specific autoregulation such as the G_1 chalone mechanism.

The situation is apparently different for the G_2 chalone. It has been shown that neonatal (Krieg, 1975) as well as hyperplastic (Frankfurt, 1971) epidermis does in fact respond to this factor. Therefore, a simple feedback system which is controlled via the absolute level of chalone seems to exist for at least this case. However, taking into account the localization of G_2 chalone in basal cells (Elgjo et al., 1971) one may assume that there is a feedback within the stem cell population (perhaps between committed and pluripotential stem cells) rather than the classical chalone feedback between differentiated and proliferative tissue compartments. On the other hand, if Gelfant's hypothesis is correct that the G_2 chalone is a post-transcriptional repressor (Gelfant and Candelas, 1972; Candelas, 1974) or – according to Elgjo (1975; Elgjo and Edgehill, 1974)–a factor which sustains cell maturation, this inhibitor might be an *intra*cellular rather than an *inter*cellular messenger.

7.7 Epidermal chalones and carcinogenesis

Bullough (Bullough, 1965, 1972; Bullough and Deol, 1971b) has suggested that tumor growth is due to a permanent disturbance of endogeneous growth control such as the chalone mechanism. Therefore, the question of whether the chalone production (chalone level) or the chalone responsiveness of a tumor is altered in a significant manner is of crucial importance for experimental cancer research.

The three epidermal tumors investigated so far (the V $\times$ 2 carcinoma of the rabbit (Bullough and Laurence, 1968b), the Chernozemski carcinoma of the hamster (Elgjo and Hennings, 1971; Laurence and Elgjo, 1971) and the Hewitt carcinoma of the mouse (Bullough and Deol, 1971a)) were all shown to contain epidermal G_2 chalone. The tumor cells were also found to be fully responsive to the G_2 chalone in vivo and in vitro. In vitro an absolute requirement for adrenalin was observed.

As the tumor grew the mitotic activity in the normal epidermis of the tumor-bearing animal was more and more depressed. In sebaceous glands such an inhibition could not be observed. Therefore, the authors concluded that this depression could not be due to stress or another more unspecific effect but could be taken as an indication of chalone production by the tumor: as the tumor grows the chalone concentration in the whole body rises and the mitotic activity of the normal epidermis falls. The authors postulated that – due to an abnormally high rate of chalone loss into the blood – the chalone level in the tumor is permanently lowered. However, *direct* experimental evidence supporting this interesting hypothesis is still lacking.

Elgjo and Hennings (1971) reported on experiments showing that a single intraperitoneal injection of the active ethanol precipitate of pig skin extract (Hondius-Boldingh and Laurence, 1968) caused a significant depression not only of mitoses (34%) but also of DNA labelling (more than 80%) in the Czernozemski carcinoma of the hamster. Despite this massive reduction of DNA labelling no tumor regression could be observed when the animals were repeatedly injected over several days.

A similar study has been made by Bertsch and Marks (unpublished results). Using the Hewitt carcinoma of the mouse these authors found a strong inhibition of DNA labelling after a single intraperitoneal injection of the 50–70% ethanol precipitate of pig skin extract. This effect was accompanied by marked symptoms of an intoxication of the animals (a similar observation was made by Elgjo and Hennings, 1971). When the experiment was repeated with a highly purified preparation of epidermal G_1 chalone neither an inhibition of DNA labelling nor signs of illness due to a toxic effect were observed. It was concluded, therefore, that the depression of DNA synthesis caused by the impure chalone preparation was due to cytotoxic side effects or to an inhibition of pool labelling rather than to the activity of epidermal G_1 chalone. Consequently, repeated injections of high doses of highly purified G_1 chalone failed to cause any decrease of tumor growth (Marks, unpublished results).

These results can easily be interpreted if one assumes that a tumor is first of all a tissue with disturbed or altered differentiation (i.e. the sequence pluripotency → commitment → adolescence; see, for example, Fiala, 1968 or Raick, 1974). It has been pointed out above that G_1 chalone responsiveness is an expression of the mature, fully differentiated epidermis which is thought to be regenerated by committed stem cells and that neonatal or hyperlastic (dedifferentiated) tissue is obviously not controlled by G_1 chalone. This means that a tumor is the less responsive to G_1 chalone the more it is dedifferentiated. The availability of epidermal tumors with different degrees of malignancy like the Morris hepatomas would be very suitable to resolve this problem. In contrast to G_1 chalone the epidermal G_2 chalone has been shown to inhibit cell division equally well in adult, neonatal and hyperplastic epidermis. The inhibition of tumor cell division by this factor can, therefore, easily be understood and is in accordance with the hypothesis developed above.

The effect of chemical carcinogens on epidermal G_2 chalone was studied in two laboratories. Bishai et al. (1971) reported that after treatment of mouse skin with labelled dimethylbenzanthracene the hydrocarbon was found to be bound to several soluble proteins which could be precipitated with 70–80% ethanol. Since the authors did not determine the actual chalone activity of this fraction or of any of the binding proteins some doubts may be raised on their conclusion that DMBA was covalently bound to epidermal G_2 chalone and that this reaction has something to do with carcinogenesis.

Recently Rohrbach and Laerum (1974) observed a diminished antimitotic activity of extracts from methylcholanthrene-treated mouse epidermis which might be due to a transient inactivation of the epidermal G_2 chalone. Whether this may be considered to be a parameter of carcinogenesis or was due to more unspecific effects of the hydrocarbon such as cytotoxicity or irritating activity remains to be established.

References

Abercrombie, M. (1957) Localized formation of new tissue in an adult mammal. Symp. Soc. Exp. Biol. 11, 235–254.

Baden, H. P. and Sviokla, S. (1968) The effect of chalone on epidermal DNA synthesis. Exp. Cell Res. 50, 644.

Bertsch, S. (1975) Untersuchungen zur Wachstumskontrolle in embryonaler, neonataler und regenerierender Epidermis. Ph. D. Thesis. University of Heidelberg.

Bertsch, S. and Marks, F. (1974) Lack of an effect of tumor-promoting phorbol esters and of epidermal G_1 chalone on DNA synthesis in the epidermis of newborn mice. Cancer Res. 34, 3283–3288.

Bichel, P. (1971) Autoregulation of ascites tumour growth by inhibition of the G-1 and the G-2 phase. Europ. J. Cancer 7, 349–355.

Bichel, P. (1973) Self-limitation of ascites tumor growth: a possible chalone regulation. Natl. Cancer Inst. Monogr. 38, 197–203.

Bishai, I. S. M., Moscarello, M. A. and Ritchie, A. C. (1971) Dimethylbenzanthracene binding to epidermal chalone. Nature 232, 114–116.

Brønstad, G. O., Elgjo, K. and Øye, I. (1971) Adrenalin increases cyclic 3′, 5′-AMP formation in hamster epidermis. Nature New Biol. 233, 78–79.

Brugal, G. and Pelmont, J. (1974) Présence, dans l'intestin du Triton adulte *Pleurodeles waltlii* Michah., de deux facteurs antimitotiques naturels (chalones) actifs sur la proliferation cellulaire de l'intestin embryonnaire. C. R. Acad. Sci. Paris, D 278, 2831–2834.

Bullough, W. S. (1962) The control of mitotic activity in adult mammalian tissues. Biol. Rev. 37, 307–342.

Bullough, W. S. (1964) The production of epidermal cells. Symp. Zool. Soc. London 12, 1–23.

Bullough, W. S. (1965) Mitotic and functional homeostasis: a speculative review. Cancer Res. 25, 1683–1727.

Bullough, W. S. (1967) The evolution of differentiation. (Academic Press, London and New York).

Bullough, W. S. (1972) The control of epidermal thickness. Brit. J. Dermatol. 87, 187–199 and 347–354.

Bullough, W. S. (1973) Epidermal chalone mechanism. Natl. Cancer Inst. Monogr. 38, 99–107.

Bullough, W. S. and Deol, J. U. R. (1971a) Chalone-induced mitotic inhibition in the Hewitt keratinising epidermal carcinoma of the mouse. Europ. J. Cancer 7, 425–431.

Bullough, W. S. and Deol, J. U. R. (1971b) The pattern of tumor growth. Symp. Soc. Exp. Biol. 25, 255.

Bullough, W. S. and Deol, J. U. R. (1972) Chalone control of mitotic activity in eccrine sweat glands. Brit. J. Dermatol. 86, 586–592.

Bullough, W. S., Hewitt, C. L. and Laurence, E. B. (1964) The epidermal chalone: a preliminary attempt at isolation. Exp. Cell Res. 36, 192–200.

Bullough, W. S. and Johnson, M. (1951) A simple technique for maintaining mammalian epidermal mitosis in vitro. Exp. Cell Res. 2, 445–453.

Bullough, W. S. and Laurence, E. B. (1960a) The control of epidermal mitotic activity in the mouse. Proc. Roy. Soc. B 151, 517–536.

Bullough, W. S. and Laurence, E. B. (1960b) The control of mitotic activity in mouse skin. Dermis and hypodermis. Exp. Cell Res. 21, 394–405.

Bullough, W. S. and Laurence, E. B. (1961a) The study of mammalian epidermal mitosis in vitro. A critical analysis of technique. Exp. Cell Res. 24, 289–297.

Bullough, W. S. and Laurence, E. B. (1961b) Stress and adrenalin in relation to the diurnal cycle of epidermal mitotic activity in adult male mice. Proc. Roy. Soc. B 154, 540–556.

Bullough, W. S. and Laurence, E. B. (1964) Mitotic control by internal secretion: the role of the chalone–adrenalin complex. Exp. Cell Res. 33, 176–194.

Bullough, W. S. and Laurence, E. B. (1966) The diurnal cycle in epidermal mitotic duration and its relation to chalone and adrenalin. Exp. Cell Res. 43, 343–350.

Bullough, W. S. and Laurence, E. B. (1968a) The role of glucocorticoid hormones in the control of epidermal mitosis. Cell Tissue Kinet. 1, 5–10.

Bullough, W. S. and Laurence, E. B. (1968b) Control of mitosis in rabbit V × 2 epidermal tumours by means of epidermal chalone. Europ. J. Cancer 4, 587–594.

Bullough, W. S. and Laurence, E. B. (1968c) Control of mitosis in mouse and hamster melanomata by means of the melanocyte chalone. Europ. J. Cancer 4, 607–615.

Bullough, W. S. and Laurence, E. B. (1970a) The lymphocytic chalone and its antimitotic action on a mouse lymphoma in vitro. Europ. J. Cancer 6, 525–531.

Bullough, W. S. and Laurence, E. B. (1970b) Chalone control of mitotic activity in sebaceous glands. Cell Tissue Kinet. 3, 291–300.

Bullough, W. S., Laurence, E. B., Iversen, O. H. and Elgjo, K. (1967) The vertebrate epidermal chalone. Nature 214, 578–580.

Bullough, W. S. and Van Oordt, G. J. (1950) The mitogenic actions of testosterone propionate and of estrone on the epidermis of the adult male mouse. Acta Endocrinol. 4, 291–305.

Cameron, I. L. and Cleffman, G. (1964) Initiation of mitosis in relation to the cell cycle following feeding of starved chickens. J. Cell Biol. 21, 169.

Candelas, G. C. (1974) Analysis of induced mitotic activity in mouse ear epidermis under in vitro conditions. In: Cell Cycle Controls (eds.: G. M. Padilla, I. L. Cameron and A. Zimmerman) Academic Press, New York, pp. 61–76.

Chopra, D. P., Yu, R. J. and Flaxman, B. A. (1972) Demonstration of a tissue-specific inhibitor of mitosis of human epidermal cells in vitro. J. Invest. Dermatol. 59, 207–210.

Chopra, D. P. (1973) Regulation of mitosis in the embryonic kidney *(Xenopus laevis)* by kidney growth inhibitor (chalone). Natl. Cancer Inst. Monogr. 38, 189–196.

Christophers, E. (1971) Cellular architecture of the stratum corneum. J. Invest. Dermatol. 56, 165–169.

Christophers, E. and Laurence, E. B. (1973) Regional variations in mouse skin: quantitation of epidermal compartments in two different body sites. Virchows Arch. B. Zellpathol. 12, 212–222.

Clarkson, B., Ota, K., Ohkita, T. and O'Connor, A. (1965) Kinetics of proliferation of cancer cells in neoplastic effusions in man. Cancer 18, 1189–1213.

Cohen, S. and Taylor, J. M. (1972) Epidermal growth factor: chemical and biological characterization. In: Epidermal Wound Healing (eds.: H. I. Maibach and D. T. Rovee) Year Book Medical Publ., Inc., Chicago, pp. 203–218.

Dahl, M. C. G. and Shuster, S. (1972) A rapid in vitro assay of epidermal chalone. J. Invest. Dermatol. 58, 253.

DeCosse, J. J. and Gelfant, S. (1968) Noncycling tumor cells: mitogenic response to anti-lymphocytic serum. Science 162, 698–699.

Delescluse, C. and Pruniéras, M. (1971) Effet sur cellules épidermiques en culture d'un extrait aqueux d'épiderme type chalone Ann. Derm. Syph. (Paris) 98, 533–535.

Delecluse, C., Régnier, M. and Pruniéras, M. (1972a) Inhibition spècifique de la synthèse de DNA dans des cultures primaires de cellules épidermiques. Ann. Derm. Syph. (Paris) 99, 291–293.

Delescluse, C., Régnier, M. and Pruniéras, M. J. (1972b) Specific effect of epidermal extract on DNA synthesis in tissue culture. J. Invest. Dermatol. 58, 253–254.

Duell, E. A., Voorhees, J. J., Kelsey, W. H. and Hayes, E. (1971) Isoproterenol-sensitive adenyl cyclase in a particulate fraction of epidermis. Arch. Dermatol. 104, 601–610.

Elgjo, K. (1969) Epidermal cell proliferation during the first 24 h after injection of an aqueous skin extract (chalone). Virchows Arch. B. Zellpath. 4, 119–125.

Elgjo, K. (1974a) Reversible inhibition of epidermal G_1 cells by repeated injections of aqueous skin extracts (chalone). Virchows Arch. B. Zellpath. 15, 157–163.

Elgjo, K. (1974b) Evidence for presence of the epidermal G_2 inhibitor (epidermal chalone) in dermis. Virchows Arch. B. Zellpath. 16, 243–247.

Elgjo, K. (1975) Epidermal chalone and cyclic AMP: an in vivo study. J. Invest. Dermatol. 64, 14–18.

Elgjo, K. and Edgehill, W. (1973) Epidermal growth inhibitors (chalones) in dermis and serum. Virchows Arch. B. Zellpath. 13, 14–23.

Elgjo, K. and Hennings, H. (1971) Epidermal chalone and cell proliferation in a transplantable squamous cell carcinoma in hamsters. I. In vivo results. Virchows Arch. B. Zellpath. 7, 1–7.

Elgjo, K., Hennings, H. and Edgehill, W. (1971) Epidermal mitotic rate and DNA synthesis after injections of water extracts made from mouse skin treated with actinomycin D: two or more growth-regulating substances? Virchows Arch. B. Zellpath. 7, 342–347.

Elgjo, K., Laerum, O. D. and Edgehill, W. (1971) Growth regulation in mouse epidermis. I. G_2 inhibitor present in the basal cell layer. Virchows Arch. B. Zellpath. 8, 277–283.

Elgjo, K., Laerum, O. D. and Edgehill, W. (1972) Growth regulation in mouse epidermis. II. G_1 inhibitor present in the differentiating cell layer. Virchows Arch. B. Zellpath. 10, 229–236.

Evans, L. S. and Van 't Hof, J. (1974) Promotion of cell arrest in G_2 in root and shoot meristems in *Pisum* by a factor from the cotyledons. Exp. Cell Res. 87, 259–264.

Fiala, S. (1968) The cancer cell as a stem cell unable to differentiate. A theory of carcinogenesis. Neoplasma 15, 607–622.

Finegold, M. J. (1965) Control of cell multiplication in epidermis. Proc. Soc. Exp. Biol. Med. 119, 96–100.

Flesch, P. and Esoda, E. C. J. (1964) Chemical anomalies in pathological horny layers. In: The Epidermis (eds.: W. Montagna and W. C. Lobitz) Academic Press, New York and London, pp. 539–550.

Florentin, R. A., Nam, S. C., Janakidèvi, K., Lee, K. T., Reiner, J. M. and Thomas, W. A. (1973) Population dynamics of arterial smooth muscle cells. II. In vivo inhibition of entry into mitosis of swine arterial smooth muscle cells by aortic tissue extracts Arch. Pathol. 95, 317–320.

Frankfurt, O. S. (1968) Effect of hydrocortisone, adrenalin and actinomycin D on transition of cells to the DNA synthesis phase. Exp. Cell Res. 52, 220–232.

Frankfurt, O. S. (1971) Epidermal chalone. Effect on cell cycle and on development of hyperplasia. Exp. Cell Res. 64, 140–144.

Froese, G. (1971) Regulation of growth in Chinese hamster cells by a local inhibitor. Exp. Cell Res. 65, 297–306.

Fujii, T. and Mizuno T. (1969) The relation between wound repair process and early changes of skin carcinogenesis. Proc. Japan Acad. 45, 925–930.

Gelfant, S. (1963) Symp. Intern. Cell Biol. 2, 229.

Gelfant, S. (1966) Patterns of cell division: the demonstration of discrete cell populations. In: Methods in Cell Physiology (ed.: D. M. Prescott) Academic Press, New York, vol. II, pp. 359–395.

Gelfant, S. and Candelas, G. (1972) Regulation of epidermal mitosis. J. Invest. Dermatol. 59, 7–12.

Gradwohl, P. (1973) Tissue-unspecificity of skin extracts tested for the presence of chalones. Experientia 29, 772.

Grimes, P. and Sallmann, L. v. (1972) Possible cyclic adenosine monophosphate mediation in isoproterenol-induced suppression of cell division in rat lens epithelium. Invest. Ophthalmol. 11, 231–235.

Hall, R. G. (1970) DNA synthesis in organ cultures of the hamster cheek pouch. Inhibition by a homologous extract. Exp. Cell Res. 58, 429–431.

Hanna, C. (1965) Changes in DNA, RNA and protein synthesis in the developing lens. Invest. Ophthalmol. 4, 480–491.

Hell, E. (1970) A stimulant to DNA synthesis in guinea pig ear epidermis. Brit. J. Dermatol. 83, 632–636.

Hell, E. and Cooper, J. (1973) Short life stimulant released from ground skin slices. Brit. J. Dermatol. 88, 369–372.

Hennings, H. and Elgjo, K. (1970) Epidermal regeneration after cellophane tape stripping of hairless mouse skin. Cell Tissue Kinet. 3, 243–252.

Hennings, H. and Elgjo, K. (1971) Hydrocortisone: Inhibition of DNA synthesis and mitotic rate after local application to mouse epidermis. Virchows Arch. B. Zellpath. 8, 42–49.

Hennings, H., Elgjo, K. and Iversen, O. H. (1969) Delayed inhibition of epidermal DNA synthesis after injection of an aqueous skin extract (chalone). Virchows Arch. B. Zellpath. 4, 45–53.

Holtzer, H. (1972) The cell cycle, myogenesis and psoriasis. J. Invest. Dermatol. 59, 33–34.

Holzmann, H., Morsches, B., Krapp, R., Hoffman, G. and Oertel, G. W. (1972) Zur Therapie der Psoriasis mit Dehydroepiandrosteron-Oenanthat. Zeitschr. Haut- u Geschl.-Krankh. 47, 99.

Hondius-Boldingh, W. and Laurence, E. B. (1968) Extraction, purification and preliminary characterization of the epidermal chalone. A tissue-specific mitotic inhibitor obtained from vertebrate skin. Europ. J. Biochem. 5, 191–198.

Hooker, C. W. and Pfeiffer, C. A. (1943) Effects of sex hormones upon body growth, skin, hair and sebaceous glans in the rat. Endocrinology 32, 69.

Huijing, F. and Lee, E. Y. C. (eds.) (1973) Protein phosphorylation in control mechanisms. Miami Winter Symp., Vol. 5. Academic Press, New York and London.

Iversen, O. H. (1960a) In: Proc. First Int. Congr. Cybernetic Med. (ed.: A. Masturo) Società Internazionale di Medicina Cibernetica. Naples, pp. 420–430.

Iversen, O. H. (1960b) Cell metabolism in experimental skin carcinogenesis. Acta Pathol. Microbiol. Scand. 50, 17–24.

Iversen, O. H. (1961) The regulation of cell numbers in epidermis. A cybernetic point of view. Acta Pathol. Microbiol. Scand. Supp. 148, 91–96.

Iversen, O. H. (1968) Effect of epidermal chalone on human epidermal mitotic activity in vitro. Nature 219, 75.

Iversen, O. H. (1969) Chalones of the skin. In: Homeostatic regulators (eds.: G. E. W. Wolstenholme and J. Knight) J. & A. Churchill, London, pp. 29–56.

Iversen, O. H. and Bjerknes, R. (1963) Kinetics of epidermal reaction to carcinogens. Acta Pathol. Microbiol. Scand. Suppl. 165, 1–74.

Iversen, O. H. and Evensen, A. (1962) Experimental skin carcinogenesis in mice. Acta Pathol. Microbiol. Scand. Suppl. 156, 1–184.

Iversen, O. H., Aandahl, E. and Elgjo, K. (1965) The effect of an epidermis-specific mitotic inhibitor (chalone) extracted from epidermal cells. Acta Pathol. Microbiol. Scand. 64, 506–510.

Iversen, O. H., Bhangoo, K. S. and Hansen, K. (1974) Control of epidermal cell renewal in the bat web. A study of the cell number, cell size and mitotic rate in the epidermis on both sides of the web after the removal of the epidermis on the ventral side only, with special emphasis on growth control theories. Virchows Arch. B. Zellpath. 16, 157–179.

Iversen, O. H., Bjerknes, B. and Devik, F. (1968) Kinetics of cell renewal, cell migration and cell loss in the hairless mouse epidermis. Cell Tissue Kinet. 1, 351–367.

Karasek, M. A. (1972) Dermal factors affecting epidermal cells in vitro. J. Invest. Dermatol. 59, 99–101.

Karatschai, M., Kinzel, V., Goerttler, K. and Süss, R. (1971) 'Geography' of mitoses and cell division in the basal cell layer of mouse epidermis. Z. Krebsforsch. 76, 59.

Kligman, A. M. (1964) The biology of the stratum corneum. In: The Epidermis (eds.: W. Montagna and W. C. Lobitz) Academic Press, New York and London, pp. 387–433.

Krieg, L. (1975) Zur Wachstumskontrolle in Mäuseepidermis nach Einwirkung hyperplasiogener und tumorpromovierender Reize. Ph. D. Thesis. University of Heidelberg.

Krieg, L., Kühlmann, I. and Marks, F. (1974) Effect of tumor-promoting phorbol esters and of acetic acid on mechanisms controlling DNA synthesis and mitosis (chalones) and on the biosynthesis of histidine-rich protein in mouse epidermis. Cancer Res. 34, 3135–3146.

Kumar, R., Tao, M. and Solomon, L. M. (1971) Cyclic 3′, 5′-adenosine monophosphate-stimulated protein kinase from human skin. J. Invest. Dermatol. 57, 312–315.

Kumar, R., Tao, M. and Solomon, L. M. (1972) Adenosine 3′, 5′-cyclic monophosphate-stimulated protein kinase from human skin. II. Isolation and properties of multiple forms. J. Invest. Dermatol. 59, 196–201.

Lajtha, L. G. (1973) Review on leucocytes. Natl. Cancer Inst. Monogr. 38, 111–115.

Laurence, E. B. (1973a) Experimental approach to the epidermal chalone. Natl. Cancer Inst. Monogr. 38, 37–46.

Laurence, E. B. (1973b) The epidermal chalone and keratinizing epithelia. Natl. Cancer Inst. Monogr. 38, 61–68.

Laurence, E. B. and Elgjo, K. (1971) Epidermal chalone and cell proliferation in a transplantable squamous cell carcinoma in hamsters. II. In vitro results. Virchows Arch. B. Zellpath. 7, 8–15.

Laurence, E. B. and Randers-Hansen, E. (1971) An in vivo study of epidermal chalone and stress hormones on mitosis in tongue epithelium and ear epidermis of the mouse. Virchows Arch. B. Zellpath. 9, 271–279.

Laurence, E. B. and Randers-Hansen, E. (1972) Regional specificity of the epidermal chalone extracted from two different body sites. Virchows Arch. B. Zellpath. 11, 34–42.

Laurence, E. B., Randers-Hansen, E., Christophers, E. and Rytömaa, T. (1972) Systemic factors influencing epidermal mitosis. Rev. Europ. Études Clin. Biol. 17, 133–139.

Lenfant, M., Kren-Proschek, L., Verly, W. G. and Dugas, H. (1973) Thymidine as one of the factors in a beef liver extract decreasing [³H]thymidine incorporation into DNA. Canad. J. Biochem. 51, 654–665.

Locke, M. (1967) The development of patterns in the integument of insects. Adv. Morphogenesis 6, 33–88.

Mackenzie, I. C. (1969) Ordered structure of the stratum corneum of mammalian skin. Nature 222, 881.

Mackenzie, I. C. (1972) The ordered structure of mammalian epidermis. In: Epidermal wound healing (eds.: H. I. Maibach and D. T. Rove) Year Book Medical Publ. Inc., Chicago, pp. 5–25.

Marks, F. (1971) Direct evidence of two tissue-specific chalone-like factors regulating mitosis and DNA synthesis in mouse epidermis. Hoppe-Seylers Z. Physiol. Chem. 353, 1273–1274.

Marks, F. (1973a) A tissue-specific factor inhibiting DNA synthesis in mouse epidermis. Natl. Cancer Inst. Monogr. 38, 79–90.

Marks, F. (1973b) The second messenger system of mouse epidermis. III. Guanyl cyclase. Biochim. Biophys. Acta 309, 349–356.

Marks, F. (1974) Attempts to purify and characterize a factor inhibiting epidermal DNA synthesis ('G_1 chalone'). Hoppe-Seylers Z. Physiol. Chem. 355, 1228.

Marks, F. and Grimm, W. (1972) Diurnal fluctuations and beta-adrenergic elevation of cyclic AMP in mouse epidermis in vivo. Nature New Biol. 240, 178–179.

Marks, F. and Raab, I. (1974) The second messenger system of mouse epidermis. IV. Cyclic AMP and cyclic GMP phosphodiesterase. Biochim. Biophys. Acta 334, 368–377.

Marks, F. and Rebien, W. (1972) Cyclic 3′, 5′-AMP and theophylline inhibit epidermal mitosis in G_2 phase, Naturwissenschaften 59, 41.

Marks, F. and Rebien, W. (1972) The second messenger system of mouse epidermis. I. Properties and β-adrenergic activation of adenylate cyclase in vitro. Biochim. Biophys. Acta 284, 556–567.

Marks, R., Fukui, K. and Halprin, K. (1971) The application of an in vitro technique to the study of epidermal replication and metabolism. Brit. J. Dermatol. 84, 453–460.

Marrs, J. M. and Voorhees, J. J. (1971a) A method for bioassay of an epidermal chalone-like inhibitor. J. Invest. Dermatol. 56, 174–181.

Marrs, J. M. and Voorhees, J. J. (1971b) Preliminary characterization of an epidermal chalone-like inhibitor. J. Invest. Dermatol. 56, 353–358.

Mazia, D. (1961) Mitosis and the physiology of cell division. In: The Cell (eds.: J. Brachet and A. Mirsky) Academic Press, New York, vol. III, chapter 2.

McGuire, J. and Arensen, S. (1972) Control of keratinocyte division in vitro. J. Invest. Dermatol. 59, 84–90.

Melbye, S. W. and Karasek, M. A. (1973) Some characteristics of a factor stimulating skin epithelial cell growth in vitro. Exp. Cell Res. 79, 279–286.

Mercer, E. H. (1961) Keratin and keratinization. Pergamon Press, London.

Mier, P. D. and Urselmann, E. (1970) The adenyl cyclase of skin. I. Measurements and properties. Brit. J. Dermatol. 83, 359–363.

Mier, P. D. and Urselmann, E. (1972) Adenosine 3′, 5′-cyclic monophosphate phosphodiesterase in skin. I. Measurement and properties. Brit. J. Dermatol. 86, 141–146.

Mier, P. D. and Van der Hurk, J. (1972) Cyclic 3′, 5′ adenosine monophosphate-dependent protein kinase of skin. I. Measurement and properties. Brit. J. Dermatol. 87, 571–576.

Mizuno, T. and Fujii, T. (1969) Analysis of the two processes, wound repair and early changes in carcinogenesis by the use of Millipore filter implanting: the possible role of a heparin-like compound in cell interactions. J. Fac. Sc. Univ. Tokyo, Sec. IV, 11, 475–495.

Montagna, W., Kenyon, P. and Hamilton, J. B. (1949) Mitotic activity in the epidermis of the rabbit stimulated with local applications of testosterone. J. Exp. Zool. 110, 379–396.

Mueller, G. C. (1971) Biochemical perspectives of the G_1 and S intervals in the replication cycle of animal cells. In: The Cell Cycle (ed.: R. Baserga) M. Dekker, New York, pp. 270–308.

Nam, S. C., Florentin, R. A., Janakidevi, K., Lee, K. T., Reiner, J. M. and Thomas, W. A. (1974) Population dynamics of arterial smooth muscle cells. III. Inhibition by aortic tissue extracts of proliferative response to intimal injury in hypercholesterolemic swine. Exp. Mol. Pathol. 21, 259–267.

Nome, O. (1974) Tissue-specificity of the epidermal chalones. M. D. Thesis, University of Oslo.

Ohashi, M., Sawada, Y. and Makita, R. (1973) Odland bodies and intercellular substances. Acta Dermato-Venerol (Stockholm), Suppl. 73, 47–54.

Orfanos, C. E. (1972) Feinstrukturelle Morphologie und Histopathologie der verhornenden Epidermis. Georg Thieme Verlag, Stuttgart, pp. 44–54.

Pederson, T. and Gelfant, S. (1970) G2-population cells in mouse kidney and duodenum and their behaviour during the cell division cycle. Exp. Cell Res. 59, 32–36.

Philpott, G. W. (1971) Tissue-specific inhibition of cell proliferation in embryonic stomach epithelium in vitro. Gastroenterology 61, 25–34.

Pilgrim, C., Lennartz, K. J., Wegener, K., Hollweg, S. and Maurer, W. (1965) Autoradiographische Untersuchungen über tageszeitliche Schwankungen des H-3-Index und des Mitose-Index bei Zellarten der ausgewachsenen Maus, des Ratten-Fetus sowie bei Ascites-Tumorzellen. Z. Zellforsch. 68, 138–154.

Pinkus, H. (1951) Examination of the epidermis by the strip method of removing horny layers. J. Invest. Dermatol. 16, 383–386; 19, 431–446.

Potten, C. S. (1974) The epidermal proliferative unit: the possible role of the central basal cell. Cell Tissue Kinet. 7, 77–88.

Potten, C. S. and Allen, T. D. (1975) The fine structure and cell kinetics of mouse epidermis after wounding. J. Cell Sci. 17, 413–447.

Raick, A. N. (1973) Ultrastructural, histological, and biochemical alterations produced by 12-O-tetradecanoyl-phorbol-13-acetate on mouse epidermis and their relevance to skin tumor promotion. Cancer Res. 33, 269–286.

Raick, A. N. (1974) Cell differentiation and tumor-promoting action in skin carcinogenesis. Cancer Res. 34, 2915–2925.

Rohrbach, R. and Laerum, O. D. (1974) Variations of mitosis-inhibiting chalone in epidermis and dermis after carcinogen treatment. Cell Tissue Kinet. 7, 251–257.

Rothberg, S. and Arp, B. C. (1973) Epidermal chalone and inhibition of DNA synthesis. Natl. Cancer Inst. Monogr. 38, 93–98.

Rothberg, S. and Arp, B. C. (1975) Inhibition of epidermal and dermal DNA synthesis by mouse and cow-snout epidermal extracts. J. Invest. Dermatol. 64, 245–249.

Saetren, H. (1956) A principle of auto-regulation of growth. Production of organ-specific mitose-inhibitors in kidney and liver. Exp. Cell Res. 11, 229–232.

Schäfer, E. A. (1916) The endocrine organs. Longmans Green & Co., London.

Seiji, M., Nakano, H., Akiba, H. and Kato, T. (1974) Inhibition of DNA and protein synthesis in melanomata by a melanoma extract. J. Invest. Dermatol. 62, 11–19.

Simnett, J. D. and Chopra, D. P. (1969) Organ specific inhibitor of mitosis in the amphibian kidney. Nature 222, 1189–1190.

Simnett, J. D., Fisher, J. M. and Heppleston, A. G. (1969) Tissue-specific inhibition of lung alveolar cell mitosis in organ culture. Nature 223, 944–946.

Stumpf, W. E., Sar, M. and Joshil, S. G. (1974) Estrogen target cells in the skin. Experientia 30, 196–198.

Teel, R. W. (1972) Inhibition of DNA synthesis in hamster cheek pouch tissue in organ culture by dibutyryl cyclic AMP and a homologous extract. Biochem. Biophys. Res. Commun. 47, 1010–1014.

Teir, H., Lahtiharju, A., Alho, A. and Forsell, K. J. (1967) Autoregulation of growth by tissue breakdown products. In: Control of Cellular Growth in Adult Organisms (eds.: H. Teir and T. Rytömaa) Academic Press, London and New York, pp. 67–81.

Tomkins, G. M., Levinson, B., Baxter, J. D. and Dethlefsen, L. (1972) Further evidence for posttranscriptional control of inducible tyrosine aminotransferase synthesis in cultured hepatoma cells. Nature New Biol. 239, 9–14.

Tsanev, R. (1963) Role of nucleic acids in wound healing process. Symp. Biol. Hungarica 3, 55–73.

Tsanev, R. and Sendov, B. (1966) A model of the regulatory mechanism of cellular multiplication. J. Theoret. Biol. 12, 327–341.

Tsanev, R. and Sendov, B. (1968) Computer studies on the mechanism controlling cellular proliferation. In: Effects of Radiation on Cellular Proliferation and Differentiation. International Atomic Energy Agency. Vienna.

Tutton, P. J. M. (1973) Control of epithelial cell proliferation in the small intestinal crypt. Cell Tissue Kinet. 6, 211–216.

Tutton, P. J. M. and Helme, R. D. (1973) Stress induced inhibition of jejunal crypt cell proliferation. Virchows Arch. B. Zellpath. 15, 23–34.

Tutton, P. J. M. and Helme, R. D. (1974) The influence of adrenoreceptor activity on crypt cell proliferation in the rat jejunum. Cell Tissue Kinet. 7, 125–136.

Tvermyr, E. M. F. (1969) Circadian rhythms in epidermal mitotic activity. Virchows Arch. B. Zellpath. 2, 318–325.

Tvermyr, E. M. F. (1972) Circadian rhythms in hairless mouse epidermal DNA synthesis as measured by double labelling with H3-thymidine (H3Tdr). Virchows Arch. B. Zellpath. 11, 43–54.

Voaden, M. J. (1968) A chalone in the rabbit lens? Exp. Eye Res. 7, 326–331.

Voaden, M. J. and Leeson, S. J. (1970) A chalone in mammalian lens. Exp. Eye Res. 9, 57–72.

Voorhees, J. J. and Mier, P. D. (1974) The epidermis and cyclic AMP. Brit. J. Dermatol. 90, 223–227.

Voorhees, J. J., Duell, E. A., Kelsey, W. H. (1972) Dibutyryl cyclic AMP inhibition of epidermal cell division. Arch. Dermatol. 105, 384–386.

Voorhees, J. J., Duell, E. A., Bass, L. J. and Harrell, E. R. (1973) Role of cyclic AMP in the control of epidermal growth and differentiation. Natl. Cancer Inst. Monogr. 38, 47–59.

Voorhees, J. J., Duell, E. A., Stawiski, M. and Harrell, E. R. (1974) Cyclic nucleotide metabolism in normal and proliferating epidermis. In: Advances in Cyclic Nucleotide Research (eds.: P. Greengard and G. A. Robison) Raven Press, New York, Vol. 4, pp. 117–162.

Weiss, P. and Kavanau, J. L. (1957) A model of growth and growth-control in mathematical terms. J. Gen. Physiol. 41, 1–47.

Wiley, C. L., Williams, W. W. and McDonald, C. J. (1973) The effects of the epidermal chalone on DNA synthesis in mammalian epidermal cells. J. Invest. Dermatol. 60, 160–165.

Winter, G. D. (1972) Epidermal regeneration studied in the domestic pig. In: Epidermal Wound Healing (eds.: H. I. Maibach and D. T. Rovee) Year Book Medical Publ. Inc., Chicago, pp. 71–112.

Yamada, T. (1972) Control mechanisms in cellular metaplasia. In: Cell Differentiation (eds.: R. Harris, P. Allin and D. Viza) E. Munksgaard, Copenhagen, pp. 56–60.

Yamaguchi, T., Hirobe, T., Kinjo, Y. and Manaka, K. (1974) The effect of chalone on the cell cycle in the epidermis during wound healing. Exp. Cell Res. 89, 247–254.

Young, J. M., Lawrence, H. S. and Cordell, S. L. (1975) In vitro epidermal cell proliferation in rat skin plugs. J. Invest. Dermatol. 64, 23–29.

Zil, J. S. (1972) Vitamin A effects on epidermal mitotic activity. J. Invest. Dermatol. 59, 228–232.

CHAPTER 8

Epidermal chalone in experimental skin carcinogenesis*

KJELL ELGJO

Institute of Pathology, University of Oslo, Rikshospitalet, Oslo 1, Norway

Most studies of skin carcinogenesis have been performed in mice. Mouse skin was also used in the first chalone experiments done by Bullough and Laurence (1964). Later investigations have confirmed that the mouse epidermis – used either in vivo or in vitro – is perhaps the most expedient tissue in studies of the epidermal chalone and its characteristics. In this chapter I will try to relate some of the alterations found in the mouse epidermis during chemical carcinogenesis to what is known about the epidermal chalone and its role in the regulation of epidermal cell renewal. No attempt will be made to evaluate the possible role of growth-regulating substances such as chalone in the development and growth of the final result of skin carcinogenesis – carcinoma of the skin.

8.1 Histology of the mouse skin

Most agents used in chemical skin carcinogenesis affect at least two different types of tissue; the epidermis and the dermis. The dermis consists mainly of connective tissue with fibroblasts in varying amounts of intercellular material. It also contains vessels, nerves, smooth muscle fibres, and several epidermal appendages such as sweat glands, sebaceous glands, and hair follicles.

The epidermis in mice is fairly thin with only 3–4 layers of cells. In the normal epidermis cell divisions take place only among cells situated deepest

* This paper was written during the tenure of an American Cancer Society – Eleanor Roosevelt – International Cancer Fellowship awarded by the International Union Against Cancer.

in the epidermis and separated from the dermal tissue by a basement membrane. These cells constitute the basal layer of the epidermis. The more superficial cells are no longer capable of division and represent the differentiating, or keratinizing, cell layer. Only the most superficial of these cells are fully keratinized; the deeper cells are in different stages of keratinization. The surface of epidermis is covered by a horny layer of varying thickness.

In most text-books and articles, designations of 'keratinizing', 'maturing', and 'differentiating' are used synonymously to describe post-mitotic epidermal cells. A certain proportion of the basal layer cells also belong to the post-mitotic cell population since they will not divide again but move out into the differentiating cell layer after an interval of time that is determined by their degree of maturation. This has been discussed in detail by Iversen et al. (1968).

8.2 Growth regulation in epidermis

Keratinized cells are continuously lost from the surface of epidermis. Lost cells must be replaced by new cells at the same rate as the cell loss to maintain a constant thickness of epidermis. It is therefore natural to assume that there exists a monitoring of the rate of cell division among the basal layer cells to keep it adjusted to the rate of cell loss from the surface.

Studies on wound healing (Bullough and Laurence, 1960; Finegold, 1965; Iversen et al., 1974) and on the regenerative reaction seen after damaging epidermal cells with various hyperplasia-inducing agents (Iversen and Evensen, 1962; Elgjo, 1968a, b) have demonstrated that the normal epidermal cell renewal is probably regulated according to a negative feedback principle, as outlined by Weiss and Kavanau (1957). In such a system it is assumed that the post-mitotic, differentiating cells give continual information to the dividing cells (the progenitor cell population) about the need for new cells. This is effected by means of a signal substance(s) that is produced by the differentiating cells, and that inhibits the rate of cell proliferation among the progenitor cells (for discussion, see Iversen and Bjerknes, 1963).

8.3 Epidermal growth regulators

The first systematic attempt to find a chemical substance that could act as a signal in a negative feedback regulation of epidermal cell renewal revealed that water extracts of epidermis contain some agent that inhibits epidermal mitoses both in vitro and when injected intraperitoneally in mice (Bullough and Laurence, 1964; Iversen et al., 1965). The early investigations by

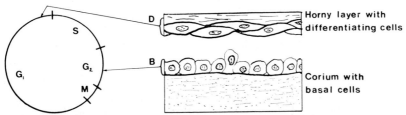

Fig. 8.1. Water extracts of isolated differentiating cells inhibit epidermal cells from starting DNA synthesis; while similar extracts made from basal layer cells inhibit epidermal G_2 cells from starting mitotic division. Water extracts of whole epidermis contain both inhibitors. (Reproduced from Elgjo et al., 1972.)

Bullough et al. (1964) showed that the signal substance was non-dialysable and thermolabile. Further experiments also demonstrated that it was tissue-specific but was not species specific (Bullough et al., 1967).

Later, some investigators have tried to purify the signal substance (named 'chalone' by Bullough in 1962), while others have attempted to evaluate its mode of action. Work on purification of the epidermal chalone is reported elsewhere in this book. Some other characteristics will be mentioned here.

The first chalone experiments showed that water extracts of mouse skin contained some substance(s) that inhibited epidermal cells in the premitotic, post-synthetic G_2 phase (Bullough and Laurence, 1964). Later, it was found that such extracts of epidermis would also inhibit epidermal cells in the presynthetic (prereplicative) part of the G_1 phase of the cell cycle at the time of injection (Hennings et al., 1969). This double effect of the extracts on both G_2 and G_1 cells in the epidermis seems to be caused by two different substances (Elgjo and Hennings, 1970). One of the substances is present in, and possibly produced by, the basal layer cells and acts on epidermal cells in the G_2 phase (Elgjo et al., 1971). The other substance is mainly present in and probably produced by the differentiating cells (Elgjo et al., 1972). Fig. 8.1 illustrates this situation diagramatically. Furthermore, the dermal connective tissue contains a water-soluble substance that inhibits epidermal cells in the same ways as the epidermal G_2-inhibitor (Elgjo and Edgehill, 1973; Elgjo, 1974). Thus, the regulation of normal cell renewal in epidermis is apparently fairly complex, although all findings referred to above are compatible with the original hypothesis assuming that the regulation takes place according to a negative feedback principle.

In the following, the term 'epidermal chalone' is used to indicate the complete set of tissue-specific growth-regulating substances in epidermis. The terms 'G_1-inhibitor' and 'G_2-inhibitor' are used to designate the two epidermal growth-regulators known so far.

In addition to the epidermal chalone, various exogeneous and endogeneous factors can modify the rate of cell proliferation in the normal epidermis.
Thus, several hormones can influence epidermal cell renewal even though
epidermis is not regarded as a target tissue for those hormones (Bullough,
1962; Epifanova, 1971). In their early experiments Bullough and Laurence
(1964) noted that adrenalin seemed to be necessary for the epidermal chalone
to be active in vitro. Later investigations have shown that both normal and
synthetic catecholamines have a profound effect on epidermal cell division,
mainly on epidermal cells in the G_2 phase (Voorhees et al., 1973). As
discussed by Voorhees et al. (1973) this effect of catecholamines is probably
mediated by cyclic $3',5'$-adenosine monophosphate (cyclic AMP). The
precise way in which the epidermal chalone and hormones interact is not
known. Also unknown is the way in which cyclic AMP interacts with the
epidermal chalone. It appears, however, that a certain level of epidermal
cyclic AMP is required for the epidermal chalone to be effective (Elgjo, 1975).

8.4 Epidermal growth alterations induced by hyperplasia-inducing agents

Topical application of carcinogenic or non-carcinogenic hyperplasia-inducing substances is accompanied by alterations in both the epidermal
metabolism and the epidermal growth pattern. This complex reaction to
topical treatment is to some extent dependent on the type and the dose of
hyperplasia-inducing agents which is applied, as discussed below. However,
the series of alterations that occur after topical application of such agents
can be divided into several more or less well-defined phases, independent
on the chemical compound that is applied:

1) Immediately after treatment with some hyperplasia-inducing agents,
epidermal DNA synthesis (Iversen and Evensen, 1962; Hennings and Boutwell, 1969; Hennings and Boutwell, 1970) and the mitotic rate (Elgjo, 1968a,
b) are depressed for several hours, while epidermal RNA and protein
syntheses usually increase rapidly after the application (Baird et al., 1971;
Raick, 1973). Also, the epidermal level of cyclic AMP is decreased for
several hours (Belman and Troll, 1974; Grimm and Marks, 1974).

2) The second phase is characterized by a rapid rise in epidermal DNA
synthesis (Iversen and Evensen, 1962; Hennings and Boutwell, 1969, 1970)
and in the mitotic rate (Elgjo, 1968a, b). Epidermal RNA and protein
syntheses are usually still above the normal level (Baird et al., 1971; Raick,
1973). The epidermal cyclic AMP level increases significantly during this
phase (Grimm and Marks, 1974).

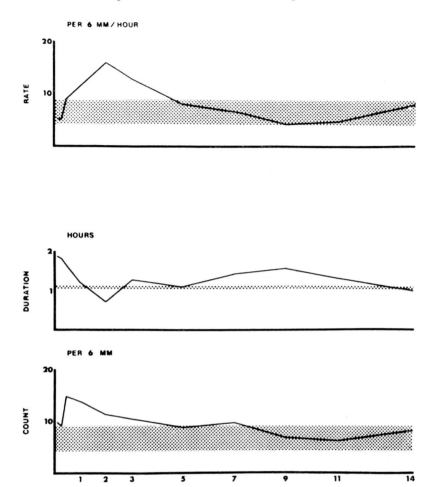

Fig. 8.2. Hairless mouse dorsal skin was treated topically with 0.03 ml of a 0.06% solution of cantharidin in benzene. The mitotic rate (= the number of cells starting their division per hour per 6 mm of interfollicular epidermis) was estimated by means of Colcemid. The mitosis counts were made in mice that did not receive Colcemid. The mitotic duration was calculated from the equation: (number of cells in mitosis) = (mitotic rate per hour) × (mitotic duration). For details, see Elgjo 1968a. (Reproduced from Elgjo, 1968a.)

3) The third phase is dependent on the dose and the type of agent applied to the skin. After a single application of most substances the epidermal mitotic rate and epidermal DNA synthesis return to normal levels again without any further significant alterations (Iversen and Evensen, 1962;

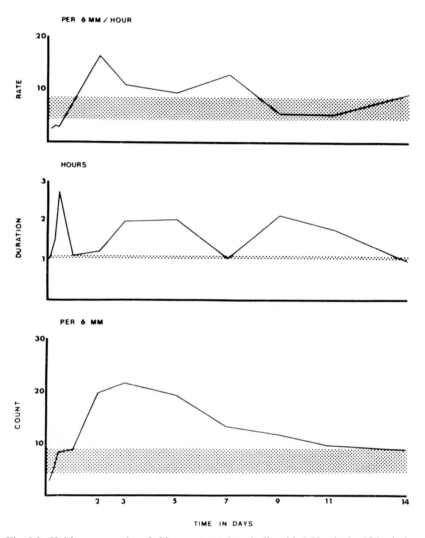

Fig. 8.3. Hairless mouse dorsal skin was treated topically with 0.03 ml of a 1% solution of methylcholanthrene in benzene. The growth parameters were estimated as described in fig. 8.2. (Reproduced from Elgjo, 1968a.)

Elgjo, 1968a). After application of some hyperplasia-inducing agents such as methylcholanthrene there is a second peak of increased mitotic rate in epidermis (Elgjo, 1968a). The various phases of the induced alterations in the epidermal growth pattern are illustrated in figs. 8.2 and 8.3.

In all three phases a high mitotic rate is generally accompanied by a short mitotic duration (figs. 8.2 and 8.3). The mitotic duration tends, however, to be longer after application of methylcholanthrene than after treatment with benzene or cantharidin. Likewise S-phase duration in the epidermis is also prolonged after treatment with carcinogens (Iversen and Evensen, 1962).

When mouse skin is treated with repeated topical applications of hyperplasia-inducing substances the initial growth pattern is similar to that found

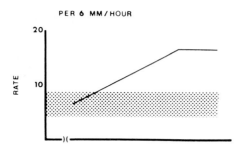

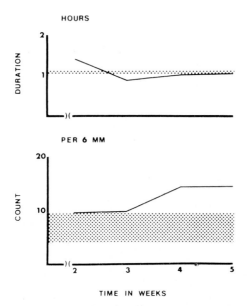

Fig. 8.4. Hairless mouse dorsal skin was treated topically 3 times weekly with 0.02 ml of benzene. The growth parameters were estimated as described in fig. 8.2. (Reproduced from Elgjo, 1968b.)

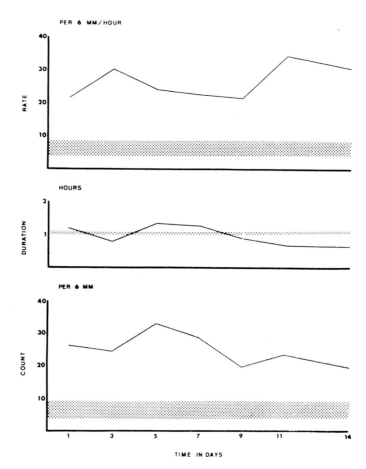

Fig. 8.5. Hairless mouse dorsal skin was treated topically 3 times weekly with 0.02 ml of a 0.06% solution of cantharidin in benzene. The growth parameters were estimated as described in fig. 8.2. (Reproduced from Elgjo, 1968b.)

after a single application. The long-term alterations are, however, different in many ways after several applications. Thus, when mouse epidermis is treated with repeated topical applications of methylcholanthrene the mitotic rate is consistently but moderately increased with some fairly rhythmic fluctuations. This increased mitotic rate is accompanied by long mitotic durations (Elgjo, 1968b). This is in contrast to the alterations found after repeated applications of the weak tumour promoter cantharidin or of benzene (figs. 8.4, 8.5 and 8.6). These agents induce a very high mitotic rate accompanied by a short mitotic duration (Elgjo, 1968b).

The hypothesis that epidermal cell renewal is regulated according to a

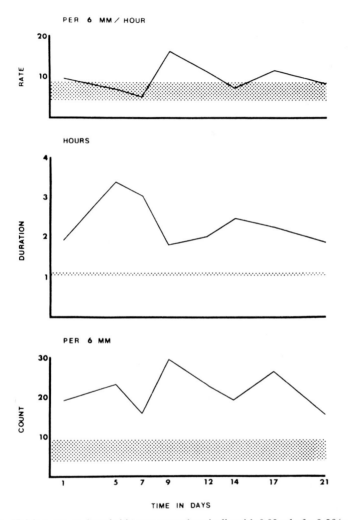

Fig. 8.6. Hairless mouse dorsal skin was treated topically with 0.02 ml of a 0.5% solution of methylcholanthrene in benzene. The growth parameters were estimated as described in fig. 8.2. (Reproduced from Elgjo, 1968b.)

negative feedback principle was originally based on results obtained from experiments with hyperplasia-inducing agents and from wounding experiments. The alterations in epidermal growth parameters observed in such experiments can to some extent be accounted for in other ways (for detailed discussion of this, see Iversen et al., 1974). However, the simplest and most satisfactory explanation is that the regulation of epidermal cell proliferation is mediated by chemical inhibitors produced by mature or maturing cells and acting on the dividing cells, as discussed above. It should therefore be possible to view the chemically induced growth alterations as transient disturbances in the production and breakdown of the epidermal chalone. Some experiments have been done to examine chalone concentrations in chemical carcinogenesis. Before reviewing these data, let us consider which changes one can expect to find in epidermal chalone content during treatment with hyperplasia-inducing agents.

When a hyperplasia-inducing chemical substance is applied topically to the skin some epidermal cells are usually damaged and others killed. Most probably the more superficial, differentiating cells receive a higher dose of the applied agent. In the first hours there is also an unspecific toxic effect on all cells in epidermis that causes a temporary arrest of cell division. In the following days the dead and damaged cells are sloughed off, or they can disintegrate in situ. According to the negative feedback theory such a sudden drop in the number of differentiating cells should be followed by a sudden drop in inhibitor production and concentration. This loss of inhibition would allow the basal cells to proliferate at a high rate. This burst of proliferative activity results in the production of a cohort of new cells of about the same age (for discussion of this, see Iversen and Evensen, 1962; Elgjo, 1968a).

It is probable that the ability to produce epidermal chalone is a function of cell age and thus of differentiation, at least within a certain span of the life of an epidermal cell (Iversen and Bjerknes, 1963). The G_1-inhibitor, which seems to regulate the rate with which cells enter the S phase is thus found in the differentiating cell layer in mouse epidermis (Elgjo et al., 1972). Because of the low average age of the epidermal cells the first few days after the first mitotic peak the content of epidermal chalone should be expected to be lower than normal for some time after the treatment.

As the cohort of new cells differentiate, the epidermal chalone concentration should increase correspondingly until the time when these cells become fully keratinized and are shed. When this happens the inhibitor concentration should again drop and the basal layer cells be allowed to proliferate at above the normal rate. Since the cells of the first cohort produced during the initial wave of mitoses are not of exactly the same age, and as maturation time most probably varies within a certain range of time, the drop in chalone concentration should not be so dramatic when the first cohort of cells is shed as it was immediately after the treatment. The second wave of mitoses can therefore not be expected to be as high and as sharp as the first wave. This assumption agrees well with the experimental data shown in figs. 8.2 and 8.3. Probably for the same reasons there is usually no third wave of mitoses after a single topical treatment with a hyperplasia-inducing agent.

However, as the cells produced during the second peak of mitoses differentiate a second and less pronounced increase in the epidermal chalone concentration would be expected.

Before looking at the available data on chalone concentration in topically treated epidermis some apparent discrepancies between theory and results should be discussed.

It is obvious that the peaks of epidermal cell proliferation last only for a relatively short time and that the mitotic rate decreases before the new cells produced during that same proliferative peak can be expected to make enough epidermal chalone to stop further cell divisions. This phenomenon is at first difficult to reconcile with the hypothesis that epidermal cell renewal is regulated according to a negative feedback theory.

The relatively short duration of the proliferative peaks is probably related to the mode of action of the epidermal chalone. The alterations found in epidermal growth parameters after application of a hyperplasia-inducing agent indicate that the basal layer cells react not only to the actual concentration of chalone but also to the rate with which the concentration changes (Elgjo 1968a, b). This would correspond to what is called a derivative type of control in a cybernetic system (Iversen and Bjerknes, 1963). In such a system the sudden loss of many inhibitor-producing cells with a correspondingly sudden fall in chalone concentration would trigger a wave of cell divisions. The actual concentration of chalone at the time of treatment is of less importance in this context, as it is the speed with which the chalone concentration changes that determines the reaction. When the chalone concentration stops decreasing and becomes fixed at a new and transiently lower level the basal cells react by decreasing their proliferative activity again. As more cells again reach a sufficient degree of differentiation to produce epidermal chalone the concentration of this signal substance should increase with a corresponding decrease in the mitotic activity. When the new cohort of cells is shed the same series of events would be repeated.

Several factors could modify the predicted fluctuations in epidermal chalone concentrations after topical treatment. As mentioned above, such treatment of epidermis is usually followed by increased RNA and protein syntheses. Thus, application of aromatic hydrocarbon carcinogens induces the synthesis of the set of drug-metabolizing enzymes now called aryl hydrocarbon hydroxylase (AHH) (Gelboin et al., 1970; Bowden et al., 1974). The concentration of AHH in normal, untreated epidermis is low. Even though it is not known how the epidermal chalone is broken down in the target cells it is quite possible that an induction of a wide range of enzymes could also affect the stability of the epidermal chalone.

Application of some tumor-promoting phorbol esters is followed by fluctuations in the epidermal level of cyclic AMP (Grimm and Marks, 1974). The activity of the epidermal chalone is in some way dependent on the epidermal cyclic AMP levels (Elgjo, 1974). Changes in the epidermal cyclic AMP levels could therefore interact with the epidermal chalone in such a way that the alterations in the epidermal mitotic rate are modified in some situations and cannot be directly related only to the epidermal chalone concentration.

Recently, Krieg et al. (1974) reported that topical application of tumor promoting phorbol esters to mouse skin alters the reaction to injection of extracts containing the epidermal G_1-inhibitor. During the period of increased epidermal DNA synthesis following the application of such phorbol esters the basal layer cells seemed to be refractory to treatment with epidermal G_1-inhibitor. The normal reaction to chalone treatment reappeared simultaneously with an increase in epidermal synthesis of histidine-rich protein. However, extracts made of mouse skin treated with the phorbol esters contained normal amounts of G_1-inhibitor even at the time when the dividing epidermal cells did not respond to the injected chalone. This altered response to the epidermal G_1-inhibitor was seen even after removal of keratinizing cells with cellophane tape. It is therefore not likely that this phenomenon is related to the tumor promoting effect as such. On the other hand, periods of altered response to chalone could well result in a discrepancy between the actual chalone concentration in epidermis and the expected values.

There is evidence that some chalones are counteracted or neutralized by chalone antagonists or 'anti-chalones' (Rytömaa and Kiviniemi, 1968; Laurence et al., 1972). The possible ways such a chalone antagonist could act in the skin has recently been discussed by Bjerknes and Iversen (1974). The mitosis-inhibiting activity of dermal connective tissue extracts could thus represent a binding of epidermal chalone to components in the corium (Elgjo and Edgehill, 1973; Elgjo, 1974). Topical treatment of the skin with hyperplasia-inducing substances is followed by alterations even in dermis. Such alterations could well influence the local chalone concentration and metabolism, either by changing dermal components or by altering the blood flow to the area and thus the removal of growth-regulating substances by the blood (Houck and Cheng, 1973).

Repeated applications of methylcholanthrene to mouse epidermis induce a state in which the mitotic rate is moderately increased and the epidermis considerably thicker than normal. The fact that the mitotic rate is high would indicate that the inhibitor concentration in the basal layer is low, even though the number of cells per unit epidermis is increased. However, it is probable that each application of methylcholanthrene is followed by a sudden loss of cells and a corresponding fall in chalone concentration even in the hyperplastic epidermis. The high but fluctuating mitotic rate in epidermis could therefore be a result of a derivative type of negative feedback, as discussed above. It is therefore natural to expect a changing chalone concentration in the methylcholanthrene-treated epidermis but it is not possible to predict whether the base-line chalone concentration will be low, normal, or increased as long as the average age and the average differentiation time are not known in this epidermis. Since the mitotic duration is greatly prolonged after repeated methylcholanthrene applications (fig. 8.4) (in contrast to what is found after a similar treatment with non-carcinogenic agents) it is possible that topical carcinogen-treatment alters growth-regulating mechanisms in ways different from the action of non-carcinogens. No direct estimates have been made of the epidermal chalone concentration after repeated topical applications of hyperplasia-inducing agents. The various possible interpretations must therefore be regarded as speculative until we get experimental data in this area.

8.5 *Chalone activity in topically treated epidermis*

Only one systematic series of experiments has been done to examine the variations in extractable chalone activity after application of a carcinogenic agent to mouse skin (Rohrbach, 1972; Rohrbach et al., 1972; Rohrbach and Laerum, 1974). In this study the complete carcinogen methylcholanthrene was applied to hairless mouse skin and water extracts of the treated area tested for their content of chalone activity at different intervals of time after the application. These extracts were tested by injecting a fixed dose of lyophilized water extract of the treated mouse skin into normal mice. The content of G_2-inhibitor was estimated by means of the mitosis-arresting agent Colcemid. Epidermal DNA synthesis was estimated by injecting tritiated thymidine 12 h after injection of the skin extract to test the concentration of G_1-inhibitor.

The observed fluctuations in epidermal chalone content were in very good agreement with the predicted values. The first 12 h after the application the chalone content of the treated epidermis was normal. From 24 h until day 3 the treated epidermis contained no inhibiting activity when tested in the doses used in the experiment. The following days the chalone content increased and reached a maximum on day 5 (G_1-inhibitor) or on day 7 (G_2-inhibitor). Thus, on day 7 the concentration of extractable G_2-inhibitor was 25% higher than that usually found in normal epidermis. The content of G_2-inhibiting activity in the dermis of the treated skin was also increased on this day (Rohrbach and Laerum, 1974).

The only exception from the predicted values was found in the days following the peak chalone concentration on days 4 and 7. Instead of the expected high chalone concentration that should follow a partially synchronous maturation of a cohort of cells the content of epidermal G_1-inhibitor was lower than normal and the content of G_2-inhibitor about normal (fig. 8.7).

On the whole, the agreement between the estimated chalone concentrations in the treated epidermis and the predicted changes was surprisingly good when the crude nature of the assay system is taken into account. Probably, only fairly great variations can be evaluated in such a system. Moreover, it is probable that the mitotic rate in an epidermis that has been

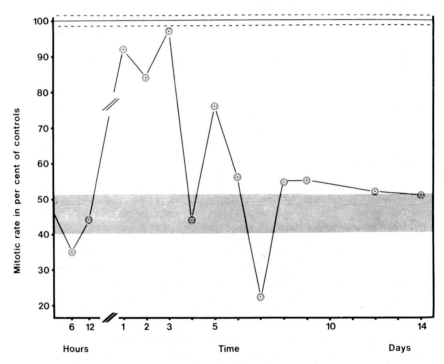

Fig. 8.7. Hairless mouse skin was treated topically with a single application of a 0.5% solution of methylcholanthrene in acetone. Water extracts were made of the treated area of skin (as described in Hennings et al., 1969) at intervals after the carcinogen treatment. The extracts were tested in untreated hairless mice. The mitosis-inhibiting activity (e.g., the content of G_2-inhibitor) is expressed as per cent of the mitotic rate in controls injected with saline. For details, see Rohrbach et al., 1972, from which paper the figure is reproduced.

damaged by local application of a hyperplasia-inducing agent is dependent on other factors than chalone alone, as discussed briefly above. An additional factor which is difficult to evaluate is the relative concentration of epidermal chalone in a certain dose of lyophilized skin extract. After treatment with hyperplasia-inducing substances the altered skin metabolism could well result in qualitatively different protein synthesis, so that the injected dose of skin extract would contain less chalone per mg protein without a corresponding decrease in chalone concentration per living epidermal *cell*. This has been discussed by Rohrbach (1972).

Rohrbach (1972) also estimated the chalone concentrations in epidermis treated with croton oil. After application of this substance the epidermal chalone concentration fluctuated the first days with minimum values on days 2, 3, and 6. These times of no or minimal chalone content had the same temporal relationship to peaks and troughs in the epidermal mitotic rate as that found after treatment with methylcholanthrene.

The few experiments done so far give good support for the assumption that the alterations in epidermal growth parameters seen after treatment with carcinogenic or non-carcinogenic hyperplasia-inducing substances can be directly related to variations in epidermal chalone concentrations. Further experiments are obviously needed to examine the later phases of skin carcinogenesis in the same way, especially after repeated applications of a carcinogen or during a two stage skin carcinogenesis experiment. This could give some indication whether the growth alterations found at these later stages could be accounted for by simple variations in the chalone content, or if other mechanisms are involved.

In this short survey I have tried to correlate the data we have on experimentally induced growth alterations in epidermis with the still very little information available regarding the variations in epidermal chalone content during the development of hyperplasia. I have intentionally used the somewhat imprecise term 'epidermal chalone'. Even though we know that at least two different factors are involved we have almost no knowledge about the metabolism of these tissue-specific growth regulators. With an increasing knowledge of how chalones influence normal growth we will, however, hopefully better understand how and why the normal growth regulation breaks down during carcinogenesis.

References

Baird, W. M., Sedgwick, J. A. and Boutwell, R. K. (1971) Effects of phorbol and four diesters of phorbol on the incorporation of tritiated precursors into DNA, RNA, and protein in mouse epidermis. Cancer Res. 31, 1434–1439.

Belman, S. and Troll, W. (1974) Phorbol-12-myristate-13-acetate effect on cyclic adenosine 3′, 5′-monophosphate levels in mouse skin and inhibition of phorbol-myristate-acetate-promoted tumorigenesis by theophylline. Cancer Res. 34, 3446–3455.

Bjerknes, R. and Iversen, O. H. (1974) 'Antichalone'. A theoretical treatment of the possible role of antichalone in the growth control system. Acta Path. Microbiol. Scand. Sect. A. Suppl. 248, 33–42.

Bowden, G. T., Slaga, T. J., Shapas, B. G. and Boutwell, R. K. (1974) The role of aryl hydrocarbon hydroxylase by 7,12-dimethylbenz(a)anthracene and 1,2,5,6-dibenzanthracene using DNA binding and thymidine-^{3}H incorporation into DNA as criteria. Cancer Res. 34, 2634–2642.

Bullough, W. S. (1962) The control of mitotic activity in adult mammalian tissues. Biol. Rev. 37, 307–342.

Bullough, W. S. and Laurence, E. B. (1960) The control of epidermal mitotic activity in the mouse. Proc. Roy. Soc. B 151, 517–536.

Bullough, W. S. and Laurence, E. B. (1964) Mitotic control by internal secretion. The role of the chalone-adrenalin complex. Exp. Cell Res. 33, 176–194.

Bullough, W. S., Hewett, C. L. and Laurence, E. B. (1964) The epidermal chalone: a preliminary attempt at isolation. Exp. Cell Res. 36, 192–200.

Bullough, W. S., Laurence, E. B., Iversen, O. H. and Elgjo, K. (1967) The vertebrate epidermal chalone. Nature 214, 578–580.

Elgjo, K. (1968a) Epidermal cell population kinetics after a single application of some hyperplasia-producing substances. Europ. J. Cancer 3, 519–530.

Elgjo, K. (1968b) Epidermal cell population kinetics after repeated applications of some hyperplasia-producing substances. Europ. J. Cancer 4, 183–192.

Elgjo, K. (1974) Evidence for presence of the epidermal G_2-inhibitor ('epidermal chalone') in dermis. Virchows Arch. B Cell Path. 16, 243–247.

Elgjo, K. (1975) Epidermal chalone and cyclic AMP: An in vivo study. J. Invest. Dermatol. 64, 14–18.

Elgjo, K. and Hennings, H. (1971) Epidermal mitotic rate and DNA synthesis after injection of water extracts made from mouse skin treated with actinomycin D: Two or more growth-regulating substances? Virchows Arch. B Cell Pathol. 7, 342–347.

Elgjo, K. and Edgehill, W. (1973) Epidermal growth inhibitors (chalones) in dermis and serum. Virchows Arch. B Cell Pathol. 13, 14–23.

Elgjo, K., Laerum, O. D. and Edgehill, W. (1971) Growth regulation of mouse epidermis I. G-2 inhibitor present in the basal cell layer. Virchows Arch. B Cell Pathol. 8, 277–283.

Elgjo, K., Laerum, O. D. and Edgehill, W. (1972) Growth regulation of mouse epidermis II. G-1 inhibitor present in the differentiating cell layer. Virchows Arch. B Cell Path. 10, 229–236.

Epifanova, O. I. (1971) Effects of hormones on the cell cycle. The Cell Cycle and Cancer (ed.: R. Baserga) Marcel Dekker, New York, pp. 145–190.

Finegold, M. J. (1965) Control of cell multiplication in epidermis. Proc. Soc. Exp. Biol. (N.Y.) 119, 96–100.

Gelboin, H. V., Wiebel, F. and Diamond, L. (1970) Dimethylbenzanthracene tumorigenesis and aryl hydrocarbon hydroxylase in mouse skin: Inhibition by 7,8-benzoflavone. Science 170, 169–171.

Grimm, W. and Marks, F. (1974) Effect of tumor-promoting phorbol esters on the normal and the isoproterenol-elevated level of adenosine 3′, 5′-cyclic monophosphate in mouse epidermis in vivo. Cancer Res. 34, 3128–3134.

Hennings, H. and Boutwell, R. K. (1969) The inhibition of DNA synthesis by initiators of mouse skin tumorigenesis. Cancer Res. 29, 510–514.

Hennings, H. and Boutwell, R. K. (1970) Studies on the mechanism of skin tumor promotion. Cancer Res. 30, 312–320.

Hennings, H., Elgjo, K. and Iversen, O. H. (1969) Delayed inhibition of epidermal DNA synthesis after injection of an aqueous skin extract (chalone). Virchows Arch B Cell Path. 4, 45–53.

Houck, J. C. and Cheng, R. F. (1973) Isolation, purification, and chemical characterization of the serum mitogen for diploid human fibroblasts. J. Cell. Physiol. 81, 257–270.

Iversen, O. H. and Evensen, A. (1962) Experimental skin carcinogenesis in mice. Acta Path. Microbiol. Scand. Suppl. 156.

Iversen, O. H. and Bjerknes, R. (1963) Kinetics of epidermal reaction to carcinogens. Acta Path. Microbiol. Scand. Suppl. 165.

Iversen, O. H., Aandahl, E. and Elgjo, K. (1965) The effect of an epidermis-specific mitotic inhibitor (chalone) extracted from epidermal cells. Acta Path. Microbiol. Scand. 64, 506–510.

Iversen, O. H., Bjerknes, R. and Devik, F. (1968) Kinetics of cell renewal, cell migration and cell loss in the hairless mouse dorsal epidermis. Cell Tissue Kinet. 1, 351–359.

Iversen, O. H., Bhangoo, K. S. and Hansen, K. (1974) Control of epidermal cell renewal in the bat web. Virchows Arch. B Cell Path. 16, 157–179.

Krieg, L., Kühlmann, I. and Marks, F. (1974) Effect of tumor-promoting phorbol esters and of acetic acid on mechanisms controlling DNA synthesis and mitosis (chalones) and on the biosynthesis of histidine-rich protein in mouse epidermis. Cancer Res. 34, 3135–3146.

Laurence, E. B., Randers Hansen, E., Christopher, E. and Rytömaa, T. (1972) Systemic factors influencing epidermis mitosis. Europ. J. Clin. Biol. Res. 17, 133–139.

Raick, A. N. (1973) Ultrastructural, histological, and biochemical alterations produced by 12-*O*-tetradecanoyl-phorbol-13-acetate on mouse epidermis and their relevance to skin tumor promotion. Cancer Res. 33, 269–286.

Rohrbach, R. (1972) Die Aktivität Mitose- und DNS-Synthese-inhibierender Hautextrakte (Chalone) nach carcinogenen und nichtcarcinogenen Reizen. Habilitationsschrift zur Erlangung der venia legendi an der Medizinischen Fakultät der Albert-Ludwig-Universität Freiburg im Breisgau.

Rohrbach, R. and Laerum, O. D. (1974) Variations of mitosis-inhibiting chalone activity in epidermis and dermis after carcinogen treatment. Cell Tissue Kinet. 7, 251–257.

Rohrbach, R., Elgjo, K., Iversen, O. H. and Sandritter, W. (1972) Effects of methylcholanthrene on epidermal growth regulators. I. Variations in the M-factor. Beitr. Path. 147, 21–27.

Rytömaa, T. and Kiviniemi, K. (1968) Control of granulocyte production. I. Chalone and antichalone, two specific humoral regulators. Cell Tissue Kinet. 1, 329–340.

Voorhees, J. J., Duell, E. A., Bass, L. J. and Harrell, E. R. (1973) Role of cyclic AMP in the control of epidermal cell growth and differentiation. Natl. Cancer Inst. Monogr. 38, 47–60.

Weiss, P. and Kavanau, J. L. (1957) A model of growth and growth control in mathematical terms. J. Gen. Physiol. 41, 1–47.

CHAPTER 9

Fibroblast chalone and a putative circulating anti-chalone

John C. Houck

Biochemical Research Laboratory, Research Foundation of Children's Hospital, Washington, D. C. 20009, U.S.A.

9.1 Introduction

The response of fibroblast in vivo to injury is to be 'turned on' mitotically and subsequently to be 'turned off'. The initial events of wound repair involve, besides epithelial and capillary proliferation, the proliferation of the fibroblasts until these latter cells reach a high population density within the interstices of the wound space. These cells then cease to be mitotically active but become active biochemically in terms of the synthesis of firstly glycosaminoglycans and eventually collagen.

The behavior of diploid human fibroblasts in vitro is essentially similar to their behavior in vivo in that cultivated diploid fibroblasts will proliferate until they reach a cell density sufficiently high so that they begin to impinge one upon the other. At this point in the kinetics of the proliferation of these cells, their mitotic rate seems to slow down and eventually almost ceases when the cells are touching one another in a confluent monolayer. If a 'scratch' is made in this confluent monolayer, it can be seen that those cells immediately adjacent to the wounded area become mitotically active and the daughter cells of this mitosis migrate into the open area and continue proliferating until once again a confluent monolayer is reestablished (Raff and Houck, 1969). Therefore, this in vitro model of the in vivo behavior of the fibroblast during wound repair would appear to be an excellent one for the study of factors controlling the proliferation of cells in vitro and, by implication, in vivo.

It has been shown that although fibroblasts cease to proliferate in confluent monolayer under normal culture conditions, a burst of cellular proliferation can be induced in these cells by doubling the concentration of serum in the medium from 10 to 20%. In turn, this subsequent burst of proliferation ceases with a formation of a much thicker layer of confluent cells. Larger concentrations of serum can usually not be added to the medium because above 20% serum is usually cytotoxic (Houck and Cheng, 1973).

Finally, it is important to note that although a number of materials can substitute for serum in studies involving chick or even mouse fibroblasts, no materials can be substituted for serum for the culture of *diploid* human fibroblasts in vitro (Ibid.)

This paper describes the demonstration of a fibroblast chalone and the isolation and purification of a putative fibroblast antichalone in the circulation.

9.2 *Materials and methods*

Two diploid human fibroblast cell lines derived from embryonic lung (WI-38) and from adult cutaneous biopsy (GWF) were used in the course of this study. The karyology of these cells was carefully monitored. These cells were used for no more than 35 doublings (WI-38) or 15 doublings (GWF). These cells were also constantly monitored for mycoplasma contamination and the cells which were found to be contaminated or which had doubled more than indicated above were discarded.

The diploid human fibroblasts mentioned above were cultivated in Eagle's MEM supplemented with glutamine, penicillin–streptomycin, and 10% calf serum. The cells were incubated in sealed vessels at 37°C.

The WI-38 and GWF cells were also cultivated in roller bottles under these conditions and the cells were harvested and stored in the frozen state.

The proliferation assay required seeding of Leighton tubes with 4×10^4 cells per cm^2 which were then allowed to stand at 37°C for 24 h. These cultures were then rinsed repeatedly with several portions of Earle's basal salt solution to remove both the serum and the cells that did not adhere to the glass surface. For WI-38, approximately 90% of the cells were glass-adherent; for GWF, approximately 75% of the cells were adherent. The number of cells per cm^2 was counted at least daily, using an inverted microscope and a ruled Whipple eyepiece, as has been described previously (Raff and Houck, 1969; Houck and Cheng, 1973). From the slope of the linear portion of the log plot of the cell number versus incubation time, which extended over 120 h, the rate of growth was calculated as 'population generation time' in h. This, in turn, was expressed as the percent of the cell population increase per 24 h of percent growth rate.

After rinsing, a similar collection of cells during log growth were allowed to incubate for up to 24 h with 1 μCi of [^{3}H]thymidine. After this time, the medium was removed, the cells were rinsed with serum-free MEM twice, trypsinized, harvested, counted in a hemocytometer, and then mixed with 5% cold trichloracetic acid (TCA). The resulting precipitate was rinsed once again with TCA in the cold and allowed to stand in suspension overnight with 5 ml of TCA. The next morning, the suspension was centrifuged, the supernatant removed, and three more rinsings with 5% TCA were accomplished to remove all of the non-specifically absorbed [^{3}H]thymidine from the precipitated RNA, DNA, and protein. After this final rinse, the precipitate was solubilized in NCS solubilizer at 83 °C and then mixed with a liquid scintillation cocktail and counted in a Nuclear Chicago liquid scintillation counter in the usual fashion. The results were expressed as cpm/10^6 cells (Houck et al., 1972).

Large numbers of diploid human fibroblasts which had been grown in roller bottles were collected by trypsination and, after thorough rinsing with isotonic saline, were sonically disrupted. After centrifugation, the clear supernatant was removed and dialyzed against 200 volumes of water in the cold for 24 to 48 h. After dialysis, the contents of the dialysis bag were centrifuged and the clear supernatant was lyophilized.

Amicon Diaflo ultrafiltration membrane sieving, using Model 402 chambers of the Amicon Corp. (Boston), was done in accordance with the techniques described by Zipilvan et al. (1969). The ultrafiltration was accomplished at 4 °C and essentially 5 to 6 volumes of 0.15 M sodium chloride was washed through the interconnected Diaflo cells until no further material absorbing at 220 or 280 nm could be determined in the final effluent.

Isoelectric focusing was performed in accordance with the instructions of the LKB Co., using the LKB '8100 Ampholine' refrigerated preparative electrofocusing apparatus over various pH gradients at 500 volts and 40% carrier ampholyte for 48 h, as described by Vesterberg and Svenson (1969). The sucrose gradient after isoelectric focusing was eluted through a photometric flow analyzer (280 nm) and recorder into a fraction collector. pH determinations were done, using a Radiometer pH meter and an immersion electrode immediately after collecting these fractions.

Preparative acrylamide gel electrophoresis was performed, using a refrigerated Polyprep 200 apparatus from the Buchler Institute (Fort Lee, N. J.), according to their instruction manual, at pH 9.5. The initial sample was dissolved in 6 ml of 5% sucrose and this was added to 2.8% acrylamide stacking gel, 1 cm high, on a 3 cm high separating gel (7%). The system was run at 15 mA for 1 h prior to adding the sample, and the preparative electrophoretic run was at 50 mA for 9 h, with a flow time of 2.25 ml/min.

Molecular weight determinations were performed, using both gel filtration with Bio-Gel P-200 from Calbiochem in accordance with the method of Piez (1969) and by SDS polyacrylamide gel electrophoresis (without mer-captoethanol) according to Weber and Osborne (1969). Both procedures involve a plot of the log of the molecular weight of known standards versus either elution volume (v/v) for P-200 or electrophoretic mobility for acyl-amide gels. The standards for gel filtration were blue dextran 2000, purified transferrin, albumin, ovalbumin, all from Calbiochem, and the β-chain of acid soluble gelatin. Albumin, ovalbumin, and myoglobin were used as standards for SDS electrophoresis. Gel filtration was performed in 0.05 M acetate buffer, pH 5.5, using a 200 $\times$ 2.5 cm column with 4 mg of sample in 2.0 ml of buffer. Analytical acrylamide gel electrophoresis was performed in the discontinuous system of Davis (1969) using 150 μg samples at pH 9.5 or 4.3 or 8.0 and 2.8 % stacking gel and 7 % separating gels, starting at 1 mA per column for 30 min and maintained with 3 mA per column for 1.5 h. These gels were stained with Coomassie blue in the usual fashion.

9.3 Experimental results

9.3.1 Demonstration of fibroblast chalone

The inhibitory effects of various concentrations of extracts of diploid human fibroblasts upon the incorporation of [^{3}H]thymidine by these cells in culture, as described above, is shown in table 9.1. At a concentration as low as 500 μg/ml, extracts of pure fibroblasts will inhibit 73 % of the control uptake of [^{3}H]thymidine by these cells in vitro. This particular extract of

Table 9.1

Inhibitory effects of fibroblast extract concentration on incorporation of [^{3}H]thymidine by diploid human fibroblasts.

Extract (mg/ml)	[^{3}H]thymidine uptake (cpm/10^6 cells)	% Inhibition
0	3118	—
0.250	2253	28
0.500	833	73
1.0	889	71
2.0	785	75

Table 9.2

Kinetics of [³H]thymidine uptake by diploid human fibroblasts in the presence and absence of fibroblast extract (330 μg/ml).

Hours	[³H]thymidine uptake (cpm/10⁶ cells)		% Inhibition
	Control	Inhibitor	
2	277	227	18
3	460	267	42
4	807	407	50
24	4266	2026	53

Table 9.3

Effect of rinsing inhibitor-treated fibroblasts on the subsequent incorporation of [³H]-thymidine.

	Control	Inhibitor at 0.5 mg/ml		Inhibitor at 2.0 mg/ml	
		No rinse	After rinse	No rinse	After rinse
[³H]thymidine (a)	4995	1135	4475	1205	3614
(cpm/10⁶ cells) (b)	4868	1240	4727	1234	3834
Mean	4931	1187	4601	1219	3724
% Inhibition	—	76	7	75	24

Table 9.4

The effects of various concentrations of ultrafiltered fibroblast extracts upon the time required for population doubling of WI-38, GWF, and human osteosarcoma cells during log phase growth in vitro.

μg chalone/ml	Population generation time (h)		
	WI-38	GWF	Human osteosarcoma
0	34	35	45
50	40	42	45
100	48	50	46
150	47	53	45
200	50	60	40
250	83	91	51
500	105	128	73

diploid human fibroblasts at a concentration of 1 mg/ml had no effect upon the [³H]thymidine uptake by diploid human lymphocytes when stimulated with PHA in culture and, similarly, had no effect upon the thymidine uptake by either HeLa cells or human bronchial carcinoma cells in culture. The kinetics of the inhibitory effect of this dialyzed and lyophilized extract from diploid human fibroblasts upon the uptake of [³H]thymidine into these cells in culture in log phase growth was explored, with the fibroblast extract being used at a concentration of 330 μg/ml. Within 3 h, as shown in table 9.2, there was a significant inhibition of the uptake of [³H] thymidine into the acid insoluble DNA of fibroblasts exposed to this fibroblast extract.

Two doses of the fibroblast extract, 0.5 and 2.0 mg/ml, were added to the incubation medium of diploid human fibroblasts in culture. Half of these cultures were then rinsed with MEM and 10% serum twice, and new medium with 10% serum was added along with [³H]thymidine. Most of the inhibitory activity of the fibroblast extract at 0.5 mg/ml was removed by this rinsing procedure, as shown in table 9.3. At an extract concentration of 2 mg/ml, only 2/3 of the inhibitory activity toward DNA synthesis in these cells was removed by washing the cells free of the added fibroblast extract. The morphological appearance of these inhibited cells in vitro was essentially similar to those of normal growing cells.

The population doubling time of these cells in culture was found to be 33 ± 2 h (Houck and Cheng, 1973). The population doubling time of similar cells in the presence of various amounts of fibroblast extract was also calculated, and the results are summarized in table 9.4. Since the population doubling time is a reflection of the numbers of cells recruited into the cell cycle, or the growth fraction of these cells during log phase, the effect of fibroblast inhibitor upon the population doubling time would be to prolong it considerably by virtue of inhibiting the number of cells recruited into the cell cycle. Using a technique involving autoradiographic labeling via [³H]-thymidine of cells at various hours during log phase growth after a 60-min pulse, the number of cells found to enter S phase from normal diploid human fibroblasts was about 20 to 25%. In the presence of fibroblast chalone concentrate, this number was depressed at a concentration of 330 μg/ml of fibroblast extract to less than 10%.

Diploid human fibroblasts maintained in culture in confluency for 3 to 4 days and at the end of this time the used medium was removed, dialyzed exhaustively against water, and centrifuged. The clear supernatant was lyophilized. The effect of the non-dialyzable portion of this used medium from the cultivation of diploid human fibroblasts in vitro at various concentrations upon the [³H]thymidine uptake by diploid human fibroblasts in culture in log phase growth was explored, as described above. In this series of experiments, the quantitative uptake of [³H]thymidine was about 3200 cpm/10^6 cells, and up to 77% of this uptake could be inhibited by the addition of a significant amount of the non-dialyzable portion of the used medium from other diploid human fibroblasts. See table 9.5. There was no non-dialyzable mitotic inhibitor for fibroblasts in vitro to be found in either normal MEM supplemented with 10% serum, which had been un-used, or in similar medium which had been used to cultivate human lympho-cytes for 24 h (this medium is not adequate to lymphocyte cultivation for longer periods of time than this).

This inhibitory activity of used medium upon the [³H]thymidine uptake of diploid human fibroblasts was not associated with any apparent mor-phologically demonstrable cytotoxicity, since these cells excluded vital dye and did not detach from the glass, and the inhibitory effects upon these fibroblasts was completely reversible after rinsing with medium containing 10% serum.

The crude inhibitory activity of these extracts of sonicated fibroblasts or dialyzed used medium from the cultivation of fibroblasts in vitro was subjected to Amicon Diaflo ultrafiltration, as described above. All of the inhibitory activity from either cell extracts or used medium was concentrated in a molecular weight range between 30,000 and 50,000 daltons. No in-hibitory activity could be demonstrated above 50,000 daltons or below 30,000 daltons after equilibrium ultrafiltration.

Pre-incubation of the ultrafiltered material resulting from either used medium or sonicated fibroblasts with 20 μg/ml of purified trypsin, ribonu-clease, or deoxyribonuclease was performed for 2 h per mg of lyophilized

Table 9.5

Effect of non-dialyzable portion of used medium on [³H]thymidine uptake by diploid human fibroblasts.

	Control	Dose		
		2.0 mg/ml	1.0 mg/ml	0.5 mg/ml
[³H]thymidine uptake (a)	3221	824	1160	2343
(cmp/10^6 cells) (b)	3209	684	1311	2583
Mean	3210	754	1235	2463
% Inhibition	—	77	62	23

extracts. Trypsin incubation was concluded by mixing equivalent weight amounts of soybean trypsin inhibitor into the incubation mixture and then assaying for anti-proliferative or anti-DNA synthesis effects on WI-38 and GWF fibroblasts in vitro. Incubation with trypsin, but not the nucleases almost completely destroyed the fibroblast inhibitory activity described above. Despite the fact that the UV absorbance of these extracts from both cells and used medium had a 260 to 280 nm ratio of about 1.2, neither nuclease had any effect upon the inhibitory activity of these extracts toward diploid human fibroblasts in vitro.

The dialyzed and lyophilized used medium was subjected to isoelectric focusing, as described above. This crude fraction was resolved into three major peaks with isoelectric points of 3.5 to 4.3, 4.4 to 4.9, and 5.0 to 5.7. At 330 μg/ml, only the first peak contained significant amounts of inhibitory activity against fibroblast mitosis; even at concentrations 3 times this, no inhibitory activity could be demonstrated for the latter two isoelectric peaks.

When the material from the pH 3.5 to 4.3 peak was then subjected to molecular sieving, the mitotic inhibitory activity of the 30,000 to 50,000 range could be demonstrated with as little as 50 μg of this fraction being able to inhibit 50% of the [^{3}H]thymidine uptake by diploid human fibro-blasts during log phase growth in culture.

It therefore appears that both fibroblasts and the used medium from the cultivation of these fibroblasts in culture contains a material whose mole-cular weight is between 30,000 and 50,000 daltons and with an isoelectric point between 3.5 and 4.3 which is capable of specifically inhibiting both the proliferation and the thymidine uptake into acid insoluble DNA by diploid human fibroblasts in vitro. The most highly purified material had absolutely no inhibitory effect toward the morphological transformation of human lymphocytes stimulated by PHA, nor toward the proliferative rates of human bronchial carcinoma cells, and did not inhibit the uptake of [^{3}H]thymidine into acid insoluble DNA by either stimulated lymphocytes or HeLa cells.

Further, aqueous extracts of lung were found to contain a material of the same molecular weight which would inhibit the proliferation of diploid human fibroblasts in vitro as expressed in a profound prolongation of the population doubling time from 33 h to over 100 h. This inhibitory activity toward fibroblast proliferation of 30,000-to-50,000 dalton lung extracts was also destroyed by trypsin but not by ribonuclease or deoxyribonuclease incubation. The 30,000-to-50,000-dalton ultrafiltrate from aqueous extracts of bovine, canine, and porcine lung are about equally effective against diploid human fibroblast proliferation, indicating a singular lack of species specificity. Further, the inhibited proliferation of diploid human fibroblasts in vitro was completely overcome, even after 7 days in culture, by rinsing the cultures with MEM containing 10% serum and no tissue extracts; i.e., population doubling time was restored to about 35 h. Thus, the inhibition is completely reversible.

Finally, fibroblast proliferation inhibitor obtained from ultrafiltrates of either WI-38 or GWF cells or from lung extracts after ultrafiltration were capable of completely inhibiting the proliferation of human osteosarcoma cells in vitro. Again, this inhibition of the proliferation of human osteosarcoma cells in vitro was completely reversible by rinsing the cultures free of inhibitor with MEM and 10% serum.

Conclusion   These data suggest that fibroblasts contain a cell-specific, but not species-specific, endogenous negative feedback inhibitor of mitosis, operating in the G_1 portion of the cell cycle, which is completely reversible and apparently non-cytotoxic, i.e., a fibroblast chalone.

9.3.2 Purification of fibroblast anti-chalone from serum

The effects of various concentrations of fibroblast-derived ultrafiltrate toward fibroblast (WI-38) proliferation in MEM supplemented with various amounts of calf serum is shown in table 9.6. These results indicate that as the serum concentration was increased, the prolongation of population doubling time was decreased and therefore that the inhibitory effect of fibroblast chalone was inversely related to the concentration of serum in the medium.

The effects of various concentrations of calf serum upon the growth rate (% of doubling accomplished in 24 h) for both WI-38 and GWF fibroblasts were determined, as shown in table 9.7. At low concentrations of calf serum, there was a linear relationship between the rate of cell growth and serum concentration in the medium. However, above 30% serum, an apparent toxicity toward these fibroblasts could be found. It appeared that the optimal serum concentration in chemically defined medium was between 10 and 20%.

A WI-38 cell line which had been transformed by incubation with SV_{40} (10^6 units/ml for 10 doublings) was also used. The SV_{40}-transformed WI-38 cells were karyologically heteroploid, and viral transformation of these cells was also indicated by their loss of contact inhibition. These transformed cells did not require serum in the medium in order for them to divide. However, the addition of serum to the culture medium of these cells did decrease their generation time and, hence, increase their proliferative rate.

Table 9.6

The effects of various concentrations of ultrafiltered fibroblast extract upon the population doubling time (h) of WI-38 cultures during log phase growth in MEM supplemented with different amounts of calf serum.

μg chalone/ml	Percent serum in MEM			
	5	10	20	25
0	55	34	35	135 (cytotoxic)
50	80	40	35	155
100	85	48	44	195
150	110	47	45	235
200	125	50	48	—
250	230	83	55	—
500	—	105	80	—

Calf serum was subjected to ammonium sulfate precipitation and alcohol fractionation in the usual manner in the cold. Five and four fractions resulted respectively, all of which had an essentially similar amount of growth-promoting activity toward diploid human fibroblasts in vitro. Dialyzed, lyophilized calf serum was reconstituted in 0.15 M NaCl and subjected to Diaflo ultrafiltration membrane sieving, as described above. The serum was fractionated according to molecular weight and the mitogenically active component was found exclusively in the fraction which contained serum proteins with molecular weights ranging from 50,000 to 100,000 daltons. At concentrations of ultrafiltration fraction II of 2.0 mg/ml, the rate of growth was found to be comparable to that observed with 10% serum. Higher concentrations of this ultrafiltration fraction did not inhibit fibroblast mitosis.

The rate of the passage of this serum mitogenic activity through the 100,000-dalton filter, the Diaflo XM 100A, was extremely slow. Thus, it may be assumed that the molecular weight of the component might be very close to 100,000 daltons. For preparative purposes, however, we collected the serum fraction between 50,000 and 300,000.

This ultrafiltered fraction was subjected to isoelectric focusing over a pH gradient of 3 to 10, with all of the activity being found in an isoelectric point of 5.2 to 5.4. MEM supplemented with isoelectric fraction 3 of this pH at 125 μg/ml gave population doubling times comparable to those found for WI-38 or GWF fibroblasts in medium supplemented with 10% whole calf serum.

This fraction from isoelectric focusing was subjected to preparative gel electrophoresis, as described above. Three very sharply defined peaks, which were totally separated, one from the other, were obtained. Only the middle peak contained mitogenically active fraction from serum. At a concentration of 50 μg/ml, this middle fraction from preparative electrophoresis gave population doubling times for both WI-38 and GWF fibroblasts similar to those found in medium supplemented with 10% whole calf serum. Tests with recombinations of the various fractions from preparative acrylamide gel electrophoresis confirmed that only the middle fraction was active.

On acrylamide gel electrophoresis, the fraction from isoelectric focusing which contained the mitogenic activity of serum contained three bands which could be visualized by Coomassie blue staining. After preparative acrylamide gel electrophoresis, however, only one single band at pH 9.5 could be demonstrated, even at concentrations in excess of 250 μg/gel. This mitogenically active component of serum moved as an electrophoretically homogeneous β-globulin. Acrylamide gel analytical electrophoresis was also performed at pH 8.0 and 4.3 (with the polarity reversed in the latter condition) and only one electrophoretic band could be demonstrated with 150 μg of materials per gel.

This material had been completely purified after only 132-fold purification. Therefore, it must constitute about 0.50% of the total serum proteins! Considerably smaller amounts of this protein were found in cow and horse serum, however.

For the determination of molecular weight, 8 mg of the serum-derived

Table 9.7

The effect of supplementing MEM with various concentrations (volume %) of calf serum upon the % growth rate of WI-38 and GWF diploid human fibroblasts during log phase growth in vitro.

Serum concentration	WI-38	GWF
0	0	0
2.5	31 ± 1.8	31 ± 0.6
5.0	43 ± 1.5	39 ± 1.5
7.5	51 ± 2.7	49 ± 2.2
10.0	73 ± 3.6	71 ± 2.4
20.0	67 ± 2.9	63 ± 1.8
30.0	20 ± 2.1	17 ± 0.5
40.0	detached	detached

mitogen for diploid human fibroblasts in 3 ml of 0.05 M acetate buffer at a pH of 5.5 was run through a Bio-Gel P200 column (2.5 × 100 cm). These results indicated that the fibroblast mitogen has a molecular weight of about 120,000 daltons. Further, electrophoretic elution patterns from SDS gel electrophoresis indicated firstly only one band could be demonstrated under these conditions and that this material had a molecular weight of about 56,000 daltons. From this, we conclude that the fibroblast mitogen found in serum is made up of two identical subunits which together have a molecular weight of 112,000 to 120,000. This purified serum mitogen was biologically inactivated by incubation with either trypsin or neuraminidase. Thiobarbituric acid assay for sialic acid indicated that it contained 1.2% sialic acid and the total carbohydrate content of this mitogen was 3.4% by anthrone reaction. Amino acid analysis as well as determination of free sulfhydryl groups indicated that at least 6 moles of sulfur containing amino acids remained in the mitogen molecule. Four moles of sialic acid, four moles of free SH, and 12 moles of hexose were also found per mole of purified mitogen (Houck and Cheng, 1974).

Similar purification attempts were made, using the serum from human, horse, adult cow, fetal calf, and rabbit. The general properties of the mitogenic activity from all of these species were essentially similar to that demonstrated for the material obtained from calf serum, i.e., namely a molecular weight of about 120,000 daltons and an IEP of 5.2 to 5.4. The biological activity of these fractions were also destroyed by neuraminidase or trypsin incubation but, like the purified calf serum material, was capable of surviving for 30 min at temperatures of 56 °C.

Conclusion Mammalian sera possesses a sialoprotein weighing 120,000 daltons and made up of two identical subunits of about 60,000 daltons each. These subunits are held together by hydrophobic bonds and each subunit itself contains at least one and possibly two disulfhydryl groups. Each subunit contains two moles of sialic acid and 6 moles of hexose. All of the mitogenic activity of serum toward diploid human fibroblasts resides in this molecule. All mammalian sera studied to date contain this mitogenic sialoprotein, at a concentration in calf serum of 0.5%.

9.3.3 *Nature of the interaction between fibroblast chalone and serum mitogen*

Solutions of the purified mitogenic sialoprotein from calf serum were prepared at a concentration of 50 μg/ml in MEM supplemented only with glutamine and penicillin-streptomycin. This medium would support the growth of WI-38 of GWF diploid human fibroblasts at a population doubling time of about 28 h. When 500 μg of chalone concentrate from ultrafiltrates of used medium was added to this solution of serum mitogen, this medium supported a population doubling time of about 110 h. When mixtures of fresh purified serum mitogen at 50 μg/ml and 500 μg/ml of chalone concentrate in MEM were subjected to molecular sieving through an Amicon Diaflo ultrafiltration XM 50 filter which would pass materials of molecular weights below 50,000 daltons, the population doubling time supported by the medium remaining above this filter was restored essentially to normal (32 h); thus, essentially all of the chalone activity had been easily removed from the solution containing purified serum mitogen, suggesting that there was no strong and direct interaction between fibroblast mitogen and the chalone concentrate.

Since it is clear that there is a competitive relationship, as shown in table 9.8, between the effect of chalone and the concentration of purified serum mitogen in the medium and since the interaction between purified serum mitogen and chalone is obviously energetically trivial, then the suspicion grows that the effects of serum mitogen and chalone upon the mitotic activity of fibroblasts most probably proceed from competitive interaction at the same sites on the cell by both materials. We propose (Houck et al., 1973) the control mechanism of fibroblast proliferation in vitro and probably in vivo resides in the relationship of the concentration of fibroblast chalone to fibroblast mitogen, or 'anti-chalone'. Contact-inhibition in vitro would then involve a sharing of a critical chalone concentration between cells which are essentially contiguous through crowding into confluency. The chalone could then later be displaced from the surface of these cells by the addition of fibroblast mitogen or antichalone, or by simply

Table 9.8

Effect of supplementing MEM with various amounts of purified serum mitogen upon the concentration of ultrafiltered fibroblast extract required to double the population doubling time of WI-38 during log phase growth in vitro.

μg mitogen/ml	Fibroblast ultrafiltrate (μg/ml)
12.5	175
25.0	200
50.0	235
75.0	275
100.0	315

increasing the concentration of serum in the medium. Thus, because of the decreased concentration of chalone (due to displacement from the cell surface via anti-chalone concentration), these cells would continue to proliferate in vitro. Similarly, during wound healing and repair in vivo, the normally mitotically arrested fibroblast begins to proliferate at a considerable rate in that portion of the tissue adjacent to the injury. Insuspation of serum into the wounded tissue is, of course, one of the major characteristics of the acute inflammatory response. Thus, it is probable that the fibroblast mitogen derived from serum flooding into the injured tissue area around the site of the wound would displace chalone from the fibroblast contained within this marginal area and therefore permit the entrance of these cells into the mitotic cycle. Proliferation of fibroblasts into the injured tissue would continue until such time as the biological continuity of the microcirculation was restored and the fibroblast mitogen from serum would no longer be flooding the environment around the area of injury. Therefore, the proliferation of fibroblasts into the wound would cease and the biochemical and mechanical repair of the lesion by collagenization could begin.

If the theory that purified serum mitogen functions as an 'anti-chalone' for the fibroblast chalone is correct, then one would expect that the release of chalone activity from fibroblasts in serum-free medium would be commensurable subsequent to the addition of the purified mitogen to the culture. In fact, as has been shown earlier, simply rinsing the cells for 30 min or even allowing them to stand for 24 h does not release into the used medium measurable inhibitory activity. However, it should be remembered that this used medium contains exogenous serum mitogen and is assayed for inhibitor on WI-38 in 10% serum. Therefore, we collected the medium to which had been added 50 μg/ml of purified serum mitogen and which had been allowed to stand for 30 min, 24 h, and 48 h with diploid human fibroblasts in culture which had been in mid-lof phase growth. These cells had been rinsed with serum-free MEM three times and allowed to stand for 2 h in serum-free medium to permit further dissolution of contaminating serum. It should be noted that this procedure does not necessarily remove all of the serum adhering to these cells in culture. These various used media were then subjected to molecular ultrafiltration, using a 50,000-dalton filter. The portions of the medium above 50,000 daltons were assayed for mitogenic activity on other cells while the materials which pass through the 50,000-dalton filter were assayed for their inhibitory effect upon WI-38 fibroblasts which were grown in 10% calf serum, as described above. The mitogenic activity concentration was found to have been reduced from the biological equivalent of 50 μg to about 25 μg after 1 h, but the mitotic inhibition activity below

50,000 daltons could not be assayed in the presence of 10% serum on other diploid human fibroblasts. By 24 h, the used medium contained a concentration of purified serum mitogen essentially equivalent to about 20 μg, while the mitogenic inhibitor had increased to the point where it was significantly prolonging the population doubling time of WI-38 fibroblasts in 10% supplemented MEM from 35 h to about 50 h.

After 48 h of standing in the presence of diploid human fibroblasts, the used medium was subjected to ultrafiltration, as described above, and it clearly demonstrated a very profound loss of serum mitogen activity to less than 10 μg/ml in biological equivalent activity and contained a concentration of about 300 μg of biological equivalent of the mitogenic inhibitor. We believe that this type of quantitative and reciprocal data suggests that as the cell number increases between 24 and 48 h, the concentration of chalone released goes up significantly so that it can be assayed once it has been separated by ultrafiltration from a very considerably reduced concentration of purified serum mitogen. Therefore, we suggest that the lag in the release of a commensurable inhibitory factor from the cultivation of diploid human fibroblasts in vitro is a result of the changing relationships between the concentration of chalone to that of serum mitogen. Clearly, mitogen is being consumed and chalone is being released, and the difficulties in the biological assay of these mitotic stimulating and mitotic inhibiting activities obscures this reciprocal relationship.

For technical reasons, we have been unable, as yet, to complete the obvious experiment in which chalone is added to mitotically active cells whose used medium contains a reduced amount of serum mitogen and demonstrate that as the chalone concentrate is increased, the mitogen was being released into this used medium. It is obviously possible, without the evidence of this experiment, to simply assume that the serum mitogen is being consumed in some fashion by the growing fibroblasts in vitro. None of these experiments precludes completely the possibility that the purified serum mitogen is altering the quality of the membrane of fibroblasts in culture and that these cells are then entering into the mitotic cell cycle because of the entrance of nutritional substrates into the cell.

It should be pointed out that fibroblasts do not normally live in a medium containing large amounts of circulating macromolecules in that the microcirculatory integrity restricts the nature of the molecules which flood into the ground substance in which these cells exist. In a similar fashion, epidermal cells are compartmented so that they, too, live at some distance from the macromolecular elements of the circulation. Like fibroblasts, the germinal layer of epidermis survives by picking up nutrients by diffusion rather than by direct vascular supply. Insuspation of serum during inflammation into the ground substance of the connective tissue, then, would destroy the barrier between these two cell types and the circulation. Perhaps under these circumstances, the anti-chalone activity of serum macromolecules for fibroblasts might be correlated with an anti-chalone activity toward epidermal cell proliferation. One of the experiments that suggests that this may be the case is that if purified serum mitogen or fibroblast anti-chalone were injected along with [³H]thymidine intradermally in the guinea pig and sections of tissue around the site of injection were harvested 6 and 24 h later, autoradiographically only those fibroblasts and epidermal cells within the area of injection contained many labeled nuclei.

Although this preliminary evidence does not demonstrate an anti-chalone, nor indeed indicate that the fibroblast anti-chalone has anything to do with the factor stimulating epidermal proliferation, nonetheless, it seems not unreasonable to postulate, at least tentatively, the possibility that a number of putative anti-chalones may exist in the circulation, i.e. (a) the anti-chalone for granulocyte, which has been claimed previously, (b) an anti-chalone for fibroblast, for which evidence is presented above, and (c) a possible anti-epidermal chalone. The need for a chalone and possibly anti-chalone for the granulocyte system proceeds from the unique character of circulating chalone necessary to control the proliferation of these cell types. The idea of circulating anti-chalone for both fibroblast and epidermis makes biological sense, based largely on the fact that neither of these cell types are normally exposed to significant amounts of serum, except in pathological situations such as inflammation. It would seem unlikely, then, that lymphocyte chalone would be associated with a circulating anti-chalone, since these cells are constantly bathed with plasma.

9.4 Summary

Diploid human fibroblast-rich tissues contain a macromolecule with a molecular weight between 30,000 and 50,000 daltons which will inhibit the proliferation of fibroblasts in the G_1 phase of the cell cycle (i.e., inhibit both H-thymidine uptake as well as the normal increase in cell number). This inhibitor is destroyed by trypsin but not by ribonuclease or deoxyribonuclease, and is thermolabile. It has an acid IEP. It is not cytotoxic, and its inhibitory activity appears to be completely reversible. This fibroblast endogenous inhibitor does not interfere with the proliferation of DNA synthesis by human lymphocytes, bronchial carcinoma cells, or HeLa cells. The activity does not appear to be species-specific. Therefore, we suggest that it is quite possible that the control of fibroblast proliferation resides in a fibroblast chalone.

Diploid human fibroblasts, in contrast to chicken or mouse fibroblasts or heteroploid fibroblasts in general, stringently require serum for their proliferation. All of this mitogenic activity of calf serum can be concentrated in a molecular weight range around 100,000 daltons by ultrafiltration. All of the mitogenic activity within this molecular weight class can be concentrated at a pH of 5.2 via isoelectric focusing, and all of the activity at this isoelectric point can be concentrated in one peak on preparative polyacrylamide gel electrophoresis. This latter material is homogeneous at three different pH's in analytical gel electrophoresis as well as in SDS electrophoresis. This purified serum mitogen for diploid human fibroblasts in vitro also works in vivo and represents as much as 0.5% of the serum protein of calf, albeit there is much less of this protein in adult cow or horse. It is composed of two equal subunits weighing about 60,000 daltons each and contains about 2 moles of sialic acid, one S-S bond, and 6 moles of hexose per subunit.

There is a reciprocal relationship between the biological activity of fibroblast inhibitor and serum mitogen, but there is no apparent direct interaction between these two proteins. Addition of pure serum mitogen to diploid human fibroblasts in vitro results in the release of commensurable chalone activity into the medium and a reciprocal loss of mitogen from the medium. Therefore, we propose that serum contains a single macromolecule which competes with endogenous chalone on the surface of diploid human fibroblasts and this functions as an 'anti-chalone' for the fibroblast.

References

Benesch, R. and Benesch, R. E. (1962) Determination of SH-groups in proteins, in Methods of Biochemical Analysis, Vol. 10. Interscience Publishers, Inc., New York, pp. 43–70.

Davis, B. J. (1964) Disc electrophoresis. Ann. N. Y. Sci. 121, 404.

Houck, J. C., Weil, R. L. and Sharma, V. K. (1972) Evidence for a fibroblast chalone. Nature New Biol. 240, 210.

Houck, J. C. and Cheng, R. F. (1973) Isolation, purification, and chemical characterization of the serum mitogen for diploid human fibroblasts. J. Cell. Physiol. 81, 257.

Houck, J. C., Sharma, V. K. and Cheng, R. F. (1973) Fibroblast chalone and serum mitogen (anti-chalone). Nature New Biol. 246, 111.

Pardee, A. B., de Asua, L. J. and Rozengurt, E. (1974) Functional membrane changes and cell growth: significance and mechanism, in Control of Proliferation in Animal Cells (eds.: B. D. Clarkson and R. Baserga). Cold Spring Harbor Laboratory, New York, pp. 547–561.

Piez, K. (1968) Molecular weight determination of random coil polypeptides from collagen by molecular sieving chromatography. Anal. Biochem. 26, 305.

Raff, E. C. and Houck, J. C. (1969) Migration and proliferation of diploid human fibroblasts following 'wounding' of confluent monolayers. J. Cell. Physiol. 74, 235.

Vesterberg, O. and Svenson, H. (1966) Isoelectric fractionation analysis and characterization of ampholytes in natural pH gradients. IV. Further studies on the resolving power in connection with separation of myoglobulins. Acta Chem. Scand. 20, 820.

Warren, L. (1959) The thiobarbituric acid assay of sialic acid. J. Biol. Chem. 234, 1971.

Weber, K. and Osborne, M. (1969) The reliability of molecular weight determinations by dodecyl sulfate-polyacrylamide gel electrophoresis. J. Biol. Chem. 244, 4406.

Zipilvan, E. M., Hudson, B. G. and Blatt, W. F. (1969) Separation of immunologically active fragments by membrane partition chromatography. Anal. Biochem. 30, 91.

CHAPTER 10

Current status of melanocyte chalones

A. L. Thornley and Edna B. Laurence*

Mitosis Research Laboratory, Zoology Department, Birkbeck College, University of London, Malet Street, London WC1E 7HX, U.K.

As the neural tube sinks below the ectoderm in the vertebrate embryo, a separate group of cells can be identified in the transitional region between the forming neural tube and the ectoderm. These are the neural crest cells which give rise during development to diverse neural elements as well as to branchial cartilage and perhaps to odontoblasts (Balinsky, 1970). Further, the neural crest is held to be the source of all pigment cells in the vertebrate body. These include melanocytes which are dispersed during tissue differentiation to all parts of the body, becoming associated not only with the epidermis and its derivatives, but also with internal organs (Boyd, 1960).

The mammalian pigmentary system has been intensively studied (Montagna and Hu, 1966; Kawamura et al., 1971), yet regional dispersion of melanocytes during organogenesis is still an enigmatic phenomenon, as is the process of stabilisation of melanocyte numbers in the adult tissues. Melanocytes, whether associated with epidermal derivatives or scattered in the epidermis, share a feature which is common amongst cells of neural crest origin; in normal circumstances they divide rarely or perhaps not at all. It is therefore of considerable interest to know whether the chalone concept can be applied to the mitotically quiescent pigment-forming cells and whether or not dysfunction of a self-monitoring, chalone-regulating system can in any way be correlated with the development of benign or malignant neoplasms. This article is a synopsis of experimental evidence which suggests that melanocytes synthesise chalones.

The chalone concept was broadly defined more than a decade ago (Bul-

* The authors wish to acknowledge a grant from the University of the Witwatersrand, Johannesburg (to ALT) and a grant from the Cancer Research Campaign (to EBL).

lough, 1962) and in essence still holds today (Rytömaa, 1970; Houck and Daugherty, 1974). In terms of this definition any tissue-specific endogenous molecule acting in negative feedback regulation of chemical processes, which are essential for the progression of a cell through the proliferative cycle, may be called a chalone. It is not surprising, therefore, that experimental evidence since accumulated points to at least two sites of chalone action in the cell cycle. These are the gap before S-phase (G_1 chalones) and the gap before M-phase (G_2 chalones). It has now become a convention to speak of G_1 and G_2 chalones and, indeed, there is reason to believe that epidermal G_1 and G_2 chalones are chemically different substances (Marks, 1973). However, a critical analysis of the general mass of data concerning chalones shows that in no instance is there adequate evidence to make the cell cycle phase specificity of chalone action acceptable as fact. Nevertheless, it is convenient to keep to this convention for the purpose of this discussion.

The argument for a melanocyte G_2 chalone rests on a series of experiments conducted by Bullough and Laurence (Bullough and Laurence, 1968) and on a more recent investigation by Seiji et al. (Seiji et al., 1974).

Bullough and Laurence (1968) examined both Harding–Passey melanomas innoculated into mice, and Green Fortner amelanotic tumours in hamsters, for chalone-like substances. Preliminary in vivo experiments showed that the mitotic rate (i.e. colcemid-measured M phase influx of cells) in Harding–Passey melanomas was rapidly depressed by a partially purified epidermal chalone preparation (71–80% ethanol precipitate obtained by fractionating aqueous pig skin extract), but not by an electrophoretically purified and dialysed epidermal chalone preparation (Hondius Boldingh and Laurence, 1968).

Extending this finding, Harding–Passey, Green Fortner and pig skin extracts were tested against hamster tumour tissue (3 mm cubes) maintained in a buffered glucose medium at 37 °C for 4 h. In contrast to mouse epidermal cells, which initially respond to epidermal extracts alone, hamster tumour cells remained unresponsive to melanoma and pig skin extracts in the absence of adrenalin and hydrocortisone. The reason for this difference remains unknown. When adrenalin and hydrocortisone were added together to the incubation flasks, only a small mitotic depression (about 15%) was recorded; this increased to 61–76% on the further addition of melanoma or pig skin extract. This result may indicate that a critical level of intracellular cAMP concentration in these tumour cells must be maintained before chalone regulation of mitosis becomes operational. As established in vivo, the purified epidermal chalone did not depress mitosis in melanoma tissue. The observations led to the conclusion that both melanotic and amelanotic tumours synthesised an anti-mitotic factor acting at G_2 in the cell cycle, and that this factor was also present in the 71–80% ethanol fraction obtained from pig skin. Since purified epidermal chalone no longer had the power to inhibit mitosis in the tumours, it was reasoned that the melanocyte chalone had been discarded during electrophoretic purification and dialysis of the epidermal chalone.

The melanocyte anti-mitotic factor was found to remain in the 80% supernatant when a standard ethanol fractionation procedure was applied to the water extracts of Harding–Passey and Green Fortner tumours. These supernatants, subjected to the diagnostic test for epidermal G_2 chalone (Laurence, 1973), had no inhibitory effect on ear epidermal mitosis in vitro. No other target organs were considered in this study. A subsequent publication (Bullough and Laurence, 1970), however, mentions that water extracts of Harding–Passey tumours do not depress the mitotic rate in lymphoma tissue in vitro. In the light of current progress it is debatable whether these results constitute sufficient evidence for tissue specificity of this putative melanocyte G_2 chalone, especially in view of the fact that dose-response relationships of the extract were not considered, and that the epidermal mitotic rate in melanoma-bearing mice was actually significantly depressed when compared with normal animals. (This observation was interpreted by Bullough and Laurence (Bullough and Laurence, 1968) as a tumour-induced stress condition.)

Seiji et al. (Seiji et al., 1974) have recently reported recording a 32% mitotic depression when Harding–Passey tumour extracts were tested against exponentially growing C_34_1 cells (a subline of B-16 melanoma cells) incubated for 4 h in the presence of adrenalin and hydrocortisone, but these workers have not apparently examined the cell line specificity of this reaction so that their data cannot be regarded as an independent confirmation of the existence of the melanocyte G_2 chalone.

The search for a melanocyte chalone by Bullough and Laurence (Bullough and Laurence, 1968) was in fact initiated as a result of a series of in vivo studies performed by Mohr et al. (Mohr et al., 1968), who gave repeated injections of the 71–80% ethanol precipitate obtained from pig skin to Harding–Passey tumour-bearing mice and Green Fortner tumour-bearing hamsters with spectacular results.

During these trials 5 daily doses, ranging from 25–400 mg per mouse and 100–200 mg per hamster, were administered. An optimal dosage of 100–200 mg per mouse and 200 mg per hamster caused a rapid regression of tumours in 75 mice and 200 hamsters. These figures must be compared with no spontaneous remissions in 1000 untreated control mice and 3000 control hamsters. Harding–Passey melanoma extracts produced similar effects (Mohr et al., 1968). Metastases or tumours recurred in most mice and all the hamsters.

This dramatic response to these extracts provoked much speculation but a causal relationship between epidermal and/or melanocyte chalone-induced mitotic inhibition and tumour regression was not subsequently proved. In this context it is now known that the ethanol precipitate from pig skin contains a powerful epidermal G_1 chalone (Marks, 1973), and it is also likely that the lower dosages of 25 mg per mouse caused a non-specific inhibition of DNA synthesis (our unpublished observations).

Mohr et al. (1972), having examined the components of ethanol precipitates, came to the conclusion that the real oncolytic agent was not a chalone but contaminating *Clostridium* spores. (At present there seems to be no a priori reason why a chalone-induced mitotic depression should cause tumour regression.) This opinion is not shared by Bullough (1975) who, amongst others, has suggested an invoked immune response, in conjunction with a reduced mitotic rate in tumour tissue, may have been the main element in the elimination of these tumours. Unfortunately nothing is known about the immune condition of these animals before or after injection of skin extracts, and there is no mention of an examination of tumour biopsies, so that this question remains unresolved.

The possibility that Harding–Passey melanoma cells synthesise tissue-specific and tissue non-specific inhibitors of DNA synthesis, as well as G_2 chalone mentioned earlier, is emphasised by the detailed data published by Seiji et al. (1974), who have studied the effects of melanoma extracts on exponentially growing tumour cells in culture. Acrylamide gel electrophoresis revealed 7 major protein components in a 70–95% ethanol precipitate obtained by fractionating water extracts of Harding–Passey melanomas. Of these components at least 2 contained tyrosinase activity. When the ethanol precipitate was applied to a G-100 Sephadex column 4 components were detected, 2 of which inhibited [^{14}C]thymidine and [^{3}H]leucine incorporation when tested against B-16 melanoma cells. One of the latter, a protein (MW 30,000 to 35,000 daltons), proved to be non-specific in its action, also inhibiting [^{14}C]thymidine and [^{3}H]leucine incorporation by HeLa and L (mouse fibroblast) cells. CsCl density gradient centrifugation revealed that the second inhibitory factor was bound within a heterogeneous RNA–protein complex. This inhibitor was cell line-specific, depressing only B-16 melanoma cell incorporation of [^{14}C]thymidine and [^{3}H]leucine. Trypsin and RNase digestion of the heterogeneous complex reduced inhibitory activity by 50 and 25% respectively, so that at present both moieties must be considered an integral part of the inhibitor. No mention was made of testing this substance against tumour-bearing mice (presumably there was insufficient material) and, furthermore, information regarding proliferation kinetics in their cell cultures was not offered by these authors; thus one cannot ascertain with any accuracy from their data the point in the cell cycle at which the complex acts. The possibility that the complex also retained the G_2 inhibitor present in crude extracts, and therefore the power to inhibit M phase influx of cells, was apparently not tested. The significance of the parallel inhibition of DNA and protein synthesis is as yet obscure.

Dewey (1973) has reported finding a dialysable chymotrypsin-, trypsin- and neuraminidase-sensitive chalone-like factor in water extracts of Harding– Passey melanomas. Performing cell counts over several days showed that this factor inhibited growth of Harding–Passey cultures, but not cultured hamster lung, transformed human embryo and liver cells. Although it behaved in an anomalous fashion on Sephadex columns, he was able to infer from his data that a molecular weight of less than 2000 daltons was appropriate for the inhibitory component in the extracts. More recent in- novations (Dewey, 1975) in assaying and purifying this substance, which inhibits [^{3}H]thymidine incorporation by tumour cells in short-term cultures, has revealed a small molecule which may in reality be chymotrypsin-, trypsin- and heat-stable. It has an absorbance spectrum in the region of 190 nm (amide bonds). Tissue specificity of this highly purified peptide (?) has not yet been investigated.

Until such time as more information is available concerning the tissue specificity and dose-response relationships of the substances isolated by Dewey (1973) and Seiji et al. (1974), these results should be viewed with cautious optimism. It is a matter of speculation whether these 2 groups are purifying the same or dissimilar endogenous inhibitors. The ethanol frac- tionation technique employed by the Japanese group can cause co-precipita- tion artifacts (Houck, 1975), which may explain the apparent heterogeneity of their RNA–protein complex. The same procedure was employed by Bullough and Laurence (1968), so that it must be borne in mind that these authors may have tested melanoma fractions containing both G_1 and G_2 inhibitors.

An important factor which concerns all these experiments is that in vivo tissue specificity, which forms the crux of the problem, has not been demonstrated. This is especially important in view of the cytotoxic sub- stances (for example, 4 S RNA (Adachi et al., 1971)), which some of these malignant cells may produce. The peritoneal diffusion chamber method of culturing melanocytes (Shieferstein and Laerum, 1975) would seem to offer at present a good methodological approach to this problem since a simultaneous cytofluorometric determination of G_1, S-phase, G_2 + M cell proportions in the chambers is possible, as well as an analysis of non-specific target tissues.

In conclusion, experimental evidence suggests that abnormal melanocytes derived from Harding–Passey and Green Fortner melanomas synthesise and respond to chalone-like inhibitors of DNA synthesis (more specifically, inhibitors of isotopically labelled thymidine incorporation) and mitosis.

Nothing definite is known about the chemical constitution of the endogenous chalone-like inhibitor which restricts the flow of cells into M phase (Bullough and Laurence, 1968), whereas the chalone-like inhibitors of DNA synthesis isolated so far (Dewey, 1973; Seiji et al., 1974) are both at least partly built of peptides. Whether these 2 inhibitors of DNA synthesis act in G_1 or S phase of the cell cycle has not yet been determined. Tissue specificity of all these inhibitors needs substantiating. Not unexpectedly, melanogenesis is an unrelated function of melanocytes since amelanotic tumour cells seem to produce and respond to chalone-like inhibitors.

At present there is no patent link between chalone and the regression of Harding–Passey and Green Fortner tumours caused by injecting large amounts of crude material containing epidermal chalones. The fact that the tumours did regress is, nevertheless, an important result which warrants re-examination.

Whether chalones play a role in maintaining the mitotic inactivity of normal melanocytes in a variety of vertebrate tissues remains a fascinating problem but at present the questions posed in the introductory paragraphs of this article are unanswered.

References

Adachi, K., Hu, F. and Kondo, S. (1971) A new endogenous inhibitor for mouse melanoma cells. Biochem. Biophys. Res. Commun. 45, 742.

Balinsky, B. I. (1970) An Introduction to Embryology, Philadelphia, London, Toronto, W. B. Saunders Co.

Boyd, J. D. (1960) The embryology and comparative anatomy of the melanocyte. In: Progress in the Biological Sciences in Relation to Dermatology (ed.: A. Rook) Cambridge University Press.

Bullough, W. S. (1962) The control of mitotic activity in adult mammalian tissues. Biol. Rev. 37, 307.

Bullough, W. S. (1975) Mitotic control in adult mammalian tissues. Biol. Rev. 50, 99.

Bullough, W. S. and Laurence, E. B. (1968) Control of mitosis in mouse and hamster melanomata by means of the melanocyte chalone. Europ. J. Cancer 4, 607.

Bullough, W. S. and Laurence, E. B. (1970) The lymphocytic chalone and its antimitotic action on a mouse lymphoma in vitro. Europ. J. Cancer 6, 525.

Dewey, D. C. (1973) Melanocyte chalone. Natl. Cancer Inst. Monograph 38, 213.

Hondius Boldingh, W. and Laurence, E. B. (1968) Extraction, purification and preliminary characterization of epidermal chalone: a tissue-specific mitotic inhibitor obtained from vertebrate skin. Europ. J. Biochem. 5, 191.

Houck, J. C. and Daugherty, W. F. (1974) Chalones: A Tissue-specific Approach to Mitotic Control. Medcom Medical Update Series, New York.

Kawamura, T., Fitzpatrick, T. B. and Seiji, M. (eds.) (1971) Biology of Normal and Abnormal Melanocytes, Univ. Tokyo Press.

Laurence, E. B. (1973) Experimental approach to the epidermal chalone. Natl. Cancer Inst. Monograph 38, 37.

Marks, F. (1973) A tissue-specific factor inhibiting DNA synthesis in mouse epidermis. Natl. Cancer Inst. Monograph 38, 79.

Mohr, U., Althoff, J., Kinzel, V., Süss, R. and Volm, M. (1968) Melanoma regression induced by chalone: a new tumour inhibitory principle acting in vivo. Nature 220, 138.

Mohr, U., Hondius Boldingh, W. and Althoff, T., (1972) Identification of contaminating *Clostridium* spores as the oncolytic agent in some chalone preparations. Cancer Res. 32, 117.

Montagna, W. and Hu, F. (eds.) (1966) Advances in Biology of Skin, Vol. VIII, Pergamon Press.

Rytömaa, T. (1970) Regulation of cell production by chalones. Ann. Clin. Res. 2, 94.

Schieferstein, G. and Laerum, O. D. (1975) Proliferation pattern of hamster melanoma cells cultured in diffusion chambers in pre-immunised hosts. Arch. Derm. Forsch. 251, 169.

Seiji, M., Nakano, H., Akiba, H. and Kato, T. (1974) Inhibition of DNA and protein synthesis in melanocytes by a melanoma extract. J. Invest. Dermatol. 62, 11.

CHAPTER 11

Chalone tissue specificity and the embryonic derivation of organs. An appraisal of the problems

EDNA B. LAURENCE* and ALAN L. THORNLEY**

Mitosis Research Laboratory, Zoology Department, Birkbeck College, University of London, Malet Street, London WC1E 7HX, U.K.

11.1 The evolutionary aspects

Evidence has been accumulating over the past decade for the existence of chalones but little progress has been made in the understanding of the chemical processes involved in the inhibition of cell proliferation by these substances. The complications have become even greater now that there is evidence for chalones which act at different phases of the cell cycle (G_1 and G_2 chalones) (Elgjo et al., 1971, 1972; Elgjo, 1973; Marks, 1973; Thornley and Laurence, 1975b). This may be a reflection of unrelated mechanisms regulating cell division. The property that distinguishes one chalone from another is tissue specificity, since the mechanics of cell proliferation is a process common to all tissues. The part of the molecule which regulates cell proliferation (at whatever phase of the cell cycle) may be common to all chalones and is a study in itself (Houck and Dougherty, 1974; Thornley and Laurence, 1975a), whereas the question of tissue specificity of chalone action concerns every aspect of developmental biology and is the province of this review.

It is not known at what stage in the evolutionary development of a primitive multicellular organism chalones first functioned. Chalones may have developed as a refinement of a basic anti-mitotic messenger molecule some time after the evolution of tissues. It is possible that chalones are functional in the tissues of extant Protochordates, in which case some of these molecules could have an evolutionary history as long as, for example,

We are indebted to the Cancer Research Campaign* and the University of the Witwatersrand, Johannesburg** for grants which have enabled this collaboration to take place.

the thyroid hormone. Using the same reasoning it may be supposed that those tissues which developed late in evolution have chalones with molecular structures similar to the chalones of the tissues from which they developed – e.g. hair and sebaceous gland chalones could be slight modifications of the epidermal chalone since they are formed from epidermis late in ontogeny. In contrast, the tissues formed from different germinal layers – e.g. epidermis and granulocytes – may have chalones with very different structures. It is therefore important to know how early in embryogenesis tissue-specific chalones are formed. Do embryonic chalones differ from adult chalones?

The available data relate only to fish, amphibia, birds and mammals. No fish tissues have been studied for the effects of chalones, but an epidermal G_2 chalone has been extracted from the codfish skin (Bullough et al., 1967). The epidermal chalone system, therefore, may have evolved some 350 million years ago. Here a study of the *Agnathan* forms would be of considerable interest. Amphibia are particularly suitable for the study of chalones during ontogeny since the primitive tissue form (e.g. pronephros) is functional for at least a part of the lifespan of the animal. An analysis of tissues from neotenic amphibia may provide considerable new information. No reptilian tissues have been examined for chalones while, in the birds, embryonic chick or newly-hatched chick, but not adult, tissues have been examined. The mammals have commanded most attention because of the therapeutic potential of chalones. Being viviparous, mammals present a particularly interesting case: do adult chalones pass the placental barrier? It is now becoming apparent that with refinements in purification of chalones many have low molecular weights and are probably peptides (Houck, personal communication), and there seems no reason why they should not pass through the placental barrier and influence the growth of the foetus.

This review examines information bearing on the development of chalone systems during organogenesis in an effort to crystallise some of the problems concerning tissue specificity which have arisen as a result of preliminary biological investigations on different organs.

11.2 *Chalones and organogenesis*

After cleavage of the fertilised vertebrate egg, the organised movement of cells results in the formation of a two-layered gastrula. Subsequently a third layer is demarcated. These are the three germ layers: the outer ectoderm, the middle layer or mesoderm and the inner endoderm. Throughout the vertebrates there is a common pattern of tissue derivation from these three germ layers: (1) the ectoderm gives rise to tissues such as the brain, sensory organs and nerves, the pigmentary system, the epidermis proper and its derivatives, and the lining of the extremities of the alimentary canal (2) the mesoderm gives rise to the reproductive organs and kidneys, the muscular and skeletal systems, circulatory system (blood and lymph), the fibroblasts and the dermis of the skin, the mesenteries, etc. (3) the liver, the respiratory apparatus and the alimentary canal, except the extremities, are all endodermal in origin.

11.2.1 Evidence from tissues of ectodermal origin

From the dorsal surface of the embryo the neural folds arise which subsequently close to form the neural tube. This sinks, separating completely from the overlying epidermis. An ectodermally derived irregular mass of cells between the neural tube and the overlying epidermis is the neural crest. This mass of cells gives rise to the sympathetic nerve system, the visceral skeleton, melanocytes, etc., of which only melanocytes have been examined for chalones (reviewed elsewhere in this book. Thornley and Laurence). Various parts of the brain develop as thickenings of the neural tube; ectoderm in the region of the optic cup forms a vesicle which becomes the lens, and overlying epidermis eventually forms the cornea. After all the primary organ rudiments have been formed, an invagination of the ectoderm to meet the anterior endoderm of the alimentary canal forms the lining of the mouth, while a similar inpushing posteriorly becomes the lining of the rectum.

11.2.1.1 Epithelia of ectodermal origin
Of the ectodermal epithelia, the epidermis has been most extensively studied and biochemical evidence for epidermal chalones is reviewed elsewhere in this book (Marks). Here it suffices to say that the epidermal G_2 chalone has been found in codfish and some mammals (Bullough et al., 1967). How early in embryogenesis epidermal chalones are synthesised is not known, but the fact that rats and mice at birth are immature compared with other mammals, makes the work of Marrs and Voorhees relevant here (Marrs and Voorhees, 1971a, b). They found that the newborn rat epidermis contains a G_2 chalone which inhibits mitotic activity in the adult mouse epidermis in a manner similar to that found by Bullough and Laurence (1964) who used extracts from adult mouse epidermis.

An extensive study has been made on G_2 chalones of the oral epithelia (Randers-Hansen, 1967; Laurence and Randers-Hansen, 1971, 1972). Epidermal G_2 chalone was found in pig and human gingiva and pig palate.

However, when an extract of pig palate was injected into mice it caused a greater mitotic depression in the tongue epithelium than in the ear epidermis, while a partially purified pig skin extract caused a greater mitotic inhibition in ear than in tongue epithelium. (This result is reminiscent of the work of Nome on forestomach, see p. 282.) These experiments on oral epithelium led to a complete reevaluation of the regulation of cell proliferation by a negative feedback process (Bullough, 1965; Iversen, 1969) and gave experimental evidence for the concept of chalone antagonists (Laurence et al., 1972). Hall (1969) has found that crude epidermal extracts inhibit the epithelial cells of hamster cheek pouch from entering the S-phase of the cell cycle. It is relevant to note that he detected a stimulant of DNA synthesis in his epidermal extracts.

In contrast to the keratinising epithelia of the skin and the mouth, the ectodermally-derived epithelia of the eye take two forms. These are the non-keratinising squamous epithelium of the cornea and the epithelium of the lens. Bullough and Laurence (1964) found that crude extracts of mouse epidermis inhibited mitosis in the corneal epithelium in vitro. Recently Thornley and Laurence (in preparation) have shown that a 70–80% ethanol precipitate obtained by fractionating pig skin, when injected into mice, inhibited the incorporation of $[^3H]$thymidine in corneal epithelium as well as ear epidermis. In a series of papers. Voaden (1968a, b) and Voaden and Leeson (1970), Leeson and Voaden (1970) demonstrated that γ-crystallin of lens had the properties of an epidermal G_2 chalone, reversibly inhibiting mitosis in rabbit lens epithelium and ear epidermis in vitro. Not only did this substance inhibit mitosis in the ear epidermis in a manner similar to the epidermal G_2 chalone, but it also showed some common chemical properties – for example, lack of sulphydryl groups (Hondius Boldingh and Laurence, 1968; Voaden, 1968b). In addition, the lens epithelium reacted by mitotic inhibition to a 70–80% ethanol precipitate obtained by fractionating pig skin (Voaden, 1968b).

11.2.1.2 Epidermal derivatives
The structures which develop late in ontogeny, in some cases post-natally, from the ectoderm are mainly characteristic of mammals, as for instance, the epidermal appendages. A small amount of evidence suggests that some of these derivatives have their own chalone systems. Bullough and Laurence (1970), in an extensive study using skin extracts obtained from codfish and various species of mammal as well as extracts of mammalian oral epithelia, found that mitosis in mouse sebaceous glands was depressed only by those extracts which were from organs containing sebaceous glands. This sebace-

ous gland G_2 chalone has yet to be isolated, but it appears to differ from a purified epidermal G_2 chalone which has no effect on sebaceous gland mitosis. Thornley and Laurence (in preparation) also have found that [^{3}H]thymidine incorporation by sebaceous gland cells was not affected by the epidermal G_2 chalone, which had been purified by ethanol precipitation, electrophoresis and dialysis. However, the 70–80% ethanol precipitate of pig skin from which this G_2 chalone was derived did depress [^{3}H]thymidine incorporation by sebaceous gland cells, a finding which may indicate the presence of a sebaceous gland G_1 in addition to a G_2 chalone in pig skin extracts. Thus this gland proved an excellent tissue for determining cell line specificity of epidermal chalones. Epidermally-derived sebaceous glands are formed late in embryonic development. It is possible, therefore, that epidermal and sebaceous gland chalones are very similar in chemical constitution.

As yet inhibition of mitosis in hair bulbs has not been found after treatment with pig skin extracts (Bullough and Laurence, unpublished results). This may be due to the pig skin extracts containing little hair bulb chalone. The hair is a complicated organ (Bullough and Laurence, 1958; Argyris, 1972) and the experimental procedure may have been at fault. Hair roots (bulbs) have never been extracted for chalone assay.

The eccrine sweat gland is yet another epidermal derivative. In this organ it is the difference in rates of cell proliferation, cell migration and cell loss when compared with those of the epidermis, that cause the coiling of the duct as it penetrates the epidermis (Christophers and Plewig, 1973). Bullough and Deol (1972) examined this organ for G_2 chalones. They injected human sweat (differentiation product) into mice and found no mitotic inhibition in sebaceous glands and ear epidermal cells. Eccrine sweat duct cells, by contrast, showed a dose-response mitotic inhibition. Extracts of pig palate and epidermis had no effect on the cell proliferation in this gland. That the eccrine sweat gland product inhibits the mitotic rate in the duct cells is in contrast to the results obtained by Tutton (1973) on intestine, and Elgjo et al. (1971, 1972, 1973) on epidermis, where extracts of mainly potential progenitor cells produced a G_2 chalone.

The lachrymal and salivary glands of mammals have not been examined for chalone activity and, more surprisingly, neither have mammary glands. No doubt the complications of hormonal effects have detracted from the exploration of the latter tissue for its chalone system, although clinically this chalone may be important and biologically it would be interesting because it is considered to be homologous to sebaceous glands.

11.2.2 Evidence from tissues of mesodermal origin

More is known about the chalones isolated from mesodermal tissues than from the other two germ layers. They include the chalones of the blood and lymphatic systems and the fibroblasts. These connective tissue chalones have been considered elsewhere in this book and are not reviewed here (see Bateman, Houck, Rytömaa, this book). However, blood vessels were the subject of early work (Simms and Stillman, 1936) in which an attempt was made to isolate a tissue-specific endogenous inhibitor of 'growth'. The introduction of growth inhibitors as regulators of tissue homeostasis was probably obscured by the then current work on stimulants – for example, hormones and embryonic inducers. It was not until the latter part of the 1950's that it was acknowledged that regulation of cell proliferation is a result of the interaction of many factors, including stimulants and inhibitors (Weiss and Kavanau, 1957; Teir and Rytömaa, 1967).

In 1936 Simms and Stillman (1936) described a species non-specific, heat-labile, non-dialysable substance which could be extracted by alcohol and calcium chloride from the aortae of various vertebrates. This substance inhibited the growth of chick aortic cultures, but whether it should be classified as a chalone using the accepted definition of chalones (Bullough, 1967; Rytömaa, 1970) is speculative. However, Florentin et al. in 1973 has also described a substance occurring in pig arteries, which when injected into pigs, inhibited mitosis in arterial smooth muscle cells at the G_2 phase of the cell cycle. The epidermis was used as a non-specific target to test for tissue specificity and was found to be unaffected by extracts of pig artery. Although these authors feel that the tissue and species specificity test should be more extensive before this inhibitor is classed as a chalone, these findings support the earlier observations by Simms and Stillman.

Work which has been done on kidney chalones is particularly significant since the functional vertebrate kidney develops in three phases. Firstly, the pronephros forms. This is functional in a modified form in the adults of archaic chordates, as, for instance, the hagfish (*Agnatha*). In fish and amphibia the pronephros functions only in the larva and is replaced by the mesonephros which is the functional kidney of the adult. In reptiles, birds and mammals these two forms are rudimentary and the functional adult kidney is the metanephros. Experiments performed by Chopra and Simnett (Chopra, 1973; Chopra and Simnett, 1969, 1971; Simnett and Chopra, 1969) form a good example of the way in which the evolutionary development of chalone systems may be analysed. They cultured pronephros taken from stage 32 post tail bud *Xenopus laevis* larvae and found that extracts of the adult mesonephros depressed the mitotic index of larval explants. This inhibitor was tissue-specific because epidermis accompanying the explants was unaffected. They also implanted intact larvae (functional pronephros) into the dorsal lymph sac of normal adults (functional mesonephros) and of the animals which had been partially nephrectomised. The increased mitotic rate in the nephrectomised kidney was accompanied by an abnormally high mitotic rate in the pronephros of the implanted larvae. Adult animals, with their implants, were injected with extracts of rat kidney (functional metanephros). The mitotic index in the adult and larval kidney was then found to be depressed, but in all cases the epidermis of the skin was unaffected. These experiments indicate that the G_2 chalone regulating mitosis in the higher vertebrate kidney may have remained little changed throughout the course of vertebrate evolution.

As long ago as 1956 Saetren proposed a tissue growth regulatory mechanism based on experiments with extracts of kidney. He found, as result of his experiments with subcutaneously and intraperitoneally implanted kidney tissue, that the first mitotic peak in the kidney of partially nephrectomised adult rats could be depressed by a kidney-based factor. He extracted a heat-labile, non-dialysable substance from adult kidneys which, when injected, had the same inhibitory effect. Since the second peak of mitosis in the regenerating kidney was greater than expected, he was led to believe that the inhibitory substance was short-lived. His subsequent ingenious experiments (1963), which involved substituting removed perinephrium with finely divided kidney tubules or liver tissue, indicated that the inhibitory substance diffused slowly through kidney cells. It inhibited mitosis in the vicinity of the applied kidney tubules to a greater extent than the mitosis deeper in the cortex of the adult kidney. These experiments also showed that this inhibitor was active on juvenile rat kidney. This suggests that fast-growing developing organs respond to G_2 chalone-like substances taken from adult tissues.

Dicker and Morris (1974) have confirmed the existence of inhibitors in kidney extracts by measuring 'growth' of renal cortical explants taken from week-old rats or mice. These consisted of 'fibroblast-like cells and epitheloid-type cells'. The inhibition of 'growth' occurred only when extracts of adult kidney cortex (but not of other tissues) were added to the cultures. These extracts had the same properties as those used by Saetren (1956, 1963). The presence or absence of embryonic kidney in the extracts which were made for addition to the culture medium apparently had no effect on the growth of kidney explants.

Roels (1969) also studied the effects of tissue extracts on kidneys and has pointed out inconsistencies in results which have been obtained by using kidney homogenates to investigate compensatory growth factors.

Of the other tissues of mesodermal origin it is surprising that the reproductive system has not attracted more attention from the point of view of chalones. Indeed, no information is available on chalones in the ovary, but Clermont and Mauger (1974) have studied the chalones of the rat testis. The complexity of this organ (Dym and Clermont, 1970) meant that special methods had to be used so that compensatory changes in cell proliferation, which would have masked chalone effects, were partially eliminated. Clermont and Mauger overcame this difficulty by using irradiated animals. The proliferating, renewing type A_1 to A_4 spermatogonia, had been eliminated in these animals so that the A_0 spermatogonia were the main target cells. Crude water extracts of rat testis depressed the incorporation of [^{3}H]-thymidine by A_0 spermatogonia but not by Intermediate and type B spermatogonia as measured by autoradiographic and scintillation counting methods. They regard this G_1 (?) chalone as cell line specific because the extracts did not inhibit [^{3}H]thymidine incorporation by Intermediate and type B spermatogonia. Why these cells were not affected raises problems, as crude extracts of whole testes were used and these, presumably, contain extracts of all testis cells. Liver extracts caused no inhibition of thymidine incorporation by any of the various types of spermatogonia.

11.2.3 Evidence from tissues of endodermal origin

Of the endodermal organs the respiratory system, i.e. the larynx, trachea, bronchi, and alveoli are derived from an invagination of the ventral surface of the alimentary canal. Histologically similar components are found in the respiratory epithelia, the oesophagus, forestomach epithelium and, surprisingly, the ectodermally-originating oral epithelia. Liver, which develops from the floor of the duodenum, is discussed elsewhere in the book (Verly). Pancreas, etc. has not been examined for chalones.

Simnett et al. (1969) described the presence of a lung G_2 chalone which depressed mitosis in lung explants in vitro. They used liver and kidney explants to demonstrate the tissue specificity of this inhibitor. Bullough and Laurence (unpublished results) later found that extracts of bronchus and lung contained a G_2 chalone as identified by the adrenalin wash technique (Bullough and Laurence, 1964) using ear epidermis as a target tissue. These results seem contradictory, but they may indicate that epithelia of ectodermal and endodermal origin have cross-reacting chalone systems.

Apart from the rectal and oral epithelia the remainder of the alimentary canal is endodermal, although the structure can vary from flat and squamous epithelial to glandular villiform lining. Brugal and Pelmont (1973, 1974, 1975) investigated the intestine of the amphibian *Pleurodeles waltlii* for chalone-like substances. After separating adult intestine extracts on Sephadex G-200 they injected embryos intraperitoneally. The mitotic index in the embryonic intestine 5 and 26 h after injection revealed the possibility that there were two intestinal endogenous mitotic inhibitors which were cell cycle phase-specific and, furthermore, inactive on telencephalon. One acted at G_1 phase (molecular weight 120,000 to 150,000 daltons) and the other acted at the G_2 phase (molecular weight less than 2000 daltons) of the cell cycle. They have taken these experiments further using cytophotometric and scintillation counting methods, and suggest that the G_1 inhibitor may promote differentiation of intestinal cells (Brugal and Pelmont, 1975).

In 1963 Bischoff (1964) postulated that the epithelial cells of embryonic chick duodenum may produce a substance (chalone?) which caused the differentiation and a three-fold decrease in mitotic rate in the villi during the last week of incubation. He showed that saline extracts ofd uodenum taken from 19-day chick embryos caused a depression in 14-day duodenum when injected intravenously whereas liver extracts did not. How early in development this factor(s) was synthesised is not known since duodenum from the younger embryos was not extracted.

Philpott (1971) extracted the gizzard mucosa of unhatched chick (stage 45–46) and recorded the effects of this extract on tissues of 6- to 12-day old chick embryos in vitro. At 8 days the gastric glands of the intestine are not formed and the intestinal villi are poorly developed. After treatment he found that only the mitotic rate of the stomach epithelium was depressed whereas the intestinal epithelium and the supporting mesenchyme, as well as skin explants, had normal mitotic rates. He fractionated gizzard mucosa extracts on Sephadex G-25 and calculated that the molecular weight of this heat-labile G_2 inhibitor of 'proliferative behaviour' was in the region of 20,000 daltons.

Of particular interest is the work of Tutton (1973) who has attempted to ascertain whether chalones are produced by differentiating or potential progenitor cells of the small intestine. The rat jejunum is particularly suitable for this type of investigation since these two types of cells are demarcated spatially in the villi. Tutton ethanol-extracted the isolated epithelial cells of the crypts (i.e. progenitor cells) and found that extracts inhibited mitosis in the jejunum both in vivo and in vitro, but they had no effect in the colonic crypts, oesophagus or tongue epithelium. Extracts of the differentiating jejunal villi cells had no effect on mitosis in crypts indicating that a G_2

chalone was synthesised by proliferating crypt cells (cf. epidermis, p. 277).

Nome (1974) has made a gallant attempt to solve the problem of tissue specificity of chalones by extracting various regions of alimentary canal, mesodermal organs, as well as the skin. He then determined the effect of each extract on the mitotic rate and on DNA synthesis in some of the tissues that had been extracted. In general he found that, with the exception of the forestomach, crude water extracts of the various regions of the alimentary canal and other tissues gave a slight but non-significant depression of the mitotic rate and $[^3H]$thymidine incorporation in all the tissues he examined. Water extracts of the forestomach, on the other hand, contained both G_1 and G_2 inhibitors which were active both on forestomach and on skin epidermis but were ineffective on intestinal, kidney and spleen cell proliferation. This is an important finding and illustrates the complexities of results obtained when crude extracts of tissues are used. All these extracts may contain non-specific inhibitors of cell proliferation and cytotoxic agents. It is interesting to note that he found that crude skin extract did not inhibit the cell proliferation in forestomach epithelium to the same degree as the extract of forestomach, and vice versa. Frankfurt (1971) had previously found that substances in the skin inhibit $[^3H]$thymidine labelling and mitosis in the forestomach epithelium.

Using ear epidermis as target tissue a G_2 chalone as identified by the adrenalin wash technique was found in extracts of oesophagus, which like forestomach has a squamous parakeratotic epithelial lining (Laurence, 1973a). Even so, Laurence (1973b) later found that epidermal G_2 chalone (i.e. 70–80% ethanol precipitate from pig skin) produced no mitotic inhibition in the oesophagus. There was a 68% depression in the ear epidermis of the same mice. This result is contrary to an earlier finding that oesophageal lining responds by mitotic inhibition to crude epidermal extracts in vitro.

11.3 Major problems concerning chalones and tissue organisation

This review indicates some of the many facets in chalone research which need a thorough re-investigation with more modern and precise methods in order to understand the origin and evolution of chalone systems. Accumulating data suggest that chalones act at least at two points in the cell cycle. G_1 and G_2 chalone action has been investigated in some tissues (Elgjo et al., 1971, 1972, 1973; Bichel, 1973a, b; Marks, 1973; Simard et al., 1974; Yamaguchi et al., 1974; Brugal and Pelmont, 1975; Thornley and Laurence, 1975b) and it is reasonable to expect that where one type of action is found in an organ, the other will also exist. Generalisations about actions and molecular weights have become unacceptable now unless reference is made to the point of action in the cell cycle. The relative importance of G_1 and G_2 chalones regulating cell proliferation in each organ is unknown and it is in this context that the following problems have been formulated.

It is important to know how early in embryonic development of tissues each kind of chalone mechanism is manifested. Larval and amphibian tissues seem to respond to G_2 chalones obtained from adult tissues (Bischoff, 1964; Chopra and Simnett, 1969, 1971; Simnett and Chopra, 1969; Philpott, 1971; Chopra, 1973; Brugal and Pelmont, 1974, 1975). There are no data to show that *adult* tissues respond to either G_1 or G_2 *embryonic* chalones. Is less chalone produced by an embryonic cell when compared with an adult cell? Theoretically some chalones are small enough to pass the placental barrier and thus influence embryonic growth but this has not been investigated. Is chalone action counteracted by a factor (anti-chalone, Rytömaa, 1969; Yamaguchi et al., 1974; chalone antagonist, Laurence et al., 1972; mesenchymal factor, McLoughlin, 1963; Bullough, 1975) at the level of the embryo, or is the dilution of the maternal chalones such that growth of the foetus is unhindered?

It appears that tissue specificity or cell line specificity of chalones may be traced to very early stages in vertebrate development (Brugal, 1973; Brugal and Pelmont, 1974, 1975) and in some cases may have changed very little despite the evolution of new organs (for example, metanephros) (Chopra and Simnett, 1969, 1971; Simnett and Chopra, 1969; Chopra, 1973). Some chalones may also have been synthesised late in vertebrate evolution as, for instance, the hypothetical sebaceous gland chalone(s) (Bullough and Laurence, 1970; Thornley and Laurence, in preparation). However, this does not explain why mammalian endodermal tissues respond to ectodermal chalones (Bullough and Laurence, 1964; Frankfurt, 1971; Laurence, 1973; Nome, 1974) and vice versa: a direct contradiction of the postulate that chalones are tissue-specific. The answer to this problem may lie in the fact that evidence for these cross-reacting chalone systems has been gained from experiments using crude homogenates of epidermis, intestine, lung and stomach, all of which may contain non-specific inhibitors of cell proliferation and/or cytotoxic factors. These data need verification by direct comparison of purified G_1 and G_2 preparations and their effects on homologous tissues taken from animals belonging to different classes. It is then possible that these contradictions may be eliminated.

In mammals there is as yet little evidence for regionally distinct chalone systems in the epidermis. Ectodermally-derived epithelia, such as the lens (Voaden, 1968a, b; Leeson and Voaden, 1970; Voaden and Leeson, 1970) and cornea (Bullough and Laurence, 1964; Thornley and Laurence, in preparation), react to both G_1 and G_2 epidermal chalones. Regarding the endodermal part of the alimentary canal the opposite may be true since some regional tissue specificity has been found (Philpott, 1971; Tutton, 1973). The epidermis itself is regionally demarcated by varying rates of cell proliferation (Laurence, 1973b). It has been shown that the regions in the mouse epidermis with the highest mitotic rate respond least to the G_2 inhibitor present in partially fractionated pig skin extracts (Laurence, 1973b). At face value this appears to be an anomalous result, but it has been known for a long time that cell structure and kinetic characteristics of a tissue are a result of the balanced interaction of many substances (Teir and Rytömaa, 1967; Argyris, 1972; Wolstenholme and Knight, 1969; Rytömaa, 1973; Padilla et al., 1974). Inexplicable results are common when impure extracts are used in experiments and the need for re-investigation of these chalone systems is clear.

Are chalones synthesised by potential progenitor cells or maturing cells? Two lines of evidence now suggest G_2 chalones are produced by progenitor cells (Elgjo et al., 1971, 1972; Elgjo, 1973; Tutton, 1973). These findings have to be accommodated in any theory concerning the actions of chalones.

Since epidermal chalones appear to have been found in, or react on, mucous-secreting (Frankfurt, 1971; Laurence, 1973a, b; Nome, 1974), keratinising (Marks, 1973), and non-keratinising (Bullough and Laurence, 1964; Voaden, 1968a, b; Leeson and Voaden, 1970; Voaden and Leeson, 1970; Thornley and Laurence, in preparation) epithelia, it would seem unlikely that they are the major factors concerned with terminal differentiation in each epithelium. This poses the problem of whether or not chalones are involved in differentiation, which in turn relates to the tissue specificity of chalone action.

In conclusion, it may be pointed out that these tissue-specific endogenous inhibitors of cell proliferation have been considered to act in at least four ways:

a) as primary inhibitors of cell proliferation so that the cell remains in the 'dormant' state (Simms and Stillman, 1936) which is presumably G_0 (Lajtha and Gilbert, 1967) or A phase (Smith and Martin, 1973, 1974).

b) as primary inhibitors of cells proliferation and so promoting maturation (consequently the differentiation for function) of a cell (Bullough, 1973).

c) as primarily promoting the cell to maturation and, secondarily and consequently, inhibiting cell proliferation (Bullough and Rytömaa, 1965; Laurence et al., 1972).

d) as a factor maintaining the balance in an organ between cell loss and cell gain (Bullough, 1975).

From this review it is obvious that a decision cannot be reached as to which of these four theories is correct, or if chalones only *regulate the rate* of cell proliferation, or if the true action of chalones has yet to be found. The need for further information based on experimentation with purified chalone preparations is abundantly clear. Only then will the role of chalones as tissue-specific messenger molecules become firmly established.

References

Argyris, T. S. (1972) Chalones and the growth control of normal, regenerative, and neo-plastic growth of the skin. Am. Zool. 12, 137.

Bateman, A. This book.

Bichel, P. (1973a) Further studies on the self-limitation of growth of JB-1 ascites tumours. Europ. J. Cancer 9, 133.

Bichel, P. (1973b) Self-limitation of ascites tumor growth: a possible chalone regulation. Natl. Cancer Inst. Monogr. 38, 197.

Bischoff, R. (1964) Inhibition of mitosis by homologous tissue extracts. J. Cell Biol. 23, 10A.

Bjerknes, R. and Iversen, O. H. (1974) 'Antichalones'. A theoretical treatment of the possible role of antichalone in the growth control system. Acta Pathol. Microbiol. Scan. A. suppl. 248, 33.

Brugal, G. (1973) Effects of adult intestine and liver extracts on the mitotic activity of corresponding embryonic tissues of *Pleurodeles waltlii* Michah. (Amphibia, Urodela). Cell Tissue Kinet. 6, 519.

Brugal, G. and Pelmont, J. (1974) Présence, dans l'intestin du Triton adulte *Pleurodeles waltlii* Michah., de deux facteurs antimitotiques naturels (chalones) actifs sur la pro-lifération cellulaire de l'intestin embryonnaire. C.R. Acad. Sci. Paris 278 D, 2831.

Brugal, G. and Pelmont, J. (1975) Existence of two chalone-like substances in intestinal extracts from the adult newt, inhibiting embryonic intestinal cell proliferation. Cell Tissue Kinet. 8, 171.

Bullough, W. S. (1965) Mitotic and functional homeostasis. A speculative review. Cancer Res. 25, 1683.

Bullough W. S. (1967) The evolution of differentiation. Academic Press Inc., London and New York.

Bullough, W. S. (1973) The chalones: A review. Natl. Cancer Inst. Monogr. Suppl. 38, 5.

Bullough, W. S. (1975a) Minireview. Chalone control mechanisms. Life Sci. 16, 323.

Bullough, W. S. (1975b) Mitotic control in adult mammalian tissues. Biol. Rev. 50, 99.

Bullough, W. S. and Deol, J. U. R. (1972) Chalone control of mitotic activity in eccrine sweat glands. Brit. J. Dermatol. 86, 585.

Bullough, W. S. and Laurence, E. B. (1958) The mitotic activity of the follicle. In: The Biology of Hair Growth (ed.: W. Montagna and R. A. Ellis) Academic Press, London and New York.

Bullough, W. S. and Laurence, E. B. (1964) Mitotic control by internal secretion: The role of the chalone-adrenalin complex. Exp. Cell Res. 33, 176.

Bullough, W. S. and Laurence, E. B. (1970) Chalone control of mitotic activity in sebaceous glands. Cell Tissue Kinet. 3, 291.

Bullough, W. S. and Laurence, E. B. Unpublished results.

Bullough, W. S. and Rytömaa, T. (1965) Mitotic homeostasis. Nature (London) 205, 573.

Bullough, W. S., Laurence, E. B., Iversen, O. H. and Elgjo, K. (1967) The vertebrate epidermal chalone. Nature (London) 214, 578.

Chopra, D. P. (1973) Regulation of mitosis in the embryonic kidney *(Xenopus laevis)* by kidney growth inhibitor (chalone). Natl. Cancer Inst. Monogr. 38, 189.

Chopra, D. P. and Simnett, J. D. (1969) Demonstration of an organ-specific mitotic inhibitor in Amphibian kidney. Exp. Cell Res. 58, 319.

Chopra, D. P. and Simnett, J. D. (1971) Tissue-specific mitotic inhibition in the kidneys of embryonic grafts and partially nephrectomized host *Xenopus laevis*. J. Embryol. Exp. Morphol. 25, 321.

Christophers, E. and Plewig, G. (1973) Formation of the Acrosyringium. Arch. Dermatol. 107, 378.

Clermont, Y. and Mauger, A. (1974) Existence of a spermatogonial chalone in the rat testis. Cell Tissue Kinet. 7, 165.

Dicker, S. E. and Morris, C. A. (1974) Investigation of a substance of renal origin which inhibits the growth of renal cortex explant in vitro. J. Embryol. Exp. Morphol. 31, 655.

Dym, M. and Clermont, Y. (1970) Role of spermatogonia in the repair of the seminferous epithelium following irradiation of the rat testis. Am. J. Anat. 128, 265.

Elgjo, K. (1973) Epidermal chalone: Cell cycle specificity of two epidermal growth inhibitors. Natl. Cancer Inst. Monogr. 38, 71.

Elgjo, K., Laerum, O. D. and Edgehill, W. (1971) Growth regulation in mouse epidermis. I. G_2-inhibitor present in the basal cell layer. Virchows Arch. Zellpath. 8, 277.

Elgjo, K., Laerum, O. D. and Edgehill, W. (1972) Growth regulation in mouse epidermis. II. G_1-inhibitor present in the differentiating cell layer. Virchows Arch. Zellpath. 10, 229.

Florentin, R. A., Sang, C. N., Janakidevi, K., Lee, K. T., Reiner, J. M. and Thomas, W. A. (1973) Population dynamics of arterial smooth-muscle cells. Arch. Pathol. 95, 317.

Frankfurt, O. S. (1971) Epidermal chalone. Effect on cell cycle and on development of hyperplasia. Exp. Cell Res. 64, 140.

Hall, R. G. (1969) DNA synthesis in organ cultures of the hamster cheek pouch. Exp. Cell Res. 58, 429.

Hondius Boldingh, W. and Laurence, E. B. (1968) Extraction, purification and preliminary characterisation of the epidermal chalone. Europ. J. Biochem. 5, 191.

Houck, J. C. This book.

Houck, J. C. and Daugherty, W. F. (1974) Chalones: A tissue-specific approach to mitotic control. Medcom Press.

Iversen, O. H. (1969) Chalones of the skin. In: Ciba Foundation Monograph, Symposium on Homeostatic Regulators. (ed.: G. E. Wolstenholme and J. C. Knight) pp. 29–53.

Lajtha, L. G. and Gilbert, C. W. (1967) Kinetics of cellular proliferation. Adv. Biol. Med. Physics 11, 1.

Laurence, E. B. (1973a) Experimental approach to epidermal chalone. Natl. Cancer Inst. Monogr. 38, 37.

Laurence, E. B. (1973b) The epidermal chalone and keratinising epithelia. Natl. Cancer Inst. Monogr. 38, 61.

Laurence, E. B. and Randers Hansen, E. (1971) An in vivo study of epidermal chalone and stress hormones on mitosis in tongue epithelium and ear epidermis of the mouse. Virchows Arch. B. Zellpath. 9, 271.

Laurence, E. B. and Randers Hansen, E. (1972) Regional specificity of the epidermal chalone extracted from two different body sites. Virchows Arch. B. Zellpath. 11, 34.

Laurence, E. B., Randers Hansen, E., Christophers, E. and Rytömaa, T. (1972) Systemic factors influencing epidermal mitosis. Rev. Europ. Etud. Clin. Biol. 17, 133.

Leeson, S. J. and Voaden, M. J. (1970) A chalone in the mammalian lens. II. Relative effects of adrenaline and nor-adrenaline on cell division in the rabbit lens. Exp. Eye Res. 9, 67.

Marks, F. (1973) A tissue-specific factor inhibiting DNA synthesis in mouse epidermis. Natl. Cancer Inst. Monogr. 38, 79.

Marks, F. This book.

Marrs, J. M. and Voorhees, J. J. (1971a) A method for bioassay of an epidermal chalone-like inhibitor. J. Investig. Dermatol. 56, 174.

Marrs, J. M. and Voorhees, J. J. (1971b) Preliminary characterisation of an epidermal chalone-like inhibitor. J. Invest. Dermatol. 56, 353.

McLoughlin, C. B. (1963) Mesenchymal influences on epithelial differentiation. In: Symposia of the Society for Experimental Biology XVII, 359.

Nome, O. (1974) Tissue specificity of epidermal chalones. Thesis submitted to the University of Oslo.

Padilla, G. M., Cameron, I. L. and Zimmerman, A. (eds.) (1974) Cell Cycle Controls. Academic Press, London and New York.

Philpott, G. W. (1971) Tissue-specific inhibition of cell proliferation in embryonic epithelium in vitro. Gastroenterology 61, 25.

Randers Hansen, E. (1967) Mitotic activity and mitotic duration in tongue and gingival epithelium of mice. Effect of chalone. Odont. Tids. 75, 480.

Roels, F. (1969) Influence of homogenates on compensatory renal hyperplasia: Inconsistency of results. In: Compensatory Renal Hypertrophy (eds.: W. W. Nowinski and R. J. Goss) Academic Press, New York and London, 69.

Rytömaa, T. (1969) Granulocytic chalone and antichalone Hemic Cells in vitro (ed.: P. Farnes) In vitro 4, 47.

Rytömaa, T. (1970) Regulation of cell production by chalones. Ann. Clin. Res. 2, 94.

Rytömaa, T. (1973) Control of cell division in mammalian cells. In: The Cell Cycle in Development and Differentiation (eds.: M. Balls and F. S. Billett).

Rytömaa, T. This book.

Saetren, H. (1956) A principle of growth. Production of organ specific mitose-inhibitors in kidney and liver. Exp. Cell Res. 11, 229.

Saetren, H. (1963) The organ-specific growth inhibition of the tubule cells of the rat's kidney. Acta Chem. Scand. 17, 889.

Simard, A., Corneille, L., Deschamps, Y. and Verly, W. G. (1974) Inhibition of cell proliferation in livers of hepatectomised rats by rabbit hepatic chalone. Proc. Nat. Acad. Sci. U.S. 71, 1763.

Simms, H. S. and Stillman, N. P. (1936) Substances affecting adult tissue in vitro. II. A growth inhibitor in adult tissue. J. Gen. Physiol. 20, 621.

Simnett, J. D. and Chopra, D. P. (1969) Organ specific inhibitor of mitosis in the Amphibian kidney. Nature (London) 222, 1189.

Simnett, J. D., Fisher, J. M. and Heppleston, A. G. (1969) Tissue-specific inhibition of lung alveolar cell mitosis in organ culture. Nature (London) 223, 944.

Smith, J. A. and Martin, L. (1973) Do cells cycle? Proc. Nat. Acad. Sci. U.S. 70, 1263.

Smith, J. A. and Martin, L. (1974) Regulation of cell proliferation. In: Cell Cycle Controls (eds.: G. M. Padilla, I. L. Cameron and A. Zimmerman) Academic Press, London and New York.

Teir, H. and Rytömaa, T. (eds.) (1967) Control of Cellular Growth in Adult Organisms. Academic Press, London and New York.

Thornley, A. L. and Laurence, E. B. (1975a) The present state of biochemical research on chalones. Int. J. Biochem. 6, 313.

Thornley, A. L. and Laurence, E. B. (1975b) Chalone reulation of the epidermal cell cycle. Experientia 31, 1024.

Thornley, A. L. and Laurence, E. B. Current status of melanocyte chalones. This book.

Thornley, A. L., Laurence, E. B. and Spargo, D. In preparation. Mouse ear epidermis as a chalone assay system.

Tutton, P. J. M. (1973) Control of epithelial cell proliferation in the small intestinal crypt. Cell Tissue Kinet. 6, 211.

Verly, W. G. This book.

Voaden, M. J. (1968a) Mitotic inhibitors in the rabbit lens: Sulphydryl groups and the effects of heat on the lens proteins. Exp. Eye Res. 7, 313.

Voaden, M. J. (1968b) A chalone in the rabbit lens? Exp. Eye Res. 7, 326.

Voaden, M. J. and Leeson, S. J. (1970) A chalone in the mammalian lens. I. Effect of bilateral adrenalectomy on the mitotic activity of the adult mouse lens. Exp. Eye Res. 9, 57.

Weiss, P. and Kavanau, J. L. (1957) A model of growth control in mathematical terms. J. Gen. Physiol. 41, 1.

Wolstenholme, G. E. W. and Knight, J. (eds.) (1969) Homeostatic regulators. Ciba Foundation Symposium.

Yamaguchi, T., Hirobe, T., Kinjo, Y. and Manaka, K. (1974) The effect of chalone on the cell cycle in the epidermis during wound healing. Exp. Cell Res. 89, 247.

CHAPTER 12

Biology of the granulocyte chalone

T. Rytömaa

Second Department of Pathology, University of Helsinki and
Institute of Radiation Protection, Helsinki, Finland

12.1 Introduction

In the past few years major progress has been achieved in the understanding of the mechanisms of control of granulocyte production. One, but not the only one, of the primary regulators of this system is the granulocyte chalone, a cell line-specific, species non-specific endogenous regulator substance, which inhibits cell proliferation in a reversible manner. This article reviews the present state of knowledge of the biological characteristics of the granulocyte chalone.

Owing to the complexity of the granulocyte system, the physiological role of a chalone mechanism in granulopoiesis may not be readily apparent. Therefore, a brief description of the granulocyte system, and of some other putative primary regulators than chalone, may be of value to readers not actively engaged in work in haemopoiesis.

12.2 The granulocyte system

The granulocyte system is a sequence of cell populations which starts from a pluripotential stem cell, the ancestor of most, or, in some species such as mouse, all haemic cell lineages. The pluripotential stem cell is believed to give rise to a committed granulocyte progenitor population from which cells then enter the first morphologically recognizable precursor population (myeloblasts) and, subsequently, a series of more mature precursor populations. Both the committed progenitor cells and the morphologically recognizable cells are transit populations in which the cells divide, thus amplifying cell numbers. After the last precursor population, usually considered to be myelocytes, granulocytic cells permanently loose their capability to divide; the post-mitotic cells then mature further and are stored for some time in the bone marrow (marrow granulocyte reserve) before they enter the blood and, finally, extravascular tissues. For a more detailed description of the granulocyte system, see e.g. Metcalf and Moore (1971), Craddock (1972), Fliedner (1974), and Lajtha (1975).

It is clear that a cell system of this complexity may be regulated at different stages of the chain of cell populations, and also by different mechanisms, including, besides tissue micro-environment, long- and short-term chemical signals. These signals may stimulate or inhibit the rate of cell feeding into the granulocyte system from the pluripotential stem cell population, the number of cells in the mitotic cycle in the transit populations (i.e. growth fractions), cell cycle times, maturation rates, release of cells from the place of birth, and even cell death (especially premature death of mitotic cells leading to 'ineffective granulopoiesis'). Only a few of the several putative regulators have been identified in any detail; however, the number of chemical substances with observed or postulated effect on granulopoiesis is large. Analysis of relevant literature shows that although many of these substances influence granulocyte production, they do not control it; for example, a 'neutrophil releasing factor' is not a primary regulator of granulopoiesis.

12.3 Colony stimulating factor (CSF)

It is imperative that some mechanism exists which triggers cells from the pluripotential stem cell compartment into the granulocyte system. However, the nature of the regulatory mechanism of this step is unknown, in spite of excellent assay systems for the stem cells (e.g. the spleen colony technique) and long-term intensive research (see Lajtha, 1975).

By analogy to erythropoietin, it is commonly believed that a granulopoietin exists which induces the transit from the committed progenitor population to the morphologically recognizable precursor populations. From a theoretical point of view it is not at all clear why a cell lineage should be triggered twice by different exogenous signals; however, because the reality of erythropoietin cannot be questioned, existence of a granulopoietin appears likely. Early attempts to discover such a substance suffered from insufficient knowledge in the kinetics of the granulocyte system and, therefore, the results obtained in these studies are not relevant with respect to true granulopoietin; the finding of a real candidate for this substance is a recent discovery. The substance suggested to be granulopoietin is the colony stimulating factor (CSF), which is essential for the growth and development of granulocyte and macrophage colonies in the agar culture system (see Robinson et al., 1967; Metcalf and Moore, 1971; Metcalf, 1973).

CSF extracted from human urine is a neuraminic acid-containing glyco-protein with a molecular weight of 45,000–60,000 daltons; however, physico-chemical properties of CSF's vary greatly depending upon the source from which they are obtained. CSF purified from human urine stimulates colony formation at concentrations of less than 0.1 ng/ml (see Metcalf, 1973) which indicates high biological activity. CSF seems to be produced by many tissues in the body, including white blood cells. However, it now appears that monocytes are the main source of leukocyte CSF (Chervenick and LoBuglio, 1972; Golde and Cline, 1972; Moore et al., 1973), although mitogen-stimulated lymphocytes can also elaborate a similar substance (Cline and Golde, 1974). It is of particular interest to note that mature granulocytes do not seem to produce CSF; in contrast, they have been reported to contain inhibitors of colony formation (Paran et al., 1969; Haskill et al., 1971; Chervenick and LoBuglio, 1972; see also Laerum and Maurer, 1973).

Both the number and the size of colonies developing on agar are deter-mined by the concentration of CSF. Because there also is CSF concentration-dependent lag period before the colony-forming cells start to divide, it has been suggested that CSF may not act as an inducer (see Metcalf and Moore, 1971); hence, its function would differ considerably from that of erythro-poietin.

The in vivo effects of CSF remain to be shown by future work. Indirect evidence for a physiological role of CSF, i.e. the correlation between CSF concentrations in urine, in serum, and in different tissues with spontaneous or induced changes in granulopoiesis, is clearly in favour of such a role (see Metcalf, 1973). However, results published thusfar of the effects of injected CSF (Bradley et al., 1969; Metcalf and Stanley, 1971) do not prove that a major physiological role can be ascribed to this substance with any certainty; in fact, the effects observed are not essentially different from those of specific or non-specific factors which merely cause an accelerated release of granulocytes from the bone marrow.

12.4 Theoretical value of chalone mechanism in granulopoiesis

As already indicated, an essential part of the granulocyte system consists of a series of transit populations in which cell proliferation takes place;

thus, transit populations are the apparent target of a mitotic inhibitor. Briefly, the role of chalone in granulopoiesis is to control the number of mitoses in the precursor cells when they proceed through these transit populations, i.e. granulocyte chalone controls the degree of amplification within a clone originating from a single cell fed into the system (for experimental evidence, see later).

In an exponentially growing clone one extra mitosis would double the output of post-mitotic granulocytes, and one skipped mitosis would halve it, provided that excessive premature cell death does not occur. Thus, control of granulocyte production by the chalone mechanism would be theoretically very effective.

Regulation of both the input (feeding of cells into the granulocyte system) and the amplification (proliferative activity of granulocytic cells) is, of course, superior to the regulation of either one alone. Besides obvious 'physical' advantages, double regulation is actually mandatory from the biological point of view. In particular, in the granulocyte system changes in the input can alter the output (production of functionally competent granulocytes) only after a delay of many days. In presence of fixed amplification such a delay would not only be harmful to the host organism, but it would often be fatal. Thus, the assumption sometimes made that granulopoiesis is regulated by a single mechanism changing the rate of cell feeding into the system runs against the difficulty that natural selection has accounted for the evolution of a seemingly disadvantageous situation.

12.5 Circumstantial evidence for granulocyte chalone

The existence of chalone-like inhibitors of granulopoiesis is suggested by different types of circumstantial evidence. Although these findings have little, if any, value in directly showing the reality of granulocyte chalone, it is of interest to record some of the evidence here.

Craddock and co-workers have shown that effective withdrawal of large numbers of granulocytes from the blood leads to an accelerated release of cells from dog bone marrow and, consequently, to a stimulation of granulocyte production (Craddock et al., 1956, 1959). In contrast, infusion of autologous mature granulocytes into the blood decreases cell release from the marrow granulocyte reserve which, in turn, leads to an inhibition of granulocyte production (Craddock et al., 1960).

Basically analogous results to the withdrawal of granulocytes from the blood have been obtained by killing the cells in the blood in leukaemic patients. Thus, when large numbers of leukaemic cells are destroyed by extra-corporeal irradiation of the blood, proliferative activity of the leukaemic blasts is strongly stimulated in the bone marrow (Chan et al., 1969; Chan and Hayhoe, 1971). This effect is not explicable in terms of non-specific changes in the irradiated blood, because in one patient who had no leukaemic cells in the circulation, increased proliferation of leukaemic blasts was not observed in the bone marrow. Thus, the conditions in extracorporeal irradiation of the blood, as well as in Craddock's leukapheresis and infusion experiments referred to above, are such that part of the granulocytic tissue is manipulated, whereas another part, containing proliferative cells in the bone marrow, is not subjected to any direct perturbation. The results obtained suggest strongly that a feedback mechanism operates within the granulocyte system and, as also concluded by both groups of investigators (see Chan and Hayhoe, 1971; Craddock, 1972), appears to be based on a chalone-like agent.

Numerous authors have reported partial, and even complete, remissions of leukaemia following blood transfusions (see Hayhoe and Whitby, 1955; Schöyer, 1959). On re-examination of this effect, Wetherley-Mein and Cottom (1956) observed that transfusion of fresh blood, but not of stored 'bank' blood, caused transient fall in white blood cells (in this material, actual remission of leukaemia did not occur). Remission of leukaemia has also been reported in many patients in connection with infections (Pelner et al., 1958); even this might be explained in terms of higher inhibitor concentrations arising from increased number of normal granulocytes, although other explanations, such as non-specific stimulation of the immune system, may be more appealing.

12.6 Specificity of chalones; general remarks

If a chalone is considered as an autonomous signal emanating from mature, and presumably also from immature cells of a cell system, and acting on the proliferating cells of the same system, then unequivocal demonstration of cellular specificity of source and action appears to be of utmost importance. However, it is worth noting at once that a requirement for absolute specificity is perhaps too stringent artificial criterium for any chalone; biologically active materials show rarely, if ever, *absolute* specificity. Examples to the point are enzymes, hormones, and antibodies; yet few would question the adequacy of the statement that specificity of action is a fundamental feature of these substances.

In principle, some degree of non-specificity may thus be allowed to chalones without making the specific signals ineffective or non-discriminative in vivo. It could even be desirable to have some level of background 'noise' to prevent, in part, too strong and biologically useless oscillations in cell proliferation. These theoretical considerations tend to suggest that one may, or perhaps even should, expect some degree of non-specificity in chalone experiments, especially in assays in vitro involving isolated cells cultured in an artificial, low-chalone environment. In addition, excessive non-physiological concentrations of any chalone must, of course, inhibit a variety of unrelated cell types by mere toxicity.

For an experimental demonstration of the biological specificity of a chalone one may, somewhat arbitrarily, list the requirements as follows:

i) The source of cells from which the chalone is extracted is a pure population.

ii) Control extracts are prepared from closely related tissues.

iii) The action of a chalone is tested on closely related cell lines.

iv) The comparative tests are made in identical assay conditions and with identical assay methods.

These requirements are, of course, inappropriate if the biological specificity of a particular chalone is likely to be determined by other mechanisms than by chemical characteristics of the substance. Such a situation seems to apply at least to the epidermal chalones which affect all squamous epithelia in the body (Bullough and Laurence, 1964; Frankfurt, 1971; Elgjo, 1972; Bullough, 1973; Iversen, 1973; Laurence, 1973; Marks, 1973); this is, of course, expected, because normal reactions in squamous epithelia are essentially local and not controlled from distance.

In the case of the granulocyte system, the requirements listed above are basically relevant. However, it should be born in mind that also the granulocyte chalone may have potential targets in the body which remain unresponsive in vivo because of the anatomical location of the target, or because the cells are protected from granulocyte chalone by some barrier equivalent to placenta, blood–brain barrier, etc. There is even reason to believe that in normal conditions granulocyte chalone carried in the blood does not play a major role in the regulation of granulopoiesis itself; this is suggested by the fact that mature granulocytes in the bone marrow outnumber the blood cells by a factor of about 30 (see e.g. Craddock, 1972), hence indicating that granulocyte chalone in the bone marrow is not imported.

12.7 Experimental evidence for the existence and specificity of granulocyte chalone

In the early studies the existence and biological specificity of the granulocyte chalone was tested on bone marrow cells in short-term in vitro cultures (Rytömaa and Kiviniemi, 1964, 1967, 1968a–c). Autoradiographic analyses of the cells labelled with [^{3}H]thymidine showed that extracts of granulocytes significantly decreased the number of labelled granulocytic precursor cells without detectably changing the labelling index in the other cell types of the bone marrow, and that extracts of erythrocytes decreased the labelling index of the erythroid precursor cells without marked effect on granulocyte labelling (Rytömaa and Kiviniemi, 1968a, c, 1970; Kivilaakso and Rytömaa, 1971; Rytömaa, 1969, 1973). In principle, these studies fulfilled the requirements listed above fairly well, but some doubts were later expressed as to the validity of the results obtained (see e.g. Metcalf and Moore, 1971; Lajtha, 1973; Br. J. Cancer 29, 84, 1974).

Nevertheless, subsequent studies have clearly shown that the action of granulocyte chalone is real and tissue specific. Thus, a more recent autoradiographic study made on bone marrow cells, cultured in slightly different conditions and analysed by somewhat refined techniques, confirmed strict specificity of action of partially purified granulocyte and erythrocyte extracts on their own precursor cells (Bateman, 1974). Corresponding results were obtained when guinea-pig bone marrow cells were separated into three different subpopulations by means of the Ficoll density step centrifugation; only the top layer subpopulation, mainly composed of immature granulocytic cells, responded by inhibition ([^{3}H]TdR incorporation into the cells) to the action of granulocyte extracts, whereas the other two subpopulations of bone marrow cells did not show any inhibition at all (Paukovits, 1973). Complete specificity of action of granulocyte, erythrocyte, and lymphocyte extracts on their own precursor cells in vitro has also been demonstrated by a unique technique which measures 'structuredness' of the cytoplasmic matrix, based on fluorochromasia coupled with the technique of fluorescence polarization. Changes in 'structuredness', which parallel the proliferative state of the cells (Cercek et al., 1973, 1974), showed that granulocyte extracts affected only granulocytic cells, lymphocyte extracts affected only lymphoid cells, and erythrocyte extracts affected only erythroid cells (Lord et al., 1974a). It may be of interest to note that in this study the fractions of each of the three types of cell extracts were tested at a concentration of 33 μg/ml. Owing to differences in the preparation of the crude extracts (the techniques adopted were those originally used by the proponents of each particular 'chalone'), one may estimate that the active fractions of the lymphocyte and granulocyte extracts were tested at concentrations which may have differed by a factor of 10 with respect to protein content (see p. 303).

The complicated experimental situation found in granulopoiesis in vivo did not originally allow convincing demonstration of tissue specificity of granulocyte chalone action by injecting granulocyte extracts into recipient animals; the difficulties encountered were essentially the same as those which thusfar have prevented unequivocal demonstration of the in vivo effects of the colony stimulating factor (see Metcalf, 1973). However, in the study of granulocyte chalone the main problems were resolved by making use of the closed in vivo culture system, utilizing diffusion chambers implanted in the peritoneal cavity of mice (Benestad, 1970). This system is particularly well suited for the study of granulocyte chalone, because in the diffusion chambers immature granulocytes proliferate at a very fast rate and because the effect of an inhibitor can be measured by several independent techniques. In some of the first experiments utilizing the diffusion chamber technique, extracts of granulocytes and of liver were injected into mice each carrying two different types of chamber cultures; it was observed that granulocyte extracts inhibited DNA synthesis (incorporation of $[^3H]$-TdR into the cells) in proliferating granulocytes but did not influence proliferating immunoblasts and macrophages (Benestad et al., 1973).

These results were later confirmed and extended by Laerum and Maurer (1973) who observed that granulocyte extracts, but not epidermal extracts, decreased the labelling index of proliferating granulocytes without detectable effect on macrophage labelling, provided that granulocyte extract had been obtained from blood leukocytes contaminated with lymphocytes only. Laerum and Maurer (1973) further showed that the decrease in the number of DNA synthesizing cells was genuine and not caused by non-specific interaction with $[^3H]$TdR uptake, because the effect could also be detected by measuring DNA content of single cells with automatic fluorescence cytophotometry. It may be worth noting that in both these diffusion chamber studies the effects of the granulocyte extracts were also tested by 'old-fashioned' in vitro techniques; correlation was found between the in vitro and in vivo activities. Furthermore, granulocyte extracts used by Laerum and Maurer (1973), when tested on epidermal mitotic activity in vitro, were without effect. Preliminary experiments made by Benestad (see Brit. J. Cancer 29, 84, 1974) have also shown that injection of granulocyte extracts into animals bearing diffusion chamber cultures protects the cells from the toxic effects of hydroxyurea. Because hydroxyurea is a relatively specific S phase killing agent, the protective effect of granulocyte extracts is evidently based on S phase suppression or on blocking the centry of cells into S.

With the exception of the treatment of chloroleukaemia (Rytömaa and Kiviniemi, 1969a, 1970; see also later), only a few preliminary attempts were made in the early experiments to shown the chalone effect directly in vivo (Rytömaa and Kiviniemi, 1968d). Specific inhibition of granulopoiesis was suggested, but, owing to small numbers of animals studied, the results were not fully convincing. Schütt and Langen (1972), however, confirmed a little later that granulopoiesis can be inhibited in intact animals by injections of granulocyte extracts. These authors labelled bone marrow cells with [³H]TdR and then induced an aseptic inflammation in the peritoneal cavity of rats; it was observed that granulocyte extracts, given to the rats prior to [³H]TdR labelling, reduced the DNA specific activity of the granulocytes recovered from the inflammatory focus by about 50%.

The natural experimental approach based on the injection of chalone preparations into test animals has certain disadvantages; among them is the difficulty of performing long-term studies because relatively large quantities of sufficiently well purified material and frequent injections are needed. To avoid difficulties encountered in the use of exogenous chalone, studies have also been made in experimental animals with an elevated endogenous chalone content in the body.

Granulocyte chalone is present in excess in rats suffering either from a transplanted local chloroma tumour or from a generalized leukaemia (Rytömaa and Kiviniemi, 1967, 1968c, d). If diffusion chambers are implanted into the peritoneal cavity of these rats, growth of granulocytes, both normal and leukaemic, is inhibited in a specific manner compared with non-leukaemic hosts (Vilpo et al., 1973). This inhibition of growth could be shown directly by a reduced formation of granulocytes and also indirectly by measuring the incorporation of [³H]TdR into the cells. The specificity of the growth suppression, in turn, was confirmed by culturing mastocytoma and HeLa cells in identical conditions; neither of these cell lines was affected in chloroma-bearing host rats compared with the controls. The experiments also showed that the selective inhibition of granulocyte growth in the diffusion chambers does not depend on an immunological reaction developed against granulocytic cells in the leukaemic host rats. This possibility was excluded, for example, by the finding that an equally strong growth inhibition could be detected in experiments where the control group consisted of rats with spontaneously regressed chloroma tumours – an immunological reaction against granulocytic cells is evidently as strong in the control rats showing spontaneous regression of the tumour as in then experimental rats showing progressive growth of the tumour.

The existence of a specific feedback mechanism (granulocyte chalone) originating from the chloroma cells of chamber-carrying host rats has also been reported by Ferris et al. (1973). In accordance with the results referred to above, these authors observed that proliferative activity of the chloroleukaemia cells was inhibited when grown in leukaemic host rats, as judged from the labelled mitoses curves. In contrast, Ehrlich's ascites carcinoma cells were not affected when grown in identical conditions and, conversely, chloroleukaemia cells were not inhibited when grown in diffusion chambers in mice with Ehrlich's ascites carcinoma. It may be worth noting that since Ehrlich's ascites carcinoma cells elaborate their own chalone (Bichel, 1972, 1973), chloroleukaemia cells are evidently unresponsive to this substance (both G_1 and G_2 inhibitors).

The results of these two studies with rat chloroleukaemia (Ferris et al., 1973; Vilpo et al., 1973) indicated that transplanted chalone-producing tumours provide an experimental model which may have some general value in the study of biological actions of chalones. We have therefore used this model also in the study of epidermal chalones, as Bullough and Deol (1971) have reported that the Hewitt keratinizing epidermal carcinoma of the mouse (see Hewitt, 1966) produces an elevated epidermal chalone content in the body. The results obtained (Kariniemi and Rytömaa, 1976) showed that cell proliferation (incorporation of [^{3}H]TdR) is suppressed more or less strongly essentially in all squamous epithelia of the tumour-bearing animals, but that no inhibition is detected in most other tissues, including host animal's own granulopoiesis. A few non-epidermal tissues, especially the spleen, showed an apparently non-specific inhibition, which, however, may be related to increased stress (lymphoid tissue in general seemed to be influenced in the mice suffering from the Hewitt epidermal carcinoma).

Taken together, the findings summarized above indicate that, in all probability, granulocyte chalone is a specific inhibitor of granulopoiesis. However, to demonstrate the true biological activity of this substance, it is still necessary to show that granulocyte chalone is also effective in non-artificial conditions in vivo and that it has no untoward effects on any cell system in the body.

Granulocyte chalone, administered by multiple intravenous injections, has recently been subjected to extensive testing in this respect; it seems unlikely that any other chalone has yet been studied in greater detail in vivo. The results obtained in long-term experiments using semipurified heterologous granulocyte chalone (as estimated from the wet weight of the starting material, i.e. blood cells, the substance had been purified by more than 10^5-fold; a daily dose of less than 0.5 μg/g of this material is sufficient to produce an effect detectable even without advanced techniques) have shown that granulocyte chalone causes strong inhibition in granulopoiesis, but that almost certainly it does not affect any other cell system in the body

(Rytömaa, Vilpo, Levanto and Jones, unpublished results). Direct quantitative measurements could only be made from a limited number of cell systems, such as erythrocytes, lymphocytes, and megakaryocytes, but semi-quantitative and qualitative analyses could be extended to cover virtually every organ in the body. Except the granulocyte system, no signs whatsoever were observed indicative of inhibited cell proliferation or impaired tissue function (see also later).

Like other chalones (see e.g. Bullough et al., 1967), the granulocyte chalone is not species specific in its action. According to published studies, test materials from different species (mouse, rat, guinea-pig, rabbit, ox, horse, pig, and man) have been found to be effective on granulocytic cells of other species, including man.

12.8 Point and mode of action

It is clear from all the findings summarized above that granulocyte chalone inhibits granulopoiesis in a tissue-specific manner; this effect has been detected both directly and indirectly, and in a variety of assay conditions. However, the results obtained do not give an entirely clear-cut picture of the cell cycle specificity of the granulocyte chalone or of its mode of action.

Fluorometric analysis of the DNA content of single cells after granulocyte chalone inhibition (diffusion chamber cultures) indicates that cells are arrested in the G_1 phase, but not in the G_2 and M phases (Laerum and Maurer, 1973). The G_1 effect is supported by autoradiographic analyses (Rytömaa and Kiviniemi, 1968; Laerum and Maurer, 1973; Bateman, 1974) and also by the use of hydroxyurea (Benestad, unpublished results); however, none of the studies has excluded the possibility that also cells in the S phase are influenced by the granulocyte chalone. In fact, several findings, such as decreased mean grain count (Rytömaa and Kiviniemi, 1968a; Vilpo et al., 1973; Laerum and Maurer, 1973; Bateman, 1974), suggest that S phase cells are affected, although Laerum and Maurer (1973) have concluded that granulocyte chalone does not act directly on these cells, but that cells which are not arrested in G_1 proceed through S very slowly.

Further evidence for a direct or indirect effect of granulocyte chalone on S phase may be obtained from the labelled mitoses curves reported by Ferris et al. (1973); these authors observed that S phase of chloroleukaemia cells is significantly prolonged when the cells are cultured in diffusion chambers in leukaemic hosts as compared with control hosts. According to the same study, G_2 phase was also prolonged whereas G_1 was not, and, hence, the results seem to disagree completely with those reported by others.

However, if G_1 arrest means that the arrested cells stop moving altogether
($G_1 \to$ 'G_0' transition) then the effect cannot be detected from the labelled
mitoses curves published by Ferris et al. (1973); instead, growth fraction
should be decreased. Thus, if granulocyte chalone really diverts cells from
G_1 to 'G_0', then the labelled mitoses curves are fully in line with the other
observations and the results support strongly the conclusion that it is the
granulocyte chalone, rather than some contaminant, which prolongs S
phase duration. The other seemingly discrepant finding of Ferris et al.
(1973) that also the G_2 phase was prolonged is not in obvious conflict
with the reported unresponsiveness of G_2 phase cells (Laerum and Maurer,
1973), because cells which proceed through S slowly may also do so in
G_2 (owing to the timing of the experiment, this could not have been detected
by the fluorometric analysis).

One of the criteria defining chalone is that the inhibitory effect is reversible.
Granulocyte chalone has not been extensively studied in this respect, but
reversibility of the inhibition has nevertheless been observed e.g. in short-
term in vitro cultures of rat bone marrow cells (Rytömaa and Kiviniemi,
1968b), in microplate cultures of human granulocytic cells (Rytömaa et al.,
unpublished results), in diffusion chamber cultures of mouse granulocytes
(Laerum and Maurer, 1973), and in 'long-term' in vitro cultures of mouse
granulocytes (Lord et al., 1974b). The reversibility has usually been established by showing that the reduced fraction of S phase cells returns to
normal in 3–24 h after a single chalone pulse (the time seems to depend on
the source of target cells used and on the assay conditions). In the study by
Lord et al. (1974b) the reversibility of the chalone effect, measured in terms
of 'structuredness' of the cytoplasmic matrix, was shown by washing the
treated cells.

The finding that the inhibitory effect of chalone on the cells is removed
simply by washing the cells suggests strongly that granulocyte chalone acts
at the level of cell membrane (see also Rytömaa, 1975). It seems, however,
that cyclic AMP (or cyclic GMP) is not involved in the granulocyte chalone
mechanism, because the chalone action cannot be mimiced by exogenous
cAMP, dibutyryl cAMP, or theophylline in short-term cultures of rat bone
marrow cells (Rytömaa and Kiviniemi, 1975); furthermore, adrenaline
does not potentiate the inhibitory action of granulocyte chalone in vitro
(Rytömaa and Kiviniemi, 1967, 1969b).

12.9 Toxicity of granulocyte chalone

Even crude preparations of granulocyte chalone do not seem to be detectably cytotoxic either in vitro or in vivo. Thus, DNA synthesis is inhibited in short-term cultures of rat and human bone marrow cells (Rytömaa and Kiviniemi, 1967, 1968a–c) at chalone concentrations which are much smaller than those still lacking detectable effects on cell viability, or on RNA and protein syntheses (see also Rytömaa, 1976). Accordingly, repeated intraperitoneal chalone injections into mice carrying diffusion chamber cultures with proliferating granulocytes, macrophages, and immunoblasts do not affect the viability of the cultured cells; DNA synthesis, however, is inhibited in the proliferating granulocytes but not in the other cell types (Benestad et al., 1973; Laerum and Maurer, 1973).

Further supporting evidence for the lack of cytotoxicity of granulocyte chalone is provided, for example, by the experiments in which chloro-leukaemic rats were subjected to prolonged, intensive treatment with this substance (Rytömaa and Kiviniemi, 1969a, 1970). It was observed that the treatment suppressed leukaemia cell proliferation strongly, but did not retard the growth rate of young, fast-growing animals; in fact, chalone treated rats often showed better weight gain than control animals (Rytömaa and Kiviniemi, 1970). Other evidence for the lack of cytotoxicity is provided by the activated fur renewal in the granulocyte chalone-treated chloro-leukaemic rats (Rytömaa and Kiviniemi, 1969a, 1970; see also fig. 1 in Bullough, 1973), and by the normal breeding of the animals actually cured from the leukaemia by chalone injections (Rytömaa and Kiviniemi, 1970); these rats, by the way, eventually died of 'old age'.

Multiple intravenous injections of semipurified granulocyte chalone daily for a period of several weeks have been found to lead to a strong, selective inhibition of granulopoiesis without untoward effects other than short-lasting pyrogenic reaction (Rytömaa, Vilpo, Levanto and Jones, unpublished results). It is of particular interest to note that repeated injections of effective doses of granulocyte chalone do not influence lymphocytes, although these cells are known to be sensitive to many types of biologically active agents (e.g. cytotoxic drugs), continued stress, and different physical factors (e.g. ionizing radiation), and because lymphocytes can also be used as an indicator of exposure to chromosome damaging agents. The un-responsiveness of lymphocytes to long-term in vivo treatment with granulo-cyte chalone is shown, for example, by the unaltered blood lymphocyte count, unaltered serum immunoglobulin levels (at least of IgG, IgA, and IgM), and unaltered responsiveness of the cells to phytohaemagglutinin (Rytömaa, Vilpo, Levanto and Jones, unpublished results). In view of these results, it is hardly surprising that granulocyte chalone is not clastogenic either, i.e. it does not cause chromosome aberrations in lymphocytes, detectable by conventional and banding techniques; accordingly, added granulocyte chalone does not suppress PHA-stimulated blastic transformation of lymphocytes in vitro (Stenstrand and Rytömaa, unpublished results). Finally, it may also be noted that semipurified preparations of heterologous granulocyte chalone are not strongly antigenic, because sensitization was not observed in the experiments lasting for many weeks.

12.10 Nature of granulocyte extracts

Most of the studies referred to above have been made with test preparations which were not subjected to extensive purification (for purification and chemical characteristics of the granulocyte chalone, see Paukovits in this monograph). Although it is quite clear that few, if any, of the results obtained could have been caused by non-specific impurities contaminating the chalone preparations, it may be necessary to discuss briefly the composition of a crude granulocyte extract and of the possible experimental hazards caused by the impurities. Strictly speaking all the results summarized here apply to the extracts used by the present author only, but there is no reason to assume that the extracts used by others have been drastically different, because variations in the extraction techniques are rather small.

In a typical case, crude granulocyte extract is obtained by isolating granulocytes from the blood or collecting the cells from an artificially induced inflammatory exudate. These cell populations are not pure, but often > 80% of the cells are granulocytes; in the case of blood leukocytes, the major contaminating cell type is lymphocyte, and in the case of inflammatory cells it is monocyte-macrophage. The cell population thus obtained is extracted – without homogenization – with saline or Hanks' solution for 1–2 h at 37 °C, and the 'conditioned' supernatant is collected and lyophilized.

If the cellularity of the suspension has been high (much higher than in normal blood), the amount of organic material in the crude extract may be 10–20% of the solid weight; about one third of this is protein/polypeptide and about one tenth are purine/pyrimidine bases and their derivatives (see Rytömaa, 1976). The total amount of thymidine in these extracts is less than 0.05% of the solid weight and may actually be very close to zero. In any case, it has been shown by a dilution technique that possible contamination of the extracts with minute amounts of 'cold' thymidine has no detectable effect on the incorporation of [^{3}H]TdR into the cells (see Rytömaa, 1976). Furthermore, the effect of the extracts on DNA synthesis is readily detected by other labelled precursors than thymidine, such as [^{14}C]formate and [^{3}H]deoxycytidine (Rytömaa and Kiviniemi, 1967, 1968c, d, and unpublished results), and also by several unrelated techniques not involving DNA labelling at all (cf. above).

A crude granulocyte extract of this type inhibits [^{3}H]TdR incorporation into rat and human bone marrow cells in vitro by 10–20% at a concentration of about 100 μg/ml. This is equivalent with a total protein/polypeptide concentration of about 5 μg/ml which, in turn, is less than 0.1% of the total protein content of the culture medium. It may be of interest to note for comparison that in some chalone studies crude tissue extracts have been added to the test cultures at concentrations of 1–5 mg of protein per ml (see Iversen, 1968; Volm et al., 1969; Jones et al., 1970).

Owing to the minimal amount of chemistry involved in the preparation of crude granulocyte extracts, it is highly unlikely that they are contaminated by significant quantities of non-physiological compounds. On the other hand, possibly cytotoxic large-molecular-weight substances may be present in crude granulocyte extracts, but clearly in small quantities and they probably never cause serious complications; furthermore, these substances are easily removed from the low-molecular-weight granulocyte chalone. In contrast, low-molecular-weight impurities contaminating crude granulo-cyte extracts do represent a serious potential hazard, especially in such in vitro experiments in which the inhibitory effect is measured in terms of [^{3}H]TdR incorporation. However, this hazard is rarely, if ever, based on contaminating thymidine which would lead to a spuriously low uptake of [^{3}H]TdR (cf. above); the other nucleosides and nucleotides are much more critical than thymidine. It has been shown (Rytömaa and Kiviniemi, 1975) that several of these substances, including normal and cyclic AMP, suppress [^{3}H]TdR incorporation in an essentially non-specific manner if added to the test cultures at sufficiently high concentrations ($> 10^{-5}$ M). Indeed, it can be estimated from the composition of granulocyte extracts that the 'therapeutic width' of crude preparations is very narrow. For example, if the concentration of a typical extract capable of causing 10–20% inhibition in [^{3}H]TdR uptake is increased by a factor of 10, the resulting inhibition may no more be a reliable measure of chalone action; if the concentration is increased 100-fold, most, if not all, of the effect is caused by factors other than chalone (see Rytömaa, 1976).

12.11 Granulocyte chalone and leukaemia

One of the most controversial aspects of chalone research is the possibility that these substances may have therapeutic value in the treatment of cancer. Because much of the experimental evidence suggesting this possibility has been obtained with the granulocyte chalone, the subject is briefly discussed in this article.

A necessary, but not sufficient, prerequisite for the use of chalones in the treatment of cancer is that malignant cells are responsive to the chalone of their tissue of origin. It is almost certain that this is generally the case, as judged from the numerous observations made on different malignant cell lines, including a few spontaneous human tumours (e.g. Rytömaa and Kiviniemi, 1967, 1968c, d, 1969a, 1970; Bullough and Laurence, 1968a, b, 1970; Mohr et al., 1968; Iversen, 1969; Jones et al., 1970; Bichel, 1970, 1972, 1973; Garcia-Giralt et al., 1970; Bullough and Deol, 1971; Elgjo and Hennings, 1971; Houck et al., 1971; Houck and Irasquin, 1973; Kieger et al., 1973; Dewey, 1973; Cooper and Smith, 1793; Vilpo et al., 1973; Ferris et al., 1973; Seiji et al., 1974). Some of the results obtained in these studies are, however, of dubious value (see Rytömaa, 1976) and may have nothing to do with chalone action.

With respect to the granulocyte chalone, it has been observed that in transplanted rat chloroleukaemia the tumour cells seem to contain less granulocyte chalone than the normal cells (Rytömaa and Kiviniemi, 1968c, d), but that the chalone content of the whole body is significantly increased (Rytömaa and Kiviniemi, 1967, 1968c, d; Ferris et al., 1973; Vilpo et al., 1973). The most plausible explanation for this situation is a decreased ability of the chloroleukaemia cells to retain or bind the chalone, which, owing to the large tumour mass, is produced in excess in the body. This elevated chalone content inhibits, but does not prevent, the growth of chloroleukaemia (Ferris et al., 1973; Vilpo et al., 1973), presumably because the leukaemia cells are less responsive to the action of exogenous chalone than the corresponding normal cells (Rytömaa and Kiviniemi, 1968c, d, 1969a).

Some of these findings seem to mitigate against the possibility of using granulocyte chalone for the treatment of leukaemia. However, experimental evidence shows that multiple injections of granulocyte chalone into rats suffering either from a local chloroma tumour or from a generalized leukaemia lead to a regression of the leukaemia, which sometimes results in a permanent cure (Rytömaa and Kiviniemi, 1969a, 1970). Because granulocyte chalone is a non-toxic inhibitor of cell proliferation, the therapeutic effect of chalone treatment may appear strange. However, since large numbers of chloroleukaemia cells die 'spontaneously' (12–64% of the birth rate even in a relatively well protected environment; see Vilpo and Rytömaa, 1973), there is no need to suppose that chalone has nevertheless caused cell lysis. To achieve complete regression of the tumour it is only necessary to slow down growth rate of the tumour cells strongly enough to make it smaller than the 'spontaneous' rate of cell loss. Thus, chalone treatment is oncostatic in nature and it is merely used as an adjunct to the endogenous mechanisms which lead to the destruction of leukaemia cells in the body.

Because cells from acute and chronic myeloid leukaemia in man respond by inhibition to the granulocyte chalone in vitro (Rytömaa and Kiviniemi, 1970; Rytömaa, 1976; Rytömaa et al., unpublished results), the implication of the observed therapeutic effect of granulocyte chalone in rat chloro-leukaemia is obvious. There is no real reason to assume that the suggested mechanism for cure would only apply to transplanted animal tumours and, therefore, the potential offered by chalone treatment must be examined in clinical trials. Such experiments have not yet been possible, owing to tremendous technical difficulties in the preparation of large quantities of sufficiently well purified granulocyte chalone; however, recent developments have made it likely that the first clinical trials will be made in near future.

12.12 Summary

Granulocyte chalone is a cell line-specific, species non-specific regulator substance, which inhibits cell proliferation in the granulocyte system in a reversible manner. The existence and specificity of action of this substance has been shown both in vitro and in vivo in widely different assay conditions and using a broad spectrum of assay techniques. Granulocyte chalone inhibits cell proliferation in the transit populations of the granulocyte system; it seems to act at the level of cell membrane and divert cells from the G_1 phase to the 'G_0' phase with some direct or indirect effect on S phase cells as well. The substance is non-cytotoxic and it has no detectable effect on any other tissue than normal and leukaemic granulocytes even after long-lasting in vivo treatment. Granulocyte chalone offers an exciting potential for the treatment of myeloid leukaemia and, therefore, the substance is of more than academic interest.

Acknowledgments

I wish to express my gratitude to the Weddel Pharmaceuticals Ltd., London, England, who have prepared the crude and semi-purified granulocyte extracts which I have used in all recent experiments. My original work reported in this article has been supported by grants from the Sigrid Jusélius Foundation, Helsinki, from the Hallonblad Foundation, Helsinki, from the Finnish Cancer Society, Helsinki, from the Lady Tata Memorial Trust, London, and from the Weddel Pharmaceuticals Ltd., London.

References

Bateman, A. E. (1974) Cell specificity of chalone-type inhibitors of DNA synthesis released by blood leukocytes and erythrocytes. Cell Tissue Kinet. 7, 451.

Benestad, H. B. (1970) Formation of granulocytes and macrophages in diffusion chamber cultures of mouse blood leucocytes. Scand. J. Haemat. 7, 279.

Benestad, H. B., Rytömaa, T. and Kiviniemi, K. (1973) The cell specific effect of the granulocyte chalone demonstrated with the diffusion chamber technique. Cell Tissue Kinet. 6, 147.

Bichel, P. (1970) Tumor growth inhibiting effect of JB-1 ascitic fluid. I. An in vivo investigation. Europ. J. Cancer 6, 291.

Bichel, P. (1972) Specific growth regulation in three ascitic tumours. Europ. J. Cancer 8, 167.

Bichel, P. (1973) Self-limitation of ascites tumor growth: A possible chalone regulation. Natl. Cancer Inst. Monogr. 38, 197.

Bradley, T. R., Metcalf, D., Sumner, M. and Stanley, R. (1969) Characteristics of in vitro colony formation by cells from haemopoietic tissues. In Vitro 4, 22.

Bullough, W. S. (1973) The chalones: A review. Natl. Cancer Inst. Monogr. 38, 5.

Bullough, W. S. and Deol, J. U. R. (1971) Chalone-induced mitotic inhibition in the Hewitt keratinizing epidermal carcinoma of the mouse. Europ. J. Cancer 7, 425.

Bullough, W. S. and Laurence, E. B. (1964) Mitotic control by internal secretion: The role of the chalone-adrenalin complex. Exp. Cell Res. 33, 176.

Bullough, W. S. and Laurence, E. B. (1968a) Control of mitosis in rabbit V × 2 epidermal tumours by means of the epidermal chalone. Europ. J. Cancer 4, 587.

Bullough, W. S. and Laurence, E. B. (1968b) Melanocyte chalone and mitotic control in melanomata. Nature 220, 137.

Bullough, W. S. and Laurence, E. B. (1970) The lymphocytic chalone and its antimitotic action on a mouse lymphoma in vitro. Europ. J. Cancer 6, 525.

Bullough, W. S., Laurence, E. B., Iversen, O. H. and Elgjo, K. (1967) The vertebrate epidermal chalone. Nature 214, 578.

Cercek, L., Cercek, B. and Ockey, C. H. (1973a) Structuredness of the cytoplasmic matrix and Michaelis-Menten constants for the hydrolysis of FDA during the cell cycle in chinese hamster ovary cells. Biophysik 10, 187.

Cercek, L., Cercek, B. and Garrett, J. V. (1973b) Biophysical differentiation between normal human and chronic lymphocytic leukemia lymphocytes. In: Proceedings of the 8th Leukocyte Culture Conference, Uppsala. Academic Press, New York and London. P. 553.

Chan, B. W. B. and Hayhoe, F. G. J. (1971) Changes in proliferative activity of marrow leukemic cells during and after extracorporeal irradiation of blood. Blood 37, 657.

Chan, B. W. B., Hayhoe, F. G. J. and Bullimore, J. A. (1969) Effect of extracorporeal irradiation of the blood on bone marrow activity in acute leukemia. Nature 221, 972.

Chervenick, P. A. and LeBuglio, A. F. (1972) Human blood monocytes: Stimulators of granulocyte and mononuclear colony formation in vitro. Science 178, 164.

Cline, M. J. and Golde, D. W. (1974) Production of colony-stimulating activity by human lymphocytes. Nature 248, 703.

Cooper, P. R. and Smith, H. (1973) Influence of cell-free ascites fluid and adenosine 3′5′-cyclic monophosphate upon the cell kinetics of Ehrlich's ascites carcinoma. Nature 241, 457.

Craddock, C. G. (1960) Production and distribution of granulocytes and the control of granulocyte release. In: Ciba Foundation Symposium on Haemopoiesis (eds.: G. E. W. Wolstenholme and M. O'Connor) Churchill, London. p. 237.

Craddock, C. G. (1972) Techniques for studying granulocyte kinetics. In: Hematology (eds.: W. J. Williams, E. Beutler, A. J. Erslev and R. W. Rundles) McGraw-Hill, New York, p. 593.

Craddock, C. G., Perry, S. and Lawrence, J. S. (1956) The dynamics of leukopoiesis and leukocytosis, as studied by leukopheresis and isotope techniques. J. Clin. Invest. 35, 285.

Craddock, C. G., Perry, S. and Lawrence, J. S. (1959) Control of steady state proliferation of leukocytes. In: The Kinetics of Cellular Proliferation (ed.: F. Stohlman, Jr.) Grune and Stratton, New York, p. 242.

Dewey, D. L. (1973) The melanocyte chalone. Natl. Cancer Inst. Monogr. 38, 213.

Elgjo, K. (1972) Chalone inhibition of cellular proliferation. J. Invest. Dermatol. 59, 81.

Elgjo, K. and Hennings, H. (1971) Epidermal mitotic rate and DNA synthesis after injection of water extracts made from mouse skin treated with actinomycin D: Two or more growth-regulating substances. Virchows Arch. Abt. B, Zellpath. 7, 1.

Ferris, P., LoBue, J. and Gordon, A. S. (1973) Possible feedback inhibition of leukemic cell growth: Kinetics of Shay chloroleukemia grown in diffusion chambers and intraperitoneally in rodents. In: Humoral Control of Growth and Differentiation, Vol. I (eds.: J. LoBue and A. S. Gordon) Academic Press, New York and London, p. 213.

Fliedner, Th. M. (1974) Kinetik und Regulationsmechanismen des Granulozytenumsetzes. Schweiz. med. Wschr. 104, 98.

Frankfurt, O. S. (1971) Epidermal chalone. Effect on cell cycle and on development of hyperplasia. Exp. Cell Res. 64, 140.

Garcia-Giralt, E., Lasalvia, E., Florentin, I. and Mathé, G. (1970) Evidence for a lymphocytic chalone. Europ. J. Clin. Biol. Res. 15, 1012.

Golde, D. W. and Cline, M. J. (1972) Identification of the colony-stimulating cell in human peripheral blood. J. Clin. Invest. 51, 2981.

Haskill, J. S., McKnight, R. D. and Galbraith, P. R. (1971) Possible cell to cell interaction in regulation of granulopoiesis in vitro. Blood 38, 788.

Hayhoe, F. G. J. and Whitby, L. (1955). The management of acute leukaemia in adults. Brit. J. Haemat. 1, 1.

Hewitt, H. B., Chan, D. P. S. and Blake, E. R. (1967) Survival curves for clonogenic cells of a murine keratinizing squamous carcinoma irradiated in vivo or under hypoxic conditions. Int. J. Radiat. Biol. 12, 535.

Houck, J. C., Irasquin, H. and Leikin, S. (1971) Lymphocyte DNA synthesis inhibition. Science 173, 1139.

Houck, J. C. and Irasquin, H. (1973) Some properties of the lymphocyte chalone. Natl. Cancer Inst. Monogr. 38, 117.

Iversen, O. H. (1968) Effect of epidermal chalone on human epidermal mitotic activity in vitro. Nature 219, 75.

Iversen, O. H. (1969) Chalones of the skin. In: Ciba Foundation Symposium on Homeostatic Regulators (eds.: G. E. W. Wolstenholme and J. Knight) Churchill, London, p. 29.

Iversen, O. H. (1973) The chalones. Acta Path. Microbiol. Scand. Sect. A, Suppl. 236, 71.

Jones, J., Paraskova-Tchernozemska, E. and Moorhead, J. F. (1970) In vitro inhibition of DNA synthesis in human leukaemic cells by a lymphoid cell extract. Lancet i, 654.

Kariniemi, A.-L. and Rytömaa, T. (1976). Effect of the Hewitt keratinising epidermal carcinoma on cell proliferation in different organs of the host mouse and in human psoriatic skin cultured in diffusion chambers. Brit. J. Dermatol. (in press)

Kieger, N., Florentin, I. and Mathé, G. (1973) A lymphocyte-inhibiting factor (chalone?) extracted from thymus: immunosuppressive effects. Natl. Cancer Inst. Monogr. 38, 135.

Kivilaakso, E. and Rytömaa, T. (1971) Erythrocytic chalone, a tissue specific inhibitor of cell proliferation in the erythron. Cell Tissue Kinet. 4, 1.

Laerum, O. D. and Maurer, H. R. (1973) Proliferation kinetics of myelopoietic cells and macrophages in diffusion chambers after treatment with granulocyte extracts (chalone). Virchows Arch. Abt. B, Zellpath. 14, 293.

Lajtha, L. G. (1973) Commentary on 'Chalone of the granulocyte system', by T. Rytömaa, and 'Granulopoiesis-inhibiting factor', by W. R. Paukovits. Natl. Cancer Inst. Monogr. 38, 157.

Lajtha, L. G. (1975) Haemopoietic stem cells. Brit. J. Haemat. 29, 529.

Lord, B. I., Cercek, L., Cercek, B., Shah, G. P., Dexter, T. M. and Lajtha, L. G. (1974a) Inhibitors of haemopoietic cell proliferation: specificity of action within the haemopoietic system. Brit. J. Cancer 29, 168.

Lord, B. I., Cercek, L., Cercek, B., Shah, G. P. and Lajtha, L. G. (1974b) Inhibitors of haemopoietic cell proliferation: reversibility of action. Brit. J. Cancer 29, 407.

Marks, F. (1973) A tissue-specific factor inhibiting DNA synthesis in mouse epidermis. Natl. Cancer Inst. Monogr. 38, 79.

Metcalf, D. (1973) The colony stimulating factor (CSF). In: Humoral Control of Growth and Differentiation, Vol. I (eds.: J. LoBue and A. S. Gordon) Academic Press, New York and London, p. 91.

Metcalf, D. and Moore, M. A. S. (1971) Haemopoietic Cells. North-Holland, Amsterdam.

Metcalf, D. and Stanley, E. R. (1971) Haematological effects in mice of partially purified colony stimulating factor (CSF) prepared from human urine. Brit. J. Haemat. 21, 481.

Mohr, U., Althoff, J., Kinzel, V., Süss, R. and Volm, M. (1968) Melanoma regression induced by 'Chalone': a new tumour inhibiting principle in vivo. Nature 220, 138.

Moore, M. A. S., Williams, N. and Metcalf, D. (1973) In vitro colony formation by normal and leukemic human hematopoietic cells: characterization of the colony-forming cells. J. Natl. Cancer Inst. 50, 603.

Paran, M., Ichikawa, Y. and Sachs, L. (1969) Feedback inhibition of the development of macrophage and granulocyte colonies. II. Inhibition by granulocytes. Proc. Natl. Acad. Sci. 62, 81.

Paukovits, W. R. (1973) Granulopoiesis-inhibiting factor: demonstration and preliminary chemical and biological characterization of a specific polypeptide (chalone). Natl. Cancer Inst. Monogr. 38, 147.

Pelner, L., Fowler, G. A. and Nants, H. C. (1958) Effects of concurrent infections and their toxins on the course of leukemia. Acta Med. Scand., Suppl. 338.

Robinson, W., Metcalf, D. and Bradley, T. R. (1967) Stimulation by normal and leukemic mouse sera of colony formation in vitro by mouse bone marrow cells. J. Cell Physiol. 69, 83.

Rytömaa, T. (1969) Granulocytic chalone and antichalone. In Vitro 4, 47.

Rytömaa, T. (1973) Granulocytic chalone. Bibl. Haemat. 39, 885 (Karger, Basel).

Rytömaa, T. (1976). The chalone concept. In: International Review of Experimental Pathology, Vol. XVI (eds.: G. W. Richter and M. A. Epstein) Academic Press, New York and London (in press).

Rytömaa, T. and Kiviniemi, K. (1964) In vitro experiments for demonstration of specific feedback factors in rat serum. In: Proceedings of the XIV Scandinavian Congress of Pathology and Microbiology. Universitetsforlaget, Oslo, p. 169.

Rytömaa, T. and Kiviniemi, K. (1967) Regulation system of blood cell production. In: Control of Cellular Growth in Adult Organisms (eds.: H. Teir and T. Rytömaa) Academic Press, London, p. 106.

Rytömaa, T. and Kiviniemi, K. (1968a) Control of granulocyte production. I. Chalone and antichalone, two specific humoral regulators. Cell Tissue Kinet. 1, 329.

Rytömaa, T. and Kiviniemi, K. (1968b) Control of granulocyte production. II. Mode of action of chalone and antichalone. Cell Tissue Kinet. 1, 341.

Rytömaa, T. and Kiviniemi, K. (1968c) Control of DNA duplication in rat chloro-leukaemia by means of the granulocytic chalone. Europ. J. Cancer 4, 595.

Rytömaa, T. and Kiviniemi, K. (1968d) Control of cell production in rat chloroleukaemia by means of the granulocytic chalone. Nature 220, 136.

Rytömaa, T. and Kiviniemi, K. (1969a) Chloroma regression by the granulocytic chalone. Nature 222, 995.

Rytömaa, T. and Kiviniemi, K. (1969b) The role of stress hormones in the control of granulocyte production. Cell Tissue Kinet. 2, 263.

Rytömaa, T. and Kiviniemi, K. (1970) Regression of generalized leukaemia in rat induced by the granulocytic chalone. Europ. J. Cancer 6, 401.

Rytömaa, T. and Kiviniemi, K. (1975) Cyclic adenosine 3':5'-monophosphate and in-hibition of deoxyribonucleic acid synthesis in vitro. In Vitro 11, 1.

Schöyer, N. H. D. (1959) The aetiology of leukaemias illustrating an alternative concept of the aetiology on malignancy in general. Lancet ii, 400.

Schütt, M. and Langen, P. (1972) Comments on granulocytic chalone action. Studia Biophys. 31/32, 211.

Seiji, M., Nakano, H., Akiba, H. and Kato, T. (1974) Inhibition of DNA and protein synthesis in melanocytes by melanoma extract. J. Invest. Dermatol. 62, 11.

Vilpo, J. A. and Rytömaa, T. (1973) Proliferation kinetics of Shay chloroleukaemia cells grown in diffusion chambers in vivo. Cell Tissue Kinet. 6, 489.

Vilpo, J. A., Kiviniemi, K. and Rytömaa, T. (1973) Inhibition of granulopoiesis by endogenous granulocyte chalone studied with the diffusion chamber technique. Europ. J. Cancer 9, 515.

Volm, M., Wayss, K. and Hinderer, H. (1969) A new model of growth regulation. Cell-specific inhibition of DNA-synthesis in HeLa cells by endometrium extract. Natur-wissenschaften 56, 566.

Wetherley-Mein, G. and Cottom, D. C. (1956) Fresh blood transfusion in leukaemia. Brit. J. Haemat. 2, 25.

CHAPTER 13

In vitro biological and chemical properties of the granulocytic chalone

W. R. PAUKOVITS

Department of Cell Kinetics, Institute for Cancer Research, University of Vienna,
Borschkegasse 8a, 1090 Vienna, Austria

In the bone marrow a population of pluripotent stem cells is present, which can generate clones which can contain erythroid, granulocytic and megakaryocytic cells as well as precursors of lymphoid cells and additional stem cells. The progeny of a single cell of this type has been shown to be able to completely repopulate the hemopoietic organs of a lethally irradiated animal. These pluripotent cells are transformed by an intramedullary differentiation event into 'committed' precursor cells, committed in the sense that their developmental capacities have been limited to a narrower range. Thus the erythroid committed precursor population apparently can only turn into the erythroid precursor cells – if so induced by the humoral factor erythropoietin (Gordon, 1973). Similarly the committed precursor cell of the myeloid series, the in vitro granulocytic colony forming cell CFU-C, following an appropriate induction event, will turn into the granulocytic or monocytic line, depending on the nature of this inductive step. Conceivably a third precursor cell of this type would be a committed megakaryocytic precursor cell, but such a cell has not yet been identified.

The nature of the primary differentiation step which transforms pluripotent stem cells into one of these committed types is not known. The nonstatistical distribution of erythroid and myeloid colonies in the spleen indicates that local milieu effects seem to be involved in this process. In the bone marrow itself the cells of the stroma seem to play an important role during these processes.

Recent studies have indicated that an early stage in the differentiation of pluripotent stem cells may be a state in which the cell is still a pluripotent one, which, however, cannot reproduce as a pluripotent stem cell, i.e. its descendants are all of the committed type. This would indicate a two-step mechanism for the primary differentiation event, and also that for the expression of differentiation-induced nuclear reprogramming a round of DNA-synthesis may be necessary (Lajtha and Schofield, 1974).

The descendants of the stem cell constitute an amplifying transit population which undergoes a number of cell-cycles, but without capability for prolonged self-maintenance. This implies that a maturation process occurs in this population: the early cells divide but this capacity is limited in the later forms. After a certain number of divisions the cells either die or are transformed into a different cell type.

The events which occur during this early period of hemopoiesis are relatively well understood in the case of erythropoiesis. There the early forms apparently cannot differentiate into pronormoblasts, the capacity of being an erythropoietin responsive cell is only achieved after a number of cell cycles. Depending on the demand for production of erythrocytes a variable number of cell cycles is passed before the cell reaches the erythropoietin sensitive state and is changed into an early normoblast.

The problems of investigating the possible presence of a 'granulopoietin' are considerably greater than that of looking for stimulators of erythropoiesis since there is no specific granulocyte label known and there is no way of suppressing granulopoiesis in vivo, as in the case of polycythemia. The possibility of partially achieving this by injecting granulocytic chalone is discussed in another chapter of this book.

Two independent studies (Pluznik and Sachs, 1965, 1966; Bradley and Metcalf, 1966) indicated that when suspensions of bone marrow or spleen cells were cultured under suitable conditions in agar, cell colonies developed which were composed of granulocytes and/or macrophages (Bradley and Metcalf, 1966; Ichikawa et al., 1966). This culture system provided a means for studying the proliferation and differentiation of cells which appear to be committed to the granulocytic/monocytic series. Each of these colonies is a clone arising from a single 'in vitro colony forming unit (CFU-C)', which seems to have an absolute requirement for (a) humoral factor(s) which has been called colony stimulating factor (CSF), or colony stimulating activity (CSA) because of the possibility of several different substances having this ability. CFU-C is not identical with the pluripotent stem cell nor with the morphologically identifiable members of the granulocytic series (Moore and Metcalf, 1970).

The evidence for CSA being a physiological stimulator of granulopoiesis is fairly strong. There is a good general correlation between situations in which granulocyte and monocyte productions are increased and situations in which elevated serum CSA levels have been observed. This view is furthermore supported by the observation of Muller-Berat and Laerum (1975) that CSF and the granulocyte chalone which is known to play an important regulatory role in vivo apparently compete for the same regulatory sites on the surface membrane of bone marrow cells.

13.1 Specific inhibitors of granulopoiesis

Bone marrow contains a considerable number of mature granulocytes which are now known to release substance(s) which are able to inhibit granulo-poietic proliferation. These substances are obviously also present in the blood serum, which has been widely used as a medium constituent in bone marrow cultures. To achieve optimal growth of the cells many investigators have dialyzed the sera used which resulted in the apparent removal of inhibitors of bone marrow growth (Bradley and Sumner, 1968; Chan and Metcalf, 1970; Stanley et al., 1972).

An inhibitory activity for bone marrow growth has been demonstrated to be present also in the bone marrow itself (Evans, 1972; Haskill et al., 1972). While these inhibitory properties of bone marrow cells and blood serum on granulopoietic proliferation were known for quite a long time, T. Rytömaa of Helsinki was the first to take a closer look at the causes of this inhibition. He was able to demonstrate the presence of an inhibitor of granulopoiesis in blood serum (Rytömaa and Kiviniemi, 1964). This factor exhibited a set of properties – as e.g. absolute specificity for granulopoietic inhibition, reversibility of action, non-toxicity, species-non-specificity – which allowed its classification as the granulocytic chalone.

When mature peripheral granulocytes are incubated for one or several hours the conditioned medium contains inhibitory substances for the pro-liferation of bone marrow cells (Rytömaa and Kiviniemi, 1968, 1973, Paukovits, 1971, 1972, 1973). Chalones in general have been defined by Bullough (1965) as inhibitors of cellular proliferation which originate from the mature cells of a given cell system and which specifically act on the immature dividing precursor cells of that same system.

Further evidence of granulocyte-derived factors which play a role in granulopoietic regulation has been presented recently by Heit (1975). If granulocytic colonies are formed in agar culture, the presence of sufficiently large numbers of mature granulocytes in a second agar layer leads to a reduction of the colony number which is correlated to the number of mature cells in the underlay.

13.2 Preparation of granulocytic chalone

Granulocytic chalone is released by mature granulocytes into the surrounding medium. It is thus possible to detect chalone activity in media conditioned by mature granulocytes. The incubation of peripheral white blood cells has been used as a chalone source (Rytömaa and Kiviniemi, 1967; Paukovits, 1971; Laerum and Maurer, 1973; McVittie and McCarthy, 1974) and incubation of exudate cells in a suitable medium. In some cases also the ascitic fluid has been used as chalone source (Laerum and Maurer, 1973). Although high yields of inhibitory activity can be obtained in this way, it has been shown (Paukovits, 1971) that this ascitic fluid contains a large variety of small molecular weight inhibitors. These substances can only be separated from the chalone itself when chromatographic techniques of sufficient resolving power are applied.

Another way to obtain granulocyte-conditioned medium is by incubation of bone marrow cells. Since bone marrow contains a considerable number of mature granulocytes this appears at present to be one of the best methods for the preparation of crude chalone extracts (Paukovits, 1973; Paukovits and Paukovits, 1975). Blood serum can also be regarded as a 'granulocyte conditioned medium' and chalone has been found there long ago (Rytömaa and Kiviniemi, 1967, 1968; Paukovits, 1971). However, the problem of the presence in the preparation of other inhibitors occurs also here, but chalone may be separated from these by chromatographic techniques.

A further possibility to obtain large amounts of granulocytic chalone is to prepare chalone from splenic homogenates (Paukovits, 1973). Although large amounts of spleen are available, the problem here is that only a minor fraction of the cells in the spleen are mature granulocytic cells. Furthermore the crude extracts from this source are really 'crude' in the sense that they contain all sorts of materials which usually are present in tissue homogenates. In addition to these increased difficulties in purification of granulocytic chalone there is also the possibility of the presence of hydrolytic enzymes which may reduce the yield considerably.

The inhibitors prepared from these different sources have identical properties, the most important of which is complete specificity for granulocytic cells. Rytömaa has made a detailed investigation on the elution properties of chalone prepared by gel-filtration on Sephadex G-75 from intact and from homogenized peripheral granulocytes. Complete identity of the chalones prepared in the two ways was found (Rytömaa, 1968).

The relative elution volume of granulocytic chalone from Sephadex G-75 has been found to be $V_e/V_o = 2.73$ which would be consistent with a molecular weight of approximately 4000. These investigations also revealed that the biological activity of granulocytic chalone may be extremely high. Preparations have been obtained with a protein content below 20 μg/ml which still were biologically fully active, but none of the chemical properties of these fractions correlated with chalone activity. A molecular weight of granulocytic chalone well above the level of monomeric aminoacids has also been deduced from the electrophoretic mobility at low pH-values. Paper electrophoresis at pH 1.9 results in a good separation from the monomeric aminoacids. The mobility of e.g. Leucine is twice that of granulocytic chalone (Paukovits, 1973) at this pH, where all amino groups are charged and all carboxyls are in the uncharged condition. This allows correlation (as a very crude estimate) of molecular weight with mobility.

The ultrafiltration characteristics of granulocytic chalone are also consistent with a molecular weight of several thousands. It has been found (Laerum and Maurer, 1973; Paukovits, 1973) that chalone passes quantitatively through membranes with a cutoff limit of 10,000 daltons whereas it is retained by membranes with a cutoff limit of 500 daltons.

When, however, granulocytic chalone is chromatographed on small pore gels as Sephadex G-25, deviations from the 'several thousands' hypothesis are found, which have been analysed in detail recently (Paukovits and Paukovits, 1975).

From G-25 chalone is eluted at $V_e/V_o = 2.06$ between leucine ($V_e/V_o = 1.98$) and thymidine ($V_e/V_o = 2.26$). Leucine is known to emerge just before the salt peak at V_i which is mainly due to ion exclusion effects, whereas thymidine is retarded considerably due to the presence of an extended aromatic π-electron system. The elution position of granulocytic chalone seems to exactly coincide with V_i. Thus chalone would seem to be a rather small molecule, however the large molecule interpretation is not ruled out since it might contain a sufficiently large number of aromatic structure elements in it, to be retarded to a high degree on Sephadex G-25. Some polypeptides are known which show just this behaviour. To resolve this molecular weight – retardation problem, chromatography on Sephadex G-15 was performed. Here the interactions between solutes and the gel matrix are qualitatively the same as on Sephadex G-25. However quantitative differences in the elution behaviour could be expected due to the higher matrix density of Sephadex G-15. A shift in the elution position of granulocytic chalone relative to leucine, V_i, and thymidine would thus lend some support to the large-molecule-hypothesis. The relative elution volumes on G-15 columns of leucine and thymidine are 1.78 and 2.5 respectively, which is in accordance with the theoretical expectations.

However granulocytic chalone still elutes at $V_e/V_o = 2.06$ which is very near to V_i. This behaviour would be consistent with chalone being a small molecule. Biogel P-6, which chemically is polyacrylamide, interacts with the molecules of the solute in quite a different way than the dextran matrix of Sephadex, but the qualitative characteristics of the interaction are not too different from Sephadex. Again leucine can be expected to emerge before V_i and thymidine to be retarded somewhat due to ion exclusion effects and aromatic electron interactions respectively. The elution position of leucine is $V_e/V_o = 2.18$ and that of thymidine is 2.48. Granulocytic chalone elutes at $V_e/V_o = 2.3$ which again is very near to V_i. The gel filtration properties of granulocytic chalone on gels with a high matrix density would thus strongly suggest a low molecular weight which however is in contrast to other observations mentioned above. This peculiar behaviour of the granulocytic chalone renders any estimates of the molecular weight unreliable. Other methods will have to be used for this purpose.

The extensive use of gel-filtration on different matrix types does not lead to a final purification of granulocytic chalone. The peaks of absorbance at 215 nm, 240 nm and 280 nm do not coincide with the elution position of the biological activity. The preparation of pure granulocytic chalone will thus need the application of other purification methods. Gel chromatography however leads to the removal of considerable amounts of impurities, and preparations obtained by these methods may eventually be useful for biological investigations where ultimate chemical purity seems not to be obligatory.

13.3 Chemical nature of granulocytic chalone

The chemical nature of granulocytic chalone has never been demonstrated conclusively. Although the chalone might be a peptide, the evidence for this is weak (Paukovits, 1973) and has been obtained with rather impure samples. Chalone seems to be susceptible to the action of trypsin; however, a rather prolonged treatment is necessary. The degradation of chalone by trypsin seems to demonstrate the presence of lysine or arginine peptide bonds. This, however, is inconclusive since trypsin also can hydrolyze ester bonds of a certain type.

Granulocytic chalone is soluble in aqueous solvents irrespective of the pH and also in organic solvents of sufficient polarity (Paukovits, 1975). This would indicate that chalone is a rather polar molecule, which eventually may contain also some hydrophobic groups. The solubility of chalone in organic solvents could eventually be used to extract the inhibitor from the crude starting material without coextracting larger proteins (enzymes) and the bulk of salt present there. The experiments show, however, that despite the good solubility of purified chalone in ethanol-acetone or chloroform-methanol mixtures, no inhibitory activity can be extracted by these solvents from the lyophilized starting material. A similar behaviour has been observed with other biologically active substances (Burgus et al., 1975) and was interpreted as being the result of the binding of the active peptide to macromolecular carriers.

The most stringent problem in chemical investigations with granulocytic chalone is the exceedingly low amount of material which can be obtained from the sources discussed above. This may be due partly to the losses during the preparation and purification. Maurer (1973) has estimated that 1000 kg of spleen would be necessary to prepare 1 mg of chalone, which still is a very small amount for the determination of the chemical nature and structure of a completely unknown molecule.

13.4 Chalone and thymidine metabolism

In many in vitro studies [³H]TdR was used as the main indicator of cell proliferation. It must be emphasized, therefore, that the chalone effects are not explicable in terms of interaction with thymidine metabolism per se, although the contrary opinion may at first seem to be supported by the studies of Perry and Marsh (1964). These authors demonstrated that preparations from intact and homogenized leucocytes may cause virtually complete inhibition of [³H]TdR incorporation in human leukaemic leucocytes and in dog thoracic duct lymphocytes in vitro. It was suggested that this effect is attributable to thymidine phosphorylase which rapidly converts thymidine to thymine and thus prevents uptake of [³H]TdR in the DNA.

However, such an effect is distinctly different from the chalone action: (i) the effect of chalone is readily demonstrable by means of other indicators besides [³H]thymidine: these include [¹⁴C]formate (Rytömaa and Kiviniemi, 1967), [³H]adenine (Rytömaa and Kiviniemi, 1968b), and such substances as [³⁵S]sulphate and even amino acids (Niskanen, 1967; Rytömaa and Kiviniemi, 1967); (ii) thymidine phosphorylase is not present in the chalone-containing fractions obtained by gel filtration on Sephadex; (iii) it would be very strange if these or other comparable enzymes were target tissue specific (Rytömaa and Kiviniemi, 1968a).

Another problem which has been discussed extensively is the isotope dilution effect which may result from any cold thymidine which eventually was present in the original extracts or conditioned medium. The problem of thymidine contaminating the chalone preparations has been discussed by several authors (Laerum and Maurer, 1973; Lenfant et al., 1973; Paukovits, 1973) since any cold thymidine present in the samples would cause an apparent inhibition in a [^{3}H]thymidine incorporation assay. However, thymidine is clearly separated from granulocytic chalone if columns of sufficient resolving power are used (Paukovits and Paukovits, 1975a). The problems discussed by the authors mentioned above, could easily be avoided if such columns are used for the preparation of chalone. A simple thymidine dilution effect could be ruled out also on the basis of the specificity of the inhibitory action. Furthermore an isotope dilution effect would not show a plateau in the dose-response curve.

13.5 Specificity of action on granulopoiesis

Laerum and Maurer (1973) have summarized the criteria of a cell specific chalone action in the following way:

1) The preparation must first of all show a defined biological activity on cells of a specific target tissue.

2) The inhibitory effect on the progression of cells through the cycle must be non-toxic, with no immediate reduction of cell number. Moreover the inhibition must be reversible.

3) To be relevant for the regulation of cell proliferation it must be expected that corresponding to the lower rate of progression through the cell cycle, a lower cell yield is found after a certain time.

4) The inhibitory effect should not be species-specific, this is, however, not an a priori requirement for a chalone, but has been observed in all cases investigated so far.

5) A chalone should act exclusively on the target cells which must belong to the same cell line as the cells producing chalone. The granulocytic chalone should therefore only inhibit the proliferation of immature myeloid cells.

6) Furthermore a given chalone should have no effect on the cells of another organ system where the same type of regulatory principles has been shown to operate. The granulocytic chalone should thus not act on erythropoiesis, lymphocyte-proliferation and e.g. cell growth in the epidermis.

7) An analogous extract from another organ should have no inhibitory action in the cell system under investigation; e.g. erythrocyte or epidermal chalone extracts should have no effect on granulopoietic proliferation.

8) Other, non-specific ('non-chalone') effects on the target cells must be excluded. An example would be the reduction of [^{3}H]thymidine incorpora-

tion by the cold thymidine which might be present in the extracts.

The first indication for the cell specific action of granulocytic chalone has been observed by Rytömaa (Rytömaa and Kiviniemi, 1967). When bone marrow cells were incubated in the presence of granulocytic chalone and [^{3}H]thymidine and the proliferation of the cells analysed by autoradiography, the labeling index of the myeloid precursors was reduced significantly whereas the LI of the non-myeloid cells remained unchanged.

These results have however been criticised because granulocytic cells can be maintained in a reasonably healthy condition under various culture conditions, whereas erythroid cells are difficult to culture. However it is possible to conclude from such experiments that the overall direction of the chalone effect is towards a specific reduction of granulopoiesis.

Guinea pig bone marrow can be separated by the method of Evans et al. (1971) into distinct subpopulations, one of which is composed almost exclusively of immature granulocytic cells. We have been able to demonstrate that granulocytic chalone inhibited selectively the uptake of [^{3}H]thymidine into this myeloid precursor population whereas no such inhibition was found when the other subpopulations were treated with granulocytic chalone (Paukovits, 1972, 1973).

More recently Laerum and Maurer (1973) demonstrated that the proliferation of granulocytes and macrophages is inhibited by different factors. When extracts were made from suspensions of granulocytes contaminated with some macrophages, the proliferation of myeloid elements as well as macrophages is inhibited in diffusion chamber cultures. Extracts of granulocyte suspensions containing no macrophages inhibited only the granulocytic precursors. From these results the conclusion was drawn that granulocytic chalone is tissue-specific for myelopoietic cells. It should be kept in mind that macrophages are perhaps the nearest relatives to granulocytic cells, originating from the same committed stem cells (CFU-C) (Metcalf and Moore, 1971).

MacVittie and McCarthy (1974) were able to demonstrate in vitro that granulocyte conditioned medium at a concentration of 20% of the culture volume did not significantly reduce the lymphocytic response to phytohaemagglutinin, using both rat and mouse spleen cell suspensions and the rat marrow response to erythropoietin as measured by [^{3}H]thymidine and ^{59}Fe uptake respectively. In addition the chalone preparation did not significantly affect viability, plating efficiency or [^{3}H]thymidine uptake of proliferating mouse L-929 cells in monolayer culture.

A complete lack of cross-reactivity between granulocytic or erythrocytic chalone and granulopoiesis or erythropoiesis respectively has been observed by Bateman (1974). When assayed in short term in vitro cultures the erythrocyte product reduced DNA-synthesis (as measured autoradiographically) in erythroblasts present in the bone marrow but did not affect the DNA-synthesis in myeloid or lymphoid cells. The leukocyte product, under the same culture conditions, reduced DNA-synthesis only in leukocyte precursor cells.

A completely different approach to the specificity problem of the hematopoietic chalones has been used by Lord et al. (1974). They have used the method of fluorescence polarisation developed by Cercek and Cercek (1972) for the study of the structuredness of the cytoplasmic matrix (SCM).

The technique is based on the excitation of fluorescein molecules, produced by enzymatic hydrolysis of the non-fluorescing fluorescein-diacetate in the cytoplasm with polarized light and, measurement of the polarization of the emitted fluorescence. Rotational relaxation of the fluorescein molecule between absorption and emission of light depolarizes the fluorescence. Rotation of the fluorescein molecules depends on the physical state of organization of the cytoplasmic matrix of the molecular level.

Saline extracts of lymphocytes, granulocytes and erythrocytes (LNE, GCE, RCE) have been partially purified by ultrafiltration into selected molecular weight ranges and each tested against proliferative populations of lymphoid, granulocytic and erythroid cells. In all cases, complete specificity of effect on SCM was found, LNEs affecting only lymphoid cell populations, GCEs affecting only the granulocytic cell populations and RCEs affecting only erythroid cells. In each case, with the possible exception of the RCEs, the active fractions reside in the molecular weight ranges reported in the literature for cell extracts possessing proliferation inhibitory properties.

It has been demonstrated by several authors that extracts of several tissues (e.g. liver, skin, placenta) do not exert chalone-like effects upon granulopoiesis (Rytömaa, 1973; Laerum and Maurer, 1973; Paukovits, 1974a) and that granulocytic extracts have no inhibitory action on other tissues e.g. the epidermis (Laerum and Maurer, 1973) where a chalone mechanism is known to be effective.

13.6 Target cells of granulocytic chalone in the granulocytic maturation sequence

Granulocytic chalone inhibits the DNA-synthesis of bone marrow cells to a plateau of approximately 50% of the control value (Rytömaa and Kiviniemi, 1968; Paukovits, 1973; Paukovits and Paukovits, 1975a) which would indicate that chalone causes an almost complete cessation of DNA-synthesis in immature granulocytic cells. It has been shown by Rytömaa (1968) that about 50% of the [³H]thymidine incorporated in vitro into bone marrow cells in a short term incubation can be found in granulocytic precursor cells.

The question of which one(s) of the myeloid precursors is (are) the target cell(s) for the granulocytic chalone cannot be answered on the basis of these results. We have thus tried to determine (Paukovits, 1973) by means of physical separation of the myeloid cells of the bone marrow, which particular cell type(s) of the granulocytic series are inhibited by GIF. Myeloid precursor cells of the bone marrow were isolated by the ficoll density step centrifugation method of Evans et al. (1971). These cells were then further separated by means of velocity sedimentation (Miller and Phillips, 1969). The ficoll step yielded a good enrichment of myeloid precursor cells and an almost complete separation from other cell types in the bone marrow. By the velocity sedimentation step it was possible to subfractionate these myeloic precursors into myeloblasts, promyelocytes, and myelocytes. The in vitro colony-forming units are clearly separated from these cells due to their rapid sedimentation (Worton et al., 1969).

Due to the inherent variability in the sedimentation rates the control experiment and the granulocytic chalone run were performed simultaneously by using a double labeling technique. Controls were incubated with [¹⁴C]thymidine and the test cells were incubated with [³H]thymidine plus granulocytic chalone. After incubation the cells of both suspensions were combined, and velocity sedimentation was performed with this combined population. Cells which were inhibited by GCH would show up as minima in a plot of ³H/¹⁴C versus migration distance.

The results show that the DNA synthesis is inhibited by GCH in essentially the whole range of granulopoietic precursor cells. Two pronounced minima occurred in the isotope ratio curve, at 4 mm/h and 11 mm/h, respectively.

It is possible to identify the cells in the 4 mm/h region as myeloblasts and/or promyelocytes. In the myelocyte range (6–8 mm/h in our system), only weak inhibition was observed which, taken by itself, is not very indicative of an inhibitory action of GCH on myelocytes. It should be pointed out, however, that cell cycle kinetic effects should play an important role here and that myelocytes are not very active in DNA synthesis. The assumption that GCH also inhibits the proliferation of myelocytes also would be in accordance with the magnitude of the effect of GCH on the whole bone marrow population. This point, however, awaits further clarification.

The minimum in the isotope ratio curve of very large cells (11 mm/h) could possibly be due to an inhibitory action of GCH on very early cells (CFU-C) of the granulopoietic system, which have been described as being rather large cells with correspondingly high sedimentation velocity (Peterson, 1967).

These results therefore indicate that GCH inhibits the proliferation of all mitotically competent myeloid precursor cells of the bone marrow. Some points, however, of this hypothesis (CFU-C and myelocytes) require further investigation. It seems, nevertheless, that a single substance which is produced by the mature cells of the granulocytic series inhibits the mitotic activity in the entire myeloid proliferation compartment and possibly even in the committed stem cell compartment. This would further imply that the responsiveness to the regulatory influences of GCH is already expressed at a very early stage of granulocytic differentiation. It may thus be that the presence of receptor sites for GCH is one of the fundamental properties of mitotically competent myeloid precursor cells, the expression of these sites being one of the early events of myeloid differentiation.

13.7 Action of GIF on the committed stem cells of the granulocytic series

The cell separation experiments described in the previous section indicate that granulocytic chalone is effective at the committed stem cell level. A chalone inhibition of CFU-C proliferation would also provide a very efficient way of regulating the production of granulocytes. The agar colony formation assay allows the investigation of this problem more closely.

An effect of GCH on the unipotent committed stem cells would also be compatible with the findings of Metcalf (1971) which demonstrate that colony formation in agar by bone marrow cells is inhibited by (a) dialyzable substance(s) from bone marrow-conditioned medium. It is very probable that this substance, the molecular weight of which is less than 10,000 daltons, may be identical with the GCH.

MacVittie and McCarthy (1974) found that granulocytic chalone at a concentration which reduced the total [³H]thymidine incorporation into bone marrow cells in liquid culture by about 10 percent inhibited the formation of agar colonies between 50 and 70 percent, depending on the source of the CSF used.

This result is consistent with those reported by other investigators (Chan, 1971; Chan et al., 1971; Metcalf, 1971; Paran et al., 1971) describing the action of dialysable and non-dialysable molecules found in some sera and in spleen, bone marrow, and granulocyte conditioned media which are capable of blocking the in vitro action of CSF in agar culture of bone marrow cells.

The inhibitory action of granulocytic chalone on agar colony formation and possible mechanisms of action of chalone in bone marrow cells were also investigated by Muller-Bérat et al. (1975). If the granulocytic chalone preparation was added to the cultures at day 4 after plating (with CSF) no influence on the number of colonies was found at day 7. Also, when granulocytic chalone was assayed on day 1, without preincubation, no inhibition was observed. The chalone which apparently is bound only weakly to the cell surface can be removed by washing the cells repeatedly, and no inhibitory effect is observed after this manipulation. These phenomena were interpreted to suggest that an active membrane process takes place during the action of granulocytic chalone on the granulopoietic committed stem cells.

The inhibition of colony formation could already be observed as soon as the recording of small cellular aggregates (> 5 cells) was possible. There was no reversion of the effect and even at day 9–10 the number of colonies was decreased as compared with the controls. The action of granulocytic chalone leads therefore to a decrease in the number of small aggregates as well as the number of colonies. The mean cell number per colony was not influenced by granulocytic chalone. Finally the granulocyte/macrophage distribution factor was not altered by the action of chalone.

Granulocytic chalone leads to a rapid decrease in the number of aggregates. Prior to plating the inhibitory effect is reversible by washing the cells whereas no such reversibility was noted at later times. The authors however suggest that this does not reflect an irreversibility of the chalone effect but rather a property inherent to the test system itself. It has been shown by Metcalf (1970) that the absence of CSF for only 24 h leads to a 50 % decrease in the number of colonies. This lead to the suggestion that granulocytic chalone prevents the cells from dividing for approximately the same time (24 h), then releasing the cells for normal mitotic function too late for the stimulating action of CSF. Since some type of recruitment takes place in the agar during the first days of culturing, those cells which are ready to be triggered into proliferation by CSF are probably also those which are ready to be inhibited by the chalone. The cells triggered at day 2 and 3 escape the action of chalone because this action is relatively short lived.

These results by Muller-Bérat et al., also suggest the possibility of a competition between CSF and granulocytic chalone for certain sites on the cell surface, with CSF being the dominating molecule.

13.8 Cell-surface receptor of granulocytic chalone

A great variety of cell types in vitro responds to mild proteolytic treatment by an increased rate of proliferation. The changes in cell surface brought about by this procedure are thus believed to be involved in the regulation of cell growth. A mild treatment of confluent resting cells in culture with proteases, in particular the serine proteases, can promote the initiation of cell proliferation and result in release from density inhibition of growth (Burger, 1970; Sefton and Rubin, 1970).

Recent publications have strongly implicated the increased proteolytic activity in cultures of transformed cells with alteration of cell surface components and a resulting perturbed regulation of cell growth (Schnebli and Burger, 1972; Ossowski et al., 1973; Teng and Lan Bo Chen, 1975). Several authors (Hynes, 1974) have described an extremely trypsin sensitive component of the external cell membrane which is heavily labeled by lactoperoxidase catalyzed iodination in normal cells and is only weakly labeled or not present in transformed cells. These results have encouraged the speculation that this protein (as well as other protease sensitive membrane components) and its removal by proteolysis may play a direct role in the control of growth of cells.

A large number of growth regulating factors and polypeptide hormones exert their effects on the target cells by specifically interacting with receptor sites on the external surface of these cells (Roth, 1973). Some of these receptor sites are susceptible to proteolytic attack (Kono, 1969; Chang et al., 1974) which can be used for their demonstration.

The sigmoid dose-response curve of granulocytic chalone on myeloid cells (Paukovits, 1972b) has led to the interpretation that granulocytic chalone may act by interacting with membrane components of the target cells. The same hypothesis has been developed from the results of the influence of granulocytic chalone on the colony formation of bone marrow cells in soft agar culture. In order to test for the possible existence of granulocyte chalone receptors on the bone marrow cell membrane we have treated intact bone marrow cells for very short times with very low concentrations of trypsin. This type of treatment was used before by Chang et al. (1974) for the demonstration of erythropoietin receptor sites on the bone marrow cell surface. In principle we have measured the action of granulocytic chalone on trypsin-treated bone marrow cells in the presence of cycloheximide to prevent the regeneration of degraded membrane components (Paukovits and Paukovits, 1975). Since cycloheximide itself has been found to inhibit DNA-synthesis in bone marrow cells a rather low concentration of 0.5

μg/ml has been used, which was a compromise between reduced protein synthesis (i.e. receptor regeneration) and still enough DNA-synthesis to permit the observation of the chalone effect. The results obtained show that the inhibitability of trypsin-treated bone marrow cells is significantly reduced when protein synthesis is inhibited by cycloheximide. No such reduction is observed when protein synthesis is permitted after trypsin treatment.

Since granulocytic chalone itself is not significantly destroyed by this short trypsin treatment (Paukovits and Paukovits, 1975b), this result leads to the conclusion that there is a protein on the external surface of the granulocytic chalone-responsive cells in the bone marrow which is accessible to trypsin and which is required for the inhibitory effect of granulocytic chalone on granulopoietic DNA-synthesis. After destruction by trypsin this protein receptor is rapidly resynthesized when the cells are able to synthesize protein at a normal rate in the absence of cycloheximide.

That chalones might act via a membrane receptor mechanism has been suggested by several authors (Iversen, 1969; Marks, 1972; Voorhees et al., 1972; Houck and Irausquin, 1973) but no detailed investigations have been reported about this primary step in chalone action. The above results of Paukovits and Paukovits allow the conclusion that at least the granulocytic chalone exerts its effect upon bone marrow cells by interacting with a receptor protein located on the cell membrane. The possibility may be discussed that the high cell-type specificity of granulocytic chalone and other chalones, as well as the altered response of the target cells in the neoplastic state might have its molecular basis in this interaction (Paukovits and Paukovits, 1975b).

13.9 Granulocyte chalone and cyclic AMP

This demonstration of chalone receptors on the outer membrane of immature granulocytic cells almost immediately brings into consideration the role of cyclic AMP in the process of growth regulation. The interaction of chalone with receptor sites which govern the enzymatic activity of adenylate cyclase, as a possible mechanism of chalone action has been proposed by Iversen (1969). On the background of the results described above, which seem to demonstrate the existence of surface chalone receptors on bone marrow cells, this would seem to be a reasonable hypothesis, although the existence of a chalone receptor does not necessarily mean that this is a receptor associated with the adenylate cyclase system.

Low concentrations of cAMP exert a stimulatory effect on the DNA-synthesis of haemopoietic cells and on thymic lymphocytes (MacManus and Whitfield, 1969; Byron, 1973; Tisman and Herbert, 1973; Whitfield et al., 1973), whereas higher concentrations (above 10^{-4} M) are strongly inhibitory to bone marrow cell proliferation (Tisman and Herbert, 1973; Rytömaa and Kiviniemi, 1975). The latter authors have furthermore demonstrated that this inhibitory effect is not specific for the cyclic nucleotide since also AMP, cGMP, dibutyryl-cAMP, and deoxycytidine are efficient inhibitors of bone marrow DNA-synthesis in this concentration range. It has been concluded that although the modes of inhibitory action of these substances are probably different from one case to another, they almost certainly are all pharmacological in nature.

It remains to be shown, if there is any correlation between the interaction of chalone and its receptor sites and the stimulatory action of low (physio-logical) concentrations of cAMP on bone marrow cells. Also the effects which cGMP may eventually have in this system will have to be evaluated. It will be very interesting to know whether there are any changes in the intracellular cAMP of cGMP concentrations as a consequence of the chalone-receptor interaction.

13.10 Regulation system of granulopoiesis

A successful functional organization of a multicellular organism is evidently only possible, when simultaneously with the regulation of functional differentiation into different types of cells also the proliferative activity of these cells is subjected to a very exact control.

All the regulating factors under discussion directly or indirectly modify gene activity and induce differentiation and/or modulate the development of the differentiated state. As a result of the differentiation process, which has been defined as '. . . the sum of processes by which acquisition of specific metabolic consequences (or loss thereof) distinguishes daughter cells from each other or from the parental cell' (Gross, 1968), each cell causes charac-teristic changes in its environment and also maintains these changes. The proliferative activity of a given cell depends to a large extent on influences which are exerted by the immediate environment of this cell. In this way in any multicellular organism, an extremely complex system of cellular interactions and communication is formed, in which the differentiative status strongly influences the proliferative activities and vice versa. This is the case also in the haematopoietic system, where starting with aggregates of stem and progenitor cells scattered throughout the body, a regular and controlled supply of short lived end cells must be delivered to the peripheral blood. This situation is inherently a very complex one, and an almost unlimited number of influences have been found which – together – constitute what is called the regulation system of haematopoiesis (Metcalf and Moore, 1971).

In the granulopoietic system several distinct types of cells have to be distinguished. The pluripotent stem cells themselves certainly have their own regulatory systems, but there must be a certain kind of feedback signal which tells about the functional and population state of the more mature compartments.

The in vitro colony forming cells, which are the first functionally recognizable cells of the myeloid series, are subject to several regulatory influences as far as their proliferative activity is concerned. Several types of 'colony stimulating factors' have been described, which seem to be an in vitro prerequisite for the development of granulocytic colonies in agar culture. The proposition that CSF might be the true 'in vivo granulopoietin' (Robinson and Mangalik, 1975) has been questioned by other workers (Quesenberry et al., 1974). Recently evidence has been presented (Niho et al., 1975) that certain types of colony stimulating activities might play some regulatory role during granulopoiesis, and that membrane phenomena are involved in the production and action of CSF.

In addition to these stimulatory influences the committed stem cells are also subject to the granulocytic chalone, which is a specifically acting feedback inhibitor of granulopoiesis. As discussed in other sections of this paper CSF and the granulocytic chalone compete for the same sites on the membrane of the CFC's (Muller-Bérat et al., 1975).

Since granulocytic chalone has been found to be fully and specifically active also in vivo (Benestad et al., 1973; Laerum and Maurer, 1973; MacVittie and McCarthy, 1974) this adds much to the hypothesis that also CSF might play a role in the physiological regulation of granulopoiesis.

Originating from the myeloid committed stem cells a number of morphologically identifiable cells are produced which together constitute the proliferation compartment of granulopoiesis. These cells have been found to be under chalone control (Paukovits, 1973). A stimulatory role of CSF or CSF-like factors on these cells is questionable but cannot be ruled out completely.

After leaving the proliferation compartment the myeloid progenitors enter the maturation compartment, where cell divisions no longer take place, but maturation proceeds through several morphologically distinguishable cell types. Lastly mature polymorphonuclear cells are formed which stay in the bone marrow storage compartment until they enter the peripheral functional pool of granulocytes. This process is governed by a factor, called 'leukocytosis inducing factor' which can be found in the blood serum and which induces the transit of mature granulocytes from the bone marrow into the peripheral blood. Whether this LIF also plays a regulatory role on the transit time through the maturation compartment is not known.

The regulation system of granulopoiesis thus seems to consist of (at least) three control loops which may constitute a temporal hierarchy. A deviation from the normal number of granulocytes e.g. a reduction would thus lead to the following processes: (a) increase of the 'LIF' concentration; (b) increase in the 'CSF' concentration, (c) decrease in the peripheral chalone concentration.

For reasons discussed below, only the first two events lead to direct changes in the bone marrow. Firstly there is a rapid release of mature granulocytes from the storage compartment into the peripheral blood, and the peripheral granulocyte number is increased within a rather short time. Secondly the increased 'CSF'-concentration induces a higher rate of production in the very early myeloid cell types. The result of this process however will have no influence on the peripheral situation before a considerable time has passed. The storage compartment remains depleted of mature granulocytes for a considerable period of time. Two aspects are important here: (a) It would be desirable to reach normal storage levels in as short a time as possible. It takes rather long until the wave of increased production induced by CSF reaches this point. (b) Due to the rather drastic and sudden reduction of the number of mature cells in the bone marrow the intramedullar chalone concentration decreases.

This second event provides a mechanism by which the emptied storage pool can be filled faster than by the CSF mechanism, since the lack of chalone releases the proliferation block of the cells of the proliferation pool and within a relatively short time (on the order of the duration of a cell cycle) the output of the proliferative compartment is increased. The changes of serum chalone concentration will play almost no role here since the population density of mature granulocytes (which is directly correlated to the local chalone concentration) is far higher in the bone marrow than in the peripheral blood. Such a cascade mechanism of granulopoietic controls has been discussed by Paukovits (1974) and recently by Fliedner (1975), Heit (1975), and Heit et al. (1975). Only specific humoral regulators have been mentioned here; there are however a large number of other factors – of endocrinological or nutritional origin – which exert a very important influence on the differentiative and/or proliferative state of the haematopoietic system. The adrenal and other steroid hormones shall be mentioned here together with the experimental difficulties to cleanly separate hormonal effects from those of specific humoral regulators.

References

Bateman, A. (1974) Cell Tissue Kinet. 7, 451.

Benestad, H B , Rytömaa, T. and Kiviniemi, K. (1973) Cell Tissue Kinet. 6, 147.

Bradley, T. R. and Metcalf, D. (1966) Austr. J. Exp. Biol. Med. Sci. 44, 287.

Bradley, T. R. and Sumner, M. A. (1968) Austr. J. Exp. Biol. Med. Sci. 46, 607.

Bullough, W. S. (1965) Cancer Res. 25, 1683.

Burger, M. M. (1970) Nature 227, 170.

Burgus, R., Nelson, J. and Amoss, M. (1973) Meth. Enzymol. 37, 402.

Byron, J. W. (1973) Nature New Biol. 241, 152.

Cercek, L. and Cercek, B. (1972) Int. J. Radiat. Biol. 21, 445.

Chan, S. H. and Metcalf, D. (1970) Nature 227, 845.

Chan, S. H. (1971) Austr. J. Exp. Biol. Med. Sci. 49, 553.

Chan, S. H., Metcalf, D. and Stanley, E. R. (1971) Brit. J. Haematol. 20, 329.

Chang, S. C. S., Sikkema, D. and Goldwasser, E. (1974) Biochem. Biophys. Res. Commun. 57, 399.

Evans, W. H., Wilson, S. and Mage, M. G. (1971) J. Reticuloendoth. Soc. 9, 209.

Fliedner, T. M. (1975) Proc. 3rd Int. Workshop Myeloprolif. Diseases, Vienna (in press).

Gordon, A. S. (1973) Vitamines and Hormones 31, 105. Academic Press, New York.

Gross, P. R. (1968) Ann. Rev. Biochem. 37, 631.

Haskill, J. S., McKnight, R. D. and Galbraith, P. R. (1972) Blood 40, 394.

Heit, W. (1975) Proc. 3rd Int. Workshop on Myeloprolif. Diseases, Vienna (in press).

Heit, W., Kern, P., Heimpel, H. and Kubanek, B. (1975) Scand. J. Haematol. (in press).

Houck, J. C. and Irausquin, H. (1973) Natl. Cancer Inst. Monogr. 38, 117.

Hynes, R. O. (1974) Cell 1, 147.

Ichikawa, Y., Pluznik, D. H. and Sachs, L. (1966) Proc. Natl. Acad. Sci. U.S. 56, 488.

Iversen, O. H. (1969) In: Homeostatic Regulators (ed.: G. Wolstenholme and J. Knight) Ciba Fdn. Sympos. p. 29.

Kono, T. (1969) J. Biol. Chem. 244, 1772.

Laerum, O. D. and Maurer, H. R. (1973) Virchows Archiv, Abt. B, Zellpathol. 14, 293.

Lajtha, L. G. and Schofield, R. (1974) Differentiation 2, 313.

Lenfant, M., Kren-Proschek, L., Verly, W. G. and Dugas, H. (1973) Canad. J. Biochem. 51, 654.

Lord, B. J., Cercek, L., Cercek, B., Shah, G. P., Dexter, T. M. and Lajtha, L. G. (1974) Int. J. Cancer 29, 168.

MacManus, J. P., Whitfield, J. F. (1969) Exp. Cell Res. 58, 188.

MacVittie and McCarthy (1974) Exp. Hematol. 2, 182.

Marks, F. (1973) Natl. Cancer Inst. Monogr. 38, 79.

Maurer, H. R. (1973) 2nd Int. Chalone Conf., Lane End/Bucks.

Metcalf, D. (1970) J. Cell Physiol. 76, 89.

Metcalf, D. (1971) Austr. J. Exp. Biol. Med. Sci. 49, 351.

Metcalf, D. and Moore, M. A. S. (1971) Haemopoietic Cells, North Holland Publ. Comp., p. 163.

Miller, R. G. and Phillips, R. A. (1969) J. Cell Physiol. 73, 191.

Moore, M. A. S. and Metcalf, D. (1970) Brit. J. Haematol. 13, 256.

Muller-Bérat, C. N., Laerum, O. D. and Maurer, H. R. (1975) Scand. J. Haematol. (in press).

Niho, Y., Till, J. E. and McCulloch, E. A. (1975) Blood 45, 811.

Niskanen, E. (1967) Acta Pathol. Microbiol. Scand. 70, Suppl. 90.

Ossowski, L., Quigley, J. P., Kellerman, G. M. and Reich, E. (1973) J. Exp. Med. 138, 1056.

Paran, M., Ichikawa, Y. and Sachs, L. (1969) Proc. Nat. Acad. Sci. 62, 81.

Paukovits, W. R. (1971) Cell Tissue Kinet. 4, 539.

Paukovits, W. R. (1972a) Studia Biophys. 31/32, 301.

Paukovits, W. R. (1972b) In: Leukämien und maligne Lymphone (ed.: A. Stacher) p. 62.

Paukovits, W. R. (1973) Natl. Cancer Inst. Monogr. 38, 147.

Paukovits, W. R. (1974a) Österr. ZS. f. Onkologie 1, 51.

Paukovits, W. R. (1973) 8th Paterson Symp., Manchester, Reviewed in Brit. J. Cancer 29, 84 (1974b)

Paukovits, W. R. (1974c) Blut 27, 217.

Paukovits, W. R. (1975) Experientia (in press 1975).

Paukovits, W. R. and Paukovits, J. B. (1975a) Bolletino Ist. Sierother. Milan. (in press).

Paukovits, W. R. and Paukovits, J. B. (1975) Exp. Pathol. (in press).

Perry, S. and Marsh, J. C. (1964) Proc. Soc. Exp. Biol. 115, 51.

Peterson, E. A. and Evans, W. H. (1967) Nature 214, 824.

Pluznik, D. H. and Sachs, L. (1965) J. Cell. Comp. Physiol. 66, 319. Exp. Cell Res. 43, 553.

Quesenberry, P. J., Ryan, B. and Stohlman, F. jr. (1974) Int. J. Haematol. 28, 531.

Robinson, W. A. and Mangalik, A. (1975) Seminars Hematol. 12, 7.

Roth, J. (1973) Metabolism 22, 1059.

Rytömaa, T. and Kiviniemi, K. (1964) Proc. XIV. Scand. Congr. Path. Microbiol. p. 169, Universitetsforlaget Oslo.

Rytömaa, T. and Kiviniemi, K. (1967) In: Control of Cellular Growth in Adult Organisms (eds.: H. Teir and T. Rytömaa) Academic Press, p. 106.

Rytömaa, T. and Kiviniemi, K. (1968a) Cell Tissue Kinet. 1, 329.

Rytömaa, T. and Kiviniemi, K. (1968b) Cell Tissue Kinet. 1, 340.

Rytömaa, T. and Kiviniemi, K. (1970) Europ. J. Cancer 6, 401.

Rytömaa, T. and Kiviniemi, K. (1973) Natl. Cancer Inst. Monogr. 38, 143.

Rytömaa, T. and Kiviniemi, K. (1975) In vitro 11, 1.

Sefton, B. M. and Rubin, H. (1970) Nature 227, 843.

Schnebli, H. P. and Burger, M. M. (1972) Proc. Natl. Acad. Sci. 69, 3825.

Stanley, E. R., Metcalf, D., Maritz, J. S. and Yeo, G. F. (1972) J. Lab. Clin. Med. 79, 657.

Teng, N. N. H. and Lan Bo Chen (1975) Proc. Natl. Acad. Sci. 72, 413.

Tisman, G. and Herbert, V. (1973) In vitro 9, 86.

Whitfield, J. F., Mac Manus, J. P. and Gillan, D. J. (1973) J. Cell. Physiol. 81, 241.

Wilson, S. M. and Evans, W. H. (1972) J. Reticuloendoth. Soc. 12, 514.

Worton, R. G., McCulloch, E. A. and Till, J. E. (1969) J. Exp. Med. 130, 91.

Voorhees, J. J., Duell, E. A., Lawrence, J. B., Powell, J. A. and Harrell, E. R. (1972) J. Invest. Dermatol. 59, 114.

CHAPTER 14

Granulocyte chalone testing: a critical review

H. R. Maurer and O. D. Laerum

Pharmazeutisches Institut der Freien Universität, 1 Berlin 33, W. Germany, and The Gade Institute, Department of Pathology, University of Bergen, Norway

In this chapter we have tried to critically examine the relationships between the commonly applied criteria for a chalone effect and the evidence for fulfilment of these by the currently used assay systems for the granulocyte chalone.

14.1 Granulopoiesis: essential characteristics with respect to the regulatory control

The testing of granulocyte chalone is extremely difficult because of the complexity of the system. It starts with the multipotent stem cells, being capable of giving rise to granulopoiesis as well as the other bone marrow cell types. About 90% of these are not in the cell cycle. After entering the committed stem cell compartment, most of these cells are in the cycle. This is followed by the differentiating pool of blasts, promyelocytes and myelocytes, ending with non-proliferative metamyelocytes. Except the latter two types, most of these cells are in the cycle. (For details, see e.g. Lajtha, 1975; Lajtha and Schofield, 1974; and Robinson and Mangalik, 1975.)

In regulatory terms, the proliferation of stem cells giving increased stem cell numbers is of greatest importance for the eventual yield of mature cells. Thus a slight increase of the stem cell renewal probability gives a highly increased total number of granulocytes (Vogel et al., 1968, 1969).

The other target of regulation is on the proliferation of the differentiating cells, including all maturation stages from blasts to myelocytes. These different cell types do not necessarily react identically, and there is in fact some indirect evidence that the earlier stages are more strongly inhibited by granulocyte extracts than the later ones (Paukovits, 1972).

In this presentation we purposely restrict to the testing of a possible granulocyte chalone action on the different compartments of myelopoiesis. However, the granulocyte chalone may be only one of many messengers exerting regulatory influences. One should, therefore, always bear in mind the many different factors which may be of importance for granulopoietic proliferation, such as colony stimulating factor (CSF; see Robinson and Mangalik, 1975), which may be a larger protein as well as a smaller peptide (Price et al., 1973; Ito and Moore, 1969), diffusible granulocytopoietic stimulator (Rothstein et al., 1973), renal granulopoietic factor (GPF; Delmonte, 1974), vitamin B_{12}-binding protein (BBP; Gibson et al., 1974), and more generally stimulating or inhibitory factors, such as cyclic AMP (Byron, 1972), the different somatomedins (Van Wyk et al., 1973; Fryklund et al., 1974) as well as serum factors (Frank et al., 1972; Houck and Cheng, 1973; Temin et al., 1974). It should also be remembered that serum contains inhibitors of the CSF action, probably lipoproteins of high molecular weight (Metcalf, 1971; Granstrøm et al., 1972; Moore, 1975), of which the relation to granylocyte chalone is unknown.

Local factors in the bone marrow, such as the stroma as well as peripheral nerve endings may also be of importance for the regulation of myelopoiesis (Fliedner et al., 1970). Furthermore, there is evidence that proliferative regulation may occur by direct cell to cell interactions (Haskill et al., 1972). Thus, thymocytes may stimulate the proliferation of stem cells (Frindel and Croizat, 1973), as well as the later stages of myelopoiesis (Dexter et al., 1973). However, it can not be excluded that this interaction is mediated by local production of CSF in lymphocytes (Parker and Metcalf, 1974) as well as monocytes and other cells (Chervenick and LoBuglio, 1972).

The existence and possible interactions of all these factors may explain why there are so many difficulties in finding a reliable test system for the granulocyte chalone and especially the standardization of an assay.

14.2 Some theoretical considerations on the inhibition of cell proliferation by chalones

The essential feature of a chalone is its ability to inhibit cell proliferation. This phenomenon deserves a close inspection. What does that mean in kinetic terms? Two main characteristics of cell proliferation should be considered: the number of cells involved in proliferation and the rate at which the cells proceed through the cell cycle. Thus, a depression of proliferation may mean either that less cells per unit volume are dividing or that they do so at a slower rate, or a combination of both, i.e. less cells proliferate at reduced speed. It seems worthwhile to discuss several situations which may possibly exist from a theoretical point of view.

14.2.1 Synchronisation at constant growth fraction

If the inhibition does not affect the number of cycling cells (growth fraction being constant), but one particular phase of the cell cycle, a given cell population is synchronized. The cells accumulate in front of the block and when the block is released, they proceed at an increased number through the cycle. Example: cars stopped at a red traffic light and released at green. Result: a temporary block of proliferation is followed by an increase of proliferation ('rebound effect'). Ultimately, the result is a delay in obtaining the same cell number as that of the untreated cells.

14.2.2 Retardation of the cell cycle at constant growth fraction

If the inhibition does not affect the number of cycling cells (growth fraction being constant), but more than one or even all phases of the cell cycle, the overall cell proliferation is delayed. Example: cars retarded by speed limit. Result: cell proliferation is delayed.

14.2.3 Transfer of proliferative cells into the G_0 (Q) state: reduction of the growth fraction

If the inhibition affects the number of cells (without killing or rendering them 'sick'), but not the cell cycle phases, it follows that less cells are dividing and cell production is reduced. It is well known that most tissues contain a proliferative (P) and a non-proliferative (Q) pool of cells. Some of the apparently non-proliferating cells can be triggered back into the P-pool by regenerative or functional needs. The cells are able to re-enter the cell cycle and are therefore considered as reserve cells capable to restore the population subsequent to increased loss. On the other hand, there seems some agreement that cells may enter the Q pool immediately after mitosis from which they are released at random to reenter the P-compartment (see Rajewsky, 1974). Example: cars forced to enter the garage. Result: lower cell production per time unit.

*14.2.4 Prolongation of the cell cycle combined with reduction of the growth
      fraction*

If the inhibition affects both the number of cells and the rate at which the
cells proceed through the cycle, a very efficient retardation of proliferation
should result. Indeed evidence is accumulating that such a combination
exists and regulates proliferation in developing and aging tissues, be it
normal or neoplastic (Houck and Daugherty, 1974). Thus, even in growing
tumours two major factors are found to operate: although the tumour
mass increases, the growth rate decreases due to a prolongation of the
cell cycle and a concomitant reduction of the growth fraction (Bichel
and Dombernowsky, 1973). With decreasing growth rate an increasing
proportion of cells are transferred to the resting stage. Example: cars
retarded by speed limit and cars forced to enter garages. Result: an efficient
reduction of the overall cell proliferation yielding a lower number of cells
which are cycling at reduced rate.

14.3 Requirements of a granulocyte chalone test system

14.3.1 General characteristics

The following 4 principal characteristics have been attributed to chalones:
(1) A chalone inhibits cell proliferation, ultimately resulting in a lower
number of mitoses. (2) The inhibition of proliferation is not cytotoxic, but
reversible. (3) A chalone is cell- or tissue-specific, but not species-specific.

Therefore, a test system for the granulocyte chalone must meet the following requirements: (1) it must measure, qualitatively and quantitatively, the
inhibition of myelopoietic proliferation by a suspected chalone fraction,
(2) it must prove that a suspected chalone fraction is not toxic and does
not impair the functional state of the cells; (3) it must demonstrate the
reversibility of the proliferation inhibition by the suspected chalone fraction;
(4) it must show that a suspected chalone fraction is granulocyte-specific,
but not species-specific.

Moreover, since evidence is increasing that a physiological inhibition of
proliferation takes place in the G_1 and/or G_2 phases of the cell cycle (Elgjo
et al., 1971, 1972) a test should demonstrate the phase specificity of a suspected
chalone fraction.

For assaying a granulocyte chalone activity, the target cells should not
be in a state of proliferative inhibition on beforehand, i.e. they should be
capable to respond to it at full power. That a cell should react to an offered
chalone at full strength, is not self-evident: some tumor cells, while still

producing chalone molecules, appear to lack the capacity to retain the chalone molecules and, equally important, appear to respond less efficiently to the inhibitor (Rytömaa and Kiviniemi, 1968c).

14.3.2 Reversibility of granulocyte chalone action

What is a reversible inhibition of cell proliferation? Reversibility is certainly attributed to a chalone effect. In fact, the reversibility of proliferation inhibition is generally considered to exclude the possibility that the chalone effect is simply cytotoxic. However, one should not forget that in terms of cell proliferation in multicompartment systems, the word is ambiguous. Firstly, when the inhibitory effect of granulocytic chalone is released, cells can again progress into the cell cycle at normal or perhaps even an accelerated rate. Secondly, cells might also become forced into G_0, which is a physiological state for many tissue and blood cells. There they could stay infinitely unless they are specifically triggered into the P compartment by some stimulating factor (e.g. CSF). Still the chalone effect must be called reversible, or at least potentially reversible.

At the other end of granulopoiesis, the chalone may inhibit the proliferation of late differentiating cells. At the stage of metamyelocyte the cells automatically lose their ability to proliferate ('end cells'). If the effect at any time is potentially reversible, but the cells are thereby withheld from proliferation so long, that they become metamyelocytes, then finally non-proliferative cells should come out. Therefore, the word 'reversible' should in this connection always be related to the physiological state of the target cells.

For a complex system as granulopoiesis, where cell proliferation has to undergo tremendously strong variations to meet the functional demands of the body, a proliferative inhibition which only lasts for a short period and thereafter automatically returns to the same rate as previously, is almost non-efficient. It follows from these considerations that a granulocyte chalone regulatory system must also lead to more or less irreversible, secondary changes of the cells.

14.3.3 Cytotoxicity of granulocyte extracts in the test systems

The problem of discriminating between a true chalone and a cytotoxic effect is particularly difficult to solve for in vitro test systems, since in vitro systems are usually much less capable than in vivo systems to neutralize and eliminate toxic factors by means of dilution through the body fluids and by metabolism. It follows that a chalone effect demonstrated in vivo may be accepted with greater confidence than an in vitro effect. (For a detailed discussion and methods for demonstration of cytotoxicity see Houck and Daugherty, 1974).

14.4 Artifacts resulting from the use of [³H]thymidine in chalone test systems

The incorporation of [³H]thymidine ([³H]TdR) into DNA is widely used as a measure of DNA synthesis. The availability of [³H]TdR of high specific activity, the exclusive presence of this nucleotide in DNA and the perfection of methods for radioactivity assay have favoured the wide spread application of the DNA precursor in proliferation studies. Although some pitfalls involved in the use of [³H]TdR are known for quite a while, numerous investigators have, rather uncritically, based their conclusions on methods measuring the uptake and incorporation of [³H]TdR in the cells by autoradiography and liquid scintillation spectrometry. It seems, therefore, worthwhile to recall some of the artifacts, resulting from the careless application of the nucleotide, which may render conclusions at least questionable.

14.4.1 Enzymes of [³H]TdR metabolism

[³H]TdR added to intact animal cells is only minimally incorporated into DNA. Several enzymes of TdR metabolism may be involved. The uptake and incorporation of TdR into DNA requires phosphorylation by TdR synthetase and TdR kinase which may be constantly inactivated by the usual absence of TdR (Kit et al., 1965). TdR phosphorylase is known to degrade [³H]TdR to [³H]T, thus greatly depressing [³H]TdR utilization for DNA-labelling of normal bone marrow (Rubini, 1966) and leukemic blood cells (Marsh and Perry, 1964). Moreover, alkaline phosphatase, found in mature granulocytes in considerable quantity, can dephosphorylate [³H]TdR-P, thus reducing [³H]DNA synthesis from [³H]TdR. Other degrading enzymes can attack [³H]T to give [³H]dihydrothymine (DHT) and [³H]ureidoisobutyric acid as shown with dog bone marrow cells incubated in the presence of [³H]TdR (Rubini, 1966).

14.4.2 Enzymes of DNA replication

Mammalial tissues, particularly of lymphatic origin, contain a terminal deoxynucleotidyltransferase which catalyzes the terminal incorporation of single nucleotides into existing DNA. Thus, the calf thymus enzyme manages a chain elongation of primer DNA or small oligonucleotides by 50 to 600 nucleotides using the free terminal 3'hydroxyl group to start with (Bollum, 1963). It follows that the incorporation of labelled precursors into DNA must not necessarily mean a true DNA de novo synthesis.

14.4.3 Metabolism of ³H-label

In most cases [³H]CH$_3$-5-TdR is used. In the course of degradation the labelled methyl group may be transferred to activated methionine which via specific and unspecific methyl transferases may label proteins and other substrates. This metabolism should be kept in mind, particularly when applying continuous [³H]TdR labelling for hours and days.

14.4.4 Unspecific [³H]TdR binding to proteins

Houck and Daugherty (1974) have pointed out that various tissue proteins may unspecifically bind TdR thus spuriously indicating TdR incorporation into DNA. The adsorption of [³H]TdR onto tissue proteins leads not only to a TCA precipitable complex but also reduces the quantity of unbound [³H]TdR available for DNA incorporation.

14.4.5 Pool size dilution by unlabelled TdR

Autoradiographic studies have shown that the apparent pool size of TdR of in vitro bone marrow systems is quite small and readily perturbed by small amounts of added nucleosides (Rubini, 1966). Unlabelled TdR contained in the chalone extract to be tested or in the test cell suspension can severely depress the number of [³H]TdR molecules that can be incorporated into DNA.

Changes in the intracellular TdR pool were attributed to the apparent lack of correlation between [³H]TdR labelling index and rate of [³H]TdR incorporation into DNA of newborn rat lung explants (Simnett and Fisher, 1973), whereas mature rat lung explants take up [³H]TdR corresponding with the rate of cell proliferation. Simnett and Fisher (1973) stress that measurements of [³H]TdR incorporation by liquid scintillation counting must not necessarily correlate with the rate of cell proliferation.

14.4.6 [³H]TdR transport through the cell membrane

Alkylating agents like triethyleneiminobenzoquinone (Treminon) in concentrations that cause a drastic and instant reduction of the uptake of [^{3}H]TdR into DNA of Ehrlich- and Yoshida ascites tumor cells, do not inhibit DNA synthesis. Instead Grunicke et al. (1975) have convincingly shown that the reduced [^{3}H]TdR uptake into DNA is due to a decreased transport of the nucleoside into the cell and that the alkylating agent does neither inhibit transition of cells from G_1 to S nor progression through S, but arrests the cells at the G_2 stage. Similarly, the inhibition of [^{3}H]TdR incorporation by several compounds including p-chloromercuribenzoate, persantin and cytochalasin B has been shown to be due to an interference with TdR transport rather than DNA synthesis; this may also be true for chlorambucil which inhibits TdR uptake into DNA, but not DNA synthesis. It should be mentioned that the conclusions with Treminon are based on rather low doses of the alkylating agent that are just sufficient to completely inhibit cell division due to a block at the G_2 stage (Grunicke et al., 1975). However, among the many processes involved in DNA synthesis, the TdR transport most probably at the membranes, seem to be most susceptible to the attack by agents that are able to alkylate sulfhydryl groups involved in the transport reactions.

14.4.7 Kinetics of [^{3}H]TdR incorporation into DNA

A compound may reduce the incorporation of [^{3}H]TdR into DNA because less cells enter DNA synthesis or cells already in S proceed at a reduced rate. Simple liquid scintillation spectrometry to measure [^{3}H]TdR uptake cannot distinguish between these possibilities. Instead, kinetic studies including determination of cell cycle parameters are needed to answer the question.

14.4.8 Periodic DNA amplification and [^{3}H]TdR reutilization

In mammalian cells the rate of DNA synthesis is not constant and the DNA content does not increase as a simple linear or exponential function of time (Klevecz et al., 1974). Differential replication (amplification) of part of the genetic material, e.g. ribosomal DNA, has been observed in several cell types. Early replicating DNA, measured by [^{3}H]TdR incorporation, may subsequently be catabolized and the nucleotides reutilized. Interference with added compounds (including chalone extracts) must be taken into account. Reutilization of [^{3}H]TdR via the salvage pathway following catabolism of the DNA of dead cells is a significant process in bone marrow cells (Heiniger et al., 1971).

14.4.9 [³H]TdR incorporation into mycoplasma

A number of mycoplasma strains that are able to infect mammalian cell cultures possess pyrimidine nucleoside phosphorylase leading to utilization and cleavage ('scavenger effect') of TdR and uridine (Ur) to thymine and uracil, respectively, and thereby preventing the uptake of [³H]TdR and [³H]Ur into the nucleic acids of mycoplasma-infected cells. Such cells incorporate up to 4 times less [³H]TdR into their nuclear DNA than non-infected cells (Grüneisen et al., 1975). More important, hydroxyurea, a potent inhibitor of DNA synthesis, in concentrations of $\leqslant 10^{-2}$ M fails to reduce the overall rate of [³H]TdR incorporation into the acid-insoluble material of infected cells in spite of an effective block of cellular DNA replication. Consequently, [³H]TdR and probably other DNA precursors, will fail to reveal reduced incorporation into cellular DNA when inhibitory compounds (including chalone extracts) are added to mycoplasma infected test cells.

14.4.10 DNA repair processes using [³H]TdR

Mammalian cells are capable to repair damaged DNA pieces using the known nucleotides including [³H]TdR. Repair processes occur in non-proliferating cells. Hence uptake of [³H]TdR into the DNA of such cells must not necessarily be correlated with cell division.

14.4.11 Cell density

Addition of phytohemagglutinin (PHA) to cultured lymphocytes elicits a number of transport and synthetic processes associated with the transition of the cells from their resting G_0 state through the cell cycle. The uptake of [³H]TdR into the DNA of PHA stimulated lymphocytes was therefore considered to be a valuable in vitro test of the capacity of a chalone extract to reduce or inhibit lymphocyte proliferation. However doubts were raised as to the significance of blast transformation, DNA synthesis and extent of cell division following PHA stimulation, since neither the number of cells (Polgar and Kibrick, 1970; Rogers et al., 1972) nor the amount of DNA were increased at the end of PHA cultures (Schellekens and Eysvoogel, 1968). Moreover, [³H]TdR incorporation was depressed up to 50% in PHA-stimulated lymphocytes and yet the [³H]TdR labelling index in autoradiograms of the same cells was unchanged (Soren, 1973) which could result from a prolongation of the S phase or from non-premitotic DNA synthesis. Recently, Bernheim and Mendelsohn (1975) presented conclusive evidence that it is the concentration of lymphocytes in the cultures that determines whether the blast transformation is followed by cell proliferation or not. Lymphocytes at a cell density of 2×10^6/ml culture show blast transformation and [^{3}H]TdR incorporation, but no increase of cell number and DNA content and reveal in addition, considerable cell death. In contrast, when the lymphocytes are cultured at $1–5 \times 10^5$/ml, they readily divide and show low cell death.

14.4.12 Repetituous DNA, redundant for cell division

A chalone extract may inhibit [^{3}H]TdR incorporation into the DNA of cells other than those from which the extract was obtained. Thus, one essential characteristic of a chalone, its tissue-specificity may not be verified. Garcia-Giralt and Macieira-Coelho (1974) found that lymphocyte extracts not only depress [^{3}H]TdR uptake by lymphocytes but also by established fibroblast cells (BHK). However, mitosis was only reduced in normal lymphocytes. Even in human and mouse cells of lymphoblastic leukemia a decreased [^{3}H]TdR incorporation is not necessarily followed by inhibition of cell replication of corresponding degree. These findings could be explained by the inhibition of the synthesis of repetitious DNA, redundant for cell division. In any case, it is stressed that the 'measurement of DNA synthesis alone by [^{3}H]TdR is not a valid criterion to detect a chalone effect; cell division must also be measured'.

14.5 Survey on the presently used granulocyte chalone systems

Any chalone assay must measure cell proliferation. It seems worthwhile to summarize briefly the methods that are used and available for this purpose.

14.5.1 Methods for assaying the proliferation of granulocytic cells

14.5.1.1 Cell count
Following incubation of the test cells for the period of at least one cell cycle (t_c) a cell count should indicate the degree of cell proliferation. Cell counting can be combined with a cell viability test (dye exclusion test).

14.5.1.2 Mitotic activity
The relative number of mitoses per hour (mitotic rate) is generally used as a

measure of cell proliferation. Mitotic counts may be combined with the autoradiographic [³H]thymidine labelling technique (see below) for kinetic measurements (labelled mitoses). It should be noted that the mitotic rate is the result of all processes preceding mitoses: i.e. an inhibition in G_2 phase is also detected.

14.5.1.3 *[³H]thymidine uptake*
The degree of uptake and incorporation of [³H]thymidine into the acid-insoluble material of test cells is generally considered to be a measure of cell proliferation. However a number of artifacts may invalidate the experimental conclusions raised by means of this technique and should therefore be taken into account (see sect. 14.4).

14.5.1.4 *Micro-flow-fluorometry*
This method measures the relative amount of the DNA of single cells in suspension, thereby indicating the cell cycle distribution at a particular stage. The method does not determine the actual flow of the cells through each cell cycle phase, but indicates percentage of cells of a given population at the chosen time ('snap shot') that are in the G_1, S, G_2 and M phase of the cell cycle (see Laerum and Maurer, 1973).

14.5.1.5 *Fluorescence polarization*
This method measures changes of the structuredness of the cytoplasmic matrix (SCM) which has been related to the proliferative status of the cells (Cercek et al., 1973a, b, c). Changes of SCM seem to be related to early events of entry into the cell cycle and correlated with changes of intracellular cAMP level (Cercek et al., 1973). However, whether a particular structuredness of the cytoplasmic matrix is always characteristic for proliferation remains to be shown.

14.5.2 *Granulocytic test cells*

Obviously an ideal chalone test system for myelopoiesis should consist of a cell population that is (1) actively proliferating i.e. going through the whole cell cycle, (2) homogeneous as to the granulocyte species and stage of differentiation and (3) virtually free of contamination from other blood or bone marrow cells. Unfortunately such a system is not available and each of the following approaches suffers from the lack of one or more of these properties. It seems, therefore, worthwhile to evaluate the features of each system and to indicate where it needs improvement and refinement. Principally one can distinguish the following cell systems:

1) Myelopoietic cells in free suspension culture for short (a few h) or long term (several days) incubation.

2) Bone marrow stem cells committed for granulopoiesis grown during 3–10 days in agar colonies, dependent on colony stimulating factor (CSF).

3) Myelopoietic cells grown from bone marrow cells (during 5 days) in microdiffusion chambers that are implanted into the peritoneal cavity of rodents.

14.5.3 Short term in vitro cultures of rat bone marrow cells

Rytömaa and Kiviniemi (1967) were the first to introduce a short term in vitro culture of rat bone marrow cells as a granulocyte chalone test. In essence, the cells are suspended in Hank's balanced salt solution (with 20% serum), allowed to settle from the suspension and become attached to the upper surface of a coverslip hanging from the top of a test tube. Following incubation with [³H]thymidine for 2–10 h, the cells on the coverslips are fixed in situ and their radioactivity determined by liquid scintillation spectrometry, followed by autoradiography to determine the [³H]TdR labelling index. Cell count, mitotic index and cell morphology are assayed in a few cases.

Rytömaa and Kiviniemi have looked into the kinetics of their test: continuous (cumulative) labelling with [³H]TdR and [¹⁴C]formate up to 50 h using liquid scintillation counting and autoradiography revealed a rapid increase of labelling, leveling around 12 h and decreasing after 25 h. Although the total cellularity was found decreased in time with a curvilinear slope, the authors claimed that 'new cells do in fact continue to enter DNA synthesis for a long time after the start of the culture (up to 20 h)'. However, no data were given to prove this statement (Rytömaa and Kiviniemi, 1967).

In a subsequent paper Rytömaa and Kiviniemi (1968a) attempted to rule out any non-specific, toxic inhibition by measuring the cellularity following granulocyte chalone administration. The cellularity remained unchanged, although the labelling index was reduced by 60% following granulocyte chalone administration. Unfortunately no data were given as to the incubation time. The experiment could not exclude any toxic effects which would not immediately effect the cell number but rather render the cells into an impaired functional state. Subsequently, Rytömaa and Kiviniemi (1968b) found a rapid decrease of the absolute in vitro proliferation of normal bone marrow cells using pulse labelling with [³H]TdR. Unfortunately, the implications of this finding on the validity of the in vitro test of a granulocyte chalone were not fully recognized and not discussed.

A similar short term in vitro culture was introduced by Paukovits (1971) for screening the presumed biological activity of chromatographic fractions. In contrast to the above method by Rytömaa, where only the glass-attached cells are measured, this technique determines the uptake of $[^3H]TdR$ into total rat bone marrow cells suspended in a tube (for 5 h). As for Rytömaa's test, the inhibition of $[^3H]TdR$ uptake is taken to be a measure of the capacity of a fraction to inhibit the proliferation of granulocyte precursor cells. Later Paukovits and Paukovits (1975) refined the test by using RPMI-1640 medium at pH 6.7 and a preincubation period of 90 min with the chalone extract, followed by 30 min of incubation with $[^3H]TdR$.

Similar in vitro suspension cultures of bone marrow cells using $[^3H]TdR$ were adopted by Laerum and Maurer (1973), Maurer et al. (1975), MacVittie and McCarthy (1974) and Bannerjee et al. (1974) mainly for the purpose of granulocyte chalone screening.

However, doubts were raised as to the validity and specificity of such tests (Lajtha, 1973): depression in total $[^3H]TdR$ uptake exceeding about 20% must mean that besides G_1-myelocytes also S-myelocytes and other cycling bone marrow cells (e.g. erythroblasts) are inhibited. Thus, the specificity for both the cell cycle phase and the cell types may not be proven by such tests. Moreover, Maurer and Laerum (1973) expressed warnings as to the viability of the in vitro incubated bone marrow cells and presented evidence to indicate that, under these particular conditions the cells do no more proliferate since (1) no new cells enter the S phase in vitro ($[^3H]TdR$ continuous and pulse labelling experiments). (2) cells die (cell viability tests) and (3) practically no cells proceed through G_2 and mitosis (Colcemide experiments using microflow fluorometry). It was concluded that this test is likely to screen for an unspecific S-phase inhibitor and must be supplemented by another test to prove the chalone nature of an extract or fraction. Similar findings were made by several authors using such bone marrow cell cultures (De Munk et al., 1971; Morgan et al., 1974) which are dying cell systems unless they are stimulated by a source of CSF.

There are still other problems that may complicate the in vitro tests: (1) Pseudosynchronization. As mentioned by Rytömaa and Kiviniemi (1967) the time between killing of the rat and the start of the bone marrow cultures may pile up the cells in the S-phase, thereby disturbing the normal DNA-synthesis. (2) Artifacts resulting from the use of $[^3H]TdR$ (see 14.4). (3) Cytotoxicity. The in vitro short term test cannot exclude cytotoxicity and in the present literature this problem is not satisfactorily solved. In conclusion, the in vitro short term cultures of bone marrow cells fail to meet most of the requirements for valid granulocyte chalone tests and need considerable refinement.

14.5.4 Long term in vitro cultures of bone marrow cells

14.5.4.1 Liquid suspension cultures

Since short-term in vitro bone marrow cultures are characterized by a cell population which is more or less dying, it would be a great advantage to prolong the culture period until they could be replaced by new, truly proliferating and differentiating cells originating from stem cells in the explanted suspension. In fact, several such systems have been described during the last years (Sumner et al., 1972; Golde and Cline, 1973; Dexter et al., 1973, 1974). Most of these methods are dependent on special stimulating procedures, such as co-culture with thymus cells (Dexter et al., 1973, 1974), the addition of a CSF extract (Sumner et al., 1972) or conditioned medium (Morgan et al., 1974).

To our knowledge, the only case where such a long-term culture has been used for assaying granulocyte chalone activity was that by Lord et al. (1974a) who presented evidence for a cell specific effect on the structured cytoplasmatic matrix (SCM). In a later study on short-term incubations of bone marrow cell suspensions, Lord et al. (1974b) showed that the effects on the SCM induced by granulocyte extracts appeared within half an hour. After washing the cells and another hour of incubation the effects were reversed, but could be induced again on the same cells by new addition of the extracts. However, it remained to be shown that the changes of SCM only occurred in the true proliferating cells, and that there really was a proliferative inhibition as measured by a lower cell production in the system.

Generally, the different long-term suspension culture procedures need a more thorough investigation from a cell kinetic point of view before they can be used for granulocyte chalone testing. Otherwise a truly proliferating in vitro system of normal myelopoietic cells might be of great importance for the progress of granulocyte chalone research.

14.5.4.2 Myeloid leukemia cells in liquid suspension cultures

There exist only very few myeloid leukemia cell lines that grow in liquid suspension cultures under defined conditions and show signs of myeloid differentiation in vitro.

Ichikawa (1969) has established such a cell line in vitro from a spontaneous myeloid leukemia of SL strain mice. He found that this cell line, named M1, could differentiate to yield either macrophages or neutrophil granulocytes when exposed to conditioned medium from embryo cell cultures. Preliminary experiments by Laerum and Maurer have suggested that these cells still respond to granulocyte extracts with cell cycle specific inhibition of proliferation.

The recent report by Yunis et al. (1975) suggests permanent rat chloroma cell lines as possible test systems. Their suitability, however, remains to be shown.

14.5.4.3 Cultures in semisolid agar medium

This in vitro method was originally described by Bradley and Metcalf (1966) and Pluznik and Sachs (1966) and consists of Petri dishes with semisolid agar medium. By the addition of a so-called 'colony stimulating factor' (CSF), committed stem cells in a bone marrow cell suspension plated into agar will develop into granulocyte and macrophage colonies under in vitro conditions. CSF is a protein which can be extracted from endotoxin stimulated mouse serum, human urine or serum, embryonal fibroblasts, human monocytes and other sources (for literature, see Metcalf, 1971, 1973). Human bone marrow cells can also be cultured in agar, using a modified procedure (Pike and Robinson, 1970), and the technique has proven to be a valuable diagnostic tool in hematologic diseases (Metcalf, 1973; Moore, 1975; Muller-Bérat, personal communication, 1975; see also Laerum and Rajewsky, 1975). Agar culture gives information on the relative number of stem cells committed for granulo- and macrophagopoiesis in a given bone marrow cell suspension, as measured by the number of colonies. Further, it gives information on the proliferative capacity of the progeny of these cells (see Testa and Lord, 1973), and also the ability for differentiation into normal granulocytes and macrophages.

In a series of experiments, we were able to show that partially purified extracts of rat granulocytes in the low molecular range ('granulocyte chalone') inhibited the formation of granulopoietic colonies in agar (Muller-Bérat et al., 1973, 1975). The inhibitory effect was dose-dependent down to a colony number of 30% of the controls (see table 14.1), and this could not be explained by cytotoxicity as tested by the trypan blue exclusion test in the presence of complement. There was a direct antagonism between the chalone extract and CSF.

A short exposure of the cells to the chalone extract (1 h at 37 °C) prior to plating was sufficient to inhibit the subsequent colony formation in agar, and the inhibitory effect was easily reversed by simply washing the target cells with excess of medium before plating. When the cells were exposed to CSF (endotoxin-stimulated serum) before the contact with the chalone

Table 14.1

Effects of granulocyte (chalone) extract (ultrafiltrate from rat ascitic fluid) on the number of myelopoietic colonies in soft agar culture (murine bone marrow cells, $5 \cdot 10^4$ per dish; 0.3 % agar in McCoy's medium; ten days of culture). Each number represents the mean of three replicate dishes expressed as % deviation from untreated controls. The bone marrow cells were incubated for 1 h at $37 \,^\circ$C with different concentrations of the extract (10–60 %) prior to plating in agar.

A pronounced depression of the colony formation is seen at 10–20 % concentration of the extract which is reversed at higher concentrations, probably because of the presence of stimulating factors in the same molecular range. Epidermal extract (chalone) in corresponding doses had no inhibitory effect (above: right columns). The inhibitory effect could be reversed if the bone marrow cells were washed with excess of medium after the preincubation and before plating (below). From Muller-Bérat et al., 1975.

Expt.	Granulocyte extract (batch A)				Epidermis extract		
No.	10%	20%	50%	60%	10%	20%	50%
1	− 58	− 78	− 70	+ 3	− 6	− 8	− 11
2	− 36	− 43	− 14	+ 4	− 7	− 2	− 11
3	− 45	− 41	− 20	+ 4			

Expt.	GE	Preincubated cells *not washed*			Preinc. cells *washed*	
no.	batch	10% GE	20% GE	50% GE	10% GE	20% GE
4	B	− 40	− 47	+ 12	+ 1	+ 4
5	C	− 47	− 55	+ 11	− 4	− 1
6	D	− 17	− 46	+ 8	− 3	− 20

extract, no inhibitory effect was found, suggesting competition for a common membrane receptor (table 14.1).

However, in these experiments only an effect on the colony number and not on their size was found. Therefore, the agar method as standard technique only showed an effect at the committed stem cell level, although the same extracts also inhibited the later stages of differentiation i.e. myelopoietic cells in diffusion chambers (Laerum and Maurer, 1973).

Other workers have shown that mature phagocytes in high numbers depress the colony formation in agar (Ichikawa et al., 1967; Paran et al., 1969; Haskill et al., 1972). MacVittie and McCarthy (1974) obtained similar results using crude extracts of granulocytes.

The great advantage with the agar technique is a simple test system in vitro with rapidly proliferating myelopoietic cells resulting in mature granulocytes and macrophages. The method is not dependent on indirect measurements of proliferation, such as thymidine incorporation. Comparative investigations of cell line specificity under similar culture conditions can be done, since PHA-stimulated human lymphocytes can be grown in agar (unpublished observations) and erythropoietic cells in methylcellulose in the presence of erythropoietin (Iscove et al., 1975; Cooper et al., 1974) as well as megakaryocytes in a modified agar medium (Metcalf et al., 1975).

As a recent improvement (Maurer and Henry, 1975), we have been able to use agar colony formation in capillary tubes as a rapid screening for granulocyte chalone activity on large scale with automatic reading of the colony numbers, using a modified method originally described by Bowman et al., 1967 and applied to myelopoiesis by Abrams et al., 1973.

However, it is important to note that the agar technique in the present version is a test for the committed stem cell activity more than for the differentiating cells. Unless the washing procedure is done prior to plating as described above, reversibility of the effect is not proven and a toxic effect can not be excluded. Another disadvantage is that the method is solely dependent on the source of CSF, and the biological activity of this can vary greatly from preparation to preparation.

It should also be borne in mind that the agar technique is a biochemically very impure system. It requires the presence of crude serum (serum factors needed for cell proliferation, Frank et al., 1972; Holley, 1974; Temin et al., 1974) as well as CSF, which usually is another source of crude serum. The employment of sophisticated methods for biochemical purification of granulocyte chalone may then be abolished by adding the purified fractions to a system containing all the possibly interacting substances in serum. Therefore, the ideal test would be to add purified granulocyte chalone to agar culture containing purified CSF as well as purified serum factors.

14.5.5 In vivo cultures of myelopoietic cells in diffusion chambers

This in vivo culture system consists of a plastic ring with a cellulose acetate membrane on each side, making a cell impermeable chamber which can be implanted into the peritoneal cavity of different host animals (rats, mice). A great variety of different cell types have been successfully cultured in these chambers during the twenty years this method has been in current use (see Benestad and Breivik, 1972; and Laerum et al., 1973). It was discovered that myelopoietic cells proliferated exponentially in these chambers (Benestad, 1970) and it was also shown that the technique could be used to measure the number of stem cells implanted into the chamber from a given bone marrow cell suspension (Bøyum and Borgstrøm, 1970).

Benestad et al. (1973) found that granulocyte extracts reduced the uptake of [³H]thymidine into myelopoietic cells in diffusion chambers. However, other proliferative parameters were not studied and the subsequent cell yield was not significantly reduced, so that thymidine artifacts could not be excluded (see sect. 14.4).

By combining autoradiography ([³H]thymidine) and micro-flow fluoro-metry, we were able to show that granulocyte extracts inhibited the cell proliferation in diffusion chambers. The inhibitory effect was not due to cell death and was reversed after 8 h. Corresponding to this, a significantly reduced cell yield was found after a time period of at least one cell cycle, i.e. when the proliferative inhibition resulted in a lower number of cells leaving mitosis. The inhibition seemed to occur in G_1, but a prolongation of the subsequent S-phase was also indicated (Laerum and Maurer, 1973).

Reduced cell yield with leukemic cells in diffusion chambers, as reported by Vilpo (1973), will be described otherwhere in this book.

When chalone extracts are administered to chamber-bearing mice at 3–5 days after bone marrow cell implantation, the effect is on differentiating myelopoietic cells (Laerum and Maurer, 1973).

MacVittie and McCarthy injected crude granulocyte extracts during the first day after implantation and obtained a lower cell yield as measured on day 7 of culture. This indicated an effect also on the committed stem cells (diffusion chamber progenitor cells, DCPC), which proliferate very rapidly during the first day of culture. The finding was further confirmed by a reduced number of stem cells in the chambers, as estimated by colony formation upon subculture in agar (MacVittie and McCarthy, 1974).

The diffusion chamber method offers an exponentially proliferating culture system for myelopoietic cells in vivo and should thus be an ideal method for chalone testing. Effects on the committed stem cell level can also be observed by injection of extracts during the early phase of the culture.

However, the method is very laborious; the cells cannot be directly observed as can cells in vitro. For mass screening during a fractionation procedure of granulocyte chalone the method requires very large amounts of extracts, as the doses should be given per g body weight of the host animals. Different interactions from the host animal cannot be excluded, and this is certainly known to occur when its own bone marrow has been destroyed by X-rays (Bøyum et al., 1972). Otherwise, for the time being we consider the diffusion chamber technique to be the best available method for in vivo testing of granulocyte chalone.

14.6 Final assessment

When a crude biological fluid, such as blood, serum or ascites, is used as a source of granulocytic chalone, this is isotonic and isoosmolar. All kinds of substances, including the chalone are present in physiological concentrations. A toxic effect of such a fluid in the assay system is not to be expected. However, during the different concentration and purification steps, a certain range of molecular size is selected. For the granulocyte chalone this will be below 3000 daltons. At the same time the relative concentration of unwanted substances, i.e. peptides of similar molecular weight is correspondingly increased. Substances which otherwise are harmless in low concentrations may perhaps give toxic side effects in extremely high concentrations. At all steps of purification toxicity must, therefore, be avoided, and it follows from this that increased purity of the chalone may even increase the risk of unwanted side effects. Finally, one hopes to end up with the chemically pure chalone which should exert a physiological effect on the target cells. The testing of this, however, requires that it is added in physiological concentrations, since several physiological substances in the organism are either toxic or have other effects in high concentrations (cyclic AMP, adrenalin, cortisone, etc.).

Testing of a granulocytic chalone should only be carried out on a true proliferating system. Several proliferative parameters and different assay systems should be used in combination. Because of the complexity of granulopoiesis not only one, but all cellular compartments should be tested.

The demonstration of a cell cycle specific effect of an extract may give the possibility to distinguish between this and a moderate, reversible toxic effect on the cells.

Reduction of $[^3H]$thymidine incorporation into DNA alone following addition of a tissue extract as measure for proliferative ('chalone'!) inhibition should be avoided. If a 'chalone' extract is not able to reduce the net cell production in the system as observed at least one cell cycle period (t_c) after exposure, the relevance of the extract as a proliferative inhibitor in vivo should be considered as unproven.

At the present moment the progress of granulocyte chalone research is more dependent on reliable and rapid assay systems than on biochemical purification procedures.

References

Abrams, L., Carmeci, P., Bull, J. M. and Carbone, P. P. (1973) Capillary tube scanning applied to in vitro mouse marrow granulocyte growth. J. Nat. Cancer Inst. 50, 267–270.

Bannerjee, R., Lajtha, L. G. and Pillinger, D. J. (1973) Further studies on the inhibitory effect of granulocyte extracts on granulocytopoiesis. Paterson Lab. Annual Report (Manchester) p. 117–119.

Benestad, H. B. (1970) Formation of granulocytes and macrophages in diffusion chamber cultures of mouse blood leucocytes. Scand. J. Haematol. 7, 279–288.

Benestad, H. B. and Brevik, H. (1972) Murine haematopoiesis studied with the diffusion chamber technique. Norwegian Def. Res. Estab. Rep. No. 61.

Benestad, H. B., Rytömaa, T. and Kiviniemi, K. (1973) The cell specific effect of the granulocyte chalone demonstrated with the diffusion chamber technique. Cell Tiss. Kinet. 6, 147–154.

Bernheim, J. and Mendelsohn, J. (1975) Kinetics of DNA synthesis and cell proliferation of in vitro stimulated human leucocytes. 7th Meeting Europ. Study Group for Cell Prolif. Amsterdam, Abstracts p. 15–16.

Bichel, P. and Dombernowsky, P. (1973) On the resting stages of the IB-1 ascites tumor. Cell Tissue Kinet. 6, 359–367.

Bollum, F. J. (1963) 'Primer' in DNA polymerase reactions. Progr. Nucleic Acid Res. 1, 1–26.

Bowman, R. L., Blume, P. and Vurek, G. G. (1967) Capillary tube scanner for mechanized microbiology. Science 158, 78–83.

Bøyum, A. and Borgstrøm R. (1970) The concentration of granulocytic stem cells in mouse bone marrow, determined with diffusion chamber technique. Scand. J. Haemat. 7, 294–303.

Bøyum, A., Carsten, A. L., Laerum, O. D. and Cronkite, E. P. (1972) Kinetics of cell proliferation of murine bone marrow cells cultured in diffusion chambers: Effect of hypoxia, bleeding, erythropoietin injections, polycythemia, and irradiation of the host. Blood 40, 174–188.

Bradley, T. R. and Metcalf, D. (1966) The growth of mouse bone marrow cells in vitro. Aust. J. Exp. Biol. Med. Sci. 44, 287–299.

Byron, J. W. (1972) Evidence for a β-adrenergic receptor initiating DNA synthesis in haemopoietic stem cells. Exp. Cell Res. 71, 228–232.

Cercek, L. and Cercek, B. (1973a) Effect of centrifugal forces on the structuredness of cytoplasm in growing yeast cells. Biophysik 9, 105–108.

Cercek, L. and Cercek, B. (1973b) Relationship between changes in the structuredness of cytoplasm and rate constants for the hydrolysis of FDA in Saccharomyces cerevisiae. Biophysik 9, 109–112.

Cercek, L., Cercek, B. and Garrett, J. V. (1973c) Biophysical differentiation between normal human and chronic lymphocytic leukemia lymphocytes. 8th Leucocyte Culture Conf. Uppsala, Academic Press.

Chervenick, P. A. and LoBuglio, A. F. (1972) Human blood monocytes: Stimulators of granulocyte and mononuclear colony formation in vitro. Science 178, 164–166.

Cooper, M. C., Levy, J., Cantor, L. N., Marks, P. A. and Rifkind, R. A. (1974) The effect of erythropoietin on colony growth of erythroid precursor cells in vitro. Proc. Nat. Acad. Sci. U.S. 71, 1677–1680.

Delmonte, L. (1974) Hemopoietic cell line-specific effects of renal granulopoietic factor (GPF) on transplantable mouse marrow stem cells: Comparison with erythrocyte stimulating factor (ESF) and endotoxin. Cell Tissue Kinet. 7, 3–18.

De Munk, F. G., Sumner, M. A. and Bradley, T. R. (1971) Tritiated thymidine uptake by mouse bone marrow cells in liquid culture. Exp. Cell Res. 69, 228–231.

Dexter, T. M., Allen, T. D., Lajtha, L. G., Schofield, R. and Lord, B. I. (1973) Stimulation of differentiation and proliferation of haemopoietic cells in vitro. J. Cell Physiol. 82, 461–474.

Dexter, T. M. and Lajtha, L. G. (1974) Proliferation of haemopoietic cells in vitro. Brit. J. Haemat. 28, 525–530.

Elgjo, K., Laerum, O. D. and Edgehill, W. (1971) Growth regulation in mouse epidermis I. G_2-inhibitor present in the basal cell layer. Virchows Arch. Abt. B 8, 277–283.

Elgjo, K., Laerum, O. D. and Edgehill, W. (1972) Growth regulation in the mouse epidermis. II. G_1-inhibitor present in the differentiating cell layer. Virchows Arch. Abt. B 10, 229–236.

Fliedner, T. M., Calvo, W., Haas, R., Forteza, J. and Bohne, F. (1970) Morphologic and cytokinetic aspects of bone marrow stroma. In: Hemopoietic cellular proliferation. Stohlman, F. (ed.) Grune and Stratton, New York–London, pp. 67–86.

Frank, W., Ristow, H. J. and Schwalb, S. (1972) Untersuchungen zur wachstumsstimulierenden Wirkung von Kälberserum auf Kulturen embryonaler Rattenzellen. Exp. Cell Res. 70, 390–396.

Frindel, E. and Croizat, H. (1973) The possible role of the thymus in CFU proliferation and differentiation. Biomedicine 19, 392–394.

Fryklund, L., Uthne, K. and Sievertsson, H. (1974) Isolation and characterization of polypeptides from human plasma enhancing the growth of human normal cells in culture. Biochem. Biophys. Res. Commun. 61, 950–956.

Garcia-Giralt, E. and Macieira-Coelho, A. (1974) Differential effect of a lymphoid chalone on the target and non-target cells in vitro. 8th leucocyte culture conference. Academic Press.

Gibson, E. L., Herbert, V. and Robinson, W. (1974) Granulocyte colony stimulating activity and vitamin B_{12} binding proteins in human urine. Brit. J. Haemat. 28, 191–197.

Golde, D. W. and Cline, M. J. (1973) Growth of human bone marrow in liquid culture. Blood 41, 45–57.

Granström, M., Wahren, B., Killander, D. and Foley, G. E. (1972) Inhibitors of the bone-marrow colony formation in sera of patients with leukemia. Int. J. Cancer 10, 482–488.

Grüneisen, A., Rajewsky, M. F., Remmer, I. and Uschkoreit, J. (1975) Inhibition of ^{3}H-thymidine incorporation by hydroxyurea: Atypical response of mycoplasma-infected cells in culture. Exp. Cell Res. 90, 365–373.

Grunicke, H., Hirsch, F., Wolf, H., Bauer, U. and Kiefer, G. (1975) Selective inhibition of thymidine transport at low doses of the alkylating agent triethyleneiminobenzoquinone (Trenimon) Exp. Cell Res. 90, 357–346.

Haskill, J. S., McKnight, R. D. and Galbraith, P. R. (1972) Cell-cell interaction in vitro: Studied by density separation of colony-forming, stimulating and inhibiting cells from human bone marrow. Blood 40, 394–399.

Heiniger, H. J., Feinendegen, L. E. and Bürk, K. (1971) Reutilization of thymidine in various groups of rat bone marrow cells. Blood 37, 340–348.

Holley, R. W. (1974) Serum factors and growth control. In: Control of Proliferation in Animal Cells (eds.: B. Clarkson and R. Baserga) Cold Spring Harbor Lab. pp. 13–18.

Houck, J. C. and Cheng, R. F. (1973) Isolation, purification and chemical characterization of the serum mitogen for diploid human fibroblasts. J. Cell Physiol. 81, 257–270.

Houck, J. C. and Daugherty, W. F. (1974) Chalones: A tissue-specific approach to mitotic control. Medcom Press, New York.

Ichikawa, Y. (1969) Differentiation of a cell line of myeloid leukemia. J. Cell Physiol. 74, 223–234.

Ito, T. and Moore, G. E. (1969) The growth-stimulating activity of peptides on human hematopoietic cell cultures. Exp. Cell Res. 56, 10–14.

Iscove, N. N. and Sieber, F. (1975) Erythroid progenitors in mouse bone marrow detected by macroscopic colony formation in culture. Exp. Hemat. 3, 32–43.

Kit, S., Dubbs, D. R. and Frearson, D. M. (1965) Decline of thymidine kinase activity in stationary phase mouse fibroblast cells. J. Biol. Chem. 240, 2565.

Klevecz, R. R., Kapp, L. N. and Remington, J. A. (1974) Intermittent amplification and catabolism of DNA and its correlation with gene expression. In: Control of Proliferation in Animal Cells (eds.: B. Clarkson and R. Baserga) Cold Spring Harbor Lab. pp. 817–831.

Lajtha, L. G. (1973) Commentary on 'Chalone of the Granulocyte System', by T. Rytömaa, and 'Granulopoiesis-Inhibiting Factor' by W. R. Paukovits. Nat. Cancer Inst. Monogr. 38, 157–158.

Lajtha, L. G. (1975) Annotation: Haemopoietic stem cells. Brit. J. Haematol. 29, 529.

Lajtha, L. G. and Schofield, R. (1974) On the problem of differentiation in haemopoiesis. Differentiation 2, 313–320.

Laerum, O. D. and Maurer, H. R. (1973) Proliferation kinetics of myelopoietic cells and macrophages in diffusion chambers after treatment with granulocyte extracts (chalone). Virchows Arch. Abt. B. Zellpath. 14, 293–305.

Laerum, O. D. and M. F. Rajewsky (1975) In: Hämatologie und Bluttransfusion Bd. 16, W. Stich und G. Ruhenstroth-Bauer (eds.), pp. 41–60.

Lord, B. I., Cercek, L., Cercek, B., Shah, G. P., Dexter, T. M. and Lajtha, L. G. (1974a) Inhibitors of haemopoietic cell proliferation? Specificity of action within the haemopoietic system. Brit. J. Cancer 29, 168–175.

Lord, B. I., Cercek, L., Cercek, B., Shah, G. P. and Lajtha, L. G. (1974b) Inhibitors of haemopoietic cell proliferation: Reversibility of action. Brit. J. Cancer 29, 407–409.

MacVittie, T. J. and McCarthy, K. F. (1974) Inhibition of granulopoiesis in diffusion chambers by a granulocyte chalone. Exp. Hemat. 2, 182–194.

Marsh, J. C. and Perry, S. (1964) Thymidine catabolism by normal and leukemic human leukocytes. J. Clin. Invest. 43, 267–278.

Maurer, H. R., Heitsch, J., Weiß, G. and Laerum, O. D. (1975) Assessment of procedures for the isolation and determination of granulocyte chalone activities. Virchows Arch. Abt. B, submitted.

Maurer, H. R. and Henry, R. (1975) Automatized scanning of the growth of myelopoietic colonies in agar and its control by specific inhibitors (chalones). Manuscript in preparation.

Maurer, H. R. and Laerum, O. D. (1973) Granulocyte chalone extraction and in vitro testing. Internat. Symp. Chalone Control Mechan., Lane End, Bucks., England, abstract p. 14.

Metcalf, D. (1971) Clinical applications of the agar culture technique for haematopoietic cells. Europ. J. Clin. Biol. Res. 16, 855–859.

Metcalf, D. (1973) The discrimination of leucemic from normal cells. Biomedicine 18, 264–271.

Metcalf, D., MacDonald, H. R., Odartchenko, N. and Sordat, B. (1975) Growth of mouse megakaryocyte colonies in vitro. Proc. Nat. Acad. Sci. U.S. 72, 1744–1748.

Moore, M. A. S. (1975) Cellular interaction in granulocytic differentiation. Proc. XI Internat. Cancer Congr. Florence Oct. 1974, Excerpta Medica Amsterdam-Amer. Elsevier Publ. Co. N.Y. vol. 1, 72–78.

Moore, M. A. S., Williams, N. and Metcalf, D. (1973) In vitro colony formation by normal and leukemic human hematopoietic cells: Interaction between colony-forming and colony-stimulating cells. J. Nat. Cancer Inst. 50, 591–602.

Morgan, D. A., McCredie, K. B. and Durett, A. G. (1974) Liquid culture assays of mouse bone marrow granulopoiesis. Exp. Haemat. 2, 174–181.

Müller-Bérat, C. N., Laerum, O. D. and Maurer, H. R. (1973) Chalone inhibition of the committed stem cell to granulopoiesis in vitro. 6th Meeting Europ. Study Group for Cell Prolif. Moscow, Abstracts p. 41.

Müller-Bérat, C. N., Laerum, O. D. and Maurer, H. R. (1975) Evidence for a chalone inhibition of myelopoietic colonies in agar. Manuscript in preparation.

Paran, M., Ichikawa, Y. and Sachs, L. (1969) Feedback inhibition of the development of macrophage and granulocyte colonies. II. Inhibition by granulocytes. Proc. Nat. Acad. Sci. 62, 81–87.

Parker, J. W. and Metcalf, D. (1974) Production of colony-stimulating factor in mitogen-stimulated lymphocyte cultures. J. Immunol. 112, 502–510.

Paukovits, W. R. (1971) Control of granulocyte production: Separation and chemical identification of a specific inhibitor (chalone). Cell Tissue Kinet. 4, 539–547.

Paukovits, W. (1972) Hemmung der DNA-Synthese unreifer Knochenmarkszellen durch spezifische, physiologische Inhibitoren. In: Leukämien und maligne Lymphome (ed.: A. Stacher) Urban and Schwarzenberg, München-Berlin-Wien, pp. 62–68.

Paukovits, W. R. and Paukovits, J. B. (1975) Mechanism of action of granulopoiesis inhibiting factor (chalone). I. Evidence for a receptor protein on bone marrow cells. Exp. Pathol (in press).

Pike, B. and Robinson, W. A. (1970) Human bone marrow colony growth in agar-gel. J. Cell Physiol. 76, 77–84.

Pluznik, D. H. and Sachs, L. (1966) The induction of clones of normal mast cells by a substance in conditional medium. Exp. Cell Res. 43, 553–563.

Polgar, P. R. and Kibrick, S. (1970) Origin of small lymphocytes following blastogenesis induced by short-term PHA stimulation. Nature 225, 857–858.

Price, G. B., McCulloch, E. A. and Till, J. E. (1973) A new human low molecular weight granulocyte colony stimulating activity. Blood 42, 341–348.

Rajewsky, M. F. (1974) Proliferative properties of malignant cell systems. In: Handb. d. allgem. Pathol. Springer Verl. Berlin-Heidelberg-New York, Bd. VI/5-6, 290–325.

Robinson, W. A. and Mangalik, A. (1975) The kinetics and regulation of granulopoiesis. Seminars in Hematology 12, 7–25.

Rogers, J. C., Boldt, D., Kornfeldt, S., Skinner, S. A. and Valeri, C. R. (1972) Excretion of deoxyribonucleic acid by lymphocytes stimulated by PHA or antigen. Proc. Nat. Acad. Sci. U.S. 69, 1685–1689.

Rothstein, G., Hügl, E. H., Chervenick, P. A. and Macfarlane, J. (1973) Humoral stimulators of granulocyte production. Blood 41, 73–78.

Rubini, I. R. (1966) In vitro DNA labelling of bone marrow and leucemic blood leukocytes with tritiated thymidine. II. ^{3}H-thymidine biochemistry in vitro. J. Lab. Clin. Med. 68, 566–576.

Rytömaa, T. and Kiviniemi, K. (1967) Regulation system of blood cell production. In: H. Their and T. Rytömaa (eds.), Control of cellular growth in adult organisms, p. 106–138. London-New York: Academic Press.

Rytömaa, T. and Kiviniemi, K. (1968a) Control of granulocyte production. I. Chalone and antichalone, two specific humoral regulators. Cell Tissue Kinet. 1, 329–340.

Rytömaa, T. and Kiviniemi, K. (1968b) Control of granulocyte production. II. Mode of action of chalone and antichalone. Cell Tissue Kinet. 1, 341–350.

Rytömaa, T. and Kiviniemi, K. (1968c) Control of DNA duplication in rat chloroleukaemia by means of the granulocytic chalone. Europ. J. Cancer 4, 595–600.

Schellekens, P. T. A. and Eysvoogel, V. P. (1968) Lymphocyte transformation in vitro. III. Mechanism of stimulation in the mixed lymphocyte culture. Clin. Exp. Immunol. 3, 229–239.

Simnett, J. D. and Fisher, J. M. (1973) An assay system for humoral growth factors. Nat. Cancer Inst. Monogr. 38, 19–28.

Soren, L. (1973) Effects of removing PHA from cultures of PHA-stimulated lymphocytes. Exp. Cell Res. 79, 350–358.

Sumner, M. A., Bradley, T. R., Hodgson, G. S., Cline, M. J., Fry, P. A. and Sutherland, L. (1972) The growth of bone marrow cells in liquid culture. Brit. J. Haemat. 23, 221–234.

Temin, H. M., Smith, G. L. and Dulak, N. C. (1974) Control of multiplication of normal and Rous Sarcoma Virus-transformed chicken embryo fibroblasts by purified multiplication-stimulating activity with nonsuppressible insulin-like and sulfation factor activities. In: Control of Proliferation in Animal Cells (eds.: B. Clarkson and R. Baserga) Cold Spring Harbor Lab., pp. 19–26.

Testa, N. G. and Lord, B. I. (1973) Kinetics of growth of haemopoietic colony cells in agar. Cell Tissue Kinet. 6, 425–433.

Van Wyk, J. J., Underwood, L. E., Lister, R. C., Marshall, R. N. and Hill, C. (1973) The Somatomedins. Am. J. Dis. Child 126, 705–711.

Vilpo, J. A. (1973) Cytological characteristics, proliferation, kinetics and growth control of Shay chloroleukemia cells studied with the diffusion chamber technique. Acad. Dissert. Helsinki.

Vogel, H., Niewisch, H. and Matioli, G. (1968) The self renewal probability of hemopoietic stem cells. J. Cell. Physiol. 72, 221–228.

Vogel, H., Niewisch, H. and Matioli, G. (1969) Stochastic development of stem cells. J. Theoret. Biol. 22, 249–270.

Yunis, A. A., Arimura, G. K., Haines, H. G., Ratzen, R. J. and Gross, M. A. (1975) Characteristics of rat chloroma in culture. Cancer Res. 35, 337–345.

CHAPTER 15

Lymphocyte chalone

ABDELFATTAH M. ATTALLAH and JOHN C. HOUCK

Biochemical Research Laboratory, Research Foundation of Children's Hospital,
Washington, D. C. 20009, U.S.A.

15.1 The lymphocyte system

Immunity is a complex, heterogeneous and continuously changing biological response. The growth and differentiation of the cells which mediate this response are also complex, heterogeneous, and continuously changing (Mills and Cooperband, 1971). Small lymphocytes make up about 20% of the circulating leukocytes in man and variable proportions in other mammals (Elves, 1972).

In the peripheral lymphoid tissues, thymus-derived lymphocytes are referred to as T cells, while those derived from the bursa of Fabricius in birds (its equivalent in mammals has not yet been found) are called B cells.

The two-lymphocyte model of immunity has now been firmly established, with two distinct types of immunocompetent lymphocytes: T lymphocytes being responsible for cell-mediated immunity or delayed hypersensitivity (Roitt et al., 1969), while B lymphocytes are involved in the production of circulating protein antibodies which have the ability to bind sterically to foreign antigens (Karush, 1962) to produce humoral immunity.

The thymus plays a central role in the development of immunological reactivity in mammals. Thymectomy during the neonatal period together with irradiation primarily affects the subject's capacity to display cellular immunity such as graft rejection and delayed hypersensitivity. However, the mode of action of the thymus during the development and maturation of immunocompetence is not completely clear. There is experimental evidence that soluble extracts from the thymus can induce immunological competence in non-competent cells from thymectomized animals (Trainin and Resnitzky, 1969). On the other hand, removal at hatching of the bursa of Fabricius, a cloacal lymphoid organ unique to birds, impaired the birds' ability to make antibody but had little effect on cell-mediated immunity (Raff, 1973).

In some systems, humoral antibody formation is impaired by thymectomy. In these cases, the cell which forms humoral antibody is derived from the bone marrow but cannot synthesize antibody unless thymus-dependent cells are also present, acting as 'helper' cells (Miller and Mitchell, 1970).

Although T cells do not themselves secrete circulating or humoral antibody, the activation of B cells by certain antigens requires that T cells be present. It is generally accepted that some type of collaboration between T and B cells must occur before the B cells become activated. Thus, in these responses, T cells are referred to as helper cells and B cells as antibody-forming precursor cells. It has been suggested (Dutton et al., 1971) that both T and B cells bind antigen. As a consequence, the T cells may become activated and secrete a non-specific stimulus to B cells, which thereafter become competent to respond to the antigen by cell division and specific antibody production.

There is evidence that both types of cells have specific receptor sites for antigen so that both react with antigen in some way before the bone marrow cells are stimulated to proliferate, differentiate, and produce antibody (Makela and Cross, 1970; Roelants, 1972). The recognition site on the lymphocyte is thought to be an immunoglobulin molecule which may be buried deep in the cell membrane (Greaves and Hegg, 1971).

When B cells are activated by antigen, they divide and differentiate into blast cells with abundant endoplasmic reticulum, and some go on to become plasma cells. These cells remain in lymphoid tissues for the most part and secrete large amounts of antibody which circulate in the blood (Raff, 1973). B cells utilize serum enzyme systems to amplify their reactivity i.e., complement (Ratnoff, 1969), but the primary amplification is by production of new effector cells (see fig. 15.1).

T cells, activated by antigen, proliferate and differentiate to become blast cells without developing significant amounts of endoplasmic reticulum. They do not secrete circulating antibody but produce a variety of non-antigen-specific factors (lymphokines) which act to recruit other cells into the reaction (Waksman, 1971). T cells also release cytophilic antibody which binds to the surface of macrophages. Some lymphokines are responsible for the cytotoxicity and inflammation which is characteristic of cell-mediated immune responses; there are chemotactic factors which attract wandering phagocytic cells into the site of a cell-mediated response, migration inhibitor factors which hold these cells in the injured tissue, cytotoxic factors which cause the death of foreign cells, and mitogenic factors. The relation-

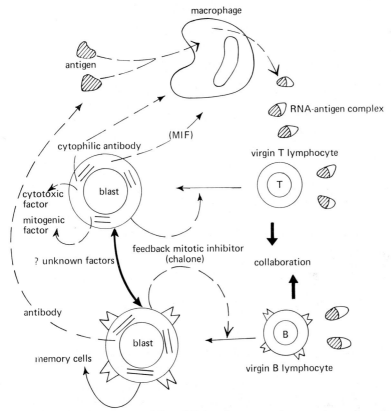

Fig. 15.1. Functional responses of T and B lymphocytes and macrophages to antigen.
From Attallah, 1975.

ship between lymphokines, their significance, and mechanisms of action are, however, not completely understood (Lawrence and Landy, 1969).

In addition, macrophages seem to play an important part in at least some immunologic reactions as nonspecific 'handlers' of antigen. Antigen is most stimulatory when it has been first phagocytized by macrophages, processed, and then presented to lymphocytes, probably as in RNA-antigen complex (Fishman and Adler, 1968).

Graft rejection is largely a cell-mediated immune reaction. In this respect, it is similar to the delayed hypersensitivity reactions that can occur after the exposure of an individual to certain antigens, such as an allograft rejection. A graft-versus-host response is a phenomenon in which injected foreign T lymphocytes respond against the antigens of the recipient host, often resulting in rejecting the host cells in vivo and the recipient's death. Table 15.1 shows the responses of lymphocytes to different stimulators.

Table 15.1

Lymphocyte responses in vitro.

Stimulator	(B) Lymphocyte	T Lymphocyte
(S) PHA	?	+
(ins) PHA	+	+
(S) conA	?	+
(ins) conA	+	+
PWM	+	+
LPS	+	−
MLC	?	+
ant-Ig	+	−

(S) = soluble; (ins) = insoluble; PHA = phytohemagglutinin; conA = concanavalin; LPS = lipopolysaccharides; MLC = mixed lymphocyte culture; + = stimulation; − = no stimulation; ? = uncertain.

15.2 Lymphocyte chalone

Moorhead et al. (1969) and Jones et al. (1970) applied the chalone concept to the lymphocyte system and were able to show that extracts of lymph node from the pig were capable of inhibiting the morphologically demonstrable transformation of PHA-stimulated human lymphocytes in vitro as well as inhibiting the ability of these cells to incorporate [^{3}H]TdR into acid insoluble DNA. This inhibition was accomplished with apparently no cytotoxicity and had a mol wt of about 50,000–75,000 daltons (Moorhead et al., 1969). The existence of a specific and endogenous mitotic inhibitor of lymphocyte transformation was confirmed by Garcia-Giralt et al. (1970, 1972) and by ourselves (Houck et al., 1971; Attallah et al., 1975). We were able to show that aqueous extracts of various lymphoid tissues contained a material which could be concentrated via ultrafiltration through Amicon Diaflo ultrafilters at a mol wt range between 30,000 and 50,000 daltons which would specifically inhibit the transformation of lectin-stimulated human lymphocytes in vitro.

This chapter explores in detail the evidence for the existence of a cell-specific but not species-specific and non-cytotoxic endogenous inhibitor of the transformation and proliferation of lymphocytes in vitro, properties which fit the initial definition offered by Bullough and Laurence (1964) for a 'chalone', the cytotoxic effect upon leukemic but not normal lymphocytes, and proposed mechanism for lymphocyte chalone action.

15.3 Specificity

The 30,000–50,000-dalton concentrates obtained from aqueous extracts of spleen, thymus, lymph node, muscle, and lung from calf were studied for their inhibitory effects upon the incorporation of [^{3}H]TdR into acid insoluble DNA of normal human lymphocytes stimulated with PHA, NC-37, diploid human fibroblasts, and Molt, human lymphoblasts, in vitro. Similarly, 10^6 mononuclear cells from bone marrow or HeLa cells were incubated with these various tissue ultrafiltrates for 24 h and the inhibitory effects upon their DNA synthesis was determined. The percent inhibition of the uptake of [H^3]TdR by these various cell systems into acid insoluble DNA was determined after incubation with 100 μg/ml of the appropriate mol wt ultrafiltrate from spleen, thymus, and lymph node and 500 μg/ml of the ultrafiltrates from brain, muscle, and lung of calf. These results are summarized in table 15.2 and indicate that ultrafiltrates of extracts from the spleen and lymph node will almost totally inhibit DNA synthesis in both lectin-stimulated normal lymphocytes and NC-37 (B cell) lymphoblastic cell lines in vitro. This same concentration of spleen and lymph node ultrafiltrate had essentially trivial effects upon the incorporation of [^{3}H]TdR into acid insoluble DNA of bone marrow and had absolutely no effect upon the DNA synthesis of either fibroblasts or HeLa cells in vitro. Thymus extracts were also capable of inhibiting DNA synthesis by either lectin-stimulated normal lymphocytes or Molt (T cell) lymphoblastic cell lines

Table 15.2

The inhibitory effects of chalone extracts obtained from various calf tissues upon the [^{3}H]thymidine uptake by various in vitro cell systems.

Extracts	Inhibition of						Chorio-carcinoma	NC-37
	PHA	Con A	MLC	Bone marrow	Fibro-blast	HeLa		
Spleen	++	++	++	+	---	---	---	++
Thymus	++	++	++	---	---	---	---	---
Lymph node	++	++	++	+	---	---	---	++
Brain	---	---	---	---	---	---	---	+
Muscle	---	---	---	---	---	---	---	---
Lung	---	---	---	---	+	---	---	NT
Kidney	---	---	---	---	---	---	---	---

++ = strong inhibition; + = weak inhibition; --- = no inhibition; NT = not tested.

in vitro but had no effect upon the DNA synthesis of NC-37 (B cell) lympho-blasts in vitro, nor any effect upon the DNA synthesis by either bone marrow, HeLa cells, or fibroblasts.

Similarly prepared extracts from brain, muscle, and lung had no effect upon the DNA synthetic rates of stimulated human lymphocytes or estab-lished lymphoblastic lines in vitro nor upon the DNA synthesis of bone marrow or fibroblasts in vitro. The lung did apparently inhibit the DNA synthesis of diploid human fibroblasts in vitro.

Similarly prepared ultrafiltrates from aqueous extracts of the lymphoid tissue from six different species were studied for their ability to inhibit the PHA transformation of lymphocytes at three different doses. These results are summarized in table 15.3 and indicate that essentially similar inhibitory activity of the ultrafiltered lymphocyte chalone concentrates from the various lymphoid tissues of these six species were demonstrated upon the DNA synthesis of human lymphocytes in vitro. An essentially linear dose response was demonstrated for all of these extracts in terms of the inhibition

Table 15.3

The percent inhibition of lymphocyte transformation in vitro demonstrated by various concentrations of chalone prepared from the lymphoid tissue of various species.

Species	Inhibition of PHA lymphocyte transformation by		
	100 μg/ml	50 μg/ml	25 μg/ml
Bovine			
thymus	+++	++	+
spleen	+++	++	+
Porcine			
thymus	+++	++	+
spleen	+++	++	+
lymph node	+++	++	NT
Canine			
spleen	+++	++	+
Rabbit			
thymus	+++	++	NT
spleen	+++	++	NT
Rat			
spleen	+++	++	+
lymph node	+++	++	+

+++ = 80–100% inhibition; ++ = 50–60% inhibition; + = 20–30% inhibition; NT = not tested.

of DNA synthesis by PHA-stimulated human lymphocytes in vitro over the range 25–100 μg/ml.

The data of table 15.2 indicates that lymphoid tissue ultrafiltrates inhibited profoundly the incorporation of $[^3H]TdR$ into the acid insoluble DNA of lymphocytes but not of bone marrow cells, diploid human fibroblasts, or HeLa cells in vitro. Other studies in this laboratory have indicated that these lymphoid tissue extracts also do not inhibit proliferation rates determined by cell counting of human colon, lung, and choriocarcinoma cells in vitro. This demonstration of cell specificity was also supported by the data of table 15.2, indicating that similar extracts from non-lymphoid tissues did not inhibit the DNA synthesis of lymphocytes. The finding that lung extracts inhibited DNA synthesis by diploid human fibroblasts in vitro is probably related to the large amount of fibroblasts in this tissue and presumably therefore a significant amount of fibroblast chalone (Houck et al., 1972). This demonstration of cell and organ specificity is further enlarged by the data of table 15.3 which indicates the complete lack of species specificity of this cell-specific inhibitor of lymphocyte DNA synthesis.

Lord et al. (1974), using the new technique of fluorescence polarization, have also shown tissue specificity of lymphocyte chalone to exist without species specificity. Garcia-Giralt et al. (1973) showed that chalone action was specific for inhibition of lymphoid cell proliferation and did not affect multiplication of erythroid, myelocytic, or megakaryotic cells present in spleen colonies. It therefore seems safe to conclude that lymphocyte chalone is not species-specific but is tissue-specific (Attallah, 1974).

15.4 Cell specificity

A rather subtle display of cell specificity has been proposed for the lymphocyte chalone vis-a-vis T, or thymus-derived, cells and B, or bone marrow-derived, cells. Florentin et al. (1973) have shown that extracts of thymus which will inhibit PHA-stimulated lymphocyte transformation, a largely T cell phenomenon, will not inhibit the function of antigen stimulation specific for B cells in vivo. Extracts of spleen which should theoretically contain both T- and B-derived lymphocytes, however, are capable of inhibiting the antigen stimulation of lymphocyte function in terms of IgM synthesis at similar concentrations. We have found that extracts of thymus will not inhibit the uptake of $[^3H]TdR$ into acid insoluble DNA by NC-37 diploid human lymphoblasts in vitro (Attallah et al., 1975). These cells are known to be B cells in that they synthesize immunoglobulins and bind the C_3 portion of the complement chain (Pattengale et al., 1973). Further, these

NC-37 cells are known to contain the genome to express Epstein–Barr virus, an important property of B cells.

An experiment which is not consistent with T and B cell specificities is that beta lipopolysaccharide from *Salmonella typhosa*, which is known to stimulate transformation of B cells (Peavy et al., 1970), can be inhibited significantly by relatively small amounts of thymus-derived chalone (Attallah et al., 1975). Normally, the endotoxin will cause about 8 to 10 times as much incorporation of $[^3H]TdR$ into acid insoluble DNA by B lymphocytes. These cells have been collected from mouse spleen via ficol–hypaque gradient (Boyum, 1968), but in the presence of as little as 50 μg/ml of the ultrafiltered extract from calf thymus over 90% of this reponse is completely inhibited. There are two separate assay systems involved in these experiments: Florentin et al. (1973), using an antigen-specific for B cells both in vitro and in vivo; and ourselves, using endotoxin which functions as a mitogen for mouse B cells in vitro. Further, the precise endpoint used in the studies of Florentin et al. (1973) was the synthesis of IgM by sensitized lymphocytes, whereas our studies concerned the uptake of tritiated thymidine into acid insoluble DNA; these two procedural differences may be of considerable significance. Thus, thymus-derived ultrafiltrates presumably containing primarily, if not exclusively, T cell-derived lymphocyte chalone could not inhibit the proliferation of an established B cell line, NC-37, but could inhibit the presumably B cell-specific transformation of mouse lymphocytes in vitro. This contradictory observation may be resolved by recent findings (Newberger et al., 1974) on the essential role of 'helper' T cells in the response of mouse lymphocytes to bacterial lipopolysaccharides. Inhibition by thymus-derived ultrafiltrate might inhibit the transformation of these 'helper' T cells and hence the transformation of mouse B cells after lipopolysaccharide stimulation.

Our data appear to confirm the original suggestion of Florentin et al. (1973) that there was a specificity of T-derived chalone for T cells as opposed to B cells in immunologically stimulated systems. It would also appear that B cell-derived chalone can effectively inhibit the lectin-stimulated transformation of T cells in vitro as well as the spontaneous mitotic activity of an established B cell lymphocyte line.

15.5 Endogenous origin

The endogenous origin of this mitotic inhibitor in the mol wt range between 30,000 and 50,000 daltons is suggested by the data of table 15.4. Large numbers of NC-37 lymphoblasts (diploid human lymphocytes obtained

Table 15.4

The inhibitory effects of sieved (30,000–50,000) used medium from NC-37 cells in vitro upon the incorporation of [³H]thymidine into DNA by PHA-stimulated human lymphocytes ('t' cell) and by NC-37 human lymphoblasts ('b' cell) in vitro.

Concentration (μg/ml)	% inhibition of	
	'T' cell (PHA)	'B' cell (NC-37)
0		
25	60**	11*
50	93**	8*
100	98** (Con. A)	40
150	99**	55
200	100**	68

* Not significantly inhibited ($P < 0.05$).
** Significantly higher for 'T' system than 'B' system.
Each number is the mean of four independent determinations carried out in triplicate.

from the peripheral blood of a patient with pneumonia), which possess the properties of a B cell type of lymphocyte, were grown as a pure established cell line. Aqueous extracts of these cells were prepared by sonication and subjected to molecular ultrafiltration. The effects of these ultrafiltrates (30,000–50,000 daltons) from pure lymphocytes upon the PHA stimulation of normal human lymphocytes in terms of the synthesis of acid insoluble DNA and upon the spontaneous mitotic activity of the NC-37 cells themselves in culture is shown in table 15.4. These data indicate that extracts of pure lymphoblasts inhibit the DNA synthesis of PHA-stimulated normal human lymphocytes in vitro. Further, this inhibitor has the same mol wt characteristics of the inhibitor extracted from whole lymphoid tissues. The inhibition of PHA-stimulated lymphocytes by B lymphoblast extract could be the result of chalone effect on B cell population, consequently altering the response to PHA stimulation. This pure lymphoblast extract inhibited the DNA synthesis of NC-37 lymphoblasts, and finally this inhibition was quantitatively much larger for PHA-stimulated normal lymphocytes than for DNA synthesis by NC-37 cells in vitro.

15.6 Properties of lymphocyte chalone

The extraction and purification of lymphocyte chalone are illustrated in fig. 15.2. The inhibitory activity of thymus- or spleen-derived chalone

PURIFICATION STEPS:

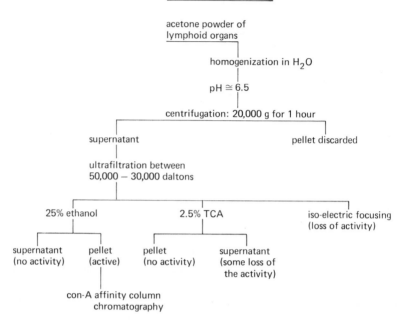

Fig. 15.2

concentrates was completely destroyed by incubation with either trypsin or chymotrypsin. This indicates that the biological activity of these extracts requires peptide bonds involving both basic and aromatic amino acids. Incubation of chalone concentrates from lymphoid tissue with either ribonuclease or deoxyribonuclease had no effect upon the inhibitory properties characteristic of these extracts in vitro. Therefore, the chalone activity resides in a peptide-containing macromolecule in which neither DNA or RNA has any significant activity.

The lymphocyte chalone activity will usually pass very slowly through a 30,000-dalton ultrafilter and will not pass at all through a 10,000-dalton filter. Preliminary evidence in this laboratory suggests that preincubation of chalone concentrates with ribonuclease, while not decreasing the total amount of inhibitory activity demonstrable, will now permit this inhibitory activity to move through a 10,000-dalton ultrafilter. Hence, the size of the lymphocyte chalone activity will be reduced by RNase treatment. Further, the ratios of the absorbance of ultrafiltered chalone concentrate at 260 to 280 nm is around 1.2, a value more appropriate for RNA than for protein. However, when this extract was subjected to column chromatography, using

Concanavalin A bound to sepharose as a column medium, all of the biological inhibitory activity remained bound to the column in 0.15 M saline or 0.01 M Tris buffer. This biologic activity could not be eluted from this Con A-sepharose column by either alpha-methyl-D-mannoside or methyl-alpha-D-glucopyranoside eluents. Therefore, the biologic activity was not specifically adherent to these columns via mannose binding to Con A. However, elution of the column with 0.5 M NaCl resulted in the complete release from the column of all the biological activity in terms of the inhibition of lymphocyte transformation in vitro. Finally, the ability of this chalone activity to adhere to the column was completely lost subsequent to ribonuclease treatment of the chalone ultrafiltered preparation.

Therefore, we postulate that the chalone could travel as a smaller mol wt material than 30,000 daltons in tight association with RNA, presumably related to the 4 S or 5 S components of ribosomes and transfer RNA respectively. We suggest that this is so because larger amounts of very large RNA molecules are available (from ribosomes) than the small mol wt RNA, presumably from transfer RNA (25,000 daltons). If chalone activity was binding to any anionic polyelectrolyte RNA, it should then be found in mol wt ranges considerably in excess of 50,000 daltons. Actual data indicates that this is not the case. Therefore, we presume that lymphocyte chalone activity resides in a molecule of mol wt less than 10,000 which is complexed by very strong ionic bonds with relatively low mol wt RNA of 20,000 daltons.

It is also possible that this large amount of contaminating 260 nm absorbing material could be due to thymidine itself. Although most of the thymidine found in large amounts in lymphoid tissue is extractable into acetone, nonetheless some thymidine could remain in the acetone powders from which the aqueous extracts of spleen and thymus have been prepared. Theoretically, the small mol wt thymidine should easily pass through the holes of the 30,000-dalton ultrafilter. However, a significant proportion of thymidine could be absorbed via low energy binding to larger macromolecules and hence not be removed during the rinsing or washing phase over a 30,000-dalton filter. This endogenous thymidine could, by pool-size dilution, decrease markedly the incorporation rate of $[^3H]TdR$ into acid insoluble DNA in these cells.

The data of table 15.5 indicate a close correlation of the inhibition of the morphologic marker of transformation (i.e., the transformation from small lymphocytes into large lymphoblasts) with the kinetics of the inhibitory effects of spleen ultrafiltrate upon the incorporation of $[^3H]TdR$ into acid insoluble DNA. This suggests that the apparent mitotic inhibition (i.e.,

Table 15.5

Inhibitory effects of spleen 'chalone' concentrate (30,000–50,000 dalton) 50 μg/ml upon the percent lymphoblastic population and [^{3}H]thymidine uptake by 10^6 PHA-stimulated human lymphocytes in vitro.

Hours after PHA	% Lymphoblasts		[^{3}H]thymidine inhibition (%)	Viability (%)
	PHA alone	PHA and chalone		
0	0	0	0	90+
24	14	2	—	90+
48	30	15	56	90+
72	60	23	51	90+
144	75	20	98	90+

inhibition of DNA synthesis by these cells) in the presence of the putative chalone concentrate was not due to either phosphorylation or pool-size dilution of the radioactive label used in these studies.

This proposed contamination of tissue ultrafiltrate by thymidine might directly inhibit lymphocyte transformation since relatively large amounts of thymidine will function as suppressors of lymphocyte function in vitro. This possibility was excluded by our finding that no inhibition of [^{3}H] cytidine uptake could be demonstrated by exogenous cold thymidine at concentrations four times larger than the actual weight of spleen ultrafiltrate used to inhibit almost 100% of the [^{3}H]cytidine uptake after PHA stimulation of lymphocyte transformation. Exogenous thymidine actually stimulated lymphocyte transformation under these conditions, as has been shown by others previously (Diddi et al., 1974).

An alternative explanation of this apparent inhibition of DNA synthesis and lymphocyte transformation by the putative lymphocyte chalone concentrate obtained from spleen might be that these extracts are capable of binding the lectin PHA so as to decrease significantly the number of cells transformed by this agent. The inhibition of established lymphocytic DNA synthesis argues against this, however. Further, the data of table 15.5 report the results of a two-way mixed lymphocyte culture experiment in which the stimulation of lymphocyte transformation was produced by membrane-bound antigenic components of these lymphocytes and not by lectins. Various amounts of chalone concentrate from thymus inhibited both the proliferation and the amount of [^{3}H]TdR taken up into acid insoluble DNA by these lymphocytes. The suggestion has been made previously (Garcia-Giralt and Macieira-Coelho, 1974) that splenic chalone concentrate was capable of inhibiting the incorporation of [^{3}H]TdR into acid insoluble DNA of leukemic lymphocytes without inhibiting the proliferation of the cells in the culture. Such does not seem to be the case for two-way mixed lymphocyte cultures, however.

15.7 Skin graft

Much attention has been focused in recent years on the T lymphocyte, since this cell is primarily responsible for allograft rejection, tumor immunity, graft-versus-host reactions, and other delayed type hypersensitivity. Garcia-Giralt et al. (1973), Kiger et al. (1971, 1973), and Houck et al. (1973) demonstrated that extracts of lymphoid tissue could partially inhibit both graft-versus-host and allograft rejection in mice.

The effects of lymphocyte chalone concentrate from the spleen upon the uptake of [^{3}H]TdR in mixed lymphocyte culture was studied. As little as 50 μg/ml will inhibit over half of the total immunologically stimulated transformation of these human cells in culture. Similar results were obtained, using extracts of thymus. This mixed lymphocyte culture incubation system has been helpful in predicting the intensity of subsequent clinical graft rejection (Houck et al. 1973).

Using a new method for the determination of macrophage migration inhibitory factor (MIF), which is extremely sensitive and quite rapid (Houck and Chang, 1973), we studied the effects of various concentrations of sieved, concentrated lymphocyte chalone from spleen upon both the PHA-stimulated transformation of human lymphocytes in culture, as judged by the uptake of [^{3}H]TdR and the release of MIF activity into the supernatant of these cultures. There was a parallel inhibition of both thymidine uptake and MIF release from transforming lymphocytes with increasing amounts of lymphocyte chalone concentrate until, at 25 μg/ml, approximately 45 % of the thymidine uptake was inhibited and no significant amount of MIF activity was released into the culture medium. Because of the considerable importance of MIF to the immunological defense mechanism of the body in terms of graft rejection, these data support the possibility of successful immunosuppression by lymphocyte chalone concentrate.

C57BL/6 mice received skin alltransplants from C3H mice. All grafts in the control and saline-treated animals were rejected by 12 days. The chalone-treated animals retained their grafts for about 29 days, with rejection occurring 8 to 10 days after cessation of chalone treatment. Thus, the survival

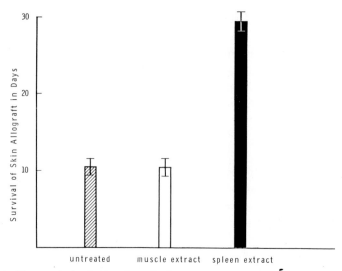

Fig. 15.3. The survival of skin allografts in C57BL/6 mice from C3H mice with and without lymphocyte chalone administration (5 mg/day for 3 days/wk).

of C3H mouse skin grafts on the chalone-treated C57BL/6 was prolonged 2.5 times that of the control mice. Only 9 doses of lymphocyte chalone were used per mouse in this study because of limitations in the amount of the partially purified and sieved spleen extract available (Houck et al., 1973).

These data suggest, first, that lymphocyte chalone concentrate from spleen could inhibit the immunologically produced transformation of human lymphocytes in mixed lymphocyte culture and, second, that this chalone concentrate could inhibit the release of MIF from transformed human lymphocytes in vitro. The in vivo demonstrations of the inhibition of allograft rejection appear quite convincing quantitatively in spite of the unknown proper dose regimen and concentration of this lymphocyte chalone.

It has been speculated that lymphocyte chalone might be used in combination with immunosuppressive drug therapy. Chung and Hufnagel (1973) suggest that chalone could be used shortly before massive antigen challenge (e.g. kidney homograft) and then continued for a certain time. Based on Burnet's clonal selection theory, the antigen would stimulate the responsive clone of cells to divide; however, not all cells of the clone would necessarily be stimulated simultaneously. Chalone would suppress cell proliferation of the excited cells and hold them in phase. An immunosuppressive drug might then be administered following chalone therapy. As repopulation of the lymphoid system takes place, new lymphoid cells would mature in the presence of antigen and would be expected, by conventional tolerance theory, to be tolerant. The result could be a stable state of tolerance and fully functioning tissue (or organ) graft.

15.8 Lymphocyte chalone and leukemia

The morphological difference between normal and leukemic cells is not clear, even at the electron microscopic level. The disease is characterized by a large number of blast cells, consequently elevating the peripheral blood lymphocyte count. These cells infiltrate the bone marrow, lymph nodes, and other tissues and eventually result in the death of the patient. It has been shown that chronic leukemic lymphocytes differ from the normal lymphocytes in their response to stimulation by PHA. These leukemic cells respond poorly to PHA, and this response was always delayed for 7 days instead of 3 days, as is the case with normal lymphocytes. This failure to transform is not known to result from a defect in the immunological capacity of the leukemic cells or from the presence of an inhibitor in the plasma of these cells (see Durant and Smalley, 1972).

Leukemia is characterized by the uncontrolled proliferation and accumulation of leukemic cells. These cells are incapable of normal maturation and are relatively unresponsive to growth regulation. When the leukemic mass reaches a critical size, the growth rate of the normal and the leukemic cells is decreased. If the number of leukemic cells is reduced sufficiently by therapy, the normal cells are released from this inhibition (Clarkson, 1972).

The effects of relatively large concentrations of the ultrafiltered spleen extract containing the putative lymphocyte chalone upon the proliferation of leukemic lymphocytes in vitro was studied (Attallah, 1975; Attallah and Houck, 1975), using four different established cell lines: (a) L-1210, a mouse leukemic lymphocyte which has been well characterized both in vivo and in vitro; (b) EL-4, a mouse leukemic lymphocyte (Gorer, 1960); (c) Molt, established from the peripheral blood of a patient during relapses of acute lymphoblastic leukemia with T cell characteristics (Minowada et al., 1973); and (d) NC-37, a permanent lymphoblastic line with B cell characteristics (Pattengale et al., 1973) which originated from the peripheral leukocytes of a patient with pneumonia.

The leukemic lymphocyte cell lines were grown in RPMI 1640 medium containing 20% fetal calf serum, glutamine, and 100 units/ml each of penicillin and streptomycin. The NC-37 human lymphoblastic cells were cultured in McCoy's medium with 20% fetal calf serum and 100 units/ml each of penicillin and streptomycin. The ultrafiltered spleen extracts were reconstituted in the appropriate medium before addition to the cultures. DNA synthesis was measured by the amount of [³H]TdR incorporation into the acid insoluble DNA fraction. Triplicate cultures were incubated at 37 °C for 18 h with the spleen extracts, followed by a 6-h pulse of [³H]TdR. The number of viable cells remaining in similar cultures was determined in triplicate by trypan blue dye exclusion, using a hemocytometer.

The effects of various concentrations of ultrafiltered spleen extracts upon the lymphoblastic cell lines is shown in table 15.6. It can be seen that (a) the spleen extracts inhibited [³H]TdR incorporation in all four established lymphocyte cell lines, and (b) many of the human and mouse lymphoblasts

Table 15.6

The effects of 24-h incubation at 37 °C of 0, 125, and 250 μg/ml of ultrafiltered spleen extracts (in triplicate) upon the mean number of viable cells (capable of excluding Trypan blue vital dye) remaining and the incorporation of [³H]Tdr (6-h pulse) into the acid insoluble DNA of four established lymphoblastic cell lines.

Cell Type	Concentration μg/ml	No. viable cells	Dead cells (%)	CPM/10⁶ viable cells	Inhibition of DNA (%)
Mouse					
1. L-1210	0	8.1×10^5/ml	<10	37,500	—
(5.5 × 10⁵/ml)*	125	4.5×10^5/ml	44	15,500	59
	250	2.8×10^5/ml	65	14,200	63
2. EL-4	0	8.0×10^5/ml	<10	13,800	—
(10.2 × 10⁵/ml)*	125	3.3×10^5/ml	59	14,400	0
	250	1.4×10^5/ml	83	8,900	33
3. Normal (PHA 48 h)	0	20.0×10^5/ml	42	18,500	—
(30 × 10⁵/ml)*	200	23.0×10^5/ml	34	930	95
Human					
1. Molt	0	7.0×10^5/ml	<10	110,000	—
(6.8 × 10⁵/ml)*	125	3.3×10^5/ml	53	12,000	89
	250	2.0×10^5/ml	72	8,000	93
2. NC-37	0	7.2×10^5/ml	<10	13,600	—
(6.2 × 10⁵/ml)	125	4.0×10^5/ml	44	1,140	92
	250	3.5×10^5/ml	51	250	98
3. Normal (PHA 72 h)	0	4.0×10^5/ml	<10	48,000	—
(5 × 10⁵/ml)*	200	3.9×10^5/ml	<10	430	99

* Number of cells seeded initially.

in these cultures were apparently killed during this incubation period. Essentially similar cytotoxicity toward leukemic lymphocytes (Molt, L-1210) in vitro was also demonstrated by ultrafiltered preparations from other dessicated, defatted calf, cow, and pig spleen powders obtained from the Viobin Corporation (Monticello, Illinois 61856). Similar ultrafiltered extracts were prepared from fresh calf spleen and 200 μg/ml of this ultrafiltered material was also found to be capable of killing 45% of the Molt cells in vitro after 24 h incubation.

These same spleen extracts were also incubated with normal human lymphocytes and normal mouse spleen cells. Triplicate cultures of 5×10^5 human lymphocytes with or without PHA were incubated with or without 200 μg/ml of ultrafiltered spleen, as described previously (Houck et al., 1971; Attallah et al., 1975). There was no reduction in the number of viable cells after 72 h, as judged by vital dye exclusion. Despite this lack of extract cytotoxicity, 50 μg/ml inhibited over 50% of the PHA-stimulated trans-formation of these cells, as measured both morphologically and by [^{3}H]TdR incorporation into acid insoluble DNA. Similary, incubation of mouse spleen cells for 48 h with or without 200 μg/ml of spleen extract showed no apparent cytotoxicity.

Ultrafiltered extracts of cow and pig kidney were prepared as described above. Neither of these extracts, at similar concentrations to that of the spleen preparations, demonstrated any inhibition of [^{3}H]TdR incorporation or cytotoxicity toward L-1210 or Molt cells after 48 h incubation in vitro. Finally, similar ultrafiltered extracts of fresh calf thymus were prepared and

Table 15.7

The cytotoxicity and DNA inhibition produced by incubating various concentrations of spleen ultrafiltered extracts with primary cultures of 5×10^5/ml EL-4 mouse lymphocytes in triplicate for 48 h in vitro.

Concentration μg/ml	Cell No. ($\times 10^5$/ml)	% viable cells	% inhibition of DNA
0	6.5	66	0
75	7.2	45*	54*
125	5.7	24*	81*
250	6.9	17*	98*
500	5.9	5*	99*

* Means found to be significantly different from 0 concentration control ($P < 0.05$).

were demonstrated to be extremely cytotoxic to Molt cells but not to normal human lymphocytes in vitro.

Thus, it would appear that 30,000–50,000-dalton extracts of lymphoid tissue, but not of non-lymphoid tissues, from cow and pig are capable of specifically inhibiting the mitotic activity of both mouse and human lympho-blastic cell lines and, more importantly, are uniquely cytotoxic to these cells in vitro.

The cytotoxicity of these extracts was also determined upon primary cultures of EL-4 lymphoblasts. The EL-4 lymphoid tumor, originally induced in C57 mice by the carcinogen 9,10-dimethyl-1,2-benzanthracine (Gorer, 1960) has been carried in several laboratories as a transplantable ascites tumor. These animals were sacrificed and the EL-4 cells removed from their in vivo peritoneal incubation medium, counted by hemocytometry in the usual fashion, and, on the basis of the exclusion of vital dye, were well over 95% viable. These primary cultures were incubated in triplicate, as described above, for 48 h with various concentrations of the dessicated, defatted ultrafiltered spleen extract. The effects of these extracts upon the incorporation of 6-h pulse of $[^3H]$TdR into acid insoluble DNA and upon the viability of these cells as determined by vital dye exclusion are presented in table 15.7. It can be seen that while the mean number of cells was not significantly reduced, the percentage of these cells remaining viable was again reduced in direct proportion to the dose of the spleen extract employed.

L-1210 murine leukemia cells (2.5×10^5 per ml) were incubated in medium containing 200 $\mu g/ml$ of ultrafiltered spleen extract. After different periods of incubation, these cells were washed twice with Hanks' solution, fresh medium was added, and the incubation continued for a total of 48 h. In the last 6 h of incubation, 1 μCi of $[^3H]$TdR was added before harvesting. The amount of $[^3H]$TdR incorporated into the acid insoluble DNA of these cells was determined by liquid scintillation counting. To be certain that there was no cell loss in the manipulation of chalone removal, un-treated cells were washed with Hanks' solution in a manner identical to the chalone-treated cultures. The data in table 15.8 shows that the cytotoxic effects paralleled DNA inhibition throughout the period of incubation with chalone and that this effect was permanent. Cells incubated with chalone for less than 6 h were found to grow subsequently at a rate similar to that of the control cells. However, irreversible cytotoxic effects were shown with those cells which had been incubated with lymphocyte chalone for longer than 6 h.

A lack of cytotoxicity of these spleen ultrafiltrates for normal lymphocytes in culture was indicated by the finding of the very large degree of reversibility

Table 15.8

L-1210 lymphoblasts 2.5 × 10⁵ per ml were incubated with 200 μg/ml of lymphocyte
chalone for various times. The cells were then washed and reincubated in fresh medium
for a total of 48 h. Viability was judged from vital dye exclusion. DNA synthesis was
determined from the amount of [³H]TdR incorporated into the acid insoluble fraction,
using a 6-h pulse after 42 h incubation at 37 °C.

Incubation time (h)	Viable cell No. (× 10⁵)	Counts/min (mean)	% DNA inhibition
0	6.1	19,392	0
8	4.6	12,643	35
16	4.4	8,302	57
26	2.9	8,029	59
48	2.9	8,664	55

of chalone-produced inhibition when the cells were rinsed prior to their
exposure to PHA stimulation in vitro. Only one rinsing of cells which had
been incubated with 100 or 200 μg/ml of spleen ultrafiltrate containing the
putative chalone activity for 48 h was sufficient to reduce the inhibition of
further PHA stimulation of these same cells from essentially 100% to
between 20 and 30%. This considerable degree of reversibility was coupled
with 100% viable cells in mixed lymphocyte culture, even after exposure to
200 μg/ml of the thymus-derived ultrafiltrate for 5 days (Attallah et al., 1975).
The recent reports by Lord et al. (1974), using a novel fluorescence polarization procedure to measure the 'structuredness' of lymphocytes when
stimulated by PHA, indicated that the inhibition of this stimulation by
similar 30,000–50,000-dalton extracts from spleen was completely reversible
and not cytotoxic toward normal lymphocytes.

The effect of lymphocyte chalone on protein, RNA, and DNA synthesis
in L-1210 leukemic cells in vitro was studied. These cells (2.5 × 10⁵/ml)
were incubated in triplicate in medium containing 250 μg/ml of sieved spleen
extract. In the last 5 h of incubation before harvesting, 1 μCi of [³H]phenyl-
alanine, [³H]uridine, and [³H]TdR were added separately to these triplicate
cultures. The uptake of these isotopes into TCA insoluble macromolecules
was determined, using liquid scintillation counting in the usual manner.
Our results show that inhibition of protein synthesis could be determined
within the first 5 h of incubation and that the degree of this inhibition increased with increasing incubation time. There was a lag of 17 h before the
inhibition of RNA and DNA synthesis could be demonstrated in these

chalone-inhibited leukemic lymphocytes. After 48 h incubation with spleen
ultrafiltrate, an equivalent inhibition of the synthesis of all three macromolecules by these cells was demonstrable.

Finally, we determined the cytotoxic effects of 100 or 200 μg/ml of ultrafiltered spleen extract upon cultures of L-1210 lymphoblasts which Garcia-
Giralt and Macieira-Coelho (1974) have shown to be inhibited in terms of
DNA synthesis but not in terms of cell proliferation and which were not
killed when cultured at 100,000 cells/ml. Therefore, we studied cultures which
had been seeded initially with varying numbers of cells and incubated for
48 h at 37 °C. These results are presented in table 15.9. Concentrations of
L-1210 from 5×10^5 to 10×10^5 cells/ml (cell concentrations used routinely
in most laboratories) incubated with both 100 and 200 μg of the spleen
ultrafiltered extract had a significant number of dead cells, as judged by
their inability to exclude vital dye. With 2.3×10^5 or less cells per ml, 100 μg/
ml of ultrafiltered spleen extract no longer demonstrated cytotoxicity, while
200 μg/ml of ultrafiltered spleen extract still killed about 40% of the cells.
However, this latter dose was without cytotoxic effect upon cultures initially
seeded with 0.8×10^5 lymphoblasts/ml and did not inhibit their proliferation.

Cultures of L-1210 were also incubated for 48 h with 10^{-4} M cytosine
arabinoside at 4 and 8×10^5 cells/ml. No significant cytotoxicity was observed in spite of this drug inhibiting 60 and 47% respectively of the [^{3}H]TdR
uptake by these cells. This finding suggests that mitotic inhibition alone
does not result in the death of these leukemic lymphocytes.

The incubation of lymphocyte chalone ultrafiltrates with murine leukemic

Table 15.9

The effects of inoculum size upon the cytotoxicity of 100 or 200 μg/ml of ultrafiltered
spleen extracts upon L-1210 mouse leukemic lymphocytes after 48 h incubation in triplicate
at 37 °C.

Number of cells seeded ($\times 10^5$/ml)	Number of viable cells ($\times 10^5$/ml) after incubation with spleen extract		
	0 μg/ml	100 μg/ml	200 μg/ml
9.5	14.0	5.3*	5.4*
5.3	6.5	3.6*	3.6*
2.3	6.4	6.3	3.7*
0.8	2.3	2.4	2.2

* Means found to be significantly different from 0 concentration control ($P < 0.05$).

lymphoblasts for less than 6 h resulted in no cytotoxic effects upon these cells in vitro. However, the quantitative cytotoxicity effect on L-1210 cells was directly correlated with the incubation time between 8 and 16 h. This cytotoxic effect was maximal after 16 h incubation, almost one complete cell cycle (Skipper et al., 1967). One interpretation of these results would be that lymphocytotoxicity for leukemic cells was specific for the G_1 phase of the cell cycle. If lymphocyte chalone concentration was maintained during this cycle, cells in S, G_2, and M phases eventually would enter the G_1 phase where they would be arrested and killed prior to S phase.

Perhaps the most important difference between crowded and sparse cultures is that most of the cells in sparse cultures are continually passing through their mitotic cycle, i.e., these cultures contained a large fraction of actively growing cells. Since DNA-specific inhibitors of replication act by interfering with cells in the S phase of the cell cycle, this large growth fraction makes these cells highly susceptible to the killing effects of such drugs as cytosine arabinoside and methotrexate (Hryniuk et al., 1969; Clarkson, 1974). Under crowded culture conditions, in contrast, a much smaller fraction of these cells are actively growing and the leukemic cell becomes much less susceptible to S phase-specific drugs (Skipper et al., 1967). Therefore, the predominant portion of these cells, being in the G_1 phase of their mitotic cycle, would presumably be most vulnerable to lymphocytic chalone.

Since many chemotherapeutic agents are most active against rapidly growing cells (Hryniuk et al., 1969; Clarkson, 1974) but not against dormant tumor cells, this finding (Attallah and Houck, 1975) of a leukemia-specific cytotoxicity for the more slowly growing crowded cell cultures (G_0 or G_1) appears to be of considerable interest, particularly since thymus-derived lymphocyte chalone cytotoxicity appears to be specific for T versus B cell-established cell lines of human lymphoblasts.

Perhaps it might be possible to introduce large amounts of the lymphocyte chalone in vivo which would arrest both normal and tumor cells in the G_1 phase of their mitotic cycle. Since lymphocyte chalone seems specifically cytotoxic for leukemic lymphocytes in their dormant state ($G_1 - G_0$), this might result in the death of a large number of these cells. A partial reduction of this in vivo concentration of lymphocyte chalone would release the 'killing resistant' leukemic cells from their G_1 inhibition and they would, in a synchronized fashion, march into S phase. At this point in their cell cycle, they would be enormously vulnerable to the various kinds of S phase chemotherapeutic agents currently used. The reduction of the in vivo concentration of the chalone would not be sufficient, however, to release the normal cell from its G_1 inhibition. Therefore, the proliferation of normal

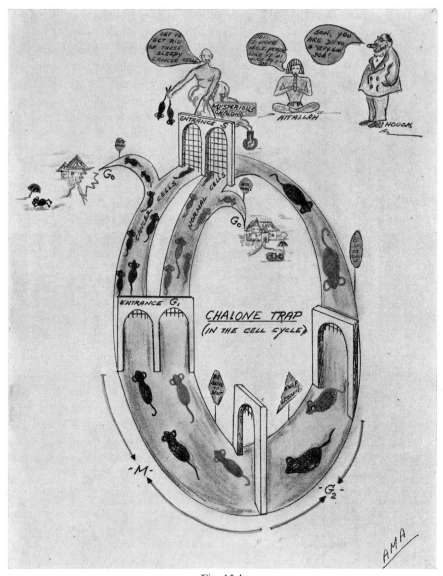

Fig. 15.4

lymphocytes would continue to be inhibited but without any cytotoxic effects from chalone and they would be protected from the cytotoxic effects of the appropriate chemotherapeutic agent.

If the fraction of all leukemic cells in the vulnerable portion of the G_1 phase is less than 100% at any given time and if cytotoxic levels of chalone were maintained for much less than the duration of a complete cell cycle, then the cytotoxic effects of a single dose of lymphocyte chalone might be expected to be suboptimal. We would expect multiple, shortly spaced doses of lymphocyte chalone to be more effective than a single dose regimen.

15.9 Proposed mechanism

Recently, Hauschka et al. (1972) have indicated that cyclic AMP is capable of significantly inhibiting the uptake of [^{3}H]thymidine into the acid in- soluble DNA fraction of Chang hamster ovary (CHO) fibroblast-like cells. They have found that this cyclic AMP inhibition of thymidine uptake by these cells was mediated through the inhibition of nucleoside kinase activity intracellularly. This inhibition of nucleoside kinase activity was not associated with an inhibition of the proliferative rates of these cells in vitro. Therefore, for at least two population doublings, the proliferative rate of CHO cells was essentially normal in the presence of sufficient amounts of dibutyryl

Table 15.10

The effects of various doses of spleen chalone concentrate, dibutyryl cyclic AMP, or cytosine arabinoside on the PHA stimulation of 10^6 human lymphocytes, as measured by [^{3}H]thymidine incorporation into trichloracetic acid soluble (DNA precursor) and insoluble (macromolecular DNA) fractions.

	% decrease in radioactive counts compared w/PHA-stimulated lymphocytes	
	Acid soluble	Acid insoluble
Spleen chalone μg/ml		
25	95	100
20	89	98
10	69	70
Cyclic AMP		
2×10^{-4} M	47	60
1×10^{-4} M	26	34
5×10^{-5} M	15	4*
2×10^{-5} M	6*	0*
Cytosine arabinoside		
5×10^{-6} M	4*	47
2×10^{-6} M	0	27
1×10^{-6} M	0	25
0.1×10^{-6} M	0	10*

* Not significantly inhibited ($P < 0.05$).

cyclic AMP to give a profound inhibition of the uptake of [^{3}H]TdR into acid insoluble radioactive counts or DNA. This finding appears similar to that of Garcia-Giralt et al. (1974) for chalone inhibition of L-1210 DNA synthesis.

The effects of various concentrations of spleen-derived lymphocyte chalone concentrate, dibutyryl cyclic AMP, and various non-cytotoxic doses of cytosine arabinoside (Chu and Fischer, 1962) upon the percent reduction of both acid soluble and acid insoluble [^{3}H]TdR counts per minute per million lymphocytes in culture is shown in table 15.10. These results demonstrate an essentially parallel inhibition of both acid soluble and acid insoluble [^{3}H]TdR in proportion to the concentration of either spleen-derived chalone or dibutyryl cyclic AMP. Similar inhibition of the incorporation of [^{3}H]TdR into acid insoluble DNA during the lectin-stimulated transformation of lymphocytes in vitro by cytosine arabinoside was not associated with a reduced amount of radioactivity in the intra-cellular acid soluble DNA precursor pool, however. Since cyclic AMP has been shown to be capable of inhibiting the nucleoside kinase activity of CHO fibroblasts in vitro and hence DNA synthesis, it is tempting to conclude that lymphocyte chalone exerts its inhibitory effect on DNA synthesis through a cyclic AMP-mediated inhibition of nucleoside kinases.

Peripheral human lymphocytes were mixed with PHA and spleen chalone extract added at various times after the start of the incubation. We have

Table 15.11

The inhibitory effects from different combinations of lymphocyte chalone and Db cAMP upon the incorporation of [^{3}H]thymidine into DNA by PHA-stimulated human lympho-cytes and by NC-37 human lymphoblasts in vitro.

Cell type	Spleen sieved (30,000–50,000)	Db cAMP*	% inhibition of [^{3}H]TdR uptake**
Normal human lymphocytes	50 μg/ml	10^{-4} M	65
	50 μg/ml	10^{-5} M	59
	50 μg/ml	5 × 10^{-6} M	74
	100 μg/ml	10^{-4} M	97
	50 μg/ml	10^{-4} M	65
	25 μg/ml	10^{-4} M	8

 * Dibutyryl cyclic AMP.
** Each number is the mean of triplicate determination.

been able to show that there is a linear fall off with time in the inhibition of PHA-induced stimulation. As DNA synthesis requires the continuous recruitment of nucleoside precursors, it is tempting to speculate that the chalone shuts off the supply of precursors for macromolecular synthesis at some stage before the incorporation of deoxynucleoside triphosphates into DNA, but this would still allow the completion of DNA synthesis from the triphosphate pool formed prior to chalone addition.

The data in table 15.11, when both cyclic AMP and chalone were given together to PHA-stimulated lymphocytes, indicate that there was no synergism of chalone and nucleotide effects but, rather, that the inhibition of stimulation was dependent solely on the concentration of chalone present. We may therefore speculate that once the chalone has acted on the cell, the cell surface and/or phosphodiasterase system are changed in such a way that they will not respond further to exogenous cyclic AMP.

Theophylline is known to inhibit lymphocyte transformation (Smith et al., 1971). Several dose combinations of lymphocyte chalone and theophylline were added to PHA-stimulated lymphocytes for 72 h. [^{3}H]TdR uptake into acid insoluble macromolecules was counted. Our results have shown that there was a synergism of chalone and theophylline inhibition of PHA transformation of normal human lymphocytes. The above results could be due to the elevation of intracellular cyclic AMP after the stimulation of its synthesis by chalone and theophylline inhibition of subsequent cyclic AMP degradation by phosphodiasterases.

Baserga (1965) has indicated the possibility that the initiation of DNA biosynthesis may be preceded by the synthesis of specific RNA and proteins. The concentration of such enzymes as thymidine kinase and DNA polymerase would increase only at the time DNA synthesis begins. We have found that the inhibition of DNA synthesis by chalone had not occurred within the shortest incubation time measured (5 h); however, protein synthesis was depressed by this time and this inhibition was followed by an inhibition of RNA and DNA synthesis at 17 and 48 h respectively.

Normal human lymphocytes were incubated with lymphocyte chalone and cyclohexamine separately for 6 h in the period between 6 and 12 h after PHA stimulation. Protein synthesis in these cells was inhibited by cyclohexamide but not by lymphocyte chalone during this period. Lymphocyte chalone, cyclohexamide, and cytosine arabinoside all demonstrated an inhibition of DNA synthesis of PHA-stimulated normal human lymphocytes between the period of 18 to 24 h after the addition of the lectin. During this period, protein synthesis was inhibited by lymphocyte chalone and by cyclohexamide but not by cytosine arabinoside. These results suggest that chalone could be inhibiting the synthesis of certain enzymes essential to DNA synthesis (thymidine kinase?).

These observations lead us to tentatively suggest a possible mechanism of action for the lymphocyte chalone in vitro: namely, that the presence of chalone maintains a high level of activity of plasma membrane adenyl cyclase sufficient to ensure a relatively high intracellular concentration of cyclic AMP. As a consequence of this cyclic AMP concentration, a long-term inhibition of nucleoside kinase activity may well be produced, as in the CHO fibroblast (Hauschka et al., 1972). In the absence of nucleoside kinase activity, little DNA synthesis would be possible to these diploid human lymphocytes in culture and, as a consequence, their proliferation would be profoundly inhibited. The proliferation of heteroploid lymphocytes might not be initially inhibited, however, since much of the redundant DNA synthesis in these cells might not be required for mitosis and unless this inhibition of DNA synthesis was complete, these cells could continue to divide.

References

Attallah, A. M. (1974) Partial purification and characterization of lymphocyte chalone. Ph. D. Thesis, George Washington University.

Attallah, A. M., Sunshine, G., Hunt, C. V. and Houck, J. C. (1975) The specific and endogenous mitotic inhibitor of lymphocytes (chalone). Exp. Cell Res., 93, 283.

Attallah, A. M. (1975) Growth regulation theories and the chalone concept: a review. II. Lymphocytes. Clin. Proc. Children's Hosp. 31, 108.

Attallah, A. M. (1975) Chalones and Cancer: a review. Clin. Proc. Children's Hosp. Nat. Med. Ctr., 31, 215.

Attallah, A. M. and Houck, J. C. (1975) Lymphocyte chalone concentrates and their effects upon leukemic cells in vitro. Proc. Internatl. Symp. Hemat., Milan, in press.

Baserga, R. (1965) The relationship of the cell cycle to tumor growth and control of cell division: a review. Cancer Res. 25, 581.

Boyum, A. (1968) Isolation of mononuclear cells and granulocytes from human blood. Isolation of mononuclear cells by one centrifugation and of granulocytes by combining centrifugation and sedimentation at 1 G. Scand. J. Clin. Lab. Invest. 21, Suppl. 97, 77.

Bullough, W. S. and Laurence, E. B. (1964) Mitotic control by internal secretions: the role of the chalone-adrenalin complex. Exp. Cell Res. 33, 176.

Chu, M. Y. and Fischer, G. A. (1962) A proposed mechanism of action of 1-B-D-arabino-furanosyl-cytosine as an inhibitor of the growth of leukemic cells. Biochem. Pharmacol. 11, 423.

Chung, A. C. and Hufnagel, C. A. (1973) Some in vivo effects of chalone (mitotic inhibitor) obtained from lymphoid tissue. Natl. Cancer Inst. Monogr. 38, 131.

Clarkson, B. D. (1972) Acute myelocytic leukemia in adults. Cancer 30, 1572.

Clarkson, B. D. (1974) The survival of the dormant state in neoplastic and normal cell populations, in Control of Proliferation in Animal Cells (eds.: B. Clarkson and R. Baserga) Cold Spring Harbor Laboratory, New York, pp. 945–973.

Diddi, M. G., Lonngi, G., Gonzales, C. R. and Gallegos, A. J. (1974) The influence of thymidine on the blastoid transformation of human lymphocytes. Proc. Exp. Biol. Med. 145, 958.

Dutton, R. W., Falkoff, R., Hirst, J. A., Hoffman, M., et al. (1971) Is there evidence for a non-antigen-specific diffusable chemical mediator from the thymus-derived cell in the initiation of the immune response?, in: Progress in Immunology (ed.: B. Amos) Academic Press, New York, pp. 355–381.

Durant, J. R. and Smally, R. V. (1972) The Chronic Leukemia. Charles C. Thomas, Springfield, Illinois.

Elves, M. W. (1972) The Lymphocytes. Year Book Medical Publisher, Chicago.

Fishman, M. and Adler, F. L. (1968) The role of macrophage RNA in the immune response. Symp. Quant. Biol. 32, 343.

Florentin, I., Kiger, N. and Mathe, G. (1973) T lymphocyte specificity of a lymphocyte inhibiting factor (chalone) extracted from the thymus. Europ. J. Immunol. 3, 624.

Garcia-Giralt, E., Lasalvia, E., Florentin, I. and Mathe, G. (1970) Evidence for a lymphocyte chalone. Eur. J. Clin. Biol. Res. 15, 1012.

Garcia-Giralt, E., Morales, H., Lasalvia, E. and Mathe, G. (1972) Suppression of graft-versus-host reaction by spleen extract. J. Immunol. 109, 878.

Garcia-Giralt, E., Rella, W., Morales, V. H., Diaz-Rubio, E. and Richard, F. (1973) Extraction from bovine spleen of immunosuppressant with no activity on hematopoietic spleen colony formation. Natl. Cancer Inst. Monogr. 38, 125.

Garcia-Giralt, E. and Macieira-Coelho, A. (1974) Differential effect of a lymphoid chalone on the target and nontarget cells in vitro, in Lymphocyte Recognition and Effector Mechanisms (eds.: K. Lindahl-Kiessling and D. Osobu) Academic Press, New York, pp. 457–474.

Garcia-Giralt, E., Diatloff, C. and Macieiro-Coelho, A. (1974) Differential inhibition of cell division by a spleen extract on normal lymphocytes and on established lymphoblastic cell lines. Ninth Leukocyte Culture Conference Program, Abstract No. 82, p. 38.

Gorer, P. A. (1960) The isoantigens of malignant cells, in Biological Approaches to Cancer Chemotherapy (ed.: R. J. C. Harris) Academic Press, London, pp. 219–230.

Greaves, M. F. and Hogg, N. M. (1971) Antigen binding sites on mouse lymphoid cells, in Cell Interactions in Immune Responses (eds.: A. Cross, T. Kosunen and O. Makela). Third Sigrid Juselius Foundation Symposium. Academic Press, New York and London.

Hauschka, P. V., Everhart, L. P. and Rubin, R. W. (1972) Alteration of nucleoside transport of Chinese hamster cells by dibutyryl adenosine $3':5'$-cyclic monophosphate. Proc. Nat. Acad. Sci. U.S. 69, 3542.

Houck, J. C., Irausquin, H. and Leikin, S. (1971) Lymphocyte DNA synthesis inhibition. Science 173, 1139.

Houck, J. C. and Cheng, R. F. (1973) Isolation, purification, and chemical characterization of the serum mitogen for diploid human fibroblasts. J. Cell. Physiol. 81, 257.

Houck, J. C., Attallah, A. M. and Lilly, J. R. (1973) Some immunosuppressive properties of lymphocyte chalone. Nature 245, 148.

Houck, J. C., Cheng, R. F. and Sharma, V. K. (1973) Control of fibroblast proliferation. Natl. Cancer Inst. Monogr. 38, 161.

Hryniuk, W. M., Fischer, G. A. and Bertino, J. R. (1969) S phase cells of rapidly growing and resting populations. Differences in response to methotrexate. Mol. Pharmacol. 5, 557.

Jones, J., Paraskova-Tchernozenska, E. and Moorhead, J. (1970) In vitro inhibition of DNA synthesis in human leukemic cells by a lymphoid cell extract. Lancet, March 28, 654.

Karush, F. (1962) Immunologic specificity and molecular structure. Adv. Immunol. 2, 1.

Kiger, N. (1971) Isolation and immunological study of thymic lymphocytic inhibitory factors. Europ. J. Clin. Biol. Res. 16, 566.

Kiger, N., Florentin, I. and Mathe, G. (1973) A lymphocyte inhibiting factor (chalone?) extracted from thymus: immunosuppressive effects. Natl. Cancer Inst. Monogr. 38, 135.

Lawrence, H. S. and Landy, M. (Eds.) (1969) Mediators of Cellular Immunity. Proceedings of an International Conference, Augusta Michigan. Academic Press, New York.

Lord, B., Cercek, L., Cercek, B., Shah, G., Dexter, T. and Lajtha, L. (1974) Inhibitors of hemopoietic cell proliferation?: specificity of action within the hemopoietic system. Brit. J. Cancer 29, 168.

Makela, O. and Cross, A. M. (1970) The diversity and specialization of immunocytes, Progr. Allerg. 14, 145.

Miller, J. F. and Mitchell, G. F. (1970) Cell-to-cell interaction in the immune response. V. Target cells for tolerance induction. J. Exp. Med. 131, 675.

Mills, J. A. and Cooperband, S. R. (1971) Lymphocyte physiology. Ann. Rev. Med. 22, 185.

Minowada, J., Ohnuma, T. and Moore, G. E. (1973) Rosette-forming human lymphoid cell lines. I. Establishment and evidence for origin of thymus-derived lymphocytes. J. Nat. Cancer Inst. 49, 891.

Moorhead, J. F., Paraskova-Tchernozenska, E., Pirrie, A. J. and Hayes, C. (1969), Lymphoid inhibitor of human lymphocyte DNA synthesis and mitosis in vitro. Nature 224, 1207.

Newberger, P., Hamaoka, T. and Katz, D. (1974) Potentiation of helper cell function in IgE antibody responses by bacterial lipolysaccharide (LPS). J. Immunol. 113, 824.

Pattengale, P. K., Smith, R. W. and Gerber, P. (1973) Selective transformation of B lymphocytes by EB virus. Lancet, July 14, 93.

Peavy, D. L., Adler, W. H. and Smith, R. T. (1970) The mitogenic effects of endotoxin and staphylococcal endotoxin B on mouse spleen cells and human peripheral lymphocytes. J. Immunol. 105, 1453.

Raff, M. C. (1973) T and B lymphocytes and immune responses. Nature 242, 19.

Ratnoff, O. D. (1969) Some relationships between hemostasis, fibrinolytic phenomena immunity, and the inflammatory response. Adv. Immunol. 10, 146.

Roelants, G. (1972) Antigen recognition by B and T lymphocytes. Curr. Topics Microbiol. Immunol. 59, 135.

Roitt, I. M., Greeves, M. F., Torrigiani, G., Brostaff, J. and Playfair, J. H. L. (1969) The cellular basis of immunological responses: a synthesis of some current views. Lancet 2, 367.

Skipper, H. E., Schnabel, F. M. and Willcox, W. S. (1967) Experimental evaluation of potential anticancer agents. XXI. Scheduling of arabinosylcytosine to take advantage of its S phase specificity against leukemia cells. Cancer Chemotherapy Reports 51, 125.

Smith, J. W., Steiner, A. L. and Parker, C. W. (1971) Human lymphocyte metabolism. Effects of cyclic and noncyclic nucleotides on stimulation by phytohemagglutinin. J. Clin. Invest. 50, 442.

Trainin, N. and Resnitzky, P. (1969) Influence of neonatal thymectomy on cloning capacity of bone marrow cells in mice. Nature 221, 1154.

CHAPTER 16

The in vivo effects of lymphoid chalone(s) and its immunosuppressive properties

ANTHONY C. CHUNG

Surgical Research Laboratory, Georgetown University Medical Center,
Washington, D. C. 20007, U.S.A.

16.1 Introduction

The immunosuppressive potentials of lymphocytic chalone(s) became apparent once Moorhead et al. (1969) and Jones et al. (1970) had reported that aqueous extracts of pig lymph nodes could inhibit the DNA synthesis and mitosis induced in vitro by phytohemagglutinin (PHA) in human lymphocytes. These observations were later extended to aqueous extracts of human lymphocytes, bovine spleen (Lasalvia et al., 1970), and thymus (Kiger, 1971). Similar effects were also observed in extracts of lymphoid tissues of rat, canine, rabbit, and guinea pig (Houck and Irausquin, 1973; Attallah et al., 1975). The action of lymphocytic chalone(s) is being reviewed extensively elsewhere. The following review will mainly be confined to the in vivo studies of lymphoid chalone and its various immunological actions.

16.2 Effects of lymphoid chalone observed in vivo

Garcia-Giralt et al. (1970) investigated the effect of a partially purified bovine spleen extract (alcohol fractionation) on DNA synthesis in spleen, bone marrow, intestine, liver, and kidney of mice. In animals received 0.05 mg/g body weight of bovine spleen chalone, the incorporation of $[^3H]TdR$ into spleen DNA was decreased to 68% of the control animals. No inhibition was observed in other organs. For animals received 0.1 mg/g body weight, the $[^3H]TdR$ incorporation rate was 49.5% for spleen and 92% for intestine as compared to respective controls.

Chung and Hufnagel (1973) reported the inhibitory effect of partially purified extracts of rabbit thymus and pig lymph nodes (molecular sieving 30,000–50,000 daltons) on thymus growth in neonatal rabbits. Neonatal rabbits (24–36 h) were given daily i.p. injection (300–350 μg/animal) of partially purified chalone from rabbit thymus or pig lymph nodes daily for 5 days, and control animals received saline. All animals were sacrificed on the 6th day. When thymus growth index was expressed as mg of thymus per g body wt, the inhibitory effect was quite evident (see table 16.1).

Studies recently carried out in our laboratory indicated that the i.p. administration in mice of partially purified chalones (30,000–50,000 daltons) from either calf thymus or bovine spleen resulted in a significant depression of circulating lymphocytes and that the effect appeared to be transient. Initial blood samples (0.05–0.08 ml) were obtained from venous plexus of orbit of mice (C57BL/6). Three blood smears were made on slides for differential cell counts and total leukocyte counts were made, using standard clinical leukocyte diluting pipets, and counted in Neubauer counting chambers. The differentials were counted on smears stained with Wright stain, counting 100 cells on each of two different slides per animal. Immediately after the initial blood samples had been taken, the mice were given

Table 16.1

Inhibition of thymus growth in neonatal rabbits by lymphoid chalones.

Treatment	Thymic growth index (mg thymus/g body wt)	
	Experimental	Control
Crude extract of rabbit	1.871	3.0
thymus 3.5 mg/animal/day	1.023	2.954
Partially purified rabbit	1.319	2.434
thymus extract (30,000–50,000	1.563	2.211
daltons) 350 μg/animal/day		
Partially purified extract from	1.554	2.769
pig lymph nodes (30,000–50,000	1.792	2.274
daltons) 300 μg/animal/day	1.524	1.824
	1.887	2.070
	1.668	1.992
	1.269	1.520
	1.166	2.770
		2.713
Mean + S.D.	1.512 $\pm$ 0.286*	2.377 $\pm$ 0.472

* Significantly different from control ($P < 0.01$).

Table 16.2

Mean ± S.D. of percent change in mouse circulating lymphocytes and neutrophils after i.p. injection of 0.1 ml (100 μg) of partially purified chalone (30,000–50,000 daltons) from calf thymus.

Time after injection (h)	Number of animals		Circulating lymphocytes percent of initial level		Circulating neutrophils percent of initial level	
	Experimental	Control	Experimental	Control	Experimental	Control
2	6	6	83.8±22.8	99.3±30.5	307±131**	352±221**
4	5	6	42.2±19.1*	93.8±12.0	175± 89.0	201± 93.3
6	5	6	49.6±20.4*	102.0±23.6	218±126	206± 87.4
24	5	6	92.0±19.2	87.4±16.2	144± 98.0	106± 71.1

  * Significantly different from control $P < 0.01$.
** Significantly different from respective 24 h levels $P < 0.05$.

i.p. 0.1 ml (100 μg) of partially purified calf thymus chalone. One group was sampled at the end of 2 h and other groups at 4, 6, and 24 h respectively after injection. Control groups were given the same material inactivated at 70 °C for 1 h.

Results indicated that no significant depression in circulating lymphocytes was observed within 2 h after injection and that there were significant depressions at 4 and 6 h after injection. No significant difference between the depressed levels of circulating lymphocytes at 4 and 6 h was observed. The circulating lymphocytes returned essentially to the initial level within 24 h after injection (table 16.2). The i.p. injection of either the active thymic chalone or inactivated control appeared to cause a transient elevation of circulating neutrophils 2 h after injection. Only the levels of circulating neutrophils at 2 h after injection were significantly higher when compared to the respective 24 h levels $P < 0.05$ (table 16.2). The thymic chalone used in this study showed a 74% depression of [³H]TdR uptake by human lymphocytes stimulated by PHA in the in vitro assay system at a concentration of 100 μg/ml (Leikin and Oppenheim, 1970).

Similar effect on circulating lymphocytes was also demonstrated with a partially purified bovine spleen chalone (30,000–50,000 daltons). Groups of mice (C57BL/6) were injected i.p. with 0.1 ml containing 10, 50, 100, or 200 μg of spleen chalone per mouse respectively resulted in marked depression of circulating lymphocytes 6 h after injection. The lymphocyte depressive effect appeared to be dose-dependent, and the effect seemed to

Table 16.3

Mean ± S.D. of percent change in circulating total leukocytes, lymphocytes, and neutrophils at 6 h after i.p. injection of 0.1 ml of bovine spleen chalone in mice (C57BL/6).

Chalone dose per mouse	No. of animals	Percent of initial value		
		Leukocytes	Lymphocytes	Neutrophils
10 μg	6	66.7±35.9	59.2±32.8	116± 68.9
50 μg	6	49.4±35.6*	34.7±26.1*	122± 65.4
100 μg	8	34.8±26.2	30.1±17.4*	208±141
200 μg	6	47.8±27.1	32.0±17.4	165±111
Control with inactivated chalone (70°C, 1 h)				
10 μg	6	99.1±23.1	95.6±23.5	128± 48.9
50 μg	5	128.0±39.5	126.0±35.3	165±120
100 μg	7	112.0±34.5	109.0±33.5	155±110

* Significantly different from respective control $P < 0.01$.

level off between 100 and 200 μg of spleen chalone per mouse (table 16.3). The spleen chalone used for this study showed an 85% depression of [^{3}H] TdR uptake by human lymphocytes stimulated by PHA in the in vitro assay system at a chalone concentration of 100 μg/ml.

The intravenous administration of 0.1 ml (100 μg) of spleen chalone to mice through tail vein produced the same effect on circulating lymphocytes as i.p. injection. The circulating lymphocytes were reduced to 35.5 ± 18.9% of the initial value 6 h after i.v. injection as compared to 30.1 ± 17.4% of initial value 6 h after i.p. injections.

Thus it appears that the administration of lymphoid chalones in mice elicits a specific though transient effect on circulating lymphocytes. It is unlikely that this effect is due to cytotoxicity since these chalone preparations did not show cytotoxicity when tested in vitro (vital dye exclusion). The effect on circulating lymphocyte counts due to specific cytotoxicity have been demonstrated in mice by Tursi et al. (1969) with anti-lymphocytic globulin injections which caused an immediate fall in circulating lymphocyte count to between 10 and 70% of its normal level. The lymphocyte counts gradually returned to normal by 2–3 weeks. The effect of lymphoid chalones on circulating lymphocyte count could not be due to specific inhibition of mitosis of lymphocytes because if it were, the maximal effect cannot be expected to be observed as early as 4 h after chalone injection. It would appear more likely that the circulating lymphocytes reacted with chalone which resulted in the transient sequestering of these lymphocytes in the lymphoid system.

Since the effect of lymphoid chalones on mice circulating lymphocyte count is dose-dependent, it is feasible to use this as an in vivo assay for preparations of lymphoid chalones. However, it is important to rule out other factors that may cause peripheral lymphocyte counts to drop. Considering that there is no in vivo assay for lymphoid chalone available at the present time, the method described above appeared to be promising.

16.3 The immunological effects of lymphoid chalones

16.3.1 Effect of lymphoid chalone on the immune response of mice to sheep red blood cells (SRBC)

Garcia-Giralt et al. (1970) demonstrated in mice that 4 daily i.v. injections of partially purified spleen chalone (alcohol fractionation) following the injection of SRBC caused a significant decrease in the number of antibody-forming cells in their spleen as compared to the control groups, one of which received bovine serum albumin instead of chalone, the other groups receiving only SRBC.

Later, Florentin et al. (1973) reported similar inhibitory effect of a partially purified chalone (alcohol fractionation) extracted from calf thymus upon the immune response of mice against SRBC. It was observed that 4 days after SRBC immunization the number of direct plaque-forming cells per spleen were significantly lowered in the group of mice treated with thymic chalone, as compared to the groups that received kidney extract ($P < 0.05$) or SRBC alone ($P < 0.02$) respectively. The results seem to indicate that this inhibitory effect of thymic chalone was not due to a non-specific action such as antigenic competition, since the simultaneous injection of kidney extract and SRBC did not change the magnitude of response to the antigen, SRBC.

16.3.2 Effect of lymphoid chalones on graft-versus-host reaction (GVHR)

The suppression of GVHR in mice by partially purified spleen chalone was first reported by Garcia-Giralt et al. (1970). The GVHR was induced by i.p. injection of parental bone marrow and lymph node (LN) cells into sublethally X-ray irradiated F_1 hybrid mice. The parental LN cells were either obtained from parental mice treated with daily i.p. injections of 6 mg of partially purified spleen chalone for 4 days or from mice treated identically with heat-inactivated spleen chalone or from untreated mice. These results indicated that the 30-day survival in F_1 mice having received LN cells from donors treated with spleen chalone was significantly better than from untreated donors or donors treated with heat-inactivated spleen chalone.

These results also indicated that spleen chalone did not influence the engraftment capacity of bone marrow (BM) stem cells as shown by the ability of BM cells from chalone-treated mice to produce colonies in lethally irradiated mice. The number of colonies observed 9 days after administration was not significantly different from the number of colonies observed with BM cells from untreated donors. Furthermore, no significant difference in the number of colonies was observed among lethally irradiated recipients given injection of normal BM cells as compared to those subsequently treated with 6 mg per day of spleen chalone from day 5 to day 9 after irradiation or in control recipient mice given saline for the same period (Garcia-Giralt et al., 1973).

In another study of GVHR, Garcia-Giralt et al. (1972) found that when the F_1 recipient mice were treated with spleen chalone plus rabbit anti-mouse-antilymphocyte serum (ALS), they showed a significantly improved survival at 60 days as compared to F_1 mice given either spleen chalone or ALS alone ($P < 0.001$).

The incubation of parental donor spleen cells in vitro with spleen chalone for 1 h at $37\,^{\circ}C$ before injecting into the F_1 recipients also resulted in significant suppression of GVHR as measured by mortality (Kiger et al., 1973).

Kiger et al. (1972) have demonstrated in mice that pretreatment of the parental donor with partially purified thymus chalone (alcohol fractionation and DEAE-Sephadex A-50 column) suppressed the capacity of spleen cells obtained from these donors to elicit GVHR in hybrid F_1 recipients. The GVHR was estimated from the splenomegally observed 14 days after the cells were injected.

The incubation of parental mice spleen cells in vitro with thymus chalone decreased the capacity of these cells to induce GVHR when injected into F_1 hybrid recipients. The inhibition was demonstrated by mortality (Kiger et al., 1972, 1973a) and also by local GVH assay expressed as lymph node index. The incubation of spleen cells with thymus chalone did not alter colony-forming unit as compared to the control (Kiger et al., 1973b).

16.3.3 Effect of lymphoid chalone on skin graft rejection

Kiger et al. (1972) reported a moderate increase in skin allograft survival time when recipient mice were given repeated injections of partially purified thymus chalone (alcohol fractionation). Recipients received 7 mg of chalone per day on days -1, $+1$, 4, 6, 7, 11, 13, 15, and 19. Skin grafting was performed on day 0.

A more substantial delay in skin allograft rejection by spleen chalone (partially purified by molecular sieving, fraction 30,000–50,000 daltons) was reported by Houck et al. (1973). The recipient mice (C57BL/6) were given 5 mg per mouse 3 times per week. The administration of chalone i.p. was started on the day of grafting and donor skin was obtained from C3H mice. The mean survival time for the control was 10.5 ± 1 days as compared to 29 ± 2 days for the group treated with chalone ($P < 0.01$).

A substantial delay in skin xenograft rejection time was reported by Chung and Hufnagel (1973) when recipient mice were repeatedly treated with partially purified lymphoid chalones (molecular sieving 30,000–50,000 daltons). Donor skin was obtained from rabbits and the mean skin xenograft survival time for the treated animals was 12.1 ± 3.5 (S.D.) days as compared to the mean survival time of the control group, 6.2 ± 1.2 (S.D.) days ($P < 0.001$).

16.4 The question of specificity of thymus and spleen chalone on T and B lymphocytes

Both spleen and thymus chalones have been shown to suppress the following immune reactions: graft-versus-host reaction (Garcia-Giralt et al., 1970, 1972, 1973; Kiger et al., 1973a, 1973b), skin graft rejection (Kiger et al., 1973b; Chung and Hufnagel, 1973; Houck et al., 1973), and phytohemagglutinin-induced lymphocyte transformation. In these cellular immune responses, mainly thymus-derived lymphocytes are involved. However, both chalones have been shown to suppress antibody formation against SRBC, which is considered to be mainly the function of non-thymus-derived lymphocytes (B lymphocytes) with the collaboration of T lymphocytes (Kiger, 1971; Garcia-Giralt et al., 1970).

The recent study by Florentin et al. (1973) has shed some light on the specificity of thymic chalone on T lymphocytes. The effect of thymic chalone on the immune responses of mice against the following antigens, dinitrophenylated human IgG (DNP-HGG), SRBC and dinitrophenylated polymerized flagellin (DNP-POL), were investigated. It was demonstrated that the administration of thymic chalone did not suppress the IgM antibody formation against DNP-POL. The immune response against DNP-POL has been shown to be independent of T lymphocytes (Feldmann and Basten,

1971). In contrast, the administration of thymic chalone markedly suppressed the IgG antibody formation against DNP-HGG, a response that was highly dependent on T lymphocytes. Thymic chalone administration moderately suppressed the IgM antibody formation against SRBC, a response that was only partly dependent on T lymphocytes. These results tend to indicate the existence of T lymphocyte specificity for the thymus chalone.

The spleen contains both T and B lymphocytes, thus it is difficult to ascertain whether chalone extracted from only B lymphocytes would act selectively on B lymphocytes or on both T and B lymphocytes. However, B lymphocytes may be obtained from bursa of Fabricius. Attallah et al. (1975) recently observed that extracts of human diploid B cell lymphoblasts from the established pure cell line NC-37 strongly inhibited the DNA synthesis in both PHA-stimulated human lymphocytes and the spontaneous DNA synthesis of NC-37 cells in vitro. In this case, it appears that extracts from B cell line has inhibited both T and B lymphocytes. However, more information is needed to define the action of extracts from pure B lymphocytes on T and B lymphocytes. The effect of extracts from pure B lymphocytes on the formation of IgM anti-DPN-POL response needs to be investigated.

References

Attallah, A. M., Sunshine, G. H., Hunt, C. V. and Houck, J. C. (1975) The specific mitotic inhibitor of lymphocytes (chalone). Exp. Cell Res., in press.

Chung, A. C. and Hufnagel, C. A. (1973) Some in vivo effects of chalone (mitotic inhibitor) obtained from lymphoid tissues. Natl. Cancer Inst. Monogr. 38, 131.

Feldmann, M. and Basten, A. (1971) The relationship between antigen structure and the requirement for thymus-derived cells in the immune response. J. Exp. Med. 134, 103.

Florentin, I., Kiger, N. and Mathe, G. (1973) T lymphocyte specificity of a lymphocyte-inhibiting factor (chalone) extracted from the thymus. Europ. J. Immunol. 3, 624.

Garcia-Giralt, E., Lasalvia, E., Florentin, I. and Mathe, G. (1970) Evidence for a lympho-cytic chalone. Europ. J. Clin. Biol. Res. 15, 1012.

Garcia-Giralt, E., Morales, V. H., Lasalvia, E. and Mathe, G. (1972) Suppression of graft-versus-host reaction by a spleen extract. J. Immunol. 109, 878.

Garcia-Giralt, E., Rella, W., Morales, V. H., Diaz-Rubio, E. and Richaud, F. (1973) Extraction from bovine spleen of immunosuppressant with no activity on hematopoietic spleen colony formation. Natl. Cancer Inst. Monogr. 38, 125.

Houck, J. C., Attallah, A. M. and Lilly, J. R. (1973) Immunosuppressive properties of the lymphocyte chalone. Nature 245, 148.

Houck, J. C. and Irausquin, H. (1973) Some properties of the lymphocyte chalone. Natl. Cancer Inst. Monogr. 38, 117.

Jones, J., Paraskova-Tchernozenska, E. and Moorhead, J. F. (1970) In vitro inhibition of DNA synthesis in human leukemic cells by a lymphoid cell extract. Lancet 25, 654.

Kiger, N. (1971) Isolation and immunological study of thymic lymphocytic inhibitory factors. Rev. Europ. Etud. Clin. Biol. 16, 566.

Kiger, N., Florentin, I. and Mathe, G. (1972) Some effects of a partially purified lympho-cyte-inhibiting factor from calf thymus. Transplantation 14, 448.

Kiger, N., Florentin, I., Garcia-Giralt, E. and Mathe, G. (1972) Lymphocyte inhibitory factors (chalones) extracted from lymphoid organs. Extraction, partial purification, and immunosuppressive properties. Transplant. Proc. 4, 531.

Kiger, N., Florentin, I., Garcia-Giralt, E. and Mathe, G. (1973) Inhibition of graft-versus-host reaction (GVHR) by in vitro incubation of donor lymphocytes with thymic or splenic chalone(s). Exp. Hemat. 1, 22.

Kiger, N., Florentin, I. and Mathe, G. (1973a) A lymphocyte inhibiting factor (chalone?) extracted from thymus, immunosuppressive effects. Natl. Cancer Inst. Monogr. 38, 135.

Kiger, N., Florentin, I. and Mathe, G. (1973b) Inhibition of graft-versus-host reaction by preincubation of the graft with a thymic extract (lymphocyte chalone). Transplantation 16, 393.

Lasalvia, E., Garcia-Giralt, E. and Macieira-Coelho, A. (1970) Extraction of an inhibitor of DNA synthesis from human peripheral blood lymphocytes and bovine spleen. Europ. J. Clin. Biol. Res. 15, 789.

Moorhead, J. F., Paraskova-Tchernozenska, E., Pirrie, A. J. and Hayes, C. (1969) Lymphoid inhibitor of human lymphocyte DNA synthesis and mitosis in vitro. Nature 224, 1207.

Supported in part by a grant-in-aid from the John A. Hartford Foundation.

CHAPTER 17

Putative bronchial chalone

John C. Houck

Biochemical Research Laboratory, Research Foundation of Children's Hospital,
Washington, D. C. 20009, U.S.A.

Simnett et al. (1969) claimed a tissue-specific inhibition of lung alveolar cell mitosis in organ culture could be demonstrated by adding lung extracts to the culture. In 1973, Giard et al. described the in vitro cultivation of a number of tumors which led to the establishment of cell lines in vitro. Included in these established cell lines were two heteroploid cell lines from two male patients in their 50's who had bronchial carcinoma. We have used one of these, A-427, as our primary system for the determination of the existence of inhibitors of the proliferation of bronchial carcinoma cells in vitro. These cells were cultivated in Dulbecco's modified Eagle's MEM supplemented with 10% heat-inactivated fetal calf serum, penicillin, streptomycin, and glutamine in the appropriate fashion. These cells have proliferated in our laboratory now for about one year at a slow but steady growth rate. The culture doubling time is approximately 96 h, a very slow proliferation rate for human tumor cells. In order to assay quantitatively for the inhibition of proliferation of these cells, 2×10^5 cells would be seeded into duplicate plastic culture flasks containing a total area of 25 cm^2. These flasks would also contain 4 ml of medium. After 24 h, the medium is changed and fresh medium containing the putative chalone concentrate is added. The numbers of cells would be determined, using an inverted microscope and a Whipple eyepiece, by counting two separate areas in each of the flasks. The total number of cells initially counted in this fashion (Raff and Houck, 1969) would average out to about 75–85% of the cells inoculated into the vessel, and over a period of 4 days, this cell number would double. These are very sparse cultures initially and the cells are widely dispersed and attach to the plastic. As the culture becomes more dense, the cells begin to pile up on

each other and defy further cell counting in this nondestructive way, with a
Whipple eyepiece and an inverted microscope.

After 4 days, the cultures were again rinsed and fresh medium containing
no putative chalone concentrate was added. The cultures were maintained
for 4 days more in order to demonstrate that any inhibition that had occurred
was completely reversible. Without exception, this reversibility was found,
even at the highest doses of ultrafiltered extracts used.

Three lung-related extracts were prepared: (1) the 10,000–50,000 dalton
fraction obtained by the ultrafiltration by Amicon Diaflo procedures
(Zipilvan et al., 1969) of aqueous extracts of the acetone powder of cow
lung (20 ml of distilled water was mixed with 1 g of lung powder for a few
minutes in a Waring blender in the cold and allowed to stand overnight at
4 °C); after centrifugation, the clear supernatant was subjected to Amicon
Diaflo ultrafiltration, using a 50,000-dalton exclusion membrane (Zipilvan
et al., 1969). This ultrafiltrate was concentrated on a 10,000-dalton exclusion
membrane and 3 to 4 volumes of water were then washed under nitrogen
pressure through the system on the 10,000-dalton membrane. In this fashion,
an essentially dialyzed ultrafiltrate was obtained which could be lyophilized;
(2) a similarly prepared ultrafiltrate from fresh dog lung: and (3) a similar
ultrafiltrate was obtained from the 'used' medium from the cultivation of
large numbers of bronchial carcinoma cells in vitro. Finally, as a control,
(4) represented a 30,000–50,000 dalton ultrafiltrate from fibroblasts which
have been shown to contain fibroblast inhibitory activity (Houck et al.,
1972, 1973).

Samples (300 μg) of each of these lyophilized ultrafiltrates were added
in duplicate to cultures of human bronchial carcinoma cells. The ultimate
concentration of these materials was 75 μg/ml. The number of cells recorded
per Whipple eyepiece field on two previously marked areas of each flask
at 1, 2, 3, and 4 days after incubation with chalone is recorded in table 17.1.
These numbers, when multiplied by a factor of 2500, give the total number
of cells per vessel, and when multiplied by 100, give the numbers of cells
per cm^2.

The data of table 17.1 indicate that (1) over a course of 96 h cultivation,
the cell number will essentially double in this assay system, (2) extracts,
after ultrafiltration, of the acetone powder of cow lung or from fresh dog
lung all give an essentially similar degree of inhibition of the increase in cell
number appropriate to this period of incubation, (3) the amount of error
in these determinations is reasonably small and it is clear that incubation
with the ultrafiltrates obtained from lung tissue will reduce by two-thirds the
proliferation rate of these cells, (4) incubation with similar amounts of the

Table 17.1

Effects of 75 μg/ml of ultrafiltered aqueous extracts of (I) bovine dessicated and defatted lung, (II) fresh dog lung, (III) 'used' medium from the cultivation of human bronchial carcinoma cells (A-427), and (IV) diploid human fibroblasts (WI-38) upon the proliferation of human bronchial carcinoma cells in vitro, as determined by cell counting in duplicate of duplicate cultures after various times of incubation.

Control I	Cell numbers/field					Increment
	Day 0	Day 1	Day 2	Day 3	Day 4	96 h
1) a	60	71	92	102	121	61
b	58	69	90	106	126	68
2) a	56	65	89	101	122	66
b	59	68	89	100	124	65
					Average	63

	Average increment (96 h)	% inhibition
I bovine lung extract	22	64
II fresh dog lung extract	26	60
III 'used' medium	11	83
IV WI-38 fibroblast extract	65	0

ultrafiltrate from the medium used in the cultivation of large numbers of these cells previously is even more effective in inhibiting the proliferation of human bronchial carcinoma cells, and (5) extracts which have been ultra-filtered in the same way and have been shown to contain fibroblast chalone had essentially no significant effect upon the numbers of cells in these cultures after various days of incubation.

All of these inhibited cultures were then rinsed with fresh medium and reincubated for 96 h more with fresh medium and serum without chalone concentrate. All of these cultures proceeded to proliferate at a rate similar to those described for the uninhibited control cultures.

These same extracts were found to be capable of inhibiting the [³H]-thymidine uptake and proliferation of diploid human fibroblasts in culture; presumably this would reflect the large number of fibroblasts and hence fibroblast chalone found in lung tissues. However, these extracts had absolutely no effect upon the [³H]thymidine uptake by PHA-stimulated lymphocytes or human colon carcinoma cell proliferation in vitro. This inhibitory activity appropriate to human bronchial cells in vitro was destroyed by preincubation with trypsin but not with ribonuclease or DNase.

Similar cultures were incubated with various amount of the ultrafiltrate from bovine lung powder, described above. The proliferation of these bronchial carcinoma cells in vitro was determined by cell counts after 96 h incubation, and the results are presented in table 17.2. The ultrafiltrate concentrations used ranged between 500 and 25 μg/ml. The reproducibility of this assay is seen in the duplication of 125 μg/ml results and the interdigitation of the data between 75 and 50 μg/ml which were done in one experiment with those of 67.5 μg/ml in another experiment may also be seen. The separate experiments are listed as A and B and they were done about two weeks apart. The point is that the assay procedure seems to be reproducible both internally and when replicated at a different time.

The results of table 17.2 indicate a dose dependency between the degree

Table 17.2

Effects of various doses of bovine lung ultrafiltrate upon the number of human bronchial carcinoma cells per field after various times of incubation.

Control II	Cell numbers/field					Increment
	Day 0	Day 1	Day 2	Day 3	Day 4	96 h
1) a	62	74	91	109	129	67
b	58	70	89	106	130	72
2) a	54	68	90	110	124	70
b	59	72	85	104	127	68
					Average	69

	Average increment	% inhibition
500 μg/ml	0	100
250 μg/ml	0	100
125 μg/ml	10	86
125 μg/ml	12	85
75 μg/ml	26	67
67.5 μg/ml	33	52
50 μg/ml	42	46
25 μg/ml	55	28

of inhibition of bronchial cell carcinoma proliferation in vitro and the concentration of the ultrafiltrate from acetone powder of cow lung. At concentrations of 250 $\mu g/ml$, essentially all of the proliferation of human bronchial carcinoma cells in vitro has been inhibited. When the cultures which had been incubated for 96 h with the largest concentrations of ultra-filtrate were rinsed and allowed to reincubate in extract-free medium, their proliferation rates were essentially returned to normal. Further, inspection of these cells which had been allowed to grow on cover slips in medium containing 250 μg of concentrate in a parallel experiment indicated that their morphology was in no way different from that of the uninhibited control cells, and they excluded vital dye (Trypan blue) and clearly were well attached to the glass. Experience with changing pH and other cytotoxic events in these cultures indicated that cells which had become 'sick' will round up and detach from the glass or plastic surface. This behavior has never been noticed for these cells in the presence of ultrafiltered lung extracts in vitro.

All the preliminary data described above suggests that there exists a macromolecule in aqueous extracts of lung which is capable of inhibiting in a non-cytotoxic fashion and in a dose-dependent manner the proliferation of human bronchial carcinoma cells in vitro. This activity was not apparently associated with RNA or DNA but with protein, as judged by the effects of the appropriate hydrolytic enzymes upon this activity in vitro. Some evidence of the cell specificity of this effect is indicated in that these extracts have no effect upon the proliferation or transformation of PHA-stimulated human lymphocytes or human colon carcinoma cells in vitro. Thus, it would seem reasonable to suggest that a species-non-specific but probably cell-specific and non-cytotoxic inhibitor is found endogenously in lung tissue which presumably relates to the number of bronchial cells in that tissue, since similar inhibitory activity of a similar molecular weight is found in pure cultures of bronchial carcinoma cells. This preliminary data, then, suggests that there might be a bronchial chalone which would be capable of affecting the mitotic control of human bronchial carcinoma cells in vitro and perhaps in vivo.

References

Giard, D., Aaronson, S., Todaro, G., Arnstein, P., Kersey, J., Dosik, H. and Parks, W. (1973) In vitro cultivation of human tumor establishment of cell line derived from a series of solid tumors. J. Natl. Cancer Inst. 51, 1417.

Houck, J. C., Weil, R. L. and Sharma, V. K. (1972) Evidence for a fibroblast chalone. Nature New Biol. 240, 210.

Houck, J. C., Sharma, V. K. and Cheng, R. F. (1973) Fibroblast chalone and serum mitogen (anti-chalone). Nature New Biol. 246, 111.

Raff, E. C. and Houck, J. C. (1969) Migration and proliferation of diploid human fibroblasts following 'wounding' of confluent monolayers. J. Cell. Physiol. 74, 235.

Simnett, J., Fisher, J. and Heppleston, A. (1969) Tissue-specific inhibition of lung alveolar cell mitosis in organ culture. Nature 223, 944.

Zipilvan, E. M., Hudson, B. G. and Blatt, W. F. (1969) Separation of immunologically active fragments by membrane partition chromatography. Anal. Biochem. 30, 91.

CHAPTER 18

The control of liver growth

WALTER G. VERLY

Biochimie, Faculté des Sciences, Université de Liège, Belgium

18.1 Liver regeneration

The liver is formed of polyhedral lobules surrounded by connective tissue containing branches of the portal vein and the hepatic artery. The lobule consists of hepatocytes forming trabeculae separated by sinusoid capillaries leading to a central vein; the blood flows from the periphery toward the center of the lobule. In adult liver, only a few hepatocytes, localized in the immediate vicinity of portal vessels, are still dividing. The cellular cycle has a G_1 of 9 h, an S of 9 h, and a $G_2 + M$ of 3–4 h. All the other hepatocytes in the lobule are stationary; they are blocked in G_0.

In the young-adult rat, about 15 h after a subtotal hepatectomy that removes 70% of the liver mass, hepatocytes which were previously blocked in G_0 resume DNA synthesis, i.e. proceed into S. These hepatocytes are localized at the periphery of the lobule. The resumption of DNA synthesis in the hepatocytes propagates as a wave toward the center of the lobule. By 24 h after the operation, 30% of the hepatocytes are in S; this percentage decreases quickly thereafter. The DNA synthesis wave is followed, after a delay of 4–5 h, by a wave of mitoses, which also propagates from the periphery toward the center of the lobule.

There is no regeneration of the removed lobes, but rather a compensatory hyperplasia of the residual lobes. Nearly all the hepatocytes are involved. If, during the 7–8 days needed for the liver to recover a normal mass, radioactive thymidine is given continuously, 95% of the hepatocytes are found to be labelled by autoradiography. During regeneration, most of the hepatocytes divide only once; a few do it twice or, at most, three times (Bucher and Malt, 1971).

When stationary cells (G_0 cells) are stimulated to resume mitosis, one always observes an activation of chromatin resulting in the production of new RNA species and new proteins. One of the first manifestations of liver regeneration, after partial hepatectomy, is an increased synthesis of nuclear RNA (Fujioka et al., 1963). The nucleotide sequences of this newly synthesized high molecular weight RNA differ from those of the RNA found in normal liver (Church and McCarthy, 1967; Mayfield and Bonner, 1972). Simultaneously, chromatin changes can be observed by circular dichroism or ethidium bromide binding; the template activity of the chromatin increases: it has doubled 6 h after the partial hepatectomy. The activated chromatin is much richer in non-histone proteins than the chromatin from the resting cells. Kostraba and Wang (1973), in reconstitution experiments, have shown that it is the non-histone protein fraction of the activated chromatin which is responsible for the production of new RNA species. The activation of chromatin, which is characteristic of the G_0–G_1 transition, is suppressed by cycloheximide, but not by actinomycin D (Baserga, 1974); it probably depends on the synthesis of a non-histone nuclear protein.

It would seem that the initial activation of chromatin by the partial hepatectomy, leads to an alternate synthesis of new RNAs and new non-histone nuclear proteins, which are responsible for the sequential activation of the genes that control the different phases of the mitotic cell cycle. Nearly all cell activities are heightened (see Bucher and Malt, 1971); there is an increase of the cell mass and a considerable enlargement of the poolsize of DNA precursors. A signal is then given to start DNA replication. Mitosis follows a few hours after the end of the S phase.

The nature of the signal which allows the cell to cross the G_1–S border is not yet well understood; its description is often an extrapolation of the known control of DNA replication in bacteria. The chromosome of *Escherichia coli*, when replicating, is attached to the cell membrane at the replication forks and at the initiation point of DNA replication. Maale (1961) has shown that the initiation of the replication of the *E. coli* chromosome depends on the synthesis of proteins: when protein synthesis is inhibited by chloramphenicol, the chromosomes which have undertaken their replication, terminate their replication, but there is no initiation of new replication cycles. The initiation of the replication of the *E. coli* chromosome is under the control of two genes: DNAA and DNAC (Hirota et al., 1970). Because of the high turnover of one of the initiation proteins coded by these genes, the initiation of the chromosome replication is linked to protein synthesis. In absence of protein synthesis, the *E. coli* chromosome, which has terminated its replication, detaches from the cell membrane (Worcel and

Burgi, 1974). In eukaryotic cells, inhibition of protein synthesis by cyclo-heximide prevents the G_1–S transition; it also stops, within 5 min, the DNA synthesis in S cells (Brown et al., 1970). Whereas, in *E. coli* the chromosome is a unique replicon, in eukaryotic cells there are several chromosomes and each of them is formed of numerous replicons; the replicons replicate by groups in an orderly fashion during the S phase of the cellular cycle. By analogy with the known mechanism of the effect of chloramphenicol in bacteria, the action of cycloheximide on DNA replication in eukaryotes could be explained by the requirement of a short-lived protein for the initiation of the replication of each group of replicons. Kumar and Friedman (1972) found, in the cytoplasm of HeLa cells in phase S, a thermolabile factor which stimulates cells in late G_1 to start DNA synthesis. Infante et al. (1973) found that DNA is attached to the internal nuclear membrane only during the S phase, and Yamada and Hanaoka (1973) observed that cyclo-heximide prevents the binding of DNA to the nuclear membrane which occurs at the G_1–S transition; this binding, which might be the starting point of DNA replication, would depend on a short-lived protein (which they called protein M) produced at the end of the G_1 phase.

The control of the preparation to mitosis (G_2 phase) and of mitosis itself (M phase) is not yet understood in molecular terms.

The division cycle thus appears as a concatenated series of events which is activated in some circumstances, and which, in principle, can be inter-rupted at any point. The G_1–S transition however seems particularly sensitive to external influences. But, logically, the control of liver growth or liver regeneration ought to be exerted on the choice between the G_0 and G_1 states. One might suppose that the hepatocyte emerging from a previous cellular division is in the G_0 state, and that it must be reactivated to become a G_1 cell ready to undertake another cellular division cycle. We should like to identify the factors necessary to promote or to stop the G_0–G_1 transition.

18.2 The control of liver regeneration

The hypothesis was made that the changes in the hepatocytes and in the plasma, resulting from the metabolic deficiency of the liver after partial hepatectomy, were responsible for the regeneration of the organ. After a 70% hepatectomy, there is a rapid decrease of the glycogen content of the liver cells, associated with a hormone-dependent mobilization of fat from adipose tissue. This leads to a rise of plasma free fatty acids, an accumulation of neutral fat in the liver remnant (which reaches 10 times the normal concentration 18 h after the operation), with a concomitant elevation of low-density lipoproteins and a decline of high-density lipoproteins in the blood. Some workers have thought that the metabolic overload of the residual liver might be the cause of the liver regeneration. But a continuous infusion of glucose, which prevents the loss of glycogen and the deposition of lipids, does not affect the regeneration of the liver (Simek et al., 1968). A 90% hepatectomy in the rat produces a rise of free fatty acids and amino-acids in the plasma. A 3-h infusion, into a normal rat, of a mixture of triiodo-thyronine, amino acids and factors (heparin, glucagon) which raise the plasma level of free fatty acids, induces in the intact liver, after a delay of 14 h, a synthesis of DNA followed by mitoses (Short et al., 1972). It is, however, doubtful if this observation gives an insight into the regulation of liver growth. No regeneration occurs after a 90% hepatectomy and, if a 70% hepatectomy is followed by a controlled liver regeneration, the changes provoked by the operation in the plasma fatty acids and amino acids are not by themselves sufficient to induce a multiplication of the hepatocytes. It is not the metabolic deficiency of the organ that regulates its regeneration; the metabolic capacity of the liver is never used to its maximum in healthy people.

Many experiments however point to a humoral factor as the cause of liver regeneration.

Repeated removal of blood from normal rats followed by reinjection of a saline suspension of the blood cells produces a dilution of the plasma proteins, but also numerous mitoses in the liver; the organ then shows a striking resemblance to regenerating liver (Glinos and Gey, 1952). Hetero-topic grafts of a liver lobe, preserving the biliary drainage, proliferate after partial hepatectomy of the host; the rates of DNA synthesis and mitosis are almost identical in the graft and the residual liver, and proportional to the extent of hepatectomy (Leong et al., 1964). Liver lobes were grafted to dogs in the neck so that the blood entered the portal vein and left via the hepatic vein (direct flow) or vice-versa (reversed flow); removal of most of the host liver produced a wave of DNA synthesis which started from the periphery of the lobules in grafts with direct flow, but from around the central vein in grafts with reversed flow (Sigel et al., 1968).

Parabiotic rats were studied by Christensen and Jacobsen (1949); they reported that partial hepatectomy of one animal resulted in an increase of hepatic mitoses in the intact partner. Similar experiments were carried out by Fisher et al. (1971). Cross-circulation was established between a normal rat and a freshly hepatectomized rat for 23 h; the rats were then separated, injected intravenously with labelled thymidine, killed after 1 h, and the specific radioactivity of the liver DNA determined. Autoradiographies showed that DNA synthesis occurred only in parenchymal cells. DNA synthesis in the liver of the normal partner increased in proportion to the amount of liver removed from the other animal; the highest stimulation was observed after total hepatectomy. This latter result shows clearly that the stimulation of the intact liver cannot be the consequence of a wound hormone released by the operated organ. On the other hand, DNA synthesis in the remaining liver of the partially hepatectomized animal was lower when it was paired with a rat having an intact liver than when it was left alone.

Goutier et al. (1965) perfused with blood liver lobes taken from rats 2 h after partial hepatectomy. They observed a 15–18-fold increase of nuclear RNA synthesis after a delay of 4–5 h when the blood came from hepatectomized rats, but not when it came from normal rats.

Serum (4 ml) from adult rats, injected intraperitoneally to animals sub-totally hepatectomized 30 h before, decreased to 3‰ the mitotic index taken 15 h later (control value 31‰: Stick and Florian, 1958). The inhibitory effect is of short duration, lasting no more than 24 h. On the contrary, serum taken 24 h after a subtotal hepatectomy increased the mitotic index; this result seemed to be due to a true stimulation of the mitotic rate, rather than to an increase of the duration of mitosis, since the distribution of pro-, meta-, ana- and telo-phases followed the normal pattern.

Glinos and Gey (1952) found that the growth of primary liver explants from 3-weeks old rats was much more stimulated by rat serum taken 24 h after a subtotal hepatectomy than by serum of normal rats. Most often no growth was observed with normal serum unless it was previously diluted. The enhancing effect on growth by dilution of the normal serum was taken as showing the presence of inhibitors of liver growth. Paul et al. (1972) used liver cells from 20-day old rat fetuses; hepatocytes were cultured for 5 days before addition of dialyzed rat serum (10%) and labelled thymidine; the radioactivity incorporated into DNA per cell was determined 24 h later. Rat serum taken 6 h after a subtotal hepatectomy produced a higher stimulation of thymidine incorporation into DNA, than serum from normal rats.

The weight of evidence is thus for the existence of humoral factors controlling liver growth and regeneration. One cannot decide, however, if the factor is an inhibitor lost after partial hepatectomy, or a growth-promoting substance produced after the operation. The safest position is probably to suppose that both kinds of factors are involved and that the state of liver growth depends on a delicate equilibrium between the two.

18.3 The chalone hypothesis

Tissue growth seems to be controlled by stimulatory and inhibitory factors.

Some stimulatory factors have a general effect on all kinds of cells; they are nutrients (such as amino acids) and hormones necessary for growth (STH, thyroid hormones, insulin, etc. . . .). Other are tissue-specific: TSH for the thyroid gland, ACTH for the adrenal cortex, erythropoietin for erythroblasts, etc . . . A factor stimulating cell division in the epidermis seems to be produced by dermal fibroblasts (Laurence et al., 1972); Houck and Cheng (1973) isolated from serum a factor which stimulates the growth of fibroblasts.

One theory proposes that the growth inhibitory factors are secreted in the extracellular fluids by the cells of the tissue on which these inhibitors exert their action. These tissue-specific inhibitors were named 'anti-templates' by Weiss and Kavanau (1957) and 'chalones' by Bullough (1962). The theory states that the extracellular concentration of chalone is related to the number of cells in the tissue. The tissue grows until the chalone reaches a concentration which maintains a dynamic equilibrium in the cell population, dying cells being replaced by cells emerging from divisions. The mass of tissues is thus controlled by a simple negative feedback mechanism.

Proving that a chalone plays a role in the control of the growth of a particular tissue needs: (1) to isolate the inhibitor from the tissue; (2) to show that the inhibitor is secreted in the extracellular fluid; (3) to prove that its physiological extracellular concentration truly regulates the cell multiplication; (4) to show that the inhibitor is tissue-specific.

A dual control of growth seems to exist for the epidermis (Laurence et al., 1972; Bullough, 1974): a stimulatory factor from the dermal fibroblasts (explaining the polarity of the epidermis with its germinative layer against the dermis), and two inhibitory factors (chalones) produced by the epidermis itself, one acting on the G_2–M transition, and the other on the G_1–S transition. A dual control has also been described for granulocytes (Rytömaa and Kiviniemi, 1968) and fibroblasts (Houck et al., 1972; Houck and Chen 1973).

In the case of liver, the arguments are conflicting. The results obtained by different authors are difficult to compare because the experimental conditions differ enormously. Many contradictions are verbal; they result from not paying sufficient attention to the experimental details. Because of that, we shall present independently the works of different laboratories with their logic, and only later see whether it is possible to draw a few conclusions.

18.4 Search for tissue-specific regulators of liver growth and regeneration

18.4.1 Growth promotors

Paul et al. (1972) have cultured liver cells from 20-day old rat fetuses in arginine-free Eagle medium supplemented with dialyzed and heat-inactivated fetal calf serum. After 5 days, the cells were transfered into a fresh medium containing labelled thymidine and the DNA radioactivity was determined 24 h later. The DNA radioactivity per cell depends on the population density, reaching a sharp maximum when there were 10^5 cells per dish (35 mm diameter; 2 ml incubation medium). This behaviour suggests the secretion by the hepatocytes, in the incubation medium, of a stimulatory and an inhibitory factor. The cells would be more sensitive to the stimulatory factor, but the stimulation could be overcome when the inhibitory factor reaches a concentration high enough. Addition to the incubation medium of rat serum taken 6 h after a subtotal hepatectomy (to replace the fetal calf serum) produced a higher stimulation of the incorporation of thymidine into the DNA and leucine into the proteins of the cultured hepatocytes, than addition of serum from normal adult rats. The difference between the two sera was not observed on 3T3 fibroblasts which suggested a tissue-specific effect. Paul and his colleagues concluded that the serum of partially hepatectomized rats contains a factor which stimulates DNA and protein syntheses in hepatocytes. It seems however that the opposite view cannot be rejected: nutrients and hormones, having a general stimulatory action on 3T3 fibroblasts as well as on hepatocytes, are present in both sera (from normal and hepatectomized rats), but normal serum moreover contains a liver-specific inhibitor of DNA synthesis.

It must be recalled that, in the experiments of Stich and Florian (1958), if the intraperitoneal injection of serum from adult rats to subtotally hepatectomized animals decreased the mitotic index in the regenerating liver, the injection of serum from subtotally hepatectomized rats actually increased the mitotic index.

Fisher et al. (1971) postulated the existence of a 'stimulatory factor' brought by the portal blood; the effect of this factor, produced at a constant rate, would depend on the number of hepatocytes. Many experiments presented by these authors could be interpreted in other ways, except, perhaps, the following one. A blood cross-circulation was established between two rats, one with an intact liver, the other with a 70% hepatectomy. Twenty-four hours after the operation, the DNA synthesis in the operated liver was lowered because of the blood exchange, whereas stimulation of DNA synthesis was observed in the liver of the intact partner. When a portacaval shunt was added to the subtotal hepatectomy, the DNA synthesis in the operated liver was decreased still further and DNA stimulation in the intact liver was as great as if the operated animal had undergone a 100% hepatectomy. The interpretation by Fisher and his colleagues of these results was that the portacaval shunt directed the portal 'stimulatory factor' from the operated liver toward the intact liver of the other parabiotic partner.

Morley and Kingdon (1972) purified from rat serum a 26,000 dalton protein which stimulated DNA synthesis specifically in hepatocytes. This protein was absent from the serum of normal adults, but appeared 12 h after a partial hepatectomy.

18.4.2 Growth inhibitors

Most of the classical paper by Saetren (1956), entitled: 'A principle of auto-regulation of growth: production of organ specific mitose-inhibitors in kidney and liver', is devoted to kidney regeneration, a few experiments are however of interest to us. In rats deprived simultaneously of 2/3 of their liver and $1^1/_2$ kidneys, 400–500 mitotic figures were observed per mg of tissue in both regenerating organs 48 h after the operation. When kidney macerate was applied intraperitoneally 30 h after the operation, the number of mitoses was reduced to 60 per mg of kidney, but no change was observed in the liver. Regretfully, the symmetrical experiment with liver macerate is not reported. The specificity of the liver macerate was tested on rats partially hepatectomized but with intact kidneys: when this macerate was introduced in the peritoneal cavity 30 h after the operation, the few mitoses remaining in the liver at the 48th hour were not in the parenchyma. Experiments performed on young rats have a more gratifying symmetry: kidney and liver macerates decreased the mitotic rate mostly in the corresponding growing organ. In these experiments, the action of the liver macerate was not on the G_0–G_1 transition, but, because 18 h separated the application of the liver macerate from the determination of the mitotic index, it is not possible to guess where the division cycle was blocked: it could be in G_1, S or G_2. Data on chemistry and metabolism are given only for the kidney inhibitor: it was heat-labile and undialysable; it was less active when applied at the time of the operation than 30 h later.

The work of Stich and Florian (1958) is more complete and centered on the control of liver regeneration; moreover, a tissue-specific inhibitor was sought not only in the liver, but also in the blood. Liver homogenates (1.8 g) from adult rats were injected intraperitoneally into 250 g rats subtotally hepatectomized 30 h earlier; the mitotic index in the liver, measured 15 h later, was 3‰ instead of 31‰ in a control which did not receive the homogenate. Homogenates from regenerating liver, testes or brain, were without effect. Serum (4 ml) from adult rats, injected intraperitoneally into rats subtotally hepatectomized 30 h before, also decreased to 3‰ the mitotic index taken in the liver 15 h later. The inhibitory effect of the serum from normal adults lasted less than 24 h. When injected into another subtotally hepatectomized rat, the serum taken 24 h after a subtotal hepatectomy did not decrease, but, on the contrary, increased the mitotic index. The authors concluded that a true stimulation of the mitotic rate, rather than an increase of the length of mitosis occurred because the distribution of the mitotic phases followed a normal pattern. Stich and Florian concluded that the liver produces a tissue-specific inhibitor of mitosis which is released into the plasma where it has a short life; after a subtotal hepatectomy, the inhibitor concentration rapidly decreases in blood which permits cell multiplication. The timing of their experiments, which is the same as that used by Saetren (1956), does not demonstrate where the inhibitor interferes with the cell division cycle. On the other hand, Stich and Florian did not explain the stimulation of hepatic mitosis by serum from subtotally hepatectomized rats; this observation would be better explained by the presence of a stimulatory substance than by the disappearance of a mitotic inhibitor.

Chopra and Simnett (1971) prepared homogenates, in saline, of kidney or liver from adult rats. After high speed centrifugation, the supernatant was lyophilized and the powder extracted with water. The administration of the liver extract together with colchicine to juvenile *Xenopus laevis* produced, within 4 h, a significant decrease of the mitotic index in the liver (from 305 to 88 arrested metaphases per 10^5 nuclei), but had no action on kidney (303 and 289 in the control and treated animals respectively). Conversely, administration of kidney extract had no effect on liver (305 and 291), but drastically reduced the mitotic index in the kidney (from 303 to 69). Chopra and Simnett concluded that rat kidney and liver contained tissue-specific mitotic inhibitors. Because of the short delay between the administration of the extract and the observed effect on mitosis, the cell cycle appears to have been inhibited in the G_2 period.

Many authors tried to isolate the inhibitors present in the crude liver extracts. The assay used differs from one worker to another; most often the effect on labelled thymidine incorporation into cellular DNA was followed, sometimes the effect on cell multiplication in vitro. Many artifacts or effects devoid of tissue-specificity were discovered. The question of whether or not a liver chalone exists is still a matter of controversy. We shall begin with the description of a few studies directed toward the discovery of tissue-specific inhibitors because the results obtained by their authors help to understand the difficulties met by others, also working with liver extracts, but who were looking for a chalone.

Otsuka and Terayama (1966) wondered why normal liver, even during regeneration, is under homeostatic control which regulates the tissue mass, while hepatoma cells can proliferate without restriction. They thought that DNA synthesis, which precedes mitosis, might be the phase where the cellular proliferation is controlled, and they studied the action of different extracts on labelled thymidine incorporation into the DNA of AH-414 hepatoma cells. These extracts were prepared by homogenization of the tissue or cells in isotonic buffer, followed by high speed centrifugation; the final supernatant was used. The AH-414 cells were cultured intraperitoneally in rats and for the assay with the tissue extract, they were suspended in Hanks' solution containing labelled thymidine and enriched with lactalbumin hydrolysate and rat serum. 'Cell-sap' from normal rat liver decreased progressively and finally stopped completely the incorporation of labelled thymidine into the AH-414 cell DNA. The incorporation of orotic acid into the DNA and, to a much lower extent, into RNA was also decreased. This different action of the extract on the incorporation of the same precursor into DNA and RNA, was interpreted by Otsuka and Terayama as showing that it was not so much the uptake of orotic acid that was interfered with, but rather the synthesis of DNA. The inhibitor did not seem to demonstrate tissue-specificity in that 'cell-saps' from kidney, brain and spleen, had the same action on incorporation rate of [^{3}H]thymidine into DNA of AH-414 cells as did liver 'cell-sap'. There was a great difference between extracts from normal and malignant tissues, however, 'Cell-sap' from ascites AH-414 hepatoma cells was devoid of inhibitory activity whereas 'cell-sap' from solid hepatoma induced in rats by 3-methyl-4-dimethyl-aminoazobenzene (MDAB) contained little activity in spite of the normal liver tissue adjacent to the tumor having a normal inhibitor content. The amount of inhibitor in the 'cell-sap' did not seem to be related to the state of proliferation since the regenerating liver, which had a higher mitotic rate than the MDAB-hepatoma, was found to have the same inhibitor content as did the normal liver. The loss of the inhibitory activity thus seemed to be characteristic of the malignant cell phenotype.

The action of this inhibitor was reversible AH-414 cells pre-incubated for 3 h with cell-sap from normal liver, after several washings, recovered the rate of incorporation of labelled thymidine into DNA found in non-exposed control cells. The inhibitor was not dialysable and was destroyed at 100 °C. It was partially purified: after precipitation of part of the proteins at pH 4.5, the inhibitor itself was precipitated between 40–60% saturation in ammonium sulfate at neutral pH; it had an isoelectric point near neutrality.

In later experiments, Otsuka (1969) used sarcoma 180 ascites cells, clearly showing that he was not interested in finding a tissue-specific inhibitor. Otsuka showed that the inhibitory activity was not due to arginase in short-term experiments. Sarcoma 180 ascites cells were incubated in Hanks' solution enriched with horse serum and supplemented with beef liver 'cell-sap' (containing 1250 arginase units) or purified arginase (3750 units) for 1 h before addition of labelled thymidine, and the DNA radioactivity measured 30 min later. Arginase had no influence on the thymidine incorporation into the DNA, whereas it was decreased to 1% of the control value by the liver extract. Chicken liver, which possesses no arginase, had the same activity as beef liver. Otsuka also found that the liver cell-sap inhibited the thymidine incorporation into the DNA of sarcoma 180 cells incubated in unsupplemented Hanks' solution. Since arginine was absent from the incubation medium, the action of the extract could not be due to arginase activity.

Otsuka (1969) further studied the beef liver 'cell-sap'. Dialysis against a solution of manganese sulfate greatly increased its inhibitory effect on the incorporation of labelled thymidine into the DNA of sarcoma 180 cells. This potentiation of inhibition could not be reversed by dialysis against manganese-free buffer unless it also contained EDTA. The inhibition of incorporation of uridine into RNA and leucine into proteins by the liver 'cell-sap' was not much enhanced by the manganese treatment. Otsuka studied the mechanism of the inhibition of thymidine incorporation into sarcoma 180 cell DNA by the Mn-treated liver 'cell-sap'. Usually the sarcoma 180 cells were preincubated for 1 h with the liver extract before addition of the labelled precursor, and the DNA radioactivity was measured 30 min later. Under these conditions, the inhibitory effect of the 'cell-sap' was much greater for thymidine (99% inhibition) than for deoxycytidine or adenine (79 and 76% respectively); the effect on thymidine incorporation into DNA was greatly reduced (from 99 to 50%) when the preincubation was suppressed and the 'cell-sap' added at the same time as the labelled precursor. After a 1-h pre-incubation with Mn-treated beef liver 'cell-sap' followed by 30 min at 37 °C with labelled thymidine, the sarcoma 180 cells were treated with 5% perchloric acid and the acid-soluble fraction submitted to paper chromatography in order to separate thymidine (dT) and the thymidine phosphates (dTMP, dTDP, dTTP). Because the presence of cell-sap decreased by around 95% the radioactivity in dTMP, dTDP and dTTP, Otsuka concluded that the extract inhibited thymidine phosphorylation; but this conclusion is incorrect because, as we shall see later (Miyamoto and Terayama, 1971), the liver extract in fact destroyed the labelled thymidine in the incubation medium. In order to see whether the Mn-treated beef liver 'cell-sap' had an action on the conversion of dTTP into DNA (polymerization step), sarcoma 180 cells were pre-incubated for 30 min with labelled thymidine, then washed thoroughly and incubated for 1 h with or without 'cell-sap'. The increase of DNA radioactivity during the second incubation period was only slightly reduced (25% maximum) by the presence of the 'cell-sap'. But, because the cell-sap had no effect on the phosphorylation of deoxycytidine while decreasing the deoxycytidine incorporation into DNA, Otsuka concluded that there was some inhibition of the polymerization step. Speculating on the cause of this inhibition, he suggested that it was the consequence of the inhibition of dTTP formation. It is intriguing that, in spite of his experimental results showing a decreased radioactivity nearly as great in dTMP and dTDP than in dTTP when the 'cell-sap' was present, Otsuka excluded the possibility of an inhibition of thymidine kinase on the ground that this enzyme commands only the minor salvage pathway which has little importance for DNA synthesis. The final conclusion of Otsuka was that cell proliferation is controlled by an inhibitor of dTTP synthesis and that tumour cells lack this regulation mechanism. What we have learned more recently permits us to say that Otsuka's results were due mainly to enzymes destroying the labelled thymidine in the incubation medium and only secondarily to a true inhibitor of DNA synthesis whose mechanism of action is still unknown.

The action of enzymes, present in the liver extract, which destroys either a cell nutrient or a labelled precursor, produces a very serious artifact in the interpretation of the results of long term in vitro experiments. But the action, on DNA synthesis for instance, of an enzyme which destroys a cell nutrient can be shown only if this nutrient is present in the incubation medium.

Miyamoto and Terayama (1971), using AH-414 hepatoma cells suspended in Hanks' solution enriched with bovine serum and lactalbumin hydrolysate, observed that 'cell-sap' from adult rat liver contained two factors inhibiting thymidine incorporation into DNA in long term experiments: one is destroyed by heating at 55°C, whereas the other is stable at this temperature. 'Cell-sap' from newborn rats contains only the heat-labile factor. Arginase is the thermostable factor in adult rat liver; its inhibition could be relieved merely by the addition of arginine. Arginine had no effect on the inhibition by 'cell-sap' from newborn rat liver which has no arginase. Miyamoto and Terayama showed that the thermolabile factor, present in newborn and adult rat livers, was constituted of thymidine hydrolase and thymidine phosphorylase; both enzymes convert thymidine into thymine which cannot be used by the cells for DNA synthesis. At the end of 3 h, the incubation medium was analyzed by thin layer chromatography and the presence of cell-sap from newborn rat liver was shown to produce a destruction of labelled thymidine sufficient to explain the reduced incorporation of this precursor into the DNA of the AH-414 hepatoma cells.

Liver extracts were found to inhibit the multiplication of cultured cells in general: arginine is an essential amino-acid for cell growth and liver contains arginase. Holley (1967) obtained an inhibition of DNA synthesis with purified liver arginase in 3T3 cells, transformed or not, and in primary mouse embryo cells. Arginase is absent from many hepatoma (Greenstein et al., 1941).

The work of Nilsson and Philipson (1968) on human liver, much better than the work of Otsuka on beef liver already described, indicates the existence of a DNA synthesis inhibitor devoid of tissue-specificity. Microsomes from human liver inhibited the incorporation of thymidine into the DNA of human diploid fibroblasts or of HeLa cells cultured in vitro. A 72-h autolysis increased the amount of inhibitor and released it from the membrane so that it was found in the supernatant after centrifugation of the liver homogenate. Nilsson and Philipson studied the properties of this solubilized inhibitor. The inhibitory activity was maintained after treatment with DNase followed by dialysis. The reduction of labelled thymidine incorporation into the HeLa cell DNA was thus not due to the presence of deoxynucleosides in the preparation (like thymidine, see later Lenfant et al., 1973). After an incubation of HeLa cells with labelled thymidine in the presence of aged liver supernatant, the radioactivity in the cellular acid-soluble fraction was nearly the same as in a control without supernatant, whereas the radioactivity incorporated into the insoluble DNA was decreased by 80%. The authors concluded that a true inhibition of DNA synthesis had occurred. The inhibition of DNA synthesis in HeLa cells appeared after a lag of 60 min and was preceded by an inhibition of leucine incorporation into proteins and uridine into RNA. The human liver supernatant inhibited the multiplication of HeLa cells but induced an increase in the amount of DNA per cell. Thus the effect did not seem to be restricted to the S phase but rather the G_2 phase could also be affected. The solubilized inhibitor was not retained by Sephadex G-200 and was destroyed at 60 °C;

its action on HeLa cells was completely reversible. A similar inhibitor was found in human spleen, kidney, but not in lung, heart or KB cells.

Hrachovec (1973) found in mouse liver microsomes an inhibitor of the growth of hepatoma in vivo and in vitro. The inhibitor decreases protein synthesis by liver ribosomes. Hepatoma microsomes contain less of this inhibitor than normal liver microsomes.

Freed and Sorof (1966) found that protein h_2 purified from rat liver supernatant by electrophoresis, inhibited the multiplication of mouse fibroblasts and other cell lines in vitro. The effect was reversibly cytostatic. Carcinogens, like aminoazo dyes, react preferentially with protein h_2, and the tumours induced by the carcinogen have a markedly reduced amount of protein h_2. Freed and Soroff speculated that protein h_2 regulates cell multiplication and that its reaction with the carcinogen might explained the oncogenesis. Holley (1967) suggested that the inhibitory effect of the h-proteins was due mostly to contaminating arginase.

Using a similar approach, Volm et al. (1969) had the fleeting hope to differentiate between liver-specific and non-specific growth inhibitors. They observed that the proteins precipitated from rat liver supernatant between 50 and 80% ethanol concentrations, inhibited thymidine incorporation into DNA of liver explants from newborn rats, and also of kidney explants, HeLa cells and other cultured tumor cells. However, when the proteins came from the liver of a rat treated with diethylnitrosamine 6 h earlier, there was no more effect on the liver explants whereas the inhibitory action persisted on the other kinds of tissues. At that time, Volm and his colleagues concluded that the liver contained two inhibitors of DNA synthesis, one of which was specific for liver and inactivated by diethylnitrosamine. This conclusion was later denied by Wayss et al. (1973) on the basis of in vivo experiments. Liver proteins prepared as above were administered to 150 g rats with partial hepatectomy: an inhibition of thymidine incorporation into DNA was observed not only in the regenerating liver, but also in the kidneys. When the proteins came from a rat treated with diethylnitrosamine 12 or 16 h before, a reduction of the inhibitory activity was observed not only for the regenerating liver, but also for the kidneys. The final conclusion is that the carcinogen deactivated non-specific inhibitory factors.

We shall now pass to a few studies which were more oriented toward the search for a liver-specific growth inhibitor. It is however difficult to know where to place the results of Henderson (1971) since no test of tissue-specificity was performed. This author purified from rat liver a factor which inhibited leucine incorporation into proteins and adenine incorporation into nucleic acids in normal, regenerating and neoplastic livers. After acid hydrolysis, the inhibitory fraction was prepared by extractions with ethyl acetate and carbon tetrachloride, followed by chromatography. The inhibitor concentration was found to be decreased in regenerating liver and absent from neoplastic liver.

Chany and Frayssinet (1971) found, in the supernatant of homogenates from rat, mouse, hamster or beef liver, a factor which inhibited the in vitro multiplication of rat, mouse or hamster hepatoma cells. The inhibitory factor was not dialysable. It was not arginase because the addition of arginine did not suppress the inhibition. The liver supernatant had no immediate action on the growth of rat, mouse or hamster fibroblasts as it had on hepatoma cells, although a delayed inhibition could be shown. The supernatant from regenerating liver had nearly as much activity as the supernatant from normal liver, whereas the supernatant of hepatomas had no inhibitory effect. Aujard et al. (1973) have shown that the inhibitor in the liver supernatant was a 100,000 dalton protein. Rat liver was perfused with MacEven fluid and the perfusate concentrated by ultrafiltration; the concentrated perfusate inhibited the in vitro multiplication of hepatoma LF20 cells (Molimard et al., 1975) but the effect on other kinds of cells was not tested. The perfusate inhibitor was destroyed by trypsin or pronase, or by heating at 100 °C; Sephadex G-100 and G-150 chromatography indicated a molecular weight around 100,000, analogous to the molecular weight of the inhibitor found in liver supernatant (Aujard et al., 1973). It is not known whether the inhibitors in liver and perfusate are identical; even if they were, the authors feel that proof should be given that this inhibitor is secreted by the hepatocytes under physiological conditions.

Injecting casein in 0.3% NaOH subcutaneously to 20 g baby rats produces a synchronized DNA synthesis in hepatic cells involving 20% of the population (Nadal, 1973). Serum of adult rats exhibits two activities on this biological system; (1) it inhibits the G_1–S transition and (2) induces the formation of binucleate hepatocytes. These activities are absent from the serum of baby rats or of subtotally hepatectomized adults. Nadal and Boffa (1974) found that the serum factor is an α_1-globulin; its mass is similar to the mass of the inhibitory factor for hepatoma cell growth found in liver by Aujard et al. (1973) and in liver perfusate by Molimard et al. (1975).

Liver or kidney were homogenized in water and submitted to high speed centrifugation. Having observed that the liver supernatant inhibited the incorporation of labelled thymidine into the DNA of regenerating liver in vivo and in vitro, whereas an equivalent amount (containing the same amount of proteins) of kidney supernatant was without action, Verly et al. (1971) devised a quantitative in vitro assay for the liver supernatant inhibitor. Male rats (70 g) were subtotally hepatectomized and the remaining liver lobes taken 24 h later, i.e. at the peak of DNA synthesis. The regenerating liver was cut into slices which were incubated in Hanks' solution. The liver preparation (assay) or an equal volume of solvent (control) was added together with labelled thymidine, and the incubation carried out at 37 °C for 2 h. The DNA specific radioactivity was then determined in each sample, and the fractional decrease of radionuclide incorporation into DNA, due to the inhibitor, calculated: I.F. (inhibited fraction) = ((control) − (assay))/ (control), where (control) and (assay) are the DNA specific radioactivities in the control and the assay respectively. A linear relationship between $1/(1 - I.F.)$ and the amount of supernatant was found, and the unit of inhibition was defined as the amount of inhibitor necessary to reduce by 50% the incorporation of labelled thymidine into DNA in the standard test. The number of inhibitory units (U) in the incubation medium was calculated with the equation: $U = I.F./(1 - I.F.)$. Good accuracy was obtained as long as I.F. remained between 0.3 and 0.8. Adult rabbit supernatant contains, per mg of proteins, six times as much inhibitor as adult rat liver supernatant. The inhibitor of rabbit liver supernatant was purified by ethanol fractional precipitation (most of the activity was found in the precipitate formed between 70 and 87% in ethanol), followed by ultra-filtration through a Diaflo UM-2 membrane (pore size 1.2 nm). Most of the inhibitor was found in the ultrafiltrate. Assuming a spherical shape, this indicated a molecular weight below 2000, which was confirmed by the elution position of the inhibitor from a Sephadex G-50 column. The purified preparation had an activity of 180 units per mg of protein-like substances (determined by Lowry's method with bovine serum albumin as standard). One unit of the purified inhibitor (I.F. = 0.50 for regenerating liver slices) had very little action on slices of rat spleen (I.F. = 0.08) or kidney (I.F. = 0.01).

Beef liver supernatant was also found to decrease the incorporation of labelled thymidine into DNA of regenerating rat liver slices. To attempt a more complete purification of the inhibitor, beef liver was chosen instead of rabbit liver and the method was changed to deal with larger amounts of material. Lenfant et al. (1973) sonicated the beef liver in water with a Polytron at room temperature. The suspension was warmed 5 min at 50 °C, then cooled to 4 °C before addition of ethanol to reach a 60% concentration; the precipitated proteins were discarded by filtration through a Whatman #4 paper. The filtrate was reduced to a tenth of its original volume and the concentrate was centrifuged; the clear solution between the fatty layer and the sediment was taken and filtered through a Diaflo UM-2 membrane. The ultrafiltrate was lyophilized and the resulting powder extracted with 0.02 M ammonium acetate, pH 7 buffer. Chromatography on Sephadex G-15 separated two inhibitors: inhibitor I appeared rather specific for hepatocytes, whereas inhibitor II was much more active on HeLa cells. Inhibitor II was completely purified and found to be thymidine. High concentration of thymidine (2 mM) are known to block DNA synthesis (Xeros, 1962), but this is not the case in the situation which is considered here; i.e., it can be calculated that one inhibitory unit corresponds to a thymidine concentration of only 0.003 mM in the incubation medium. Thymidine decreases the labelled thymidine incorporation into DNA simply by diluting the radioactive precursor. Surprisingly, the quantitative effect of the addition of unlabelled thymidine is different from one kind of cell to another. In the reported experiments, the 5 ml incubation medium contained 0.16 μg of radioactive thymidine; to reduce by half the radioactivity incorporated into DNA, it was necessary to add 0.27 μg of unlabelled thymidine to HeLa or Ehrlich cells, 0.62 μg to Novikoff cells (Chevalier and Verly, 1975), 0.77 μg to lung or regenerating liver slices, and a much larger amount to kidney slices (Lenfant et al., 1973). Such differences might be explained if the tissue behaviour can vary between two extremes. At the one extreme, the amount of exogenous thymidine incorporated into DNA is proportional to the exogenous thymidine concentration; the dilution of labelled thymidine by unlabelled thymidine has no apparent inhibitory action. At the other extreme, the amount of exogenous thymidine incorporated into DNA is constant; on addition of unlabelled thymidine to the labelled thymidine of the incubation medium, the radioactivity incorporated into DNA is decreased by a factor equal to the dilution factor. The different action of unlabelled thymidine on cells of different origin might wrongly be taken as an indication for the presence of a tissue-specific growth inhibitor. Indeed thymidine was found to be, in an endometrial extract, the main inhibitor of labelled thymidine incorporation into HeLa cell DNA (Chevalier and Verly, 1975). Because HeLa cells have an endometrial origin and are more sensitive to the addition of unlabelled thymidine than other kinds of cells, one might have drawn the wrong conclusion that the observed effect was due to a tissue-specific growth regulator present in endometrium.

Thymidine, in the beef liver extract prepared by Lenfant et al. (1973) was likely an artifact resulting from autolysis during the processing, at room temperature, of large batches of beef liver, and perhaps also during the heating at 50 °C to precipitate part of the proteins. This interpretation is supported by the observation that, in the beef liver extract, most of the inhibitor was soluble in 87% ethanol (Lenfant et al., 1973), which was not the case for the rabbit liver supernatant prepared at 4 °C. On the other hand, it was not likely that the purified rabbit liver inhibitor prepared by Verly et al. (1971) contained thymidine because only the fraction precipitated between 70 and 87 % ethanol concentrations was retained for further purification; any thymidine in the supernatant would have been discarded at this step. Indeed, Deschamps and Verly (1975) found that Sephadex G-15 chromatography of the purified rabbit liver preparation gave a single peak of inhibitory activity whose elution volume was different from that of thymidine; the peak occupied approximately the same position as the beef liver inhibitor I of Lenfant et al. (1973).

As we have now shown many times, a decreased incorporation of labelled thymidine into cellular DNA is not necessarily related to an inhibition of DNA replication. Many other causes can be suspected: (1) a factor, maybe an enzyme (thymidine hydrolase, thymidine phosphorylase) which converts the labelled thymidine into thymine in the incubation medium; (2) the factor may be thymidine diluting the DNA labelled precursor; (3) the factor may interfere with the transport of the exogenous thymidine through the plasma membrane, or reduce the activity of thymidine kinase; (4) the factor may stimulate the endogenous pathway of thymidine phosphate synthesis, changing the size of the deoxynucleotide pool, so that the salvage pathway utilizing the exogenous thymidine would be relatively less important. In the case of the purified inhibitor from rabbit liver (Verly et al., 1971), the two first possibilities can be ignored: as a small molecular weight compound the factor cannot be an enzyme which destroys thymidine, and it was shown not to be thymidine. The situation could be further clarified by measuring the specific radioactivity of the thymidine phosphates in the cellular pool to be able to calculate, from the radioactivity incorporated in the macromolecule, the amount of DNA synthesized. Deschamps and Verly (1975) incubated slices of regenerating rat liver in the presence of labelled thymidine with or without addition of one unit of the purified inhibitor; after 15, 30, 60 or 120 min, the slices were separated from the incubation medium, rinsed with Hanks' solution containing unlabelled thymidine, treated with 5 % trichloracetic acid (TCA) and the TCA-soluble fraction chromatographed on Dowex-50 to isolate the thymidine phosphates. The results showed that the specific radioactivity of the thymidine phosphates, at any time, was the same whether the inhibitor was there or not, while the radioactivity found in DNA at the end of the 2 h incubation was reduced by 50 % in the presence of the inhibitor. This clearly shows that none of the four factors enumerated above was involved in the reduction of labelled thymidine incorporation into DNA, but that the purified rabbit liver factor truly inhibited DNA synthesis. In this experiment, the specific radioactivity of the thymidine phosphates was stabilized in less than 30 min, therefore it could be calculated that, when the system had reached such a steady state, the contribution of the exogenous thymidine to the formation of the intracellular thymidine phosphates was less than 1/5000. This very low value stresses the great danger in using the incorporation of labelled thymidine as a measure of DNA synthesis, as one may then be monitoring a minor route in nucleotide metabolism. The usefulness of the determination of the thymidine phosphate specific radioactivity can be stressed by comparing the results obtained with the purified rabbit liver inhibitor to those given by the endometrial extract where the inhibitor was found to be thymidine. Using HeLa cells, Chevalier and Verly (1975) found that the endometrial extract decreased the radio-activity in the thymidine phosphates to the same extent as the incorporation of the radionuclide into DNA, thus showing that the endometrial extract had no effect on DNA synthesis in HeLa cells.

Deschamps and Verly (1975) have studied different properties of the purified inhibitor of rabbit liver (see also Verly, 1973). When 0.2 unit of the preparation was added to regenerating rat liver slices, the maximum inhibition of DNA synthesis occurred only after 30 min and the inhibition had completely disappeared after 75 min; the inhibitor was however still there, but the slices had lost their sensitivity probably because they were incubated in a poorly nutritive medium (Hanks' solution). The preparation (0.2 unit) also produced a transient inhibition of RNA synthesis whose maximum occurred only after 45 min, and an inhibition of protein synthesis which was immediately maximal. This led Deschamps and Verly to suppose that protein synthesis was the target of the inhibitor, and that inhibition of DNA synthesis might be the consequence of the absence of a needed protein. As mentioned in the introduction, Brown et al. (1970) have shown that cycloheximide, an inhibitor of protein synthesis in eukaryotic cells, prevents the G_1–S transition and stops, after a short delay, DNA synthesis in S cells. As the inhibition of protein synthesis also prevents the activation of chromatin necessary for the G_0–G_1 transition (Baserga, 1974), Deschamps and Verly speculated that the factor might also stop this transition which is the step most likely controlled to regulate liver growth and regeneration. The purified rabbit liver inhibitor decreased DNA synthesis in DAB hepatoma and Novikoff hepatoma cells, although much less than in regenerating liver slices. Its action on DNA synthesis in slices from spleen, kidney, lung, or ear skin, was very low. The purified preparation was not toxic for cultured hepatocytes. The inhibitor was hydrolyzed by pronase and trypsin, stable at 75 °C but slowly destroyed at 100 °C, and had an isoelectric point near neutrality. The small molecular weight inhibitor purified by Verly et al. (1971) from adult rabbit liver thus appeared to be a peptide.

The same preparation was used in the autoradiographic studies of Simard et al. (1974). Slices from livers of 60 g male rats subtotally hepatectomized 24 h earlier were incubated for 2 h at 37 °C in Hanks' solution in the presence of tritiated thymidine, with or without the rabbit liver purified inhibitor. The same reduction of the percentage of labelled nuclei (36 and 39%) was observed whether 1 or 2 units of inhibitor were used, whereas the reduction of labelled thymidine incorporation into DNA was 50 and 66% respectively. It thus appeared that 1 unit of inhibitor in 5 ml of incubation medium was sufficient to block completely the G_1–S transition, and that larger amounts of inhibitor acted also on S phase DNA synthesis. In vivo experiments were then carried out. Subtotally hepatectomized male rats of 60 g were injected intraperitoneally with 0.5 unit of purified inhibitor per g of body weight 21 h after the operation; the animals received tritiated thymidine by the same route 3 h later, and were sacrificed after 1 more hour. Control animals were similarly treated except that they received saline instead of the inhibitor solution. Specimens of regenerating liver, duodenal and tongue epithelia were examined. The inhibitor provoked a 38% reduction of the DNA specific radioactivity in the liver, a 40% reduction of labelled nuclei and practically no change in the number of silver grains per labelled nucleus in the autoradiograms (from 22.5 to 19.5); this indicated that, at the dose used, the main site of the inhibitor action was on a step prior the initiation of chromosomal DNA synthesis, whereas the effect on S phase synthesis was very low. Simard and his colleagues also observed a doubling of the ratio of metaphases to anaphases as if the inhibitor also blocked the cells at metaphase. The purified inhibitor had comparatively little action on the number of labelled nuclei in the duodenal and tongue epithelia. This tissue-specificity was not observed with the liver supernatant, showing clearly that data obtained with such crude extracts cannot be used to criticize results obtained with purer preparations.

Although Deschamps and Verly (1975) had observed that the inhibition, by the purified rabbit liver inhibitor, of labelled thymidine incorporation into DNA was much lower with Novikoff hepatoma cells than with slices from regenerating liver, Vinet and Verly (1975) decided to use Novikoff cells for the biological test (because it was less time-consuming) in an attempt to completely purify the hepatic inhibitor. The relationship between dose and inhibition with Novikoff cells was found to be similar to that observed with regenerating rat liver slices. The equation given by Verly et al. (1971) could thus be used to calculate the number of Novikoff inhibitory units in a given preparation. The liver of an adult rabbit was homogenized in water, the homogenate centrifuged at high speed, and the supernatant lyophilized. The resulting powder was extracted with Tris–NaCl, pH 7.4 buffer, and the solution chromatographed on Sephadex G-200. Two peaks (A and B) of inhibitory activity and a region of small molecular weight stimulatory substances were separated. Peak B contained enzymes which converted thymidine into thymine; this activity was shown to be responsible for the decreased incorporation of labelled thymidine into the DNA of Novikoff cells. Inhibitor A, which was eluted at the void volume and thus had a molecular weight above 200,000, did not show this enzymic activity; inhibitor A was proved to increase the radioactivity of the thymidine phosphates while decreasing the radioactivity incorporated into the DNA of Novikoff cells and therefore it was a true inhibitor of DNA synthesis. The pooled fractions of peak A were chromatographed on DEAE-Sephadex; the biological activity was again separated in two peaks (A-I and A-II). Inhibitor A-I had a proteolytic activity and its specific activity (inhibitory units per mg of proteins) was lower than that of A-II; therefore A-II was used for further purification. With the aim of concentrating A-II, the pooled fractions of the corresponding peak were desalted by filtration on Sephadex G-200 in water; the inhibitor appeared as a single peak (A-II-G$_w$) between the void volume and the total volume of the column. The amount of protein associated with this peak was very low: inhibitor A-II-G$_w$ was found pure by gel electrophoresis. Inhibitor A-II-G$_w$ had a molecular weight of 40,000. It is worthwhile to recall that, on the first Sephadex G-200 chromatography, the inhibitor appeared to have a mass larger than 200,000 daltons. The most probable explanation is that, in the crude extract, the inhibitor was part of a high molecular weight complex which was subsequently dissociated; this peculiar behaviour would explain why the inhibitor was so easily purified. Inhibitor A-II-G$_w$ was destroyed by pronase; it is not arginase since glucose was the only nutrient in the incubation medium (Hanks' solution). Inhibitor A-II-G$_w$ was active on Novikoff hepatoma cells and cultured hepatocytes from newborn rats, and had little effect on HeLa or Ehrlich cells. Surprisingly, it had nearly no action on DNA synthesis in regenerating rat liver slices. This would explain why, when the inhibition of labelled thymidine incorporation into the DNA of regenerating rat liver slices was used for the assay, a small molecular weight compound was followed (Verly et al., 1971), whereas, when Novikoff cells were used, a 40,000 dalton protein was isolated. During the first step of purification on Sephadex G-200, the small molecular weight inhibitor (which has little action on Novikoff cells) would have been in the region of stimulatory substances where a small peak of less stimulation could be observed. It is possible that the high molecular inhibitor does not diffuse easily through the layers of cells in a tissue slice and that its inhibitory effect can be observed only when the cells are separated and in direct contact with the incubation medium.

To come back to the small molecular weight inhibitor of rabbit liver, it must be said that the method of purification described by Verly et al. (1971) had been repeated successfully many times. It cannot however be reproduced now in the same laboratory: the inhibitor is precipitated between 60 and 87% in ethanol, and most of the redissolved precipitate does no more filter through a Diaflo UM-2 membrane. Arnberg and Proschek (unpublished) have suppressed the ethanol precipitation; they begin with a continuous diafiltration through a Diaflo PM-10 membrane before a chromatography on Sephadex G-25. They seem to have retraced the small molecular weight inhibitory peptide which they obtain however with a much lower yield.

Although most of their work was done with crude extracts so that the results cannot be used to criticize those obtained with purer preparations, recent experiments by German authors cannot be omitted because they took a strong position against the concept of a liver chalone. Spielhoff (1971) homogenized adult rat liver in an isotonic buffer; after centrifugation, the supernatant was lyophilized. The resulting powder was extracted with water, and the extract precipitated by steps with ethanol. Total extracts or re-dissolved ethanol precipitates were injected subcutaneously to 22-day old rats, labelled thymidine was given 10 h later and the animals were killed after 2 h. Total liver extracts decreased thymidine incorporation into the DNA of liver and, to a lesser extent, of kidney; but kidney extracts gave the same results. The 50–65% ethanol precipitate of the liver extract had an action on liver and nearly none on kidney; an analogous preparation from kidney extract acted on both kidney and liver. The author concluded that the extracts did not contain tissue-specific inhibitors.

Volm et al. (1973) followed the first step of the method used by Verly et al. (1971); i.e., livers from adult rats were homogenized in water, centri-fuged and the 105,000 g supernatant used for in vivo and in vitro experi-ments. The supernatant was injected intraperitoneally into rats 18 h after a subtotal hepatectomy. Labelled thymidine was given 23 h after the operation, the animals were killed 1 h later and the DNA specific radioactivities were determined in several tissues. The liver supernatant decreased the DNA specific radioactivity in the regenerating liver, but not in the kidneys; but kidney and lung supernatants had the same effect as liver supernatant on the regenerating liver. Liver supernatant decreased labelled thymidine incorporation into the DNA of liver, kidney and spleen explants from 21-

day old rats; kidney and lung supernatants were also active on these explants. Liver extracts suppressed the mitoses and the weight increase in the liver remaining after a subtotal hepatectomy, but kidney and lung extracts had the same inhibitory effects. For Volm and his colleagues, tissue-specificity must be tested not only by looking for the effect of a given organ extract on different tissues, but also by comparing its action to that of extracts from other organs. They concluded that the liver supernatant does not contain tissue-specific growth inhibitors. This conclusion appears excessive since the presence of a specific inhibitor could be masked by non-specific ones in a crude extract. It is nevertheless understandable that Volm and his colleagues were not encouraged by their results to look further for liver-specific growth inhibitors.

18.5 Conclusions

In vivo and in vitro tests were used to identify growth-inhibitors in liver extracts. The in vitro tests measured either the action on cell multiplication, or the action on the incorporation of labelled thymidine into cellular DNA.

To observe cell multiplication it is necessary to use a rich culture medium and the growth can be prevented by the destruction of a required nutrient. Arginase was found to inhibit the multiplication of many kinds of cells and arginase is an enzyme of the adult mammalian liver. Some authors have nevertheless found in liver a protein, different from arginase, which inhibits rather specifically the growth of hepatoma cells (Chany and Frayssinet, 1971; Aujard et al., 1973). When the incorporation of labelled thymidine into cellular DNA is followed in a poorly nutritive medium (like Hanks' solution) which does not contain arginine, arginase cannot influence the result. When using a rich medium containing arginine, arginase does interfere with DNA synthesis in long term experiments.

Reduction of labelled thymidine incorporation into DNA by a tissue extract can result from other causes than a decreased DNA synthesis. Enzymes are present in the liver (thymidine hydrolase, thymidine phosphorylase) which convert thymidine into thymine which is not used for DNA synthesis; the effect of these enzymes is more important in long term experiments. For example, Otsuka and Terayama (1966) observed that liver supernatants progressively decreased the incorporation of thymidine into the DNA of hepatoma cells and finally stopped it completely. This delayed effect was later shown to be due to arginase and enzymes destroying thymidine (Miyamoto and Terayama, 1971). Moreover, the extract may contain thymidine which reduces, by isotope dilution, the amount of labelled thymidine incorporated into DNA (Lenfant et al., 1973).

Crude liver extracts inhibit labelled thymidine incorporation into cell DNA in vitro. Because there are so many possible interferences, it is not surprising that the crude extract was generally found not to be specific for hepatocytes. Some purification is necessary to discard arginase, the enzymes destroying thymidine and thymidine itself. It is also necessary to show that the purified preparation really inhibits DNA synthesis: the specific radioactivity of the cellular thymidine phosphates must remain unchanged while the labelled thymidine incorporation into DNA is decreased. Such inhibitors of DNA synthesis (different from arginase) purified from liver appear to have a fair specificity for hepatocytes; Verly et al. (1971) have obtained a small inhibitory peptide (see also Deschamps and Verly, 1975), whereas Vinet and Verly (1975) have isolated a 40,000 dalton protein inhibitor.

Artifacts due to the presence of thymidine or enzymes in the extract ought to be less important when the experiment is carried out in vivo. Indeed, a tissue-specificity of the crude liver extract was claimed by people who followed its effect on the mitotic index (Saetren, 1956; Stich and Florian, 1958). But, when the incorporation of labelled thymidine into DNA was studied chemically or autoradiographically, the crude extract of liver appeared to act on other organs than liver even if a delay of several hours separated the injections of extract and labelled thymidine (Volm et al., 1973; Simard et al., 1974); a better tissue-specificity was observed with a purified preparation (Simard et al., 1974).

Blood serum is, at the same time, a simpler and a more complicated system than a liver homogenate. Simpler because only part of the molecules produced by the liver are exported in the blood plasma so that enzymes interfering with the biological tests are absent. More complicated because the serum may contain a mixture of inhibitors coming from all kinds of tissues so that specificity tests will be of no avail during the first steps of purification. Paul et al. (1972) observed a different action of normal rat serum and serum from hepatectomized animals on labelled thymidine incorporation into DNA of liver cells, but not into DNA of 3T3 fibroblasts. Nadal and Boffa (1974) purified a serum α_1-globulin inhibiting the G_1–S transition in hepatocytes.

A possible relationship between the inhibitors found in liver and in serum was studied by perfusion of adult livers (Molimard et al., 1975). Such a perfusate might be a source of very pure hepatic inhibitor. The possibility also exists to find this inhibitor in the incubation medium of hepatocyte cultures (Paul et al., 1972).

The existence of liver-specific growth inhibitors must not lead to rejecting the possibility of the presence of liver-specific growth promoters. Stich and Florian (1958) observed an increase of the mitotic index in the liver after injection of serum from partially hepatectomized rats. Paul et al. (1972) reported a stimulation of DNA synthesis in hepatocyte cultures as long as the population density was not too high. Morley and Kingdom (1972) purified from serum a 26,000 dalton protein which specifically stimulates DNA synthesis in hepatocytes.

References

Aujard, C., Chany, E. and Frayssinet, C. (1973) Inhibition of DNA synthesis of synchronized cells by liver extracts acting in vitro. Exptl. Cell Res. 78, 476–478.

Baserga, R. (1974) Non-histone chromosomal proteins in normal and abnormal growth. Life Sci. 15, 1057–1071.

Brown, R. F., Umeda, T., Takai, S. I. and Lieberman, I. (1970) Effect of inhibitors of protein synthesis on DNA formation in liver. Biochim. Biophys. Acta 209, 49–53.

Bucher, N. L. R. and Malt, R. A. (1971) Regeneration of liver and kidney. Little, Brown and Co, Boston.

Bullough, W. S. (1974) Chalone control mechanisms. Life Sci. 16, 323–330.

Bullough, W. S. (1962) The control of mitotic activity in adult mammalian tissues. Biol. Rev. 37, 307–342.

Chany, E. and Frayssinet, C. (1971) Présence dans le foie normal de substances inhibant précocement la croissance de cultures de cellules cancéreuses. C.R. Acad. Sci. Paris 272 (série D), 2644–2647.

Chevalier, S. and Verly, W. G. (1975) About the existence of an endometrial chalone. Eur. J. Cancer.

Chopra, D. P. and Simnett, J. D. (1971) Tissue-specific mitotic inhibition in the kidneys of embryonic grafts and partially nephrectomized host *Xenopus laevis* J. Embryol· Exp. Morphol. 25, 321–329.

Christensen, B. G. and Jacobsen, E. (1949) Studies on liver regeneration. Acta Med. Scand., suppl. 234, 103–108.

Church, R. B. and McCarthy, B. J. (1967) Ribonucleic acid synthesis in regenerating and embryonic liver. I. The synthesis of new species of RNA during regeneration of mouse liver after partial hepatectomy. J. Mol. Biol. 23, 459–475.

Deschamps, Y. and Verly, W. G. (1975) The hepatic chalone. II. Chemical and biological properties of the rabbit liver chalone. Biomedicine 22.

Fisher, B., Szuch, P. and Fisher, E. (1971) Evaluation of a humoral factor in liver regeneration utilizing liver transplants. Cancer Res. 31, 322–331.

Freed, J. J. and Sorof, S. (1966) Reversible inhibition of cell multiplication by a small class of liver proteins. Biochem. Biophys. Res. Commun. 22, 1–5.

Fujioka, M., Koga, M. and Lieberman, I. (1963) Metabolism of ribonucleic acid after partial hepatectomy. J. Biol. Chem. 238, 3401–3406.

Glinos, A. D. and Gey, G. O. (1952) Humoral factors involved in the induction of liver regeneration in the rat. Proc. Soc. Exp. Biol. Med. 80, 421–425.

Goutier, R., Gerber, G., Rémy-Defraigne, J. and Baes, C. (1965) Synthèse de RNA nucléaire dans le foie de rat en régénération perfusé in vitro. Arch. Int. Physiol. Bioch. 74, 517–518.

Greenstein, J. P., Jenrette, W. V., Mider, G. B. and White, J. (1941) The relative arginase activity of certain tumors and normal control tissues. J. Biol. Chem. 137, 795–796.

Henderson, I. W. D. (1971) Inhibition of protein synthesis in normal, regenerating, and neoplastic rat liver. Fed. Proc. 30, 1253.

Hirota, Y., Mordoh, J. and Jacob, F. (1970) On the process of cellular division in *Escherichia coli*. Thermosensitive mutants of *Escherichia coli* altered in the process of DNA initiation. J. Mol. Biol. 53, 369–387.

Holley, R. V. (1967) Evidence that a rat liver 'inhibitor' of the synthesis of DNA in cultured mammalian cells is arginase. Biochim. Biophys. Acta 145, 525–527.

Houck, J. C. and Cheng, R. F. (1973) Isolation purification, and chemical characterization of the serum mitogen for diploid human fibroblast. J. Cell Physiol. 81, 257–270.

Houck, J. C., Weil, R. L. and Sharma, V. K. (1972) Evidence for a fibroblast chalone. Nature New Biol. 240, 210–211.

Hrachovec, J. P. (1973) Chalone-like substances inhibitory for hepatoma growth and for protein synthesis by liver ribosomes. Fed. Proc. 32 (3). 858 (Abs no 3612).

Infante, A. A., Nauta, R., Gilbert, S., Hobart, P. and Firshein, W. (1973) DNA synthesis in developing sea urchins: role of a DNA-nuclear membrane complex. Nature New Biol. 242, 5–8.

Kostraba, N. C. and Wang, T. Y. (1973) Non-histone proteins and gene activation in regenerating rat liver. Exp. Cell Res. 80, 291–296.

Kumar, K. V. and Friedman, D. L. (1972) Initiation of DNA synthesis in HeLa cell-free system. Nature New Biol. 239, 74–76.

Laurence, E. B., Randers-Hansen, E., Christophers, E. and Rytömaa, T. (1972) Systemic factors influencing epidermal mitosis. Rev. Europ. Et. Clin. Biol. 17, 133–139.

Lenfant, M., Kren-Proschek, L., Verly, W. G. and Dugas, H. (1973) Thymidine as one of the factors in a beef liver extract decreasing [^{3}H]thymidine incorporation into DNA. Can. J. Biochem. 51, 654–665.

Leong, G. F., Grisham, J. W., Hole, B. V. and Albright, M. L. (1964) Effect of partial hepatectomy on DNA synthesis and mitosis in heterotopic partial autografts of rat liver. Cancer Res. 24, 1496–1501.

Maaløe, O. (1961) The control of normal DNA replication in bacteria. Symp. Quant. Biol. 26, 45–52.

Mayfield, J. E. and Bonner, J. (1972) A partial sequence of nuclear events in regenerating rat liver. Proc. Natl Acad. Sci. U.S. 69, 7–10.

Miyamoto, M. and Terayama, H. (1971) Nature of rat liver cell sap factors inhibiting the DNA synthesis in tumour cells. Biochim. Biophys. Acta 228, 324–330.

Molimard, R., Pietu, G., Chany, E., Trincal, G. and Frayssinet, C. (1975) An inhibitor of hepatoma cell multiplication in the efferent fluid from isolated perfused rat livers. Biomedicine.

Morley, C. G. D. and Kingdon, H. S. (1972) A DNA synthesis stimulating factor from partially hepatectomized rat serum. 164th ACS meeting, Biol. Chem. Div., 209.

Nadal, C. (1973) Synchronization of baby rat hepatocytes: a new test for the detection of factors controlling DNA synthesis in rat hepatic cells. Cell Tissue Kinet. 6, 437–446.

Nadal, C. and Boffa, G. A. (1974) Activité inhibitrice des α_1-globulines du sérum de rat sur la multiplication des hépatocytes in vivo. C.R. Acad. Sc. Paris, 278 (série D), 1071–1074.

Nilsson, G. and Philipson, L. (1968) Cell growth inhibition of human cell lines by human tissue extracts. Exp. Cell. Res. 51, 275–290.

Otsuka, H. (1969) Difference of the inhibitor of DNA synthesis in liver extract from liver arginase. Cancer Res. 29, 265–266.

Otsuka, H. (1969) Mechanism of inhibition of DNA synthesis of sarcoma 180 cells by liver extract. Cancer Res. 29, 1653–1657.

Otsuka, H. and Terayama, H. (1966) Inhibition of DNA-synthesis in ascites hepatoma cells by normal liver extract. Biochim. Biophys. Acta 123, 274–285.

Paul, D., Leffert, H., Sato, G. and Holley, R. W. (1972) Stimulation of DNA and protein synthesis in fetal-rat liver cells by serum from partially hepatectomized rats. Proc. Natl. Acad. Sci. U.S. 69, 374–377.

Rytömaa, T. and Kiviniemi, K. (1968) Control of granulocyte production. I. Chalone and antichalone, two specific humoral factors. Cell Tissue Kinet. 1, 329–340.

Saetren, H. A. (1956) A principle of auto-regulation of growth. Production of organ-specific mitose-inhibitors in kidney and liver. Exp. Cell Res. 11, 229–232.

Short, J., Brown, R. F., Husakova, A., Gilbertson, J. R. and Lieberman, I. (1972) Induction of deoxyribonucleic acid synthesis in the liver of the intact animal. J. Biol. Chem. 247, 1757–1766.

Sigel, B., Baldia, L. B., Brightman, S. A., Dunn, M. R. and Price, R. I. M. (1968) Effect of blood flow reversal in liver autotransplants upon site of hepatocyte regeneration. J. Clin. Invest. 47, 1231–1237.

Simard, A., Corneille, L., Deschamps, Y. and Verly, W. G. (1974) Inhibition of cell proliferation in the livers of hepatectomized rats by a rabbit hepatic chalone. Proc. Natl. Acad. Sci. U.S. 71, 1763–1766.

Simek, J. F., Rubin, F. and Lieberman, I. (1968) Synthesis of DNA after partial hepatectomy without changes in lipid and glycogen contents of liver. Biochem. Biophys. Res. Commun. 30, 571–575.

Spielhoff, R. (1971) The specificity of the regulation of organ growth: the effect of tissue extracts on the incorporation of triated thymidine in liver and kidney. Proc. Soc. Exp. Biol. 138, 43–45.

Stich, H. F. and Florian, M. L. (1958) The presence of a mitotic inhibitor in the serum and liver of adult rats. Can. J. Biochem. Physiol. 36, 855–859.

Verly, W. G. (1973) The hepatic chalone. Natl. Cancer Inst. Monogr. 38, 175–184.

Verly, W. G., Deschamps, Y., Pushpathadam, J. and Desrosiers, M. (1971) The hepatic chalone. I. Assay method for the hormone and purification of rabbit liver chalone. Can. J. Biochem. 49, 1376–1383.

Vinet, B. and Verly, W. G.; Purification of a protein inhibitor of DNA synthesis in cells of hepatic origin. Submitted for publication.

Volm, M., Ho, A. D., Mattern, J. and Wayss, K. (1973) Non-existence of tissue-specific growth inhibitors in the liver supernatant ('hepatic chalone'). Exp. Pathol. 8, 341–348.

Volm, M., Kinzel, V., Mohr, U. and Süss, R. (1969) Inactivation of tissue-specific inhibitors by a carcinogen. Experientia 25, 68–69.

Wayss, K., Mattern, J. and Volm, M. (1973) Elimination by the carcinogen diethylnitrosamine of non-specific inhibitory factors in the regenerating liver. Exp. Pathol. 8, 384–385.

Weiss, P. and Kavanau, J. L. (1957) A model of growth and growth control in mathematical terms. J. Gen. Physiol. 41, 1–47.

Worcel, A. and Burgi, E. (1974) Properties of a membrane-attached form of the folded chromosome of *Escherichia coli*. J. Mol. Biol. 82, 91–105.

Xeros, N. (1962) Deoxyriboside control and synchronization of mitosis. Nature 194, 682–683.

Yamada, M. and Hanaoka, F. (1973) Periodic changes in the association of mammalian DNA with the membrane during the cell cycle. Nature New Biol. 243, 227–230.

CHAPTER 19

Ascites tumours and chalones

PETER BICHEL

The Institute of Cancer Research, Radiumstationen, Nörrebrogade 44,
DK-8000 Aarhus C, Denmark*

19.1 Ascites tumours

Ascites tumours are defined as neoplasms consisting essentially of suspensions of free tumour cells growing in ascitic effusion in the peritoneal
cavity. This phenomenon was initially discovered by Hesse (1927) and Koch
(1928). Assuming a protozoan aetiology of cancer they demonstrated, using a
Flexner–Jobling rat carcinoma, the possibility of transferring the tumour
by means of the carcinomatous fluid.

On the basis of this experience the widely used Ehrlich ascites carcinoma
was produced in 1932 by Loewenthal and Jahn, and in the following years a
number of reports were published dealing with this new tumour model
(Collier and Jahn, 1934; Seeger, 1937; Auler and Hohenadel, 1938; Haagen
and Krueckeberg, 1938; Kreide and Kudiche, 1938; Lettré, 1941).

The conditions for transformation of solid into ascites tumours were
investigated by Klein (1953), who demonstrated that some solid tumours
gave rise to ascites tumours immediately after transplantation into the
peritoneal cavity. Some tumours were transformed into ascites tumours
only after a few or more transplant generations and some tumours remained
solid even after series of intraperitoneal transplantations. It was concluded
that a high degree of anaplasia and/or a rapid growth rate were necessary
but not sufficient conditions for the conversion of solid into ascites tumours.
However, the basic problems concerning the ability of some tumours to
grow in the ascites form are still unknown and need further elucidation.

---

* Sponsored by the Danish Cancer Society.

19.2 Growth patterns of ascites tumours

19.2.1 The growth curve

Based on the assumption that the free cells suspended in the ascites fluid represent the majority of the tumour cells in the host, direct determination of the total number of tumour cells in the ascites fluid would appear to be a suitable method in the evaluation of the growth patterns of such tumours.

Predominantly two different methods have been used for the estimation of the number of free tumour cells in the peritoneal cavity.

These are quantitative recovery after aspiration and repeated rinsings with physiological saline (Klein and Révész, 1953), and dye dilution techniques (Patt et al., 1953; Révész and Klein, 1954). The latter method permits an estimation of the cell-free ascites volume, and after cell counts and determination of the volume ratio of cell sediment to supernatant by centrifugation, the number of free tumour cells can be calculated.

By both methods, reliable counts of free tumour cells are obtained only if correction is made for the admixture of non-tumour cells. With the Ehrlich ascites tumour the percentage of non-tumour cells in the ascites fluid was, shortly after inoculation, dependent on the inoculum dose being higher with small than with large inocula (Klein and Révész, 1953). Soon after inoculation the ascites tumour attained a 'nearly pure culture' stage, that is 70–90% of the cells in the ascites were tumour cells (Klein and Révész, 1953). In the Krebs-2 ascites tumour a decrease in the percentage of tumour cells from the inoculum value of 92 to 78% occurred on the first day after inoculation followed by a return to a fairly constant level of about 90% on the third day (Patt et al., 1953).

During the initial phase the growth rate of the ascites tumour appears to be related to the inoculum dose. With the Ehrlich (Klein and Révész, 1953; Lala, 1968) and MC1M tumours (Klein and Révész, 1953), the initial growth rate was inversely related to the number of inoculated cells, i.e. decreasing initial growth rates were observed after the inoculation of increasing cell numbers.

With increasing age of the ascites tumour a continuous deceleration of the growth rate is observed leading to a plateau phase with a constant number of free cells. The decreasing growth rate seems mainly to be a function of the total number of cells, and levelling becomes apparent when a certain maximum number of cells has been reached. It was demonstrated by Hauschka and Grinnell (1955) and Hauschka et al. (1957) that the final population size was dependent on the ploidy of the tumour. The maximum number of cells reached by a diploid Ehrlich ascites tumour was found to be about twice as high as the number reached by a tetraploid subline of the same tumour, but a comparison of the cell volumes revealed that the volume of the diploid cells was only about one half of that of the tetraploid line. Thus, the growth of an ascites tumour seems to be limited by a maximal tumour protoplasmic mass.

In fig. 19.1 is shown the growth curve of the JB-1 ascites tumour in AKR mice after intraperitoneal inoculation of 2.5×10^6 ascites tumour cells.

The JB-1 ascites tumour is a transplantable plasmacytoma maintained syngenetically in the AKR strain of mice.

It appears from fig. 19.1 that from day 2 to 6 after inoculation the growth is exponential and the doubling time, T_D, of the tumour was estimated to be 22.8 h. The doubling time of the tumour gradually increases with the time after inoculation. From day 7 to 8, T_D was estimated to be about 70 h and from day 10 to 12, 240 h (Dombernowsky et al., 1973); at this time the growth levels off at about 10^9 cells.

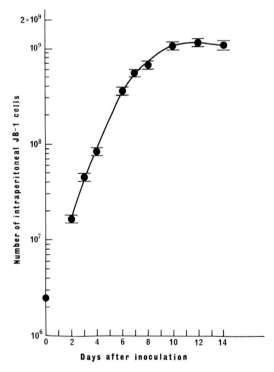

Fig. 19.1 Growth curve of the JB-1 ascites tumour after inoculation of 2.5×10^6 cells. Vectors represent standard error of the mean.

Although exceptions have been reported (Révész and Klein, 1954), several investigations of different ascites tumours have confirmed that initial rapid multiplication followed by a decreasing growth rate leading to a maximum number of cells is a general feature of ascites tumour growth (Klein and Révész, 1953; Patt et al., 1953; Patt and Blackford, 1954; Révész and Klein, 1954; Klein, 1955; Tolnai, 1965; Lala and Patt, 1966; Burns, 1968; Tannock, 1969; Frindel et al., 1969; Simpson-Herren and Lloyd, 1970; Hofer and Hofer, 1971; Dombernowsky and Hartmann, 1972).

Several mathematical models have been proposed to describe the growth curves of ascites tumours. With the Ehrlich and the MC1M ascites tumour the relationship, in the initial phase, between the number of tumour cells and time after inoculation was expressed by a cube-root transformation (Klein and Révész, 1953). With the Krebs-2 ascites tumour it was demonstrated that the initial growth pattern may be approximated to an exponential fit, especially with small numbers of cells, e.g. from 1×10^6 to 20×10^6. A cube-root transformation was found to be applicable with cell numbers from 1×10^7 to 4×10^8 (Patt and Blackford, 1954). However, neither of the two expressions could account for the entire growth pattern.

Laird (1964) and Laird et al. (1965) demonstrated that the continuous deceleration of growth in an ascites tumour is best described by a Gompertzian function, which is an exponential process limited by an exponential retardation (Laird, 1965).

19.2.2 The cell cycle

Lala and Patt (1966) were the first to point out that a major factor in the decrease in growth rate with time of an ascites tumour is a progressive increase in the duration of the mitotic cycle, and subsequent studies have confirmed these results (Frindel and Tubiana, 1967; Yankee et al., 1967; Wiebel and Baserga, 1968; Frindel et al., 1969; Peel and Fletcher, 1969; Choquet et al., 1970; Dombernowsky and Hartmann, 1972).

The mean cell cycle time T_G and the mean transit times T_{G1}, T_S, T_{G2} and T_M of G_1, S, G_2 and M, respectively, were determined in 4-, 7- and 10-day JB-1 ascites tumours by means of the labelled mitoses method, the PLM curve (Quastler and Sherman, 1959).

It appears from table 19.1 that the generation times, T_G, of the 4-, 7- and 10-day tumours were 14, 44, and 41 h, respectively. From day 4 to 7 the increase in T_G was due to an increase in the mean transit times of all phases in the cell cycle. In the 10-day plateau tumour, the decrease in T_G was due to a considerable shortening of T_{G1} while T_{G2} increased.

Table 19.1

Experimental and calculated growth parameters of the JB-1 ascites tumour at different stages of tumour development after inoculation of 2.5×10^6 cells.

	4-day tumour	7-day tumour	10-day tumour
Experimental parameters			
Cell population size $\times 10^6$	85	544	1058
T_D (h)	22.8	70	240
T_G (h)	14	44	41
T_{G_1} (h)	1	8.5	0.5
T_S (h)	11	31	31
T_{G_2} (h)	1	3	8.5
T_M (h)	1	1.5	1
Calculated parameters			
T_{Q_1} (h)	15.0	90.7	60.7
Growth fraction (per cent)	75.5	67.0	44.4
Cell production rate (per cent/h)	4.3	1.2	1.0
Cell loss rate (per cent/h)	1.3	0.2	0.7
G_1 cells (per cent)	6.5	15.3	0.6
Q_1 cells (per cent)	24.5	32.7	47.2
LI (S cells) (per cent)	60.1	46.1	34.2
G_2 cells (per cent)	4.5	3.8	8.6
Q_2 cells (per cent)	0.0	0.2	8.4
MI (per cent)	4.4	1.9	1.0

In the L1210 ascites tumour, a similar variation of T_G due to a late shortening of T_{G_1} was demonstrated by Dombernowsky and Hartmann (1972).

The results are, however, at variance with the data presented by most other authors (Lala and Patt, 1966; Yankee et al., 1967; Frindel et al., 1969; Tannock, 1969; Peel and Fletcher, 1969; Hofer and Hofer, 1971) who observed a continuous prolongation of T_G with increasing tumour mass. In the NCTC 2472 ascites tumour, Frindel et al. (1969) demonstrated a continuous increase in T_{G_1}, T_S and T_{G_2} with increasing tumour age, and similar results were obtained with the Ehrlich ascites tumour (Tannock, 1969; Peel and Fletcher, 1969) and the L1210 ascites tumour (Yankee et al., 1967). In a hypotetraploid line of the Ehrlich ascites tumour, an increase of T_S and T_{G_2} was observed, while T_{G_1} remained inappreciable during all stages of the growth (Lala and Patt, 1966).

19.2.3 The growth fraction and the cell loss

Various methods have been used to estimate the growth fraction, which is defined as the fraction of the total tumour-cell population participating in the mitotic cycle (Mendelsohn, 1960, 1962a).

With the Ehrlich ascites tumour Lala and Patt (1966) demonstrated that the decreasing growth rate with time was due not only to an increasing generation time of the ascites tumour, but also to a decreasing growth fraction.

By means of a microspectrophotometric method combined with auto-radiography, the PLM curves and a continuous labelling experiment (a CL curve) it was possible to calculate the growth fraction and the rate of cell loss in the JB-1 ascites tumour (Dombernowsky et al., 1973).

It appears from table 19.1 that the growth fraction of the JB-1 ascites tumour gradually decreases with increasing tumour age, from 76% on day 4 to 44% on day 10, which is in accordance with the observations of Lala and Patt (1966), Tannock (1969), Frindel et al. (1969) and Domber-nowsky and Hartmann (1972).

The cell loss in the 4-day tumour exceeds that in the more advanced tumours, table 19.1, probably on account of migration of cells from the peritoneal cavity. Similar results were reported in the early L1210 ascites tumour (Hofer and Hofer, 1971), while Lala and Patt (1966) calculated a relatively constant cell loss during most of the growth in the Ehrlich ascites tumour.

19.2.4 The resting compartments

The concept of a growth fraction implies that a cell population consists of two compartments, a proliferating pool of cells representing the growth fraction, and a quiescent, non-cycling or resting compartment (Lajtha et al., 1962), here designated as Q-cells.

By means of cytospectrophotometry it is possible to distinguish pre-synthetic G_1 cells with 2 N DNA content from postsynthetic G_2 cells with 4 N DNA content.

After in vivo flash labelling with $[^3H]$thymidine, the relative amounts of nuclear DNA were determined in unlabelled JB-1 tumour cells at 4, 7 and 10 days after inoculation (fig. 19.2) (Dombernowsky et al., 1973).

It appears from table 19.1 that in the 4-day tumour the number of cells having a DNA content corresponding to G_1 exceeds what can be explained from the relative duration of the G_1 phase, which means that most of these

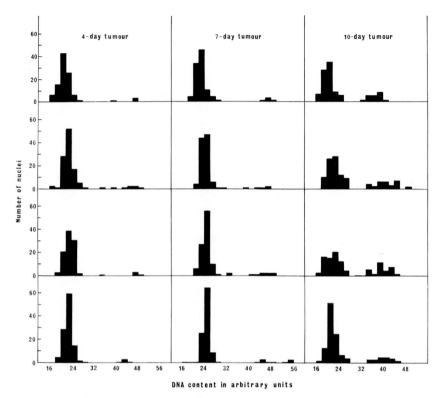

Fig. 19.2 Distribution of DNA content in unlabelled cells from four 4-, 7- and 10-day JB-1 ascites tumours, respectively, after pulse labelling with ³H-T. (Reproduced from Cell and Tissue Kinetics by kind permission of Blackwell Scientific Publications Ltd.)

cells are resting in Q_1 (Q cells with G_1 DNA content). No accumulation of cells in Q_2 (Q cells with G_2 DNA content) is observed.

In the 7-day tumour, the number of cells in G_1 and Q_1 had further increased. The vast majority of cells with G_2 DNA content were in cycle.

In the 10-day tumour, Q_1 constituted 47% of all cells, while 9% of all cells were in Q_2.

In accordance with the calculated values of Q_1 and Q_2 a considerable number of JB-1 cells with G_1- and G_2-DNA content remained unlabelled after 24 h continuous labelling of plateau tumours with [³H]TdR (fig. 19.3) which should leave most of the Q cells unlabelled (Bichel and Dombernowsky, 1973).

In the Ehrlich ascites tumour, Lala and Patt (1968) and Peel and Fletcher (1969) demonstrated that all G_0 cells had G_1 DNA contents, and based on their observations Lala and Patt concluded that decycling or recycling in

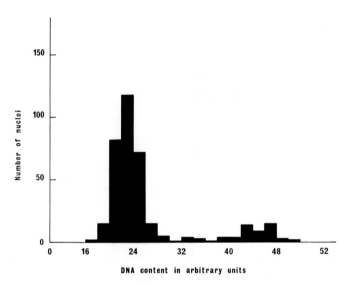

Fig. 19.3. Distribution of DNA content in unlabelled cells from JB-1 ascites tumours at the plateau after prelabelling with ³H-T for 24 h at 4-h intervals. (Reproduced from Cell and Tissue Kinetics by kind permission of Blackwell Scientific Publications Ltd.)

the Ehrlich ascites tumour occurs only after mitosis and before DNA synthesis.

However, in the NCTC 2472 ascites tumour (Frindel et al., 1969) and in the sarcoma 180 ascites tumour (DeCosse and Gelfant, 1966) an increasing percentage of cells with both G_1 and G_2 DNA contents was observed with increasing age of the tumours.

19.2.5 Recycling of resting cells

If the non-cycling cells represent true resting compartments, they would be expected to re-enter the cycle if a demand for increased growth rate occurs, such as after transplantation of old tumours to new hosts, or after aspiration of most of the tumour mass in plateau tumours.

In agreement with the observations of Baserga and Gold (1963), Lala and Patt (1968), Wiebel and Baserga (1968), Burns (1968) and Peel and Fletcher (1969), the number of cells entering the S phase increased after transplantation of 100×10^6 old JB-1 ascites tumour cells to new recipients. This was demonstrated by means of an increase in the flash labelling and continuous labelling index as well as by means of cytophotometry, in which the number of unlabelled tumour cells with S DNA content increased signifi-

cantly at the expense of unlabelled G_1 cells after transplantation of repeatedly labelled old tumour cells to new hosts (Bichel and Dombernowsky,
1973).

The observation of a resting cell population with G_1 DNA values in the
old JB-1 ascites tumour is not surprising since it is the prevailing opinion
that the decision whether a cell is going to divide or not is made in the
presynthetic period (Mueller et al., 1962; Baserga, 1965).

In mouse-ear epidermis, however, Gelfant (1962, 1966) demonstrated
that cells may be held up not only in G_1, but also in G_2 of the cell cycle, and
similar results have been reported for other tissues (Cameron and Cleffmann,
1964; Pederson and Gelfant, 1967, 1970; Post and Hoffman, 1969; Macieira-
Coelho, 1966).

A number of mice carrying JB-1 ascites tumours in the plateau phase of
growth were given five injections of tritiated thymidine at 4-h intervals.
Fifteen min after the last injection the tumours were pooled and retrans-
planted into new hosts. Every hour for the following 5 h tumour cells were
aspirated, prepared for autoradiography and the percentage of labelled
mitoses of total mitoses scored (fig. 19.4) (Bichel and Dombernowsky, 1973).

In spite of the expected labelling of all cells in cycle in the tumours used
for transplantation, only 95% of the mitotic cells were labelled. This
discrepancy might be explained by the presence of aberrant mitotic cells
unable to complete mitosis or by assuming a continuous flow of cells to a
resting compartment in Q_2 from which cells with a certain probability
return to the cycle.

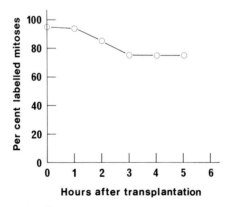

Fig. 19.4. Percentage of labelled mitoses of total mitoses after transplantation to new
hosts of plateau JB-1 ascites tumours prelabelled with ^{3}H-T in the donors for 20 h at
4-h intervals. (Reproduced from Cell and Tissue Kinetics by kind permission of Blackwell
Scientific Publications Ltd.)

From 1–3 h after transplantation the percentage of labelled mitoses gradually decreased from 95% at 1 h to 75% at 3 h after transplantation, thus indicating that some of the unlabelled, non-cycling Q_2 cells were ready rapidly to resume the cycle (fig. 19.4).

These results seem to be in accordance with the data of DeCosse and Gelfant (1966), who in the sarcoma 180 ascites tumour demonstrated a resting subpopulation of tumour cells with 4 N DNA content and, as previously mentioned, in accordance with the results of Frindel et al. (1969), who observed an increasing percentage of cells with G_2 DNA values with increasing age of the NCTC 2472 ascites tumour. On the other hand, Lala and Patt (1968) and Peel and Fletcher (1969) found that all the non-cycling cells of old Ehrlich ascites tumours had G_1 DNA values, and concluded that decycling or recycling could occur only after mitosis and before DNA synthesis.

A detailed cytokinetic study of the JB-1 ascites tumour in the regenerative phase of growth, i.e. after aspiration of most of the ascites tumour in the plateau phase, revealed a massive increase in growth rate at 24 h after aspiration. This increase was due to a release of Q_1 and Q_2 cells into the cell cycle, resulting in an increase in the growth fraction from 44 to 72% together with a marked shortening of the generation time (Dombernowsky et al., 1974).

Similar features were demonstrated in a flow microfluorometric study in which a predominance of cells with S DNA content occurred 24 h after aspiration, while the fraction of cells with 2 N and 4 N DNA content decreased (Dombernowsky and Bichel, 1975).

Thus, our present knowledge suggests that cells may pass into a true resting stage not only after completing mitosis, but also after doubling their DNA content (Epifanova and Terskikh, 1969).

19.3 Feedback regulation of growth

The recycling of resting cells after aspiration as well as after transplantation of plateau ascites tumours to new hosts, may indicate that the growth of these tumours is subject to a negative feedback regulation.

It was assumed as a working hypothesis that the cause of the low growth rate of the old ascites tumour is that the tumour cells produce a growth inhibitor which owing to the suspended nature of the ascites tumour cells is released into the ascites fluid. An increase in the number of tumour cells will therefore result in an increased concentration of the inhibitor. The increased growth rate in the recurrent growth seen after aspiration would then be a consequence of the reduced number of tumour cells leading to a decreased production and concentration of the inhibitor.

One of the necessary conditions which must be fulfilled if such a theory is to be accepted is the tissue specificity of the regulation.

Both the JB-1 and a hypotetraploid line of the Ehrlich ascites tumour will level off at an intraperitoneal tumour cell number of about 10^9. When the two tumours were simultaneously inoculated into the same mouse the number of intraperitoneal tumour cells reached 2–2.4×10^9 cells (Bichel, 1972).

These results are in accordance with the investigations of Brown (1970), who observed a complete additive growth 3 and 5 days after simultaneous inoculation of an Ehrlich ascites tumour and the Crocker ascites sarcoma 180, and a partial additive growth 9 and 14 days post-challenge.

Examination of the chromosomal pictures of the JB-1, the Ehrlich and the combined JB-1 and Ehrlich ascites tumour cells revealed that the two tumours participated almost equally in the combined growth (Bichel, 1972).

19.3.1 Arrest of JB-1 cells in G_1 and G_2

The ability of cell-free ascites fluid from old ascites tumours to inhibit the growth of the regenerating ascites tumour was investigated. Cell-free

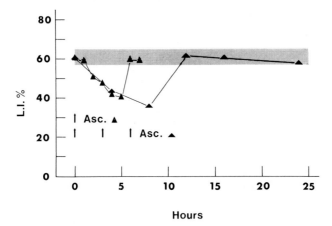

Fig. 19.5. [³H]thymidine flash-labelling index of JB-1 ascites tumour cells. Arched block: range of tumours in recurrent growth. High triangles: recurrent growth. Addition at zero hour of 2 ml of cell-free ascites fluid from JB-1 ascites tumours in their plateau phase of growth. Low triangles: recurrent growth. Addition of 2 ml of cell-free ascites fluid at 0, 3 and 6 h. (Reproduced from the European Journal of Cancer, by kind permission of Pergamon Press.)

ascites fluid obtained from AK mice bearing JB-1 ascites tumours at the plateau was injected into mice bearing JB-1 ascites tumours in the recurrent phase of growth, e.g. 24 h after aspiration. Determination of the $[^3H]$-thymidine-flash-labelling index after a single or repeated injection of the cell-free ascites fluid suggested an inhibitory step of the cell cycle located in the presynthetic period (fig. 19.5) (Bichel, 1971a).

During the first hour after a single injection of ascites fluid the flash-labelling index remained unchanged. In the next 4 h this index decreased from about 60, as usually observed in JB-1 ascites tumours in recurrent growth, to about 40. Six hours after the injection the index was again within the range of the controls.

Thus, a reversible block of the cells just prior to the DNA synthetic phase was apparently induced by the ascites fluid.

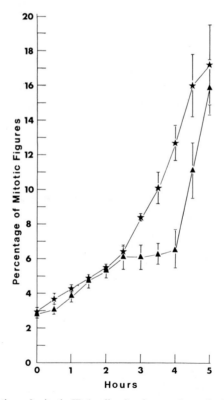

Fig. 19.6. Accumulation of mitotic JB-1 cells after intraperitoneal addition of Colcemid® at zero hour. ★—★, recurrent growth. ▲—▲, recurrent growth after addition of 2 ml of old ascites fluid at zero hour. (Reproduced from the European Journal of Cancer, by kind permission of Pergamon Press.)

Repeated injections of acellular ascites fluid were followed by a prolonged decrease in the flash-labelling index corresponding to the number of injections (fig. 19.5) (Bichel, 1971a).

Basically, similar results were obtained by Burns and Soloff (1970), who found that the attainment of a peak thymidine-^{3}H index usually seen 19 h after transplantation of 14-day old Ehrlich ascites tumour cells to new hosts was inhibited by injections of acellular ascites fluid from 14-day old Ehrlich ascites tumours.

A similar temporary arrest of JB-1 cells in G_2 was demonstrated by means of the stathmokinetic agent Colcemid ®.

By means of repeated aspirations of very small samples of the ascites tumour, the accumulation of cells in mitosis was followed for 5 h after the injection of Colcemid ® and ascites fluid (Bichel, 1971a).

It appears from fig. 19.6 that for the first 2.5 h the increase in the number of mitoses was the same in the controls only subjected to aspiration and in the mice injected with ascites fluid. From 2.5 h to 4.0 h after the injection, there was a complete cessation of the influx of cells into the mitotic phase, indicating that a block of the cell cycle had occurred about 2.5 h ahead of the mitotic phase. Four h after the injection of ascites fluid a sharp rise in the accumulation curve was observed, probably due to a release of cells which had accumulated before the block thus indicating a rapid turnover of the inhibitor. Apparently, none or at least very few cells were lost during the inhibition.

Prolonged arrest of cells was observed after repeated injections of the acellular ascites fluid at 1.5-h intervals. It was shown that the duration of the inhibition corresponded to the number of injections.

Determined with the labelled mitosis method, the duration of $G_2 + \frac{1}{2} M$ of the ascites tumour in recurrent growth is 3–4 h. The interval of about 2.5 h between the injection of ascites fluid and the cessation of the influx of tumour cells into the mitotic phase suggests that the block of the cell cycle is located to the beginning of the G_2 phase.

It was furthermore demonstrated that no inhibition of the G_1 and the G_2 phase occurred when ascites fluid from old Ehrlich ascites tumours was injected into mice carrying JB-1 ascites tumours in recurrent growth, or vice versa (Bichel, 1972). These observations lend further support to the assumption of specificity of the inhibitory reaction.

The apparent specificity of the inhibitory effect of the JB-1 ascitic fluid indicates that the inhibiting substances probably are different from the unspecific, cytotoxic polypeptide isolated from ascites fluid of Ehrlich

ascites tumours and from ascitic fluid of inoperable human ovarian carcinomata (Holmberg, 1962, 1964, 1968a, b).

Recently, it has been reported (Lala, 1972b) that although the Ehrlich
ascites tumour revealed a decreasing growth rate with time, the bone-
marrow cells of the tumour-bearing hosts seemed to escape the inhibitory
influence, which according to Lala (1972b) is due to a barrier between the
bone-marrow cells and the peritoneal cavity, which is not penetrated by the
inhibitor.

In parabiotic mice, the recurrent growth of a JB-1 ascites tumour in one
of the mice was almost completely prevented by a JB-1 ascites tumour
at the plateau carried by the parabiotic partner (Bichel, 1971b).

Consequently, it is suggested that the humoral inhibitors in the ascites
fluid are transferred to and carried by the blood and presumably reach the
bone marrow as well as a parabiotic partner. The cause of the normal and
unchanged growth of bone-marrow cells in mice with advanced Ehrlich
ascites tumours (Lala, 1972b) thus seems to be a question of specificity
rather than one of a hypothetical barrier between the bone-marrow cells
and the peritoneal cavity.

Some preliminary experiments have been carried out aiming at a characterization of the inhibitors in the ascitic fluid.

By means of stepwise ultrafiltration of the cell-free ascites fluid it was
possible to separate two fractions of the ascitic fluid, one with a molecular
weight between 10,000 and 50,000, which appeared to be responsible for
the G_1 inhibition, and another with a molecular weight between 1000 and
10,000 responsible for the G_2 inhibition (Bichel, 1973).

In the ascitic fluid of the Ehrlich ascites tumour, Hartveit (1962, 1963)
demonstrated a factor which, probably due to an immunological reaction,
was cytotoxic to Ehrlich ascites cells in vitro.

DeCosse and Gelfant (1968) demonstrated with the Ehrlich ascites tumour
that immune inhibition may restrain ascites tumour cells from cycling and
block them in G_2, and this block was apparently partly released by anti-
lymphocyte sera.

During the growth of L1210 ascites tumours in isogenic and F_1 hybrid
mice, Choquet et al. (1970) found decreased growth fractions and increased
generation times of the tumours in the F_1 hybrids as compared to the
tumours in the isogenic strain.

The possibility, however, that immune reactions could be responsible
for the G_1 and the G_2 inhibition of the cell cycle in the JB-1 ascites tumour
is probably ruled out by the fact that the JB-1 ascites tumour is carried in
the syngeneic AK/A strain of mice, and that the inhibitors in the ascites

fluid are apparently substances with molecular weights below 50,000 daltons.

A cytokinetic study of the JB-1 ascites tumour carried by mice subjected to sublethal irradiation 24 h before inoculation showed identical growth of the tumours in the irradiated and non-irradiated mice. In accordance with the observations in non-irradiated mice (Bichel and Dombernowsky, 1973; Dombernowsky et al., 1973) there was a preserved accumulation of Q_1 and Q_2 cells in the irradiated mice. These non-cycling cells re-entered the cell cycle after aspiration and after transplantation of cells from plateau tumours to new hosts (Bichel and Dombernowsky, 1975). These experiments lend further support to the assumption that the accumulation of non-cycling cells in the ageing JB-1 ascites tumour is of a non-immunological nature.

19.3.2 Conclusion

Thus, it was found that with increasing age and decreasing growth rate of the JB-1 ascites tumour, non-cycling tumour cells were accumulated at the G_1 and the G_2 level of the cell cycle. In the cell-free ascites fluid of fully developed JB-1 ascites tumours, inhibitors of the cells in the G_1 and the G_2 phase were demonstrated. The arrest of the cells in G_1 and G_2 appeared to be caused by at least two different specific substances, probably of protein nature with different molecular weights, 10,000–50,000 and 1000–10,000, respectively.

19.4 Chalones and ascites tumours

It has previously been reported that tumour extracts may contain substances with tumour-growth-inhibiting properties. Murphy and Sturm (1932a, b) observed that extracts of certain relatively slow-growing chicken tumours inhibited the growth of a mouse sarcoma, but were without effect on some other mouse tumours. Rothman (1961) demonstrated a watersoluble, dialysable substance in the necrotic fluid of old C3HBA tumours that inhibited the growth of a transplanted C3HBA mammary carcinoma. Nutini et al. (1961) showed that extracts from the sarcoma 37 and a spontaneous mammary carcinoma inhibited the growth of these tumours in mice. Horava (1954) reported that the injection of extracts of Walker 256 tumour into mice carrying the same tumours was followed by necrotizing reaction in the tumour. It is possible that mechanisms similar to those responsible for the self-limitation of growth in the JB-1 ascites tumour may have been involved in these experiments.

When the humoral inhibition of the growth of the JB-1 ascites tumour is compared with the chalone regulation of normal tissues, several similarities are revealed. The chemical messengers of the regulation appear in both cases to be endogenous tissue-specific proteins acting by reversible inhibition of the appropriate cells in the G_1 and the G_2 phase of the cell cycle, which means that the inhibitors in the ascites tumour conform to the present definition of chalones.

Although the conditions in solid tumours are much more complex than in ascites tumours and consequently more difficult to analyse, there are, as reviewed by Burns (1969), several indications of self-limitation processes regulating the growth of solid tumours as well.

On the assumption that a certain regulatory relationship might still exist between the tumour and the tissue of origin in spite of malignant transformation, most efforts have been concentrated on the investigation of the effect of normal chalones on the growth of the corresponding malignant tumours.

However, it is a well-known fact that whereas with an increasing number of transplant generations some tumours gradually transform from one histological type reminiscent of the tissue of origin to more anaplastic forms, other tumours may to a varying extent retain their original tissue structure for years.

It might be conceived that with increasing progression the tumour becomes more and more independent of the tissue of origin simultaneously with the development of a new tumour-specific feedback control determined by a new inherited physiological upper limit of size acquired during the malignant transformation.

The growth patterns of both solid and the usually very anaplastic ascites tumours, the specific feedback features of the growth of the JB-1 ascites tumour, the subnormal content in some tumours of the chalone specific for the tissue of origin and the decreased sensitivity of the tumours to their respective normal chalones (Bullough and Laurence, 1968a, b, 1970; Rytömaa and Kiviniemi, 1968; Elgjo and Hennings, 1971; Laurence and Elgjo, 1971) seem to fit in with such a hypothesis.

As pointed out by Iversen (1969, 1970), from a theoretical point of view, serious objections may be raised against treatment of malignant tumours with substances identical with the chalones of the corresponding normal tissues. Since tumour cells are apparently less sensitive to the chalones of the tissues of origin than their normal counterparts, normal cells would stop proliferation before the malignant cells.

More promising aspects emerge if in addition the tumours produce their own tumour-specific chalones. It is, however, a necessary prerequisite for future therapeutic application of chalones that their chemical constitution is known, and to my knowledge no chalones have so far been completely purified and chemically identified.

19.5 Summary

The growth curve of the JB-1 ascites tumour, a transplantable, hypotetraploid plasmacytoma, is similar to that of other hypotetraploid ascites tumours, and cytokinetic analyses of the tumour at different stages of the growth revealed that the decelerating growth with increasing tumour mass, as in most other ascites tumours, is brought about by a prolongation of the cell cycle, and a decrease in the growth fraction, while changes in the rate of cell loss is apparently of only minor importance.

Cytophotometric analyses of the tumour revealed an increasing accumulation of cells in non-cycling states, corresponding to both the G_1 and the G_2 phase of the cell cycle with increasing tumour mass. It was also shown that part of these cells were ready to re-enter the cell cycle upon transplantation of an old ascites tumour to a new host, which means that at least some of these non-cycling tumour cells represent true resting compartments.

In accordance with a negative feedback hypothesis of growth, aspiration of most of the cells from JB-1 ascites tumours at the plateau was followed by a phase of regenerative or recurrent growth, and it was shown that injections of cell-free ascitic fluid obtained from ascites tumours at the plateau into mice carrying ascites tumours in recurrent growth was followed by a transient arrest of the tumour cells in both the G_1 and the G_2 phase.

Simultaneous inoculation of two different ascites tumours into the same mouse was followed by a completely additive growth, and no block of the cell cycle was observed when old ascites fluid obtained from one of the tumours was injected into mice carrying the other ascites tumour in recurrent growth, or vice versa.

The experiments indicate that the growth deceleration is probably due to a specific feedback inhibition and is not the result of a deficient oxygen and nutrient supply or an accumulation of toxic metabolites.

By means of ultrafiltration it was possible to separate two fractions of the ascites fluid, one containing substances with molecular weights between 10,000 and 50,000 inhibiting the cells in G_1, and another containing substances with molecular weights between 1000 and 10,000 arresting the cells in G_2.

In view of the striking similarities between the effect of chalones extracted from normal tissues and the effect of the inhibitory substances contained in the cell-free ascitic fluid of the JB-1 ascites tumour, it is suggested that the growth of the JB-1 ascites tumour is, at least partially, controlled by a negative feedback regulation, exerting the effect by means of humoral, chalone-like substances.

References

Auler, H. and Hohenadel, B. (1938) Untersuchungen am Mäuseascitescarcinom. (Zugleich ein Beitrag zur Frage der Zellfreien Übertragung). Z. Krebsforsch. 48, 149.

Baserga, R. (1965) Relationship of the cell cycle to tumor growth and control of cell division: A review. Cancer Res. 25, 581.

Baserga, R. and Gold, R. (1963) The uptake of tritiated thymidine by newly transplanted Ehrlich ascites tumor cells. Exp. Cell Res. 31, 576.

Bichel, P. (1971a) Autoregulation of ascites tumour growth by inhibition of the G-1 and the G-2 phase. Europ. J. Cancer 7, 349.

Bichel, P. (1971b) Feedback regulation of growth of ascites tumours in parabiotic mice. Nature (Lond.) 231, 449.

Bichel, P. (1972) Specific growth regulation in three ascitic tumours. Europ. J. Cancer 8, 167.

Bichel, P. (1973) Further studies on the self-limitation of growth of JB-1 ascites tumours. Europ. J. Cancer 9, 133.

Bichel, P. and Dombernowsky, P. (1973) On the resting stages of the JB-1 ascites tumour. Cell Tissue Kinet. 6, 359.

Bichel, P. and Dombernowsky, P. (1975) Resting stages of the JB-1 ascites tumour in the irradiated mouse. Europ. J. Cancer 11, 425.

Brown, H. R. (1970) The growth of Ehrlich carcinoma and Crocker sarcoma ascitic cells in the same host. Anat. Rec. 166, 283.

Bullough, W. S. and Laurence, E. B. (1968a) Control of mitosis in rabbit V × 2 epidermal tumours by means of the epidermal chalone. Europ. J. Cancer 4, 587.

Bullough, W. S. and Laurence, E. B. (1968b) Control of mitosis in mouse and hamster melanomata by means of the melanocyte chalone. Europ. J. Cancer 4, 607.

Bullough, W. S. and Laurence, E. B. (1970) The lymphocytic chalone and its antimitotic action on a mouse lymphoma in vitro. Europ. J. Cancer 6, 525.

Burns, E. R. (1968) Initiation of DNA synthesis in Ehrlich ascites tumor cells in their plateau phase of growth. Cancer Res. 28, 1191.

Burns, E. R. (1969) On the failure of self-inhibition of growth in tumors. Growth 33, 25.

Burns, E. R. and Soloff, B. L. (1970) Further studies on the recurrent growth of the Ehrlich ascites tumor. Anat. Rec. 166, 285.

Cameron, I. L. and Cleffmann, G. (1964) Initiation of mitosis in relation to the cell cycle following feeding of starved chickens. J. Cell Biol. 21, 169.

Choquet, C., Chavaudre, N. and Malaise, E. P. (1970) The influence of allogeneic inhibition and tumour age on the kinetics of L1210 leukaemia in vivo. Europ. J. Cancer 6, 373.

Collier, W. A. and Jahn, G. (1934) Über die Natur des Ehrlichschen Mäusecarcinoms. Die Chemoresistenz. Z. Krebsforsch. 40, 298.

DeCosse, J. and Gelfant, S. (1966) Demonstration of subpopulations in ascites tumor cells. Proc. Amer. Ass. Cancer Res. 7, 17.

DeCosse, J. and Gelfant, S. (1968) Noncycling tumor cells: mitogenic response to anti-lymphocytic serum. Science 162, 698.

Dombernowsky, P. and Bichel, P. (1975) Cytokinetic variations during ageing and regenerative growth in the JB-1 ascites tumour studied by impulse cytophotometry. Acta Pathol. Microbiol. Scand. Sect. A 83, 222.

Dombernowsky, P. and Hartmann, N. R. (1972) Analysis of variations in the cell population kinetics with tumor age in the L1210 ascites tumor. Cancer Res. 32, 2452.

Dombernowsky, P., Bichel, P. and Hartmann, N. R. (1973) Cytokinetic analysis of the JB-1 ascites tumour at different stages of growth. Cell Tissue Kinet. 6, 347.

Dombernowsky, P., Bichel, P. and Hartmann, N. R. (1974) Cytokinetic studies of the regenerative phase in the JB-1 ascites tumour. Cell Tissue Kinet. 7, 47.

Elgjo, K. and Hennings, H. (1971) Epidermal chalone and cell proliferation in a transplantable squamous cell carcinoma in hamsters. I. In vivo results. Virchows Arch. Abt. B 7, 1.

Epifanova, O. I. and Terskikh, V. V. (1969) On the resting periods in the cell life cycle. Cell Tissue Kinet. 2, 75.

Frindel, É. and Tubiana, M. (1967) Durée du cycle cellulaire au cours de la croissance d'une ascite expérimentale de la souris C³H. C. R. Acad. Sci. (Paris) 265D, 829.

Frindel, É., Valleron, A. J., Vassort, F. and Tubiana, M. (1969) Proliferation kinetics of an experimental ascites tumour of the mouse. Cell Tissue Kinet. 2, 51.

Gelfant, S. (1962) Initiation of mitosis in relation to the cell division cycle. Exp. Cell Res. 26, 395.

Gelfant, S. (1966) Patterns of cell division: the demonstration of discrete cell populations. In: Methods in Cell Physiology, vol. 2 (ed.: D. M. Prescott) Academic Press, New York, p. 359.

Haagen, E. and Krueckeberg, B. (1938) Arbeiten am Tumorascites der Maus. III. Mitt. Beobachtungen über seine Übertragbarkeit. Z. Krebsforsch. 47, 382.

Harveit, F. (1962) Cellular injury in untreated Ehrlich's ascites carcinoma. Brit. J. Cancer 16, 556.

Harveit, F. (1963) The in vitro demonstration of a cytotoxic factor in Ehrlich's ascites carcinoma. Acta Pathol. Microbiol. Scand. 58, 10.

Hauschka, T. S. and Grinnell, S. T. (1955) Comparison of the growth curves of a diploid mouse ascites tumor and a tetraploid subline of the same tumor. Proc. Amer. Ass. Cancer Res. 2, 22.

Hauschka, T. S., Grinnell, S. T., Révész, L. and Klein, G. (1957) Quantitative studies on the multiplication of neoplastic cells in vivo. IV. Influence of doubled chromosome number on growth rate and final population size. J. Natl. Cancer Inst. 19, 13.

Hesse, F. (1927) Über experimentellen Bauchkrebs bei Ratten. Zbl. Bakt., I. Abt. Orig. 102, 367.

Hofer, K. G. and Hofer, M. (1971) Kinetics of proliferation, migration, and death of L1210 ascites cells. Cancer Res. 31, 402.

Holmberg, B. (1962) Inhibition of cellular adhesion and pseudopodia formation by a dialysable factor from tumour fluids. Nature (Lond.) 195, 45.

Holmberg, B. (1964) The isolation and composition of a cytotoxic polypeptide from tumour fluids. Z. Krebsforsch. 66, 65.

Holmberg, B. (1968a) Further biochemical studies on a dialysable polypeptide obtained from tumor fluids. Europ. J. Cancer 4, 263.

Holmberg, B. (1968b) The effects on cell multiplication in vitro of a dialysable polypeptide derived from tumor fluids. Europ. J. Cancer 4, 271.

Horava, A. (1954) Haemorrhagic necrosis induced in a transplanted malignant tumour by a biological fluid. Canad. Med. Ass. J. 70, 676.

Iversen, O. H. (1969) Chalones of the skin. G. E. W. Wolstenholme and J. Knight (Eds.): Ciba Foundation Symposium on Homeostatic Regulators. Lond.: J. A. Churchill, p. 29.

Iversen, O. H. (1970) Some theoretical considerations on chalones and the treatment of cancer: A review. Cancer Res. 30, 1481.

Klein, E. (1955) Immediate transformation of solid into ascites tumors. Studies on a mammary carcinoma of an inbred mouse strain. Exp. Cell Res. 8, 213.

Klein, G. (1953) Conversion of solid into ascites tumours. Nature (Lond.) 171, 398.

Klein, G. and Révész, L. (1953) Quantitative studies on the multiplication of neoplastic cells in vivo. I. Growth curves of the Ehrlich and MC1M ascites tumors. J. Natl. Cancer Inst. 14, 229.

Koch, J. (1928) Welche Tatsachen und Schlussfolgerungen ergeben sich aus der Infektiosität des Aszites beim Bauchfellkrebs der Ratte? Zbl. Bakt., I. Abt. Orig. 107, 332 (6).

Kreide, U. and Kudicke, H. (1938) Zellfreie Übertragung von Säugetiertumoren. Frankfurt. Z. Path. 52, 407.

Laird, A. K. (1964) Dynamics of tumor growth. Brit. J. Cancer 18, 490.

Laird, A. K. (1965) Dynamics of tumor growth: Comparison of growth rates and extrapolation of growth curve to one cell. Brit. J. Cancer 19, 278.

Laird, A. K., Tyler, S. A. and Barton, A. D. (1965) Dynamics of normal growth. Growth 29, 233.

Lajtha, L. G., Oliver, R. and Gurney, C. W. (1962) Kinetic model of a bone-marrow stem-cell population. Brit. J. Haematol. 8, 442.

Lala, P. K. (1968) Cytokinetic control mechanisms in Ehrlich ascites tumour growth. Effects of Radiation on Cellular Proliferation and Differentiation. IAEA, Vienna p. 463.

Lala, P. K. (1972) DNA-synthesis time of bone marrow cells in healthy and ascites tumor bearing mice. Cell Tissue Kinet. 5, 79.

Lala, P. K. and Patt, H. M. (1966) Cytokinetic analysis of tumor growth. Proc. Natl. Acad. Sci. 56, 1735.

Lala, P. K. and Patt, H. M. (1968) A characterization of the boundary between the cycling and resting states in ascites tumor cells. Cell Tissue Kinet. 1, 137.

Laurence, E. B. and Elgjo, K. (1971) Epidermal chalone and cell proliferation in a transplantable squamous cell carcinoma in hamsters. II. In vitro results. Virchows Arch. Abt. B 7, 8.

Lettré, H. (1941) Einige Beobachtungen über das Wachstum des Mäuse-Ascites-Tumors und seine Beeinflussung. Hoppe-Seylers Z. Physiol. Chem. 268, 59.

Loewenthal, H. and Jahn, G. (1932) Übertragungsversuche mit carcinomatöser Mäuse-Ascitesflüssigkeit und ihr Verhalten gegen physikalische und chemische Einwirkungen. Z. Krebsforsch. 37, 439.

Macieira-Coelho, A., Pontén, J. and Philipson, L. (1966) Inhibition of the division cycle in confluent cultures of human fibroblasts in vitro. Exp. Cell Res. 43, 20.

Mendelsohn, M. L. (1960) The growth fraction: a new concept applied to tumors. Science 132, 1496.

Mendelsohn, M. L. (1962) Autoradiographic analysis of cell proliferation in spontaneous breast cancer of C_3H mouse. III. The growth fraction. J. Natl. Cancer Inst. 28, 1015.

Murphy, J. B. and Sturm, E. (1932a) Properties of the causative agent of a chicken tumor. IV. Association of an inhibitor with the active principle. J. Exp. Med. 56, 107.

Murphy, J. B. and Sturm, E. (1932b) Properties of the causative agent of a chicken tumor. VI. Action of the associated inhibitor on mouse tumors. J. Exp. Med. 56, 483.

Nutini, L. G., Fardon, J. C., Cook, E. S., Perez, N. T., Medley, D. L. and Mamola, N. J. (1961) Tumors as a source of growth inhibitors and accelerators. Proc. Amer. Ass. Cancer Res. 3, 255.

Patt, H. M. and Blackford, M. E. (1954) Quantitative studies of the growth response of the Krebs ascites tumor. Cancer Res. 14, 391.

Patt, H. M., Blackford, M. E. and Drallmeier, J. L. (1953) Growth characteristics of the Krebs ascites tumor. Proc. Soc. Exp. Biol. 83, 520.

Pederson, T. and Gelfant, S. (1967) Further characterization of epidermal and renal G_2 population cells. J. Cell Biol. 35, 101A.

Peel, S. and Fletcher, P. A. (1969) Changes occurring during the growth of Ehrlich ascites cells in vivo. Europ. J. Cancer 5, 581.

Post, J. and Hoffman, J. (1969) A G_2 population of cells in autogenous rodent sarcoma. Exp. Cell Res. 57, 111.

Quastler, H. and Sherman, F. G. (1959) Cell population kinetics in the intestinal epithelium of the mouse. Exp. Cell Res. 17, 420.

Révész, L. and Klein, G. (1954) Quantitative studies on the multiplication of neoplastic cells in vivo. II. Growth curves of three ascites lymphomas. J. Natl. Cancer Inst. 15, 253.

Rothman, H. (1961) A dialyzable C3HBA tumor inhibiting factor in C3HBA tumors. Proc. Amer. Ass. Cancer Res. 3, 263.

Rytömaa, T. and Kiviniemi, K. (1968) Control of DNA duplication in rat chloroleukaemia by means of the granulocytic chalone. Europ. J. Cancer 4, 595.

Seeger, P. G. (1937) Untersuchungen am Tumorascites der Maus: Vitalfärbbarkeit der Asziteszellen. Arch. Exp. Zellforsch. 20, 280.

Simpson-Herren, L. and Lloyd, H. H. (1970) Kinetic parameters and growth curves for experimental tumor systems. Cancer Chemother. Rep. 54, 143.

Tannock, I. F. (1969) A comparison of cell proliferation parameters in solid and ascites Ehrlich tumors. Cancer Res. 29, 1527.

Tolnai, S. (1965) An analysis of the life cycle of Ehrlich ascites tumor cells. Lab. Invest. 14, 701.

Wiebel, F. and Baserga, R. (1968) Cell proliferation in newly transplanted Ehrlich ascites tumor cells. Cell Tissue Kinet. 1, 273.

Yankee, R. A., De Vita, V. T. and Perry, S. (1967) The cell cycle of leukemia L1210 cells in vivo. Cancer Res 27, 2381.

CHAPTER 20

Search for arterial smooth muscle cell chalone(s)*

W. A. Thomas, K. Janakidevi, R. A. Florentin, K. T. Lee
and J. M. Reiner

*Department of Pathology and Specialized Center of Research in Atherosclerosis,
Albany Medical College, Albany, New York 12208, U.S.A.*

Excessive proliferation of arterial smooth muscle cells (SMC) is a prominent feature in the development of atherosclerotic plaques in man and in experimental animals (Geer et al., 1961; Haust and More, 1963; Florentin et al., 1968). Mechanisms accounting for the excessive arterial SMC proliferation are complex and as yet poorly understood. Numerous drugs, hormones, and other types of therapy have been used in an attempt to modify the atherosclerotic process, but with little or no success in man. Similar efforts in experimental animals, aimed at preventing progression or causing regression of atherosclerotic lesions, have been somewhat more successful, indicating that the atherosclerotic process can be modified in a favorable direction.

Probably the most spectacular of the regression studies in experimental animals are those of Daoud et al. (1974) in swine. Advanced atherosclerotic lesions were produced in the abdominal aorta by balloon-intimal trauma and a hypercholesterolemic diet. The lesions were characterized by a great increase in arterial SMC proliferation as indicated by excessive accumulation in the intima and by a manyfold increase in [³H]TdR incorporation. Some of the swine were placed on a drastic low-fat cholesterol diet for 16 months. Swine were then sacrificed and the atherosclerotic lesions were found to have regressed until the contours of the arterial wall were almost normal. [³H]TdR studies showed that the rate of incorporation had decreased to the normal low levels of controls.

The above background material is presented to show the reason for our interest in searching for an arterial SMC chalone and perhaps to stimulate

* This study was supported by USPHS Grant HL 14177.

others to join in the search. The dietary regimens that have proved to be successful in experimental animals are too drastic to be acceptable to Western man on the long-term basis that is required. Drugs, such as some of the antimetabolites, that seem to have some effect on the atherosclerotic process in experimental animals have too many undesirable side effects to be practical for man. Obviously, an endogenous natural substance with the reputed cell-type specific characteristic of a chalone could be very useful.

Our search for arterial SMC chalones is still in an early stage and we cannot be certain as yet that one really exists. However, we do have some encouraging results that at least suggest the presence of an arterial SMC mitotic inhibitor in aqueous extracts of arterial tissue.

We decided at the outset that an inhibitor should first be demonstrated in an in vivo situation before proceeding to tissue culture methods, which are probably more practical for purification. Our experiences with arterial SMC mitotic and [^{3}H]TdR labeling indices were largely with swine (Florentin et al., 1969a, b; Thomas et al., 1971), so we chose this animal for our initial studies. Difficulties included the exceedingly low mitotic indices in arterial SMC and marked variability from swine to swine. To circumvent the latter we developed a method for comparing control and experimental tissues in the same swine. This involved use of the paired carotid arteries. We found that, at any given time, colchicine mitotic indices in the right and left carotids at corresponding anatomical points were reasonably similar (table 20.1).

Table 20.1

Comparison of mitotic counts of arterial SMC in the two carotid arteries of swine four hours after colchicine injection.

Swine	No. of mitoses/total cells counted		No. of mitoses/100,000 SMC		Difference of left carotid from right, %
	Right carotid	Left carotid	Right carotid	Left carotid	
1	86/62,030	114/93,485	139	122	12
2	176/94,084	165/92,229	187	179	4
3	165/118,869	135/89,607	139	151	9
4	220/59,658	201/68,832	368	292	21
5	173/108,351	149/103,410	160	144	10
	Mean ± SE		199 ± 38	178 ± 26	11 ± 3

Table 20.2

Mitotic counts on one carotid artery (control) four hours after colchicine divided by mitotic counts on other carotid artery two hours after colchicine*.

Swine	Mitotic counts/ total SMC counted		No. of mitoses/ 100,000 SMC		4 h counts/ 2-h counts ratio
	4 h	2 h	4 h	2 h	
1	300/174,262	203/300,340	172	67	2.57
2	426/99,250	219/73,173	429	299	1.43
3	191/206,970	83/124,635	92	66	1.39
4	251/96,600	203/187,370	259	108	2.40
5	117/82,560	64/81,825	142	78	1.82
6	222/181,270	123/177,660	122	69	1.77
7	235/173,300	109/119,730	135	91	1.48
8	9/71,385	2/54,850	13	4	3.25
9	8/88,205	3/77,065	9	5	1.80
10	7/85,680	3/55,965	8	5	1.60
	Mean $\pm$ SE		138 $\pm$ 39	79 $\pm$ 26	1.95 $\pm$ 0.18

* Swine were injected intraperitoneally with 5 ml of saline at 2 h.

Table 20.3

Mitotic counts on one carotid artery (experimental) four hours after colchicine divided by those on other carotid artery two hours after colchicine*.

Swine	Aortic extract, μg of protein	Mitotic counts/ total SMC counted		No of mitoses/ 100,000 SMC		4-h counts/ 2-h counts ratio
		4 h	2 h	4 h	2 h	
1	1,705	34/12,584	44/17,416	270	253	1.07
2	1,705	9/22,923	4/14,121	39	28	1.39
3	1,000	62/71,206	63/61,799	87	102	0.85
4	980	116/78,785	97/76,030	147	127	1.16
5	980	98/70,035	83/57,990	140	143	0.98
6	650	33/139,250	32/162,220	20	19	1.05
7	647	19/207,605	20/155,615	9	12	0.75
8	550	205/86,070	203/101,640	238	200	1.19
9	550	426/80,445	304/73,145	529	415	1.27
		Mean $\pm$ SE		164$\pm$52	144$\pm$41	1.08$\pm$0.06**

* Counts on swine given at two hours intraperitoneal injections of aortic extract containing more than 500 μg of protein.
** Difference between 1.08 $\pm$ 0.06 from this table and 1.95 $\pm$ 0.18 from table 20.2 is significant at $P < 0.001$ by the Student t-test.

We then proceeded to determine changes over a short period of time. Colchicine was given at time zero. At time 2 h, swine were anesthetized and a biopsy was taken from one carotid. A second dose of colchicine was given, and at time 4 h the other carotid was biopsied. Comparison of mitotic indices at the two times indicated that on the average there was doubling. Ratios of 4-h/2-h values are given in table 20.2.

Next we proceeded to test the effect of an injection of aqueous aortic extract on this ratio. Donor swine aortas from a slaughterhouse were extracted in a fashion similar to that used by others for skin. The extract was adjusted to 80% with ethanol, the precipitate dissolved, and the solution lyophilized. When needed for use, the powder was redissolved in saline and undissolved portions removed by centrifugation. Protein content of the solution was determined and injections were made intraperitoneally in the doses indicated in tables 20.3 and 20.4. The injections were made at time 2 h after biopsy of one carotid. The other carotid was biopsied at 4 h. Comparison of the values for the two time periods in swine receiving 500

Table 20.4

Mitotic counts on one carotid artery four hours after colchicine divided by those on other carotid artery two hours after colchicine*.

Swine	Aortic extract, μg of protein	Mitotic counts/ total SMC counted		No. of mitoses/ 100,000 SMC		4-h counts/ 2-h counts ratio	No positive/ total in subset ratio
		4 h	2 h	4 h	2 h		
1	490	62/94,205	20/67,540	66	30	2.20	
2	490	52/112,995	15/24,520	46	61	0.75	2/3
3	450	46/203,580	23/187,455	17	18	0.94	
4	290	26/107,690	16/115,375	24	14	1.71	
5	285	35/97,705	50/113,640	36	46	0.78	2/4
6	285	75/152,040	63/122,585	49	51	0.96	
7	245	80/94,265	15/59,985	85	25	3.40	
8	80	92/97,105	37/104,305	95	35	2.71	
9	80	25/103,200	22/70,370	31	24	1.29	1/3
10	49	66/117,235	12/57,105	56	21	2.67	

* Counts on swine given at two hours intraperitoneal injections of aortic extract containing less than 500 μg of protein.

Table 20.5

Comparison of effects of aortic extracts and saline intraperitoneal injections on four-hour/two-hour epidermal mitotic count values*.

Group	No. of swine	No. of paired samples	4-h value/2-h value ± S.E.**	Dose, μg
Saline-treated	10	34	1.38 ± 0.15	...
Aortic-extract treated	7	22	1.59 ± 0.15	1,050–2,650

* Aortic extracts of saline were injected two hours after colchicine. Skin samples from the two sides of the body were paired by anatomic location.

** Differences between four-hour/two-hour values for the two groups are not significant by the Student *t*-test.

Table 20.6

Comparison of extent of intimal lesions resulting from balloon-catheter trauma and a hypercholesterolemic diet in abdominal aortas of aortic extract-treated and control swine.

Pair No.	Days on diet	% of intima involved by lesions of any thickness		% of intima involved by lesions 500 μm or greater in thickness	
		Aortic extract	Control	Chalone	Control
1	8	42	53	6	20
2	15	31	30	1	6
3	20	12	56	0	4
4	57	17	26	0	0
5	60	2	26	0	0
6	62	28	38	0	0
7	78	20	34	0	10
8	82	39	35	3	3
9	100	53	51	12	42
10	100	37	61	2	16
11	104	18	46	8	3
Mean		27.2%	41.5%	2.9%	9.5%
Statistical sig. of difference*		$P < 0.005$		$P < 0.03$	

* Student's paired *t*-test.

micrograms or more showed very little increase from 2 to 4 h suggesting that a mitotic inhibitor was present (Florentin et al., 1973).

Further studies with the above approach have been made difficult by the fact that there is not only variability among swine, but also from experiment to experiment. At times, arterial SMC mitotic indices in nearly all of the swine are so low as to make studies impractical. This variation is probably on a seasonal basis, although we have not carried out sufficient studies to be certain of this point.

Attempts to demonstrate specificity have been limited to the skin. We used the same general approach as with carotids, taking skin biopsies from one side at time 2 h following colchicine injection and at time 4 h from the other side after treatment with aortic extract or saline only. Unlike those of the carotids, skin mitotic indices do not double in the second two hours. However, they do increase, and the increase after saline injections was no greater than that after aortic extract (table 20.5). This suggests at least some degree of specificity, but obviously more studies are needed.

In a second study (Nam et al., 1974) in swine we decided to test the effect of daily injections of aortic extracts on arterial SMC proliferation in an experimental situation in which there would be considerable proliferative activity. This involved use of a model in which arterial intima is traumatized with a balloon-catheter followed by feeding a hypercholesterolemic diet. Injection of the aortic extracts twice daily did not prevent proliferative activity but did appear to reduce it somewhat as shown in table 20.6. This encouraging result provided further stimulation to purify and characterize the putative aortic chalone.

We decided that the next step should be to develop a more practical method for bioassay than that provided by the paired carotid arteries method in swine. We have not as yet succeeded in developing a satisfactory bioassay in either small animals or tissue culture. However, it is unlikely that this will be an insurmountable obstacle. When a suitable bioassay method is developed we will proceed to purify the putative mitotic inhibitor and to test it for specificity. In addition, we have begun a search for a DNA synthesis inhibitor such as those that have been demonstrated in other tissues.

References

Daoud, A. S., Jarmolych, J., Fritz, K. and Augustyn, J. (1974) Regression of advanced arteriosclerosis in swine: Morphologic Study. Circulation 50, III–92.

Florentin, R. A. and Nam, S. C. (1968a) Dietary-induced atherosclerosis in miniature swine. Exp. Mol. Pathol. 8, 263–301.

Florentin, R. A., Nam, S. C., Lee, K. T. and Thomas, W. A. (1969b) Increased ^{3}H-thymidine incorporation into endothelial cells of swine fed cholesterol for 3 days. Exp. Mol. Pathol. 10, 250–255.

Florentin, R. A., Nam, S. C., Lee, K. T., Lee, K. J. and Thomas, W. A. (1969c) Increased mitotic activity in aortas of swine. Arch. Pathol. 88, 463–469.

Florentin, R. A., Nam, S. C., Janakidevi, K., Lee, K. T., Reiner, J. M. and Thomas, W. A. (1973d) Population dynamics of arterial smooth muscle cells. II. In vivo inhibition of entry into mitosis of swine arterial smooth muscle cells by aortic tissue extracts. Arch. Pathol. 95, 317–320.

Geer, J. C., McGill, H. C. and Strong, J. C. (1961) The fine structure of human atherosclerotic lesions. Am. J. Pathol. 38, 263–275.

Haust, M. D. and More, R. H. (1963) In: Evaluation of the Atherosclerotic Plaque (ed.: R. L. Jones) University of Chicago Press, p. 51.

Nam, S. C., Florentin, R. A., Janakidevi, K., Lee, K. T., Reiner, J. M. and Thomas, W. A. (1974) Population dynamics of arterial smooth muscle cells. III. Inhibition by aortic tissue extracts of proliferative response to intimal injury in hypercholesterolemic swine. Exp. Mol. Pathol. 21, 295–267.

Thomas, W. A., Florentin, R. A., Nam, S. C., Reiner, J. M. and Lee, K. T. (1971) Alterations in population dynamics of arterial smooth muscle cells during atherogenesis. I. Activation of interphase cells in cholesterol-fed swine prior to gross atherosclerosis demonstrated by 'post-pulse salvage labeling'. Exp. Mol. Pathol. 15, 245–267.

CHAPTER 21

Colon carcinoma:
its genesis and chalone control

K. KANAGALINGAM and J. C. HOUCK

Research Foundation, Children's Hospital, Washington, D. C. 20009, U.S.A.

21.1 Introduction

An analysis of the high mortality rates due to cancer reveals that carcinoma of the colon as killer ranks second only to lung cancer in men and breast cancer in women. It is generally held that a combination of factors, both intrinsic and extrinsic, or conditions secondary to occupation may be responsible in the initiation of colon cancer. Hence it is believed that 70–85% of these cancers are preventable and have the potential for management. The object of this review is to make a cursory examination of the current knowledge of carcinoma of the colon and the progress of its management at the clinical level and in the laboratory through studies in vitro and in animals in vivo. The application of the chalone concept to the regulation of human colon carcinoma cell proliferation in vitro is described.

Epidemiologic as well as pathologic studies of the disease have indicated that the occurrence of colon cancer varies not only with geographic areas but also that socioeconomic background has a strong impact on its incidence (Higginson, 1966; Burkitt, 1971; Haenszel and Correa, 1971; Stewart, 1971; Reddy, 1973). Colonic lesions appear to be associated with the environmental factors, particularly the diet. A Western diet high in animal protein and fat constitutes a high risk area (U.S. and Europe), while the populations of low risk areas (South America, Asia, and Africa) consume food high in vegetable proteins and fiber but low in fats. Thus, in Japan, where colon cancer is uncommon, unsaturated fats constitute only 12% of the average caloric intake, whereas 40–44% of the caloric intake in the U.S. is fat and carcinoma of the large bowel is much more common (Wynder and Shigematsu, 1967). Genetic factors do not seem to play a role in this distribution, as shown by the much-quoted example of the higher incidence of colon carcinoma among Japanese immigrants in the U.S. and especially their offspring born in the U.S. than for their kin who remain in Japan (Wynder et al., 1969).

It has been suggested that diet determines the composition of the intestinal flora and that they, in turn, produce carcinogenic compounds from the food and intestinal secretions (Reddy, 1973). Alfatoxin produced by *Aspergillus flavus* and aglycone methoxyazomethanol from cycasin are known carcinogens. The former was shown to induce neoplasms in Vitamin A-deficient animals (Newberne and Rogers, 1973). Bracken fern is another example of a dietary constituent known to be carcinogenic to the large bowel (Pamuku et al., 1970).

A firm correlation between a high concentration of neutral sterols and bile-acid derivatives in the feces and the incidence of colon cancer was shown by Hill et al. (1971). Aries et al. (1969) demonstrated that significantly more bacteroids and fewer streptococci and lactobacilli were found in populations with a higher incidence of colon cancer. It was postulated that some degradative products of bile salts by bacteroids may be carcinogenic. Three-methyl cholanthrene, which is a potent carcinogen, may be produced by bacterial conversion of deoxycholic acid in the large bowel. Most carcinogens of the colon were inactive in germ-free experimental animals.

Though these observations are significant, the conclusions will remain speculative until studies that demonstrate a molecular interaction of the potential carcinogens with mucosal cells of the intestinal epithelium can be accomplished. Efforts are currently being made in several laboratories to study these fundamental biochemical changes which, in turn, may lead to the development of pharmacological therapy. In order to achieve this, there is a need for the development of better experimental animal models for the carcinoma of the colon.

21.2 Histologic and subcellular organization of the mucosa

Unlike the epithelium of the small intestine, the normal colonic mucosa, when examined microscopically, appears flat without villi. In cross-section, it is made up of tubular glands called crypts of Lieberkuhn. The proliferating epithelial cells of the mucosa are restricted to the deepest one-third of these crypts. As the cells migrate upward toward the surface to replace the exfoliated cells they differentiate and mature into goblet and absorptive cells. As these upward migrating cells reach the neck of the gland, they get sloughed off into the colonic lumen (Lipkin et al., 1963; Sawicki et al., 1968).

Thereby a perfect balance of dividing cells at the base and mature cells at the surface is maintained. It has been shown by autoradiography that the lowermost cells, being mitotically active, are also active in terms of DNA synthesis, whereas the cells at the luminal surface are not (Lipkin and Bell, 1968). Also, it is known that the amounts and distribution of several enzymes and the array of isoenzymes change as these intestinal epithelial cells mature (Dahlquist and Nordstrom, 1966; Moog et al., 1966; Imondi et al., 1969; Salser and Balis, 1973). Colonic carcinomas have been observed only among the surface cells. It is not yet clear if they have a surface origin. However, it has been shown that the mature cells at the surface which do not have DNA synthetic activity assume the capacity to incorporate thymidine into DNA and engage in active proliferation when they are associated with adenomatous polyps and villous papillomas (Deschner et al., 1966; Bleiberg et al., 1972). Furthermore, the vulnerability of the surface cells to cancer has been suggested by the difference in the rates of repair of the damage caused in both surface and crypt cell DNA during the early stages by compounds known to be carcinogenic to the colon of rat. That is, after clinical damage, the crypt cell DNA was repaired whereas the DNA of those cells on the surface was not (Kanagalingam and Balis, 1974).

21.3 Target of action

When carcinogens or their active metabolic products encounter susceptible cells, they may interact covalently with all the major groups of macromolecules in the target cells, including protein, RNA, and DNA. In liver, mammary gland and skin interactions of isotopically labeled chemical carcinogens with metabolites and specific cellular targets as DNA, RNA, and protein have been demonstrated in general (Matsumoto and Higa, 1966; Shank and Magee, 1967; Miller, 1970) and, in particular, the involvement of DNA has been suggested (Warwick and Roberts, 1967; Szafarz and Weisburger, 1969). Such an association in the intestinal tract has not yet been established. This may be due to the higher and more rapid turnover of cells and subcellular components in the intestinal mucosa (Deschner and Lipkin, 1970; Lipkin et al., 1970) in relation to the other organs studied. Even in those examples where a covalent interaction of the carcinogenic metabolite with the target macromolecular element is broadly seen, the chemical or biological consequence of such a reaction is not clear, probably because versatile methods which would facilitate a study of the interaction in the intact animal are lacking. Hence, it has not been possible to establish a categoric link between the interaction and the subsequent expression of cancer. Nevertheless, an altered DNA has provided a suitable basis for speculations on the mechanism of carcinogenesis. Many consider that in most cancer systems the transformation of a normal somatic cell to a neoplastic cell is irreversible and heritable. Thus, it would appear that the influence of the carcinogenic stimulus would be to react with the basic replicable macromolecules in the cell that have the capacity to store, transfer, and get involved in the control mechanisms of growth and development of the cell. Such an interaction could be a direct one, causing the deletion or addition of bases, or the alkylation of DNA. Hence, the host cell genome itself would be altered (Brookes and Lawley, 1964), resulting in somatic mutations and producing aberrant transcription (Ames et al., 1973). If the change is virally induced, then the integration of the viral genome with the host cell genome may ensue (Temin, 1964).

21.4 Metabolism of colon carcinogens

Carcinogenesis in general may be virally induced or may arise in response to radiation or be due to the action of natural or synthetic chemicals. So far, the involvement of virus or radiation stimuli in intestinal cancer has not been demonstrated. But there is evidence of mouse leukemia virus being stimulated by chemical carcinogens (Igel et al., 1969), and the presence of virus-like particles in chemically induced rat hepatomas has been demonstrated (Weinstein et al., 1972; Orenstein and Weinstein, 1973).

Spontaneous cancer of the intestine was not found in experimental or domestic animals except for some breeds of hamsters (Fortner, 1965). Recently, in many laboratories, malignant neoplasms of the large intestine have been induced by a number of chemicals, some of them giving a high yield (Walpole et al., 1952; Laqueur et al., 1963; Spjut and Spratt, 1965; Druckrey et al., 1967) of tumors.

Two major classes of compounds have given colonic cancers consistently in vivo: derivatives of the aromatic amine, 3-methyl-4-aminobiphenyl and derivatives of 1,2-dimethylhydrazine.

2',3' dimethyl aminobiphenyl given subcutaneously to rats was found to induce a high incidence of polyps and neoplasms in rats (Walpole and Williams, 1958). Whether administered subcutaneously or orally (Cleveland et al., 1967; Spjut and Noall, 1970), the expression of cancer took about 10 months to one year after the insult was given. Male and female rats responded similarly. Many colonic carcinogens in the 4-aminobiphenyl series have methyl substituents other than at the 2',3' position (Walpole and Williams, 1958; Spjut and Noall, 1970; Spjut, 1971). 3-methyl-2-naphthylamine is another aryl amine that has been shown to induce cancer of the colon (Burdette, 1965; Hadidian et al., 1968). The effect of this compound on male rats appeared more pronounced than in the females, probably due to the latter's fatality from breast cancer. A basic characteristic of these aromatic colonic carcinogens is the presence of a CH_3 group in the ortho position to the NH_2 group (see fig. 21.1).

Regardless of the route of administration of the carcinogen to the animal, it must undergo transformation into the active metabolite. According to Weisburger (1971), the first step in the metabolism of all carcinogenic aromatic amines would be their N-hydroxylation (fig. 21.2). This occurs in the liver by the action of a number of membrane bound enzymes. As a second step, most of the N-hydroxylated derivatives become conjugated with glucoronic acid, also catalyzed by an enzyme system. This glucoronide is then released into the intestine via the bile fluids (Cleveland et al., 1967; Spjut and Noall, 1970) and finds its way to the caecum and colon, where it is split by bacterial β-glucoronidase. In germ-free rats which are devoid of this bacterial enzyme, these compounds do not induce cancer (Wynder et al., 1969). Another factor that renders the large bowel susceptible to cancer is the presence here of the enzyme N-hydroxylase which reduces the active hydroxylamine intermediate back to the precursor amine (Weisburger et al., 1970; Williams et al., 1970).

The tropical fern 'cycad' produces nuts rich in cycasin which is the β-glucoside of methylazoxymethanol. Among the aliphatics, this compound

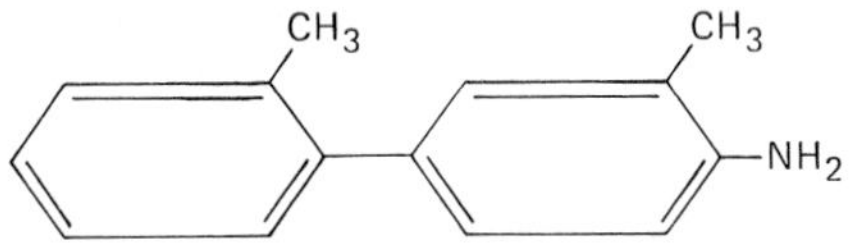

2', 3-dimethyl aminobiphenyl

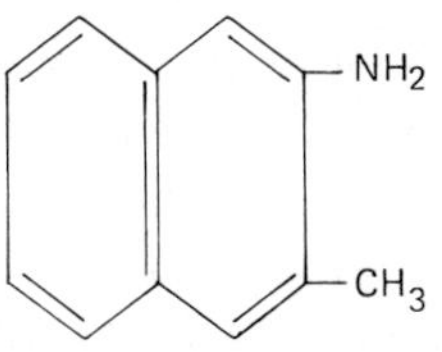

3-methyl 2-naphthylamine

Fig. 21.1. Aromatic (colon carcinogenic) amines.

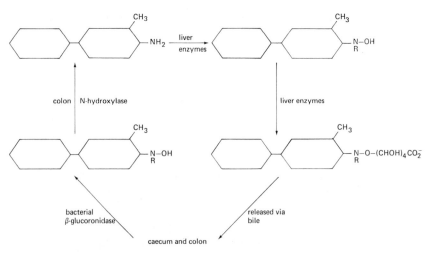

Fig. 21.2. Metabolism of 3-methyl-4-amino-biphenyl.

stands unique in its capacity to incite colonic tumors. The carcinogenicity of cycasin was first discovered by Laqueur and Spatz (Laqueur, 1965; Laqueur et al., 1967; Laqueur and Spatz, 1968; Spatz, 1969). Chronic feeding of cycasin to several strains of rats yielded many tumors in the large intestine in addition to cancers of the liver and kidney. A continual diet with 200–400 ppm cycasin was sufficient to induce colonic tumors. The more stable ester (methylazoxymethanol acetate) of cycasin produced tumors in germ-free rats of any age, whether given orally or subcutaneously (Laqueur et al., 1967), whereas the precursor cycasin was potent only in weanling or older rats.

The above findings prompted the demonstration by Druckrey (1970; Druckrey et al., 1965) of the carcinogenicity in the colon of a number of precursors of methylazoxymethanol. For example, 1,2-dimethylhydrazine yielded numerous tumors in the colon and a few in the duodenum, jejunum, and ileum. As the dose level was increased from 10 to 40 mg/kg body weight, the latent period became shorter. These tumors were demonstrated to be able to metastasize. Azoxymethane administration gave colonic as well as rectal tumors in rats. Both dimethylhydrazine and azoxymethane were effective as colon carcinogens, whether administered orally or subcutaneously. N-nitrosomethylurea is another related compound which given at a dose of 90 mg/kg induced tumors of the colon and other parts of the gut (Leaver et al., 1969). N-methyl and N-ethyl derivatives of N′-nitro-N-nitrosoguanidine were also found to induce tumors in the colon (Schoental and Bensted, 1969; Sugimura et al., 1969). Recently methyl (acetoxymethyl) nitrosamine has been demonstrated as carcinogenic to both the colon and small intestine (Rice et al., 1975).

The striking feature of these compounds is that they all have a characteristically common CH_3-N-N- configuration which may be essential for them to be metabolized to the ultimate carcinogen. Methylazoxymethanol appears to be the reactive metabolite that becomes actively carcinogenic at the site of its release in the gastrointestinal tract. It is either obtained from its corresponding β-glucoside, cycasin, as described above, in the colon, or it may be metabolized from one of its precursors, 1,2-dimethylhydrazine. The latter undergoes oxidation first to azomethane and then to azoxymethane. The hydroxylated derivative also then conjugates with glucoronic acid in the liver and is released in the bile into the duodenum. As a consequence, tumors have sometimes been found in the duodenum of rats and in the gall bladder of hamsters (Laqueur et al., 1967; Spatz, 1970). These metabolic steps are summarized in fig. 21.3.

Many investigations of the etiology and epidemiology of the disease have shed more light in the correlation of bacterial constituents in the bowel and the incidence of cancer (Aries et al., 1969; Wynder et al., 1969; Burkitt

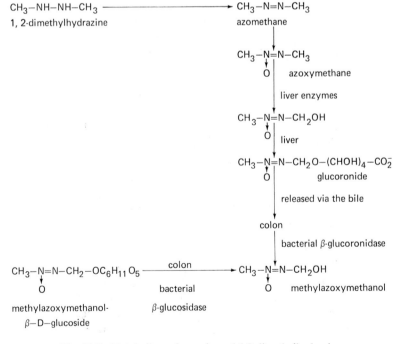

Fig. 21.3. Metabolism of cycasin and 1,2-dimethylhydrazine.

1971; Hill et al., 1971; Hill, 1974). In order for the bacterial action to be most effective, the fecal matter may be expected to remain in the large bowel for extended periods or move at a very slow pace. In fact, populations with loose feces or which exhibited frequent stools have been shown to have a lower incidence of cancer (Higginson, 1966; Walker and Walker, 1969; Wynder et al., 1969; Bremner and Ackerman, 1970; Hill et al., 1971). Though this would imply that hard stools and constipation may enhance chances of colon carcinogenesis, no difference in the production of tumors was observed in rats given both a carcinogen and a laxative (Cleveland and Cole, 1969).

21.5 Immunologic aspects

Foreign bodies which cause neoplastic changes in cells are believed to be tumor-specific antigens (Foley, 1953; Prehn and Main, 1957; Klein, 1966). Gold and Freeman (1965a, 1965b) have claimed the presence of these tumor specific antigens in the colon and other sections of the human digestive system. The response of the host to the intrusion of these antigens is to trigger the immunologic surveillance function (Burnet, 1971) of its lympho-reticular system whereby a reaction is initiated that destroys and eliminates the foreign bodies or minimizes the advent of malignancy. Tonsils, Peyer's patches, vermiform appendix, and the mesenteric lymph nodes are areas of the gastrointestinal tract with a plethora of lymphoid tissue. These may provide immunologic protection against carcinogenic agents in the alimentary canal. Immunoglobulin A, produced mainly in the small intestine (Crabbe et al., 1965), is also believed to have such a protective function (Loran and Crocker, 1963; Loran et al., 1964). It has been suggested that the rare occurrence of tumors in the small intestine may be attributed to the high concentration of IgA in this location (Lowenfels, 1973). An increased incidence of cancer associated with a deficiency in immunologic response has been demonstrated in a variety of animal models (Gatti and Good, 1971).

The tumor-specific antigen of the digestive system was present in the gut, liver, and pancreas of the fetus but was absent in other normal or cancerous adult human tissues. Hence, it was called carcinoembryonic antigen (CEA) of the human digestive system. Other antigens, the so-called non-specific cross-reacting antigen (NCA) and membrane-associated tissular auto-antigen (MTA) have been described (von Kleist and Burtin, 1969; von Kleist et al., 1974) in colonic carcinomas. Although circulating antibodies against CEA have been reported in patients with gastrointestinal cancer (Gold, 1967), the precise role of CEA, NCA, or MTA in colon carcinogenesis is unclear. After extensive study, even the detection of CEA as a diagnostic aid for colorectal carcinoma has been questioned (Miller, 1974).

21.6 Clinical management

Prognosis for the carcinoma of the colon is relatively good if it is detected and treated early. Giant strides have been made in its diagnosis since the development of fiber-optics in colonoscopy (Wolff and Shinya, 1974). Once detected at an early stage, such refined methods as 'no-touch' technique of resection (Turnbull et al., 1967), adjuvant intraluminal chemotherapy (Holden et al., 1967), and preoperative irradiation (Dwight et al., 1972) could be employed to manage or even arrest the disease. The most effective chemotherapeutic agent of colorectal carcinoma has been 5-fluorouracil (Heidelberger et al., 1957), which was first introduced for this clinical application in 1958 (Ansfield et al., 1962). The rate of tumor regression has been said to be 11–50%. The precise mechanism of its action is not known, though it appears to suppress DNA synthesis by inhibiting the enzyme thymidylate synthetase which catalyzes the methylation of 2-deoxyuridylic acid to thymidylic acid. The other chemotherapeutic agents used, namely vincristine (Horton et al., 1965), vinblastine (Al-Sarraf et al., 1972), and methotrexate (Moertel et al., 1970) have been effective only to a lesser degree. Although cytosine arabinoside and mitomycin C also show some anti-tumor activity by themselves in the large bowel, combinations of 5-fluorouracil with cytosine arabinoside (Gailani et al., 1972) or 5-fluorouracil and mitomycin C with 1, 3-bis (2-chloroethyl)-1-nitrosourea (Reitemeir et al., 1970) have not shown response rates greater than when 5-fluorouracil alone was used.

21.7 Autoregulation of epithelial cell proliferation

To maintain the normal development of the mucosal epithelium of the gastrointestinal tract a steady balance between the differentiated and mature surface cells and the actively mitotic deeper lying crypt cells must be established. This is achieved through the activation from time to time throughout life of a mechanism that regulates the proliferation of the crypt cells. Investigations in many laboratories are oriented toward an understanding of the mechanism of this type of autoregulation. Success in this area may lead to the development of controlling factors for malignant transformation of cells.

It was suggested by Weiss and Kavanau (1957) about 20 years ago that mitotic activity of most cells may be under the control of an endogenously present negative feedback inhibitor of mitosis. This led to the experimental demonstration by Bullough and Laurence (1960) of the existence of such an inhibitor for epidermal cell proliferation. They baptised this inhibitor of mitosis as 'chalone'. Since then, several laboratories have reported chalones to be found in many different systems, including granulocytes (Rytömaa and Kiviniemi, 1968), lymphocytes (Moorhead et al., 1969; Houck et al., 1971), fibroblasts (Houck et al., 1972), and crystalline lens (Voaden, 1968). Endogenous mitotic inhibitors have also been implicated in the control of cellular proliferation in such tissues as thyroid (Gary and Hall, 1970), liver (Saetren, 1956), lung (Simnett et al., 1969), and kidney (Saetren 1956, 1963; Chopra and Simnett, 1969).

A feedback inhibitor of mitosis in the gastrointestinal tract has recently become increasingly evident. Saline extracts of older embryonic duodenal mucosa were found to inhibit mitotic activity in the duodenal epithelium of younger mice in vitro and in vivo (Bischoff, 1964). Studies of Loran et al. (Loran and Crocker, 1963; Loran et al., 1964) on parabiotic rats indicated an increase in the mitotic index in the small intestine following partial resection of the ileum. They attributed this to the action of a circulating humoral factor, a growth hormone which stimulated the increased and rapid proliferation of the jejunal crypt cells. Alternatively, it has been argued that the sudden burst of cell division may have been caused by a decrease in the amount of circulating inhibitors produced by the small intestine. Tutton (1973) has since obtained an alcohol precipitable factor from the jejunal crypt cells that induced chalone-like antimitotic activity in the epithelium of the small intestine of rat. Two factors which showed inhibitory activity against mitosis have been reported in extracts of embryonic intestine (Brugal and Pelmont, 1974). Chalones in the stomach epithelium and the tissue specificity of their inhibition of cell proliferation has been evident from the work of Philpott (1971), who showed that aqueous extracts of hatching chick stomach mucosa selectively suppressed mitotic activity in younger embryonic stomach epithelia in vitro but did not have any influence on the mitosis in developing intestine, skin, or mesenchyme.

21.8 Colon chalone

We have recently found evidence that extracts of human colon carcinoma cells and also of normal colonic tissue contained such an inhibitory factor which influenced the proliferative activity of these colon carcinoma cells in vitro by exerting a regulatory control on their mitosis (Houck et al., 1975).

Human colon carcinoma cells (so-called SW-48 cells), obtained through the courtesy of Dr. Albert Liebovitz (Scott and White Clinic, Temple, Texas 76501) were cultivated at 37 °C in L-15 medium containing 10 % fetal calf serum and supplemented with gentamycin and fungizone. These cells grew readily in this medium, adhering to each other and to the growing surface in stationary culture. They produced considerable amounts of a mucinous material. They are heteroploid in karyology and have a doubling time of about 36 h in vitro.

21.9 Preparation of extracts

Large volumes of the 'used' medium were accumulated over a period of time by growing extensive populations of SW-48 cells in several 75 cm^2 Falcon tissue culture flasks and roller bottles. The L-15 growth medium containing 10 % fetal calf serum and antibiotics and incubated in the absence of cells at 37 °C for 7 days under conditions of cell cultures was the source of the 'unused' medium employed in control experiments.

After the SW-48 cells reached confluency in the flasks, they were harvested from time to time by trypsinization (0.25 % trypsin) in the presence of EDTA (0.1 %) and stored in 1 mM Tris–HCl, pH 7.4 at −80 °C. Volumes of cells accumulated in this manner were lysed by repeated freezing and thawing, followed by brief sonication. Microscopic examination showed that the suspension at this stage was largely devoid of unbroken cells. The lysate was centrifuged at 20,000 g for 1 h to obtain a clear supernatant of cell extract. All operations were performed at 4 °C.

Colon of the pig and dog and the jejunum of dog was obtained from freshly sacrificed animals. They were placed on aluminum foil spread over ice in a tray and slit open to expose the epithelium. The mucosal lining was gently rinsed with normal saline and scrapings obtained with the aid of a glass slide. These scrapings were homogenized separately in 50 mM Tris–HCl, pH 7.4 (10 ml/g) at 4 °C in a Potter–Elvehjem tissue homogenizer. Scrapings of the mucosa of aganglionic human colon from a patient with Hirschsprung's disease were made and similarly extracted. Centrifugation at 20,000 g for 1 h gave a clear supernatant of tissue extracts.

Extracts were also prepared from frozen dog lung and from bovine lung acetone powder obtained commercially. The former was minced in normal saline in a Virtis homogeniser and the latter suspended in normal saline. Both were stirred for 18 h at 4 °C and centrifuged as before to make the lung tissue extracts.

21.10 Fractionation according to molecular weight

The extracts were subjected to molecular ultrafiltration using the Amicon Diaflo ultrafiltration system (Zipilvan et al., 1969). Thus, the 'used' medium and 'unused' medium were subdivided into fractions between 1000 and 10,000 daltons, between 10,000 and 30,000 daltons, between 30,000 and 50,000 daltons, between 50,000 and 300,000 daltons and into a fraction in excess of 300,000 daltons. From the various tissue extracts, the fraction between 10,000 and 50,000 daltons was prepared also by ultrafiltration. All the molecular weight fractions were concentrated and washed on the membrane, dialyzed extensively, and lyophilized (Houck and Cheng, 1973).

21.11 Determination of cell number and thymidine uptake

One 10^5 to 4×10^5 human colon carcinoma cells were seeded into large numbers of 25 cm^2 Falcon tissue flasks containing L-15 medium supplemented with 10% fetal calf serum, gentamycin, and fungizone. One day later, when the cells had attached and established themselves, the flasks were inoculated with appropriate molecular weight fractions of the extracts and incubated at 37 °C. One, 2, and 3 days later, the cells were harvested by trypsinization in the presence of EDTA. The number of cells per flask was then estimated in triplicate by counting the cell suspension in a hemocytometer.

The mean cell number per flask was calculated and the standard deviation of these means after up to 5 days of incubation was found to lie within the range of about $\pm 7\%$. The average cell number per flask was determined after treatment with extracts and the percentage of inhibition was calculated by comparison of this figure with the cell number in the untreated controls.

Cytotoxicity was indicated by loss of cell numbers via detachment of the cells from the growing surface. Viability of the cells was established by their capacity to exclude the vital dye trypan blue.

Thymidine uptake into acid insoluble DNA was followed, using [^{3}H]TdR. Forty-two h after the incubation of the cell cultures with the extracts, 1 μCi of tritiated thymidine (0.36 Ci/mMole) was added to the medium and after 6 h, the cells were harvested in the usual manner and precipitated with cold 6% TCA. The acid insoluble fraction was collected on glass fiber filter discs and the unincorporated thymidine was eliminated by repeated washing with cold TCA. The dried filter was counted in a liquid scintillation spectrometer to determine the TdR uptake as counts per minute.

21.12 Effect of 'used' and 'unused' medium

Dose dependence studies of the inhibitory activity of the various fractions from the 'used' medium has shown that the best inhibition of SW-48 cell proliferation in vitro was exhibited by the molecular weight fraction between 10,000 and 50,000 daltons. Increasing the concentration from 1 mg/ml increased the percentage of inhibition (table 21.1). The fraction between 1000 and 10,000 daltons and the fraction in excess of 300,000 daltons were both essentially cytotoxic to the colon carcinoma cells. The fraction between 50,000 and 300,000 daltons was neither inhibitory nor cytotoxic. When the 10,000 to 50,000-dalton fraction was further subdivided into fractions between 10,000 and 30,000 daltons and between 30,000 and 50,000 daltons, it was found that after 48 h incubation in vitro, the SW-48 cell proliferation was inhibited only by 6% by the lower range fraction, whereas the higher range fraction showed a 55% inhibition after the same period. After 72 h incubation, however, at the concentration used (1 mg/ml), the inhibitory effect of the 10,000–30,000-dalton fraction was increased to 35%, while that of the 30,000–50,000-dalton fraction was increased to 100% (table 21.2).

The 10,000–30,000 dalton fraction as well as the fraction between 30,000–

Table 21.1

The effects of concentrations of various mol wt fractions of the 'used' medium from the cultivation of human colon carcinoma cells in vitro upon the number of these cells per culture (in triplicate) after 72 h incubation.

Conc. of mol wt fraction	Mean cell number ($\times 10^{-5}$)		% inhibition
	0 h	72 h	
None	1.72 ± 0.05	6.32 ± 0.14	—
Over 300,000			
(1, 2, or 3 mg/ml)	1.72 ± 0.05	reduced numbers	cytotoxic
50,000–300,000			
(1, 2, or 3 mg/ml)	4.00 ± 0.10	18.6 ± 0.23	0
10,000–50,000			
0 mg/ml	2.00 ± 0.07	5.8 ± 0.11	—
0.5 mg/ml	2.00 ± 0.07	5.4 ± 0.12	10
1.0 mg/ml	2.00 ± 0.07	4.0 ± 0.10	47
2.0 mg/ml	2.00 ± 0.07	2.8 ± 0.09	79
3.0 mg/ml	2.00 ± 0.07	2.5 ± 0.08	87
1000–10,000			
(1, 2, or 3 mg/ml)	2.00	reduced numbers	cytotoxic

50,000 daltons obtained from the 'unused' medium had very little effect on the proliferation of human colon carcinoma cells in vitro. After 48 h incubation at a concentration of 1 mg/ml or more, the fraction between 10,000 and 30,000 daltons inhibited the proliferation of these cells by only 5% and the 30,000–50,000-dalton fraction by 11% (table 21.2). Even after 72 h, the rate of proliferation of these cells in the presence of extracts from the 'unused' medium was not different from that of the control cells which had no added extract.

Table 21.2

Comparison of the inhibitory effects of the various molecular weight fractions from 'used' medium and 'unused' medium upon the number of human colon carcinoma cells per culture after 48 and 72 h incubation in vitro.

Mol wt fraction (1 mg/ml)	Mean cell numbers ($\times 10^{-5}$)			% inhibition
	0 h	48 h	72 h	
'used' medium				
A. None	0.71 ± 0.09	2.01 ± 0.06	—	—
30,000–50,000	0.71 ± 0.09	1.29 ± 0.03	—	55
10,000–30,000	0.71 ± 0.09	1.92 ± 0.05	—	6
B. None	1.72 ± 0.05	—	6.32 ± 0.14	—
30,000–50,000	1.72 ± 0.05	—	1.60 ± 0.06	103
None	3.20 ± 0.07	—	14.3 ± 0.20	—
10,000–30,000	3.20 ± 0.07	—	10.4 ± 0.12	35
'unused' medium				
None	2.09 ± 0.05	6.04 ± 0.13	—	—
30,000–50,000	2.09 ± 0.05	5.59 ± 0.22	—	11
10,000–30,000	2.09 ± 0.05	5.86 ± 0.18	—	5

Table 21.3

Inhibition of the uptake of tritiated thymidine by human colon carcinoma cells in vitro after a 6-h pulse in the presence of 10,000–50,000-dalton fraction from extracts of the 'used' medium (1 mg/ml), SW-48 cells (1 mg/ml) and colonic mucosa of dog (0.8 mg/ml).

Source	cpm/10^5 cells		% inhibition
	Control	Extract added	
used' medium	3,550	595	83
SW-48 cells	3,555	808	76
Dog colon	3,355	1,217	64

We have also found that at a concentration of 1 mg/ml, the molecular weight fraction between 10,000 and 50,000 daltons of the 'used' medium inhibited the uptake of labeled thymidine into the DNA of the SW-48 cells in vitro by about 83% after a 6-h pulse (table 21.3). A similar sized fraction of the same concentration obtained from the 'unused' medium did not affect the thymidine uptake in these cells to any appreciable extent.

21.13 *Effect of tissue extracts*

The proliferation of human colon carcinoma cells in vitro was found to be inhibited after 48-h incubation with the ultrafiltrate fraction between 10,000 and 50,000 daltons extracted from colonic tissues of different animal species. Thus, at a concentration of 1 mg/ml, this molecular weight fraction from the colonic mucosal epithelium of human showed a 95% inhibition, porcine colon extract 83% inhibition, and dog colon extract 64% inhibition. Furthermore, similar sized fractions from isolated SW-48 cell extracts were seen to cause about 84% inhibition of the growth of these cells in vitro after 48 h. These data are summarized in table 21.4. Concomitant with the inhibition of cellular proliferation, the ultrafiltrate fraction of this size range from the different sources also inhibited uptake of thymidine into the DNA of SW-48

Table 21.4

Inhibitory effects of the 10,000–50,000-dalton fractions (1 mg/ml) from extracts of SW-48 cells, of human, porcine, and dog colonic mucosa upon the number of human colon carcinoma cells per culture after 48 (or 72) h incubation in vitro.

	Mean cell number ($\times 10^{-5}$)			% inhibition
	0 h	48 h	72 h	
SW-48 cells				
control	2.52 ± 0.12	4.30 ± 0.02	12.30 ± 0.20	—
extract added	2.52 ± 0.12	3.14 ± 0.10	4.11 ± 0.21	84
Human				
control	3.20 ± 0.07	—	14.30 ± 0.18	—
extract added	3.20 ± 0.07	—	3.80 ± 0.15	95
Porcine				
control	2.09 ± 0.05	6.04 ± 0.12	—	—
extract added	2.09 ± 0.05	2.74 ± 0.20	—	83
Dog				
control	2.52 ± 0.12	4.30 ± 0.02	12.30 ± 0.20	—
extract added	2.52 ± 0.12	3.56 ± 0.11	6.00 ± 0.26	64

cells in vitro. It was found that 'used' medium inhibited thymidine uptake after a 6-h pulse by 83%, the SW-48 cell extracts by 76%, and extracts of dog colon by 64% (table 21.3). These data support the species nonspecificity of chalone action reported for other systems.

21.14 Tissue specificity

One major characteristic of chalone action is its specificity. The molecular sized fraction between 10,000 and 50,000 daltons from the 'used' medium did not have any inhibitory effect at 1 or 3 mg/ml concentration upon the PHA-stimulated transformation of diploid human lymphocytes in vitro (Houck et al., 1971) or upon the proliferation of diploid human fibroblasts, WI-38 cells (Houck and Cheng, 1973). We now have evidence that the colon chalone fraction obtained from the 'used' medium of growth of human colon carcinoma cells in vitro also had no inhibitory effect upon the proliferation of either human bronchial carcinoma cells or HeLa cells in vitro.

Furthermore, extracts of tissues other than colon, such as dog lung or bovine lung or from another section of the gastrointestinal tract, namely the jejunal mucosa, did not have any significant effect on either the proliferation (table 21.5) or thymidine incorporation of SW-48 cells in vitro. In fact, the extract of the small intestine appeared to stimulate the proliferative activity of the SW-48 cells. This finding confirms essentially the observation of Nome (1974) that the mitotic rate of both small intestine and colon was increased one-half h after the administration of unfractionated jejunal extracts to rats in vivo. He has reported that thereafter there was a non-specific depression of the mitotic rate of colon and also forestomach.

Table 21.5

Effect of various mol wt fractions from extracts of dog jejunal mucosa, dog lung, and bovine lung upon the number of human colon carcinoma cells per culture after 48-h incubation in vitro.

	Mol wt fraction (1 mg/ml)	Mean cell number ($\times 10^{-5}$)		% inhibition
		0 h	48 h	
Dog jejunum	None	1.03 ± 0.03	2.42 ± 0.05	—
	10,000–50,000	1.03 ± 0.03	3.02 ± 0.18	−43
Dog lung	None	1.53 ± 0.04	3.46 ± 0.09	—
	10,000–50,000	1.53 ± 0.04	3.30 ± 0.23	8
Bovine lung	None	1.53 ± 0.04	3.46 ± 0.09	—
	30,000–50,000	1.53 ± 0.04	3.29 ± 0.07	9
	10,000–30,000	1.53 ± 0.04	3.28 ± 0.20	9

21.15 Reversibility

When the medium containing the inhibitory factor was withdrawn from cultures of human colon carcinoma cells after 48 h and the cells were washed and resupplied with fresh (chalone) extract-free L-15 medium, they resumed the normal proliferation rate and grew like the uninhibited control cultures. This was so whatever the source of the inhibitory chalone fraction. The reversibility of action of chalone is another characteristic of this factor reported in many such systems.

21.16 Conclusions

It is evident from the foregoing overall discussion that environmental factors play a significant role in the development of colon cancer. However, after the initial exposure to carcinogens, the latent period is so long as to delay the expression of tumorgenesis to relatively older ages in humans. This complication has rendered the formulation of preventive measures difficult. Hence, it is apparent that besides colostomy, the development of other curative procedures may be rewarding.

Meanwhile, the chalone concept has gained acceptance in its potential for providing a built-in chemotherapeutic system for the control of cancer. Our experience with chalone extracts of colonic cells seems consistent with the theory that mucosal cell proliferation may be under the influence of a negative feedback control mechanism. Such a mechanism has been reported for other sections of the gastrointestinal tract. Thus, chalone-type activities were found in the stomach (Philpott, 1971), in the duodenum (Bischoff, 1964) and in the small intestine (Loran et al., 1964; Tutton, 1973; Brugal and Pelmont, 1974). We have now found reason to believe that such a system is present in the mucosal epithelium of the large bowel. Ultrafiltered extracts of the 'used' medium obtained during the cultivation of human colon carcinoma cells in vitro contained this mitotic inhibitory factor, whereas the 'unused' medium which was treated under the same conditions as the cell cultures in the absence of the SW-48 cells exhibited no significant inhibitory activity on the growth of these cells in vitro. In fact, a fraction of similar molecular size distribution that was active in the control of colon carcinoma cell proliferation was isolated from extracts of the SW-48 cells themselves, indicating the endogenous origin of this factor. The lack of inhibitory activity of the chalone-containing ultrafiltrate fraction of the 'used' medium when employed against PHA-stimulated lymphocyte trans-formation or in the in vitro proliferation of diploid human fibroblasts or of human bronchial carcinoma cells or of the HeLa cells is evidence enough of the tissue-specific activity of this inhibitor of mitosis. The proliferation of SW-48 cells in vitro was not only inhibited by the partially purified chalones obtained from their own cell population or from the 'used' medium resulting from the growth of these cells, but also extracts from the mucosal epithelium of colon of pig, dog, and man were found to have the same inhibitory influence. Therefore, it seems this inhibition does not show species specificity.

The suppression of the uptake of thymidine by the colon carcinoma cells in the presence of the ultrafiltrate fraction is strongly suggestive that the colon chalones may act in the G_1 phase of the cell cycle. However, Philpott (1971), who followed the proportion of stomach mucosal cells in a given population that entered into mitosis during a 5-h test period, found that the inhibitory effects on cell proliferation in his study were acting on cells in G_2 or S phase of the cell cycle. Though this is contrary to our finding in the colon system, it is consistent with the observation in other systems of the presence of G_1 as well as G_2 specific inhibitors of the chalone type. Thus, it would appear that accumulation of detailed knowledge of the mechanism of action of inhibitors at various phases of the cell cycle may have a potential in chemotherapeutic development.

We have found evidence that the colon chalone lies within the molecular weight range between 10,000 and 50,000 daltons. It has been previously reported that the chalone from extracts of stomach mucosa partially purified on Sephadex G-25 column had a molecular weight greater than 20,000 daltons (Philpott, 1971). Also, the colon chalone was trypsin- as well as chymotrypsin-labile, indicating the necessity of basic and aromatic peptide bonds for its activity. The activity of the chalone was unaffected by pre-treatment with ribonuclease.

The data suggest that colon mucosal cells contain a specific and endo-genous inhibitor of their own proliferation which acts in the G_1 phase of the cell cycle. It is apparently not species-specific, nor is it cytotoxic and its action appears to be completely reversible. Thus, this inhibitor exhibits all the characteristics of a colon chalone.

References

Al-Sarraf, M., Vaughn, C. B., Reed, M. L. and Vaitkevicius, V. K. (1972) Combined 5-fluorouracil and vinblastine therapy for gastrointestinal and other solid tumors. Oncology 26, 99.

Ames, B. N., Durston, W. E., Yamasaki, E. and Lee, F. D. (1973) Carcinogens are mutagens: a simple test system combining liver homogenates for activation and bacteria for detection. Proc. Natl. Acad. Sci. U.S. 70, 2281.

Ansfield, R. J., Schroeder, J. M. and Curreri, A. R. (1962) Five years' clinical experience with 5-fluorouracil. JAMA 181, 295.

Aries, V. C., Growther, J. L., Drasar, B. S., Hill, M. J. and Williams, R. E. O. (1969) Bacteria and the aetiology of cancer of the large bowel. Gut 10, 334.

Bischoff, R. (1964) Inhibition of mitosis by homologous tissue extracts. J. Cell Biol. 23, 10A.

Bleiberg, H., Mainguet, P. and Galand, P. (1972) Cell renewal in familial polyposis: comparison between polyps and adjacent healthy mucosa. Gastroenterology 63, 240.

Bremner, C. G. and Ackerman, L. V. (1970) Polyps and carcinoma of the large bowel in the South African Bantu. Cancer 26, 991.

Brookes, P. and Lawley, P. D. (1964) Reaction of some mutagenic and carcinogenic compounds with nucleic acids. J. Cell Comp. Physiol. 64, (Suppl. 1) 111.

Brugal, G. and Pelmont, J. (1974) Présence, dans l'intestin du Triton adulte pleurodeles waltii Michah., de deux facteurs anti-mutatiques naturels (chalones) actifs sur la proliferation cellulaire de l'intestin embryonaire. Compt. Rend. Acad. Sci. Paris D28, 2831.

Bull, D. M. and Tomasi, T. B. (1968) Deficiency of immunoglobulin A in intestinal disease. Gastroenterology 54, 313.

Bullough, W. S. and Laurence, E. B. (1960) The control of epidermal mitotic activity in the mouse. Proc. Royal Soc. B. 151, 517.

Burdette, W. J. (ed.) (1965) Carcinoma of the Alimentary Tract. University of Utah Press, Salt Lake City.

Burkitt, D. P. (1971) Epidemiology of cancer of the colon and rectum. Cancer 28, 3.

Burnet, F. M. (1971) Immunological surveillance in neoplasia. Transplant. Rev. 7, 3.

Chopra, D. P. and Simnett, J. D. (1969) Demonstration of an organ-specific mitotic inhibitor in amphibian kidney. Exp. Cell Res. 58, 319.

Chopra, D. P. and Simnett, J. D. (1970) Stimulation of mitosis in amphibian kidney by organ-specific antiserum. Nature 225, 657.

Cleveland, J. C. and Cole, J. W. (1969) Relationship of experimentally induced intestinal tumors to laxative ingestion. Cancer 23, 1200.

Cleveland, J. C., Litvak, S. F. and Cole, J. W. (1967) Identification of the route of action of the carcinogen 3,2'dimethyl-4-aminobiphenyl in the induction of intestinal neoplasia. Cancer Res. 27, 708.

Crabbe, P. A., Carbonara, A. O. and Heremans, J. F. (1965) The normal human intestinal mucosa as a major source of plasma cells containing γ A-immunoglobulin. Lab. Invest. 14, 235.

Dahlquist, A. and Nordstrom, C. (1966) The distribution of disaccharidase activities in the villi and crypts of the small intestinal mucosa. Biochim. Biophys. Acta 113, 624.

Deschner, E. and Lipkin, M. (1970) Study of human rectal epithelial cells in vitro. III. RNA, protein, and DNA synthesis in polyps and adjacent mucosa. J. Natl. Cancer Inst. 44, 175.

Deschner, E., Lipkin, M. and Solomon, C. (1966) Study of human rectal epithelial cells in vitro. II. H^3 thymidine incorporation into polyps and adjacent mucosa. J. Natl. Cancer Inst. 36, 849.

Druckrey, H. (1970) Production of colonic carcinomas by 1,2-dialkylhydrazines and azoxyalkanes, in Carcinoma of the Colon and Antecedent Epithelium (ed. W. J. Burdette). Charles C. Thomas, Springfield, Illinois, pp. 267–279.

Druckrey, H., Ivanković, S. and Preussmann, R. (1965) Selektive Erzeugung maligner Tumoren im Gehirn und Rückenmark von Ratten durch N-Methyl-N-mitrosoharnstoff. Z. Krebsforch. 66, 389.

Druckrey, H., Preussmann, R., Matzkies, F. and Ivanković, S. (1967) Selektive Erzeugung von Darmkrebs bei Ratten durch 1,2-Dimethylhydrazin. Naturwissenschaften 54, 285.

Dwight, R. W., Higgins, G. A., Roswit, B., LeVeen, H. H. and Keehn, R. J. (1972) Preoperative radiation and surgery for cancer of the sigmoid colon and rectum. Am. J. Surg. 123, 93.

Foley, E. J. (1953) Antigenic properties of methylcholanthrene-induced tumors in mice of the strain of origin. Cancer Res. 13, 835.

Fortner, J. G. (1965) Tumors of the alimentary tract in the hamster and cat, in: Carcinoma of the Alimentary Tract. (ed. W. J. Burdette). University of Utah Press, Salt Lake City, pp. 75–87.

Gailani, S., Holland, J. F., Falkson, G., Leone, L., Burningham, R. and Larsen, V. (1972) Comparison of treatment of metastatic gastrointestinal cancer with 5-fluorouracil (5-FU) to a combination of 5-FU with cytosine arabinoside. Cancer 29, 1308.

Gary, R. and Hall, R. (1970) Stimulation of mitosis in rat thyroid by long-acting thyroid stimulators. Lancet 1, 693.

Gatti, R. A. and Good, R. A. (1971) Occurrence of malignancy in immunodeficiency diseases – a literature review. Cancer 28, 89.

Gold, P. (1967) Circulating antibodies against carcinoembryonic antigens of the human digestive system. Cancer 20, 1663.

Gold, P. and Freeman, S. O. (1965a) Demonstration of tumor-specific antigens in human colonic carcinomata by immunological tolerance and absorption techniques. J. Exp. Med. 121, 439.

Gold, P. and Freeman, S. O. (1965b) Specific carcinoembryonic antigens of the human digestive system. J. Exp. Med. 122, 467.

Hadidian, Z., Fredrickson, T. N., Weisburger, E. K., Weisburger, J. H., Glass, R. M. and Mantel, N. (1968) Tests for chemical carcinogens. Report on the activity of derivatives of aromatic amines, nitrosamines, quinolines, nitroalkanes, amides, epoxides, aziridines, and purine antimetabolites. J. Natl. Cancer Inst. 41, 985.

Haenszel, W. M. and Correa, P. (1971) Cancer of the colon and rectum and adenomatous polyps: a review of epidemiologic findings. Cancer 28, 14.

Heidelberger, C., Chauduri, N. K., Danneberg, P., Mooren, D. and Greisbach, L. (1957) Fluorinated pyrimidines, a new class of tumor-inhibitory compounds. Nature 179, 663.

Higginson, J. (1966) Etiological factors in gastrointestinal cancer in man. J. Natl. Cancer Inst. 37, 527.

Hill, M. J. (1974) Bacteria and the etiology of colonic cancer. Cancer 34, 815.

Hill, M. J., Crowther, J. S., Drasar, B. S., Hawsworth, G., Aries, V. and Williams, R. E. O. (1971) Bacteria and the aetiology of cancer of the large bowel. Lancet i, 95.

Holden, W. D., Dixon, W. J. and Kingman, J. S. (1967) The use of triethylene thiophosphoramide as adjuvant to the surgical treatment of colorectal carcinoma. Ann. Surg. 165, 481.

Horton, J., Olson, K., Gehrt, P. and Spear, M. (1965) Combination therapy with 5-fluorouracil, mitomycin C, vincristine and thioTEPA for advanced cancer. Cancer Chemotherapy Rep. 49, 59.

Houck, J. C. and Cheng, R. F. (1973) Isolation, purification, and chemical characterization of the serum mitogen for diploid human fibroblasts. J. Cell. Physiol. 81, 257.

Houck, J., Irausquin, H. and Leikin, S. (1971) Lymphocyte DNA synthesis inhibition. Science 173, 1139.

Houck, J. C., Weil, R. L. and Sharma, V. K. (1972) Evidence for a fibroblast chalone. Nature New Biol. 240, 210.

Houck, J. C., Kanagalingam, K., Kaufman, S. L. and Sunshine, G. (1975) Evidence for a colon chalone. J. Natl. Cancer Inst. (in press).

Igel, H. J., Huebner, R. J., Turner, H. C., Katin, P. and Falk, H. L. (1969) Mouse leukemia virus activation by chemical carcinogens. Science 166, 1624.

Imondi, A. R., Balis, M. E. and Liplin, M. (1969) Changes in enzyme levels accompanying differentiation of intestinal epithelial cells. Exp. Cell Res. 58, 323.

Kanagalingam, K. and Balis, M. E. (1974) Chemically induced damage of rat intestinal DNA and its apparent repair in vivo. Proc. Amer. Assoc. Cancer Res. 15, 46.

Klein, G. (1966) Tumor antigens. Ann. Rev. Microbiol. 20, 223.

Laqueur, G. L. (1965) The induction of intestinal neoplasms in rats with the glycoside cycasin and its aglycone. Virchow. Arch. Path. Anat. 340, 151.

Laqueur, G. L. and Spatz, M. (1968) Toxicology of cycasin. Cancer Res. 28, 2262.

Laqueur, G. L., Mickelson, O., Whiting, M. G. and Kurland, L. T. (1963) Carcinogenic properties of nuts from *Cycas circinalis L.* indigenous to Guam. J. Natl. Cancer Inst. 31, 919.

Laqueur, G. L., McDaniel, E. G. and Matsumoto, H. (1967) Tumor induction in germ-free rats with methylazoxymethanol (MAM) and synthetic MAM acetate. J. Natl. Cancer Inst. 39, 355.

Leaver, D. D., Swann, P. F. and Magee, P. N. (1969) The induction of tumors in the rat by a single dose of N-nitrosomethylurea. Brit. J. Cancer 23, 177.

Lipkin, M. and Bell, B. (1968) Cell proliferation, in: Handbook of Physiology, Vol. 5 (ed. C. F. Code). American Physiological Society, Washington, D. C., pp. 2861–2879.

Lipkin, M., Deschner, E. E. and Troncale, F. (1970) Cell differentiation and the development of colonic neoplasms. Gastroenterology 59, 303.

Lipkin, M., Sherlock, P. and Bell, B. (1963) Cell proliferation kinetics in the gastro-intestinal tract of man. II. Cell renewal in stomach, ileum, colon, and rectum. Gastroenterology 45, 721.

Loran, M. R. and Crocker, T. T. (1963) Population dynamics of intestinal epithelia in the rat two months after resection of the ileum. J. Cell Biol. 19, 285.

Loran, M. R., Crocker, T. T. and Carbone, J. (1964) The humoral effect of intestinal resection on cellular proliferation and maturation in parabiotic rats. Fed. Proc. 23, 407.

Lowenfels, A. B. (1973) Etiologic aspects of cancer of the gastrointestinal tract. Surg. Gynecol. Obstet. 137, 291.

Matsumoto, H. and Higa, H. H. (1966) Studies on methylazoxymethanol the aglycone of cycasin: methylation of nucleic acids in vitro. Biochem. J. 98, 20c.

Miller, A. B. (1974) The Joint National Cancer Institute of Canada – American Cancer Society Study of a test for carcinoembryonic antigen (CEA). Cancer 34, 932.

Miller, J. A. (1970) Carcinogenesis by chemicals: an overview. G. H. A. Clowes Memorial Lecture. Cancer Res. 30, 559.

Moertel, C. G., Reitemeier, R. J. and Hahn, R. G. (1970) Oral methotrexate therapy of gastrointestinal carcinoma. Surg. Gynecol. Obstet. 130, 292.

Moog, F., Vire, H. R. and Grey, R. D. (1966) The multiple forms of alkaline phosphatase in the small intestine of the young mouse. Biochim. Biophys. Acta 113, 336.

Moorhead, J. F., Paraskova-Tchernozenska, E., Pirrie, A. J. and Hayes, C. (1969) Lymphoid inhibitor of human lymphocyte DNA synthesis and mitosis in vitro. Nature 224, 1207.

Newberne, P. M. and Rogers, A. E. (1973) Rat colon carcinomas associated with aflatoxin and marginal Vitamin A. J. Natl. Cancer Inst. 50, 439.

Nome, O. (1974) Tissue specificity of epidermal chalones. Ph. D. Thesis, Oslo.

Orenstein, J. M. and Weinstein, I. B. (1973) Filamentous forms of enveloped A particles in cell cultures from chemically induced rat hepatomas. Cancer Res. 33, 1998.

Pamuku, A. M., Yalciner, S., Price, J. M. and Bryan, G. T. (1970) Effects of the coadministration of thiamine on the incidence of urinary bladder carcinomas in rats fed bracken fern. Cancer Res. 30, 2671.

Plaut, A. G. and Keonil, P. (1969) Immunoglobulins in human small intestinal fluid. Gastroenterology 56, 522.

Prehn, R. T. and Main, M. M. (1957) Immunity to methylcholanthrene-induced carcinomas. J. Natl. Cancer Inst. 18, 769.

Philpott, G. W. (1971) Tissue-specific inhibition of cell proliferation in embryonic stomach epithelium in vitro. Gastroenterology 61, 25.

Reddy, B. S. and Wynder, E. L. (1973) Large bowel carcinomas-fecal constituents in populations with diverse incidence rates of colon cancer. J. Natl. Cancer Inst. 50, 1437.

Reitemeier, R. J., Moertel, C. G. and Hahn, R. G. (1970) Combination chemotherapy in gastrointestinal cancer. Cancer Res. 30, 1425.

Rice, J. M., Joshi, S. R., Roller, P. P. and Wenk, M. L. (1975) Methyl (acetoxymethyl) nitrosamine: a new carcinogen highly specific for colon and small intestine. Proc. Amer. Assoc. Cancer Res. 16, 32.

Rytömaa, T. and Kiviniemi, K. (1968) Control of DNA duplication in rat chloroleukemia by means of the granulocyte chalone. Europ. J. Cancer 4, 595.

Saetren, M. (1956) A principle of autoregulation of growth. Production of organ-specific mitose – inhibitors in kidney and liver. Exp. Cell Res. 11, 229.

Saetren, M. (1963) The organ-specific growth inhibition of the tubule cells of the rat kidneys. Acta Chem. Scand. 17, 889.

Salser, J. S. and Balis, M. E. (1973) Distribution of regulation of deoxythymidine kinase activity in differentiating cells of mammalian intestines. Cancer Res. 33, 1889.

Sawicki, W., Rowinski, J., Macijewski, W. and Kwarecki, K. (1968) Kinetics of proliferation and migration of epithelial cells in the guinea pig colon. Exp. Cell Res. 50, 93.

Schoental, R. and Bensted, J. P. M. (1969) Gastrointestinal tumors in rats and mice following various routes of administration of N-methyl-N-nitroso-N'-nitroguanidine and N-ethyl-N-nitroso-N'-nitroguanidine. Brit. J. Cancer 23, 757.

Shank, R. C. and Magee, P. N. (1967) Similarities between the biochemical actions of cycasin and dimethylnitrosamine. Biochem. J. 105, 521.

Simnett, J. D., Fisher, J. M. and Heppleston, A. G. (1969) Tissue-specific inhibition of lung alveolar cell mitosis in organ culture. Nature 223, 944.

Spatz, M. (1969) Toxic and carcinogenic alkylating agents from cycads. Ann. N. Y. Acad. Sci. 163, 848.

Spatz, M. (1970) Carcinogenicity of methylazoxymethanol (MAM) in guinea pigs and hamsters. Abstracts, Tenth International Cancer Congress, Houston, pp. 24–25.

Spjut, H. J. (1971) Experimental induction of tumors of the large bowel of rats. Cancer 28, 29.

Spjut, H. J. and Noall, M. W. (1970) Colonic neoplasms induced by 3,2'-dimethyl-4-

aminobiphenyl, in: Carcinoma of the Colon and Antecedent Epithelium (ed.: W. J. Burdette). Charles C. Thomas, Springfield, Illinois, pp. 280–288.

Spjut, H. J. and Spratt, J. S., Jr. (1965) Endemic and morphologic similarities existing between spontaneous colonic neoplasms in man and 3:2'-dimethyl-4-aminobiphenyl-induced colonic neoplasms in rats. Ann. Surg. 161, 309.

Stewart, H. L. (1971) Geographic pathology of cancer of the colon and rectum. Cancer 28, 25.

Sugimura, T., Fujumura, S. and Baba, T. (1970) Tumor production in the glandular stomach and alimentary tract of the rat by N-methyl-N'-nitro-N-nitrosoguanidine. Cancer Res. 30, 455.

Szafarz, D. and Weisburger, J. H. (1969) Stability of binding of label from N-hydroxy-N-2-fluorenylacetamide to intracellular targets, particularly deoxyribonucleic acid in rat liver. Cancer Res. 29, 962.

Temin, H. M. (1964) Homology between RNA from Rous sarcoma virus and DNA from Rous sarcoma virus-infected cells. Proc. Natl. Acad. Sci. U.S. 52, 323.

Turnbull, R. B., Kyle, K., Watson, F. R. and Spratt, J. (1967) Cancer of the colon – the influence of the no-touch isolation technique on survival rates. Ann. Surg. 166, 420.

Tutton, P. J. M. (1973) Control of epithelial cell proliferation in the small intestine. Cell Tissue Kinet. 6, 211.

Voaden, M. J. (1968) A chalone in the rabbit lens? Exp. Eye Res. 7, 326.

von Kleist, S. and Burtin, P. (1969) Isolation of a fetal antigen from colonic tumors. Cancer Res. 29, 1961.

von Kleist, S., King, M. and Burtin, P. (1974) Characterization of a normal tissular antigen extracted from colonic tumors. Immunochemistry 11, 249.

Walker, A. R. P. and Walker, B. F. (1969) Bowel mobility and colonic cancer. Brit. Med. J. 3, 238.

Walpole, A. L. and Williams, M. H. C. (1958) Aromatic amines as carcinogens in industry. Brit. Med. Bull. 14, 141.

Walpole, A. L., Williams, M. H. C. and Roberts, D. C. (1952) The carcinogenic action of 4-aminodiphenyl and 3:2'-dimethyl-4-aminodiphenyl. Brit. J. Industr. Med. 9, 255.

Warwick, G. P. and Roberts, J. J. (1967) Persistent binding of butter yellow metabolites to rat liver DNA. Nature 213, 1206.

Weinstein, I. B., Gebert, R., Stadler, U. C., Orenstein, J. M. and Axel, R. (1972) Type C virus from cell cultures of chemically induced rat hepatomas. Science 178, 1098.

Weisburger, J. H. (1971) Colon carcinogens: their metabolism and mode of action. Cancer 28, 60.

Weisburger, J. H., Grantham, P. H., Horton, R. E. and Weisburger, E. K. (1970) Metabolism of the carcinogen N-hydroxy-N-2-fluorenylacetamide in germ-free rats. Biochem. Pharmacol. 19, 151.

Weiss, P. and Kavanau, J. L. (1957) A model of growth and growth control in mathematical terms. J. Gen. Physiol. 41, 1.

Williams, J. R., Grantham, P. H., Marsh, H. H., III, Weisburger, J. H. and Weisburger, E. K. (1970) Participation of liver fractions and of intestinal bacteria in the metabolism of N-hydroxy-N-2-fluorenylacetamide in the rat. Biochem. Pharmacol. 19, 173.

Wolff, W. I. and Shinya, H. (1974) Earlier diagnosis of cancer of the colon through colonic endoscopy (colonoscopy). Cancer 34, 912.

Wynder, E. L. and Shigematsu, T. (1967) Environmental factors of cancer of the colon and rectum. Cancer 20, 1520.

Wynder, E. L., Kajitani, T., Ishikawa, S., Dodo, H. and Takano, A. (1969) Environmental factors of cancer of the colon and rectum. II. Japanese epidemiological data. Cancer 23, 1210.

Zipilvan, E. M., Hudson, B. G. and Blatt, W. F. (1969) Separation of immunologically active fragments by membrane partition chromatography. Anal. Biochem. 30, 91.

CHAPTER 22

Critique

JOHN C. HOUCK and CARL V. HUNT

Biochemical Research Laboratory, Research Foundation of Children's Hospital,
Washington, D.C. 20009, U.S.A.

The suggested existence of specific negative feedback inhibitors of mitosis by Weiss and Kavanau (1957) was developed by Bullough and Laurence (1960) into the concept of specific and endogenous mitotic inhibitors or chalones.

Evidence of chalones is still not totally convincing, however, because there are considerable experimental difficulties in establishing unequivocally the validity of a specific chalone for a specific cell system. This critique will therefore address itself to three of the major technical problems involved in establishing the reality of a particular chalone; namely (22.1) Bacterial and entotoxin contamination; (22.2) in vitro assay artifacts; and (22.3) cytotoxicity.

22.1 Microorganism contamination of chalone extracts

Mohr et al. (1968) reported that crude concentrates of pig skin extracts were found to have marked oncolytic activity in melanomata in hamsters and mice. While this activity was at first attributed to the action of epidermal chalone, it was later shown to be associated with *Clostridium* spores present in the skin extracts (Mohr et al., 1972a, b).

We have found evidence that bacterial contamination of tissue extracts can mimic the type of activity attributed to lymphocyte chalone. It was found that a population of gram-negative microorganisms could be isolated from dialyzates of commercially prepared bovine spleen powder extracts which had been kept in the cold and ultrafiltered to obtain a 10,000–50,000-dalton fraction. The unidentified microorganisms were cultured in nutrient medium at 4 °C, centrifuged, resuspended in distilled water, and lyophilized.

The lyophilized powder was resuspended in phosphate buffered saline, centrifuged, and the supernatant filter-sterilized. This clarified extract was added to lymphocyte cultures in the present of PHA or with other lymphocytes in a two-way mixed lymphocyte culture. Marked inhibition of $[^3H]$TdR incorporation and lymphoblast development was observed without apparent cytotoxicity. It was also found that this activity could be removed by filter sterilization prior to lyphilization. This suggests that the active material is probably an endotoxin or on the capsula of the bacterium.

It has previously been reported that a highly purified enterotoxin (choleragen) from a strain of Vibrio Cholerae (Sultzer and Craig, 1973; Hart and Finkelstein, 1975) can non-cytotoxically inhibit human and mouse lymphocyte responses to a number of mitogens and the mixed lymphocyte culture reaction. When administered in vivo, the cholera enterotoxin was found to cause a rise in cyclic AMP levels in splenic white cells, a marked depletion in the number of spleen cells, a circulating blood lymphopenia immunosuppression of skin allograft rejection, and inhibition of several other cell-mediated immunologic reactions (Warren et al., 1974). Chisari and Northrup (1974) found a severe thymic cortical atrophy after in vivo exposure of mice to choleragen. It has also been reported that cholera enterotoxin can suppress the graft-versus-host syndrome (Keast, 1973; Thomson and Julia, 1974) and depending upon the dose and time of treatment, enhance or suppress the immune response in mice to sheep erythrocytes and lipopolysaccharide (Kately et al., 1975).

Antimitogenic factors have also been found in culture filtrates (Seravalli and Taranta, 1974) and in fractionated cytoplasmic components (Malakian and Kaloustian, 1975) of group A streptococci.

One of the important criteria for establishing the reality of a chalone is tissue specificity. To what extent are bacterial endotoxins cell-specific? There does not appear to be extensive information on this point. We have found that our bacterial extracts which inhibit lymphocyte transformation do not apparently effect the mitotic activity of either WI-38 fibroblasts or SW-38 colon carcinoma cells. Keush and Dante (1975) examined the effects of a number of enterotoxins on two cell culture systems. They found a clear segregation of the enterotoxins studied into two classes. One group caused detachment of cells from glass surfaces and the other group caused an activation of the adenyl cyclase-cyclic adenosine 3′,5′-monophosphate system. Further studies on the effects of various enterotoxins on in vitro cell systems would be helpful in establishing the extent of enterotoxin specificity.

Bacterial contamination has been reported in epidermal and lymphoid tissue chalone extracts. In both cases, bacterial products and/or components have been shown to produce effects which could be ascribed to chalone activity. This potential problem has previously not received the attention it deserves by workers in the field of chalones.

22.2 Assay artifacts in vitro

There are three primary techniques for demonstrating the entrance of a cell into mitotic cycle: (1) to actually count the mitotic figures which have been trapped in metaphase by such inhibitors as colcemid or vinblastin; (2) to actually determine the number of viable cells in an attempt to determine their increase after a given incubation time; and (3) to measure the uptake of tritiated thymidine into acid insoluble DNA by these cells as they enter into the S-phase portion of the cell cycle – this latter being a prerequisite for mitosis. The determination of the mitotic index (the numbers of cells in metaphase versus the total number of cells) is extremely slow and tedious, yet reasonably reliable. Similarly, the actual counting of the number of cells in a proliferating culture is subject largely to arithmetic rather than methodological error, but, again, this technique represents a reliable method for demonstrating proliferation of cells in vitro. The most convenient and yet perhaps the most unreliable method for determining cell proliferation in vitro, however, is the uptake of [^{3}H]thymidine into the acid insoluble DNA content of these cells. There are at least two major reasons why this technique is subject to potential errors of interpretation.

Firstly, a number of tissues contain enzymes capable of phosphorylating or degrading the radioactively labeled thymidine so that it can no longer function as a precursor to DNA synthesis, either because it cannot enter the cell or because it is no longer in the metabolic pathway leading to the synthesis of DNA. The possibility exists that extracts of whole tissues could be contaminated by these normally intracellular metabolic enzymes of the thymidine pathway. Thus, the exogenous thymidine which has been labeled with tritium could be destroyed or altered by these enzymes so that they are no longer a reliable measure of the ability of these cells to synthesize DNA in vitro. For example, both the reticulo-endothelial system and the liver contain very large amounts of thymidine kinase which would be capable of phosphorylating a very high proportion of the [^{3}H]thymidine added to the cultures. In this fashion, a spurious demonstration of an apparent inhibition of mitosis could result.

This particular objection can be partially overcome by the appropriate controls as well as by the direct determination of the thymidine kinase or hydrolase activities in a given tissue extract. It is interesting to note that, from our experience, extensive dialysis against water of extracts containing these thymidine phosphorylating enzymes results in the complete disappearance of this activity, either because of their precipitation as an euglobulin or because of the loss of essential co-factors for the activity which are not found in the simplified culture medium MEM or 199.

A second problem relating to the thymidine uptake as a measure of the entrance of cell populations into the cell cycle is particularly prominent when the putative chalone activity has a small molecular weight, i.e., less than 5000 daltons, as suggested for granulocyte, melanocyte, and liver. That is, these tissue extracts could well be – and probably are – contaminated with unlabeled or cold nucleosides and nucleotides, including thymidine. These small molecular weight nucleosides could dilute out the pool size of the labeled thymidine added to the system under study. Thus, an apparent inhibition of thymidine uptake, and hence of cell entrance into the S-phase, could be a result of simply decreasing the probability of a cell incorporating labeled thymidine molecules. This 'pool-size dilution' problem can, in part, be obviated by extensive ultrafiltration of the tissue extracts to remove these small molecular weight nucleosides and nucleotides. This latter technique, however, is inappropriate when the tissue extracts being studied contain small molecular weight chalones. Further, this pool-size dilution problem cannot necessarily be solved by a demonstration of tissue specificity of the putative chalone. If the intracellular normal thymidine pool is significantly different in two different tissues, then the tissue with the larger thymidine pool shows the least effect of further pool-size dilution after the addition of cold thymidine contaminated chalone extracts and this might suggest a spurious tissue specificity of the chalone activity of these extracts.

A further complication of thymidine uptake studies is that various tissue proteins can non-specifically bind thymidine and thus spuriously indicate thymidine incorporation into DNA (Morley and Kingdon, 1972). This absorption of [3H]thymidine onto tissue proteins results not only in a TCA precipitable complex mimicking the incorporation of [3H]thymidine into macromolecular DNA but may also reduce the concentration of free or unbound labeled thymidine available for incorporation into DNA. Either way, the singular interpretation of [3H]thymidine incorporation rates under these conditions as representing the net entrance of the cell population under study into S-phase is obviously unsupportable and misleading.

Radioactive markers of macromolecular assembly of DNA during S-phase other than thymidine could be considered. For example, adenine and formate are incorporated into DNA although both are also incorporated into RNA. However, a chemical isolation of DNA from RNA is not difficult and this process, which has not been used extensively in the chalone literature to date, could establish the significance of the alteration in the incorporation rates of these precursors into acid insoluble DNA in terms of the entrance of these cells into the S phase portion of their cycle.

In summary, the primary difficulties in interpreting decreases in [³H]-thymidine incorporation rates into the acid insoluble DNA for in vitro cell populations in the presence of crude tissue extracts presumably containing a putative chalone are (1) changes in thymidine pool size by contamination of the chalone extract with tissue-derived cold thymidine, and (2) the alteration of the thymidine so as to render it unavailable for incorporation into the macromolecular synthesis of DNA.

Up until recently, this type of analysis of the possible artifacts leading to interpretation of mitotic inhibition by crude tissue extracts has not been extensively used by investigators attempting to establish the existence of chalones.

22.3 Cytotoxicity

The most fundamental criticism of experimental work attempting to establish chalone-like activity proceeds from the cytotoxicity of a wide number of tissue extracts in vitro. Probably the most important cytotoxic contaminant of tissue extracts would be the complement chain of proteins derived from the blood found in that particular tissue. The latter portion of the inter-digitated series of hydrolases (which constitute the complement system) contains a phospholipase and other hydrolases which are capable of enzymatically destroying cell membranes. Therefore, if a latter portion of the complement system was contaminating the tissue extract under study and if it could be activated during the various processes or partial purification employed, this might lead to the destruction of the cells and an apparent inhibition of their mitotic activity. This perhaps is most succinctly summed up in Houck's Law: 'Dead cells do not divide!' and its corollary, 'Dying cells divide damn slowly!'

It is almost impossible to prove a cell is not being cytotoxically rendered incapable of normal mitotic activity. Usually the evidence for cytotoxicity is based on the failure of non-viable cells to exclude a vital dye, often Trypan blue. This is, however, a rather terminal manifestation of the effects of cytotoxic materials upon cells in vitro. That is, ultimately the entrance of a vital dye into a given cell requires the destruction or loss of the integrity of the membrane systems of that cell. One could easily imagine the initially toxic events could have taken place in that cell at the time of measuring the incorporation of markers for the entrance of these cells into their mitotic cycle which would not yet have had sufficient time to associated with the loss of the integrity of the surface membrane. Obviously measures of normal mitochondrial function or of the blycolytic activity would be still quite possible in cells whose ability to exclude vital dye is considerably reduced because these enzymatic systems still maintain their function with what is clearly a dying cell. Consequently it is possible that a marginally cytotoxic agent could be applied to a given cell type and by virtue of making the cell sufficiently 'sick', inhibit thereby the enormous energetic expenditures required by these cells to enter the S phase of their cell cycle. Yet, theoretically during this period of time, the cell may not be sufficiently injured to alter the permeability of its cell membrane to a highly charged 'vital dye'. The reversibility of this phenomenon would simply mean that the cytotoxic agent was not sufficiently powerful or was not in sufficient concentration to effect, as yet, irreversible changes; yet, it was very slowly killing the cells and thereby inhibiting their entrance into the mitotic cell cycle.

The specificity of chalone activity for a particular cell type would not necessarily overcome the argument of cytotoxicity. Certain kinds of cells such as lymphocytes have a very different chemistry about their surface membranes than, say, fibroblasts, which grow attached to glass. It is possible that the fibroblasts attached to glass would not be affected by a mildly cytotoxic agent, whereas the lymphocyte in suspension culture would be. This could occur either because part of the fibroblast is masked, being absorbed to the glass upon which it is growing, whereas all the lymphocyte is equally exposed to attack, or it might also be due to the intrinsic differences in the susceptibility or the numbers of binding sites on the appropriate cell for a mildly cytotoxic agent. Therefore, it is enormously difficult, if not impossible, to rigorously exclude the possibility of cytotoxicity complicating the interpretation of in vitro data demonstrating the inhibition of mitosis in the presence of tissue extracts. Perhaps the best that can currently be done to exclude cytotoxicity as an explanation for the mitotic inhibition of putative chalone concentrates would be to demonstrate that this inhibitory action was not associated with vital dye staining of the target cells over a long period of incubation and that it was still reversible over this period.

Originally we felt that the inhibition of [³H]thymidine incorporation into cells under the influence of the putative chalone might not be associated with inhibition of the usual rate of uptake such as an amino acid or of uridine. However, this is not a definitive solution to the question of the cytotoxicity of chalone-containing tissue extracts for, as will be discussed later, it appears that the chalones which we have studied biochemically are also associated eventually with an inhibition of both protein and RNA synthesis in vitro.

In the author's opinion, it would be unfair to minimize the intellectual difficulty of the question of cytotoxicity as an alternative explanation for the apparent effects of putative chalones in vitro. The longest experience we have had with incubating the chalone-containing ultrafiltrates of lymphoid tissue extracts with lymphocytes has been for a total of seven days in mixed lymphocyte culture. All of the cells in these cultures remained viable, as judged by the exclusion of vital dye. It would have to be believed that by one week, if the chalone content of these extracts was cytotoxic, it should have manifested this cytotoxicity in terms of the exclusion of vital dyes. It is also possible, of course, that responsiveness of these cells in culture to the cytotoxic properties of chalone is distributed on a statistical basis and during this period of incubation, those cells which could be cytotoxically grossly injured have been and have disintegrated and hence are lost morphologically from the culture. Even under these conditions, however, one would expect to find other statistical portions of the population which were now dying and failing to exclude vital dye. Admittedly, this is argumentation rather than definitive experimentation, but we suggest that this is the most powerful single criticism of the chalone and it cannot easily be resolved experimentally. Finally, blood contains a number of macromolecules such as fetuin and a-fetoprotein which can non-specifically inhibit the uptake of [³H]thymidine by cells in vitro (Margita and Thomasi, 1975a, b; Yachnin, 1975). These non-specific inhibitors complicate considerably the search for real chalones.

22.4 Criticisms of in vivo studies of chalones

The major criticisms in vivo relate largely to the immunologic complications involved in injecting a variety of foreign materials into an animal and thereby greatly stimulating its immunologic rejection mechanisms. In studies of the ability of chalone extracts to inhibit in vivo tumor growth, usually a test system involves the use of transplanted tumors within an inbred mouse or rat strain. Under these conditions however, it is still possible that the added exogenous material contained in the chalone extract could stimulate the animal's immunologic defense systems so as to inhibit the tumor growth, not via inhibition of mitotic activity by chalones but rather via rejection phenomena.

This possibility may be particularly important in the studies described below in terms of granulocyte chalone activity against transplanted Shay chloroleukemia cells in rats. Here small molecular weight materials collected from the granulocytes of rodents (and presumably lymphocytes as well) are injected into an animal. This material is very similar to the 'transfer factor' described by Sherwood-Lawrence (1969). The consequences of 'transfer factor' in immunologically incompetent patients is to increase enormously the activity of the reticulo-endothelial system of these patients, permitting them to control previously intractable fungus infections. It is possible that this 'transfer factor', when injected into normal rodents, could activate their reticulo-endothelial system in a similar fashion and thereby immunologically inhibit the growth of these transplanted tumors and even destroy them in vivo. Since the experimental tumors transplanted even within a given cell strain are not homografts, then there is the real possibility that as these tumors have altered the nature of their surface membranes chemically and probably immunologically, an immunological rejection of the allograft tumor transplant could gratuitously have been stimulated by administration of the crude chalone concentrate. Whether such an immunologic stimulation could be accomplished by a 'transfer factor' contaminant of leukocyte chalone extracts in a host bearing transplanted tumor remains unknown. It seems only fair however, that this particular criticism be included in an objective critique of chalone studies.

Another difficulty in terms of long-term in vivo studies, of course, is the possibility that the host animal under study will develop antibodies against the injected chalone-containing tissue extract. One possible exception to this question of anti-chalone antibody might be the lymphocyte chalone itself, since inhibition of lymphocyte transformation might and should preclude the release of either cytophilic or circulating antibody from T and B cell type lymphocytes respectively. In this particular system, long-term exposure to lymphocyte chalone would probably not involve antibody formation to this chalone. Further, since most chalones currently known seem to be of a relatively small molecular weight, the immunogenicity of these materials may be relatively low.

References

Bullough, W. S. and Laurence, E. B. (1960) The control of epidermal mitotic activity in the mouse. Proc. R. Soc. Lond. (Biol.) 151, 517.

Chisari, F. V. and Northrup, R. S. (1974) Pathophysiological effects of lethal and immuno-regulatory doses of cholera enterotoxin in the mouse. J. Immunol. 113, 740.

Davis, B. D., Dulbecco, R., Eisen, H. N., Ginsburg, H. S. and Wood, Jr., W. B. (1973) Microbiology, 2nd ed, Harper and Rowe, p. 639.

Hart, D. A. and Finkelstein, R. A. (1975) Inhibition of mitogen stimulation of human peripheral blood leukocytes by Vibrio Choleral enterotoxin J. Immunol. 114, 476.

Kately, J. R., Kasarov, L. and Friedman, H. (1975) Modulation of in vivo antibody responses by cholera toxin. J. Immunol. 114, 81.

Keast, D. (1973) Role of bacterial endotoxin in the graft-vs-host syndrome. J. Infect. Dis. 128, suppl. s104.

Keusch, G. T. and Donta, S. T. (1975) Classification of enterotoxins on the basis of activity in cell culture. J. Infect. Dis. 131, 58.

Lawrence, H. S. (1969) Transfer factor. Adv. Immunol. 11, 195.

Malakian, A. H. and Kabastian, S. (1975) A potent antimitogenic factor from group A streptacocci. Immunology 28, 103.

Mohr, U., Althoff, J., Kinzel, V., Suss, R. and Volm, M. (1968) Melanoma regression induced by 'Chalone': a new tumor inhibiting principle acting in vivo. Nature 220, 138.

Mohr, U., Boldingh, W. H. and Althoff, J. (1972a) Identification of contaminating clostridium spores as the oncolytic agent in some chalone preparations. Cancer Res. 32, 1117.

Mohr, U., Boldingh, W. H., Emminger, A. and Behagel, H. A. (1972b) Oncolysis by a new strain of clostridium. Cancer Res. 32, 1122.

Morley, C. G. D. and Kingdon, H. (1972) Use of ^{3}H-thymidine for measurement of DNA synthesis in rat liver – a warning. Anal. Biochem. 45, 298.

Murgita, R. A. and Tomasi, Jr., T. B. (1975a) Suppression of the immune response by α-fetoprotein. I. The effect of mouse α-fetoprotein on the primary and secondary antibody response. J. Exp. Med. 141, 269.

Murgita, R. A. and Tomasi, Jr., T. B. (1975b) Suppression of the immune response by α-fetoprotein. II. The effect of mouse α-fetoprotein on mixed lymphocyte reactivity and mitogen induced lymphocyte transformation. J. Exp. Med. 141, 440.

Servalli, E. and Tarant, A. (1974) Lymphocyte transformation and macrophage migration inhibition by electrofocused and gel-filtered fractions of group A streptococcal filtrate. Cell. Immunol. 14, 366.

Sultzer, B. M. and Craig, J. P. (1973) Cholera toxin inhibits macromolecular synthesis in mouse spleen cells. Nature New Biol. 244, 178.

Thomson, P. D. and Jutila, J. W. (1974) The supression of graft-versus-host disease in mice by endotoxin-treated adherent spleen cells. J. Reticuloendothel. Soc. 16, 327.

Warren, K. S., Mahmoud, A. F., Boros, D. L., Rall, T. W., Mandel, M. A. and Carpenter, Jr., C. J. (1974) In vivo suppression by cholera toxin of cell-mediated and foreign body inflammation responses. J. Immunol. 112, 996.

Weiss, P. and Kavanau, J. L. (1957) A model of growth and growth control in mathematical terms. J. Gen. Physiol. 41, 1.

Yachnin, S. (1975) Fetuin, an inhibitor of lymphocyte transformation. J. Exp. Med. 141, 242.

CHAPTER 23

Comprehensive bibliography of chalone literature

ABDELFATTAH M. ATTALLAH and JOHN C. HOUCK

*Biochemical Research Laboratory, Research Foundation, Children's Hospital,
Washington, D.C. 20009, U.S.A.*

General

1. Weiss, P. Self-regulation of organ growth by its own products. Science 115, 487–488 (1952).
2. Bullough, W. S. Hormones and mitotic activity. Vitamins and Hormones 13, 261–292 (1955).
3. Weiss, P. and Kavanau, J. L. A model of growth and growth control in mathematical terms. J. Gen. Physiol. 41, 1–47 (1957).
4. Glinos, A. D. Environmental feedback control of cell division. Ann. N. Y. Acad. Sci. 90, 592–602 (1960).
5. Bullough, W. S. The control of mitotic activity in adult mammalian tissues. Biol. Review 37, 307–342 (1962).
6. Iversen, O. H. and Bjerknes, R. Kinetics of epidermal reaction to carcinogens. Acta Path. Microbiol. Scandinav., Suppl. 165 (1963).
7. Bullough, W. S. and Laurence, E. B. Mitotic control by internal secretion: the role of the chalone-adrenalin complex. Exper. Cell Res. 33, 176–194 (1964).
8. Bullough, W. S. Growth regulation by tissue-specific factors, or chalones, in Cellular Control Mechanisms and Cancer (Eds. Emmelot, P. and Muehlbock, O.) Elsevier, Amsterdam, pp. 124–125 (1964).
9. Iversen, O. H. The regulation of cell numbers in mouse epidermis as simulated by an analog computer – its relation to experimental skin carcinogenesis. Progress in Biocybernetics (Eds. Wiener, N. and Schade, J. P.), Elsevier, Amsterdam, Vol. 1, pp. 85–95 (1964).
10. Bullough, W. S. Mitotic and functional homeostasis: a speculative review. Cancer Res. 25, 1683–1727 (1965).
11. Bullough, W. S. and Rytomaa, T. Mitotic homeostasis. Nature 205, 573–578 (1965).
12. Poole, Brian. The stimulus to hypertrophic growth. Adv. Morphogen. 5, 93–129 (1966).
13. Tsanev, R. and Sendov, B. A model of the regulatory mechanism of cellular multiplication. J. Theoret. Biol. 12, 327–341 (1966).

14. Bullough, W. S. and Laurence, E. B. Epigenetic mitotic control, in Control of Cellular Growth in Adult Organisms (Eds. Teir, H. and Rytomaa, T.) Academic Press, London and New York (1967).
15. Bullough, W. S. The Evolution of Differentiation. Academic Press, London (1967).
16. Iversen, O. H. Some methodological remarks concerning the measurements of growth, in Control of Cellular Growth in Adult Organisms, a Sigrid Juselius Foundation Symposium (Eds. Teir, M. and Rytomaa, T.) Academic Press, London and New York, pp. 401–405 (1967).
17. Bullough, W. S. The control of tissue growth, in The Biological Basis of Medicine (Eds. Bittar, E. E. and Bittar, N.) Academic Press, London, Vol. 1, Chap. 9, pp. 311–333 (1968).
18. Ascheim, E. Epidermal homeostasis – a numerical model. Kinetics of Epidermal Cells. Experientia 24, 94–98 (1968).
19. Sendov, B. and Tsanev, R. Computer simulation of the regenerative processes in the liver. J. Theoret. Biol. 18, 90–104 (1968).
20. Grundmann, E. Intrazellulaere Steuerungsfaktoren bei der Tumorgenese. Arznei-mittelforschung 18, 970–973 (1968).
21. Loewenstein, W. R. III. Emergence of order in tissues and organs. Communication through cell junctions. Implications in growth control and differentiation. Dev. Biol. Suppl. 2, 151–183 (1968).
22. Anderson, J. M. and Jarrett, O. Chalones and cancer. Letters, The Lancet, January 4, p. 55 (1969).
23. Bullough, W. S., The chalones. Science Journal 5, 71–76 (1969).
24. Paukovits, von W. Die Regulation der Zellteilung in normalen und malignen Geweben. Krebsartz, pp. 222–223 (1969).
25. Bullough, W. S. Epithelial repair, in Repair and Regeneration (Eds. Dunphy, J. E. and van Winkle, W.) McGraw-Hill, Ch. 4 (1969).
26. Iversen, O. H. and Bjerknes, R. Growth regulation in the epidermis. A cybernetic and biologic study. Cybernetic Medicine 1, 1–17 (1969).
27. Johnson, H. A. Liver regeneration and the 'critical mass' hypothesis. Amer. J. Pathol. 57, 1–15 (1969).
28. Ripley, P. A. Heuristic model of mitotic autoregulation in cell populations. Nature 223, 1382–1383 (1969).
29. Iversen, O. H. Cybernetics and medicine. Brit. J. Hosp. Med. 10–14, Nov. 1970.
30. Kirk, J., Orr, J. S., Wheldon, T. E. and Gray, W. M. Stress cycle analysis in the biocybernetic study of blood cell population. J. Theoret. Biol. 26, 265–276 (1970).
31. Wheldon, T. E., Gray, W. M., Kirk, J. and Orr, J. S. Mitotic autoregulation of populations of normal and malignant cells. Nature 226, 547 (1970).
32. Cone, Jr., C. D. Unified theory on the basic mechanism of normal mitotic control and oncogenesis. J. Theoret. Biol. 30, 151–181 (1971).
33. Cone, Jr., C. D. Maintenance of mitotic homeostasis in somatic cell populations. J. Theoret. Biol. 30, 183–194 (1971).
34. Bullough, W. S. Ageing of mammals. Nature 229, 608–610 (1971).
35. Argyris, T. S. Chalones and the control of normal regenerative and neoplastic growth of the skin. Amer. Zool. 12, 137–149 (1972).
36. Bullough, W. S. Chalone control systems, in Humoral Control of Growth and Differentiation (Eds. Gordon, A. S. and LoBue, J.) Academic Press, New York (1972).

37. Bullough, W. S., The chalones: a review. Nat. Cancer Inst. Monogr. 38, 5–16 (1973).
38. Forscher, B. K. and Houck, J. C., eds., Chalones: Concepts and Current Researches. Proc. First Sym. International Chalone Conf. Nat. Cancer Inst. Monogr. 38 (1973).
39. Houck, J. C. and Hennings, H. Chalone, specific endogenous mitotic inhibitors. FEBS lett. 32, 1–8 (1973).
40. Bjerknes, R. and Iversen, O. H. 'Antichalones' A theoretical treatment of the possible role of antichalone in the growth control system. Acta. Path. Microbiol. Scan. A. suppl. 248, 33–42 (1974).
41. Bullough, W. S. Chalone control mechanisms. Life Sci. 16, 323–330 (1974).
42. Houck, J. C. and Daugherty, W. F. Chalones: a tissue-specific approach to mitotic control. New York: Medcom (1974).
43. Nome, O. Tissue-specificity of the epidermal chalones. M. D. Thesis University of Oslo. (1974).
44. Attallah, A. M. A proposed mechanism of chalone action. Clin. Proc. CHNMC In Press (1976).
45. Attallah, A. M. Chalones and cancer: a review. Clin. Proc. CHNMC 31 in press (1975).
46. Attallah, A. M. Growth regulation theories and the chalone concept: a review. II. Lymphocytes. Clin. Proc. CHNMC 31, 108–113 (1975).
47. Bullough, W. S. Mitotic control in adult mammalian tissues. Biol. Rev. 50, 99–130 (1975).
48. Houck, J. C. and Attallah, A. M. Chalones (specific and endogenous mitotic inhibitors) and cancer, in; Cancer: A Comprehensive Treatise, Vol. 3. Biology of Tumors. Ed. F. Becker, Plenum Press. New York. In press. (1975).
49. Thornley, A. L. and Laurence, E. B. The present state of biochemical research on chalones. Int. J. Biochem. 6, 313–320 (1975).

Epidermis

1. Nettleship, A. The effects of homologous tissue extracts on rate of epithelization. Amer. J. Clin. Path. 13, 349–351 (1943).
2. Bullough, W. S. Mitotic activity in the adult male mouse. Mus. musculus L. The diurnal cycles and their relation to waking and sleeping. Proc. Royal Soc. London 135, 212–242 (1947–48).
3. Bullough, W. S. and Laurence, E. B. The control of epidermal mitotic activity in the mouse. Proc. Royal Soc. B 151, 517–536 (1960).
4. Iversen, O. H. A homeostatic mechanism regulating the cell number in epidermis. Its relation to experimental skin carcinogenesis. Atti del 1. Congresso Internazionale di Medicina Cibernetica, Napoli, Ottobre 2–5, 1960, Giannini, Napoli, 1962.
5. Yasuda, K. and Montagna, W. Histology and cytochemistry of human skin. XX. The distribution of monoamine oxidase. J. Histochem. and Cytochem. 8, 356–366 (1960).
6. Bullough, W. S. and Laurence, E. B. The control of mitotic activity in mouse skin. Dermis and hypodermis. Exp. Cell Res. 21, 394–405 (1961).
7. Iversen, O. H. The regulation of cell numbers in epidermis. Acta Path. Microbiol. Scand., Suppl. 148 (1961).
8. Oehlert, W. and Buchner, Th. Mechanismus und zeitlicher ablauf der physiologischen

regeneration in mehrschichtigen plattenepithel und in der schleimahut des magen-darmtraktes der weissen maus. Beitr. Pathol. Anat. 125, 375–402 (1961).

9. Bullough, W. S. and Laurence, E. B. Stress and adrenaline in relation to the diurnal cycle of epidermal mitotic activity in adult male mice. Proc. Royal Soc. B. 154, 540–556 (1961).

10. Bullough, W. S. and Laurence, E. B. The control of mitotic activity in the skin, in Wound Healing (Ed. Slome, D.) Pergamon Press, London (1961).

11. Bullough, W. S. Modern research on the skin of mice and men. Proc. Royal Inst. 38, 630–639 (1961).

12. Bullough, W. S. Growth control in mammalian skin. Nature 193, 520–523 (1962).

13. Oehlert, W. and Block, P. Der mechanismus und zeitliche ablauf der reparativen regeneration in geweben mit post und intermitotischem zellbestand. Verh. Dtsch. Ges. Pathol. 46, 333–340 (1962).

14. Block, P., Seiter, I. and Oehlert, W. Autoradiographic studies of the initial cellular response to injury. Exp. Cell Res. 30, 311–321 (1963).

15. Daniels, Jr., F. Ultraviolet carcinogenesis in man. NCI Monograph No. 10. Conference: Biology of Cutaneous Cancer, pp. 407–422 (1963).

16. Sullivan, D. J. and Epstein, W. L. Mitotic activity of wounded human epidermis. J. Invest. Dermatol. 41, 39–43 (1963).

17. Bullough, W. S. and Laurence, E. B. Duration of epidermal mitosis in vitro. Exp. Cell Res. 35, 629–641 (1964).

18. Bullough, W. S., Hewett, C. L. and Laurence, E. B. The epidermal chalone: a preliminary attempt at isolation. Exp. Cell Res. 36, 192–200 (1964).

19. Bullough, W. S. and Laurence, E. B. The production of epidermal cells. Symp. Zool. Soc. London 12, 1–23 (1964).

20. Bullough, W. S. Growth regulation by tissue-specific factors, or chalones, in Cellular Control Mechanisms and Cancer (Eds. Emmelot, P. and Muehlbock, O.) Elsevier, Amsterdam, pp. 124–145 (1964).

21. Davis, J. C. The effect of cortisol on mitosis in the skin of the mouse. J. Path. Bact. 88, 247–254 (1964).

22. Skjaeggestad, Ø. Cell loss and hyperplasia. Proc. XIV Scand. Congr. Path. Microbiol., pp. 179–180 (1964).

23. Finegold, M. J. Control of cell multiplication in epidermis. Proc. Soc. Exp. Biol. and Med. 119, 96–100 (1965).

24. Iversen, O. H., Aandahl, E. and Elgjo, K. The effect of an epidermis-specific mitotic inhibitor (chalone) extracted from epidermal cells. Acta Path. et Microbiol. Scand. 64, 506 (1965).

25. Bullough, W. S. Cell replacement after tissue damage, in Wound Healing (Ed. Illingworth, C.) Churchill, London (1966).

26. Bullough, W. S. and Laurence, E. B. Tissue homeostasis in adult mammals, in Advances in Biology of Skin, VII, Carcinogenesis (Eds. Montagna, W. and Dobson, R. L.) Pergamon Press, New York (1966).

27. Bullough, W. S. and Laurence, E. B. Accelerating and decelerating actions of adrenalin on epidermal mitotic activity. Nature 210, 715–716 (1966).

28. Bullough, W. S. and Laurence, E. B. The diurnal cycle in epidermal mitotic duration and its relation to chalone and adrenalin. Exp. Cell Res. 43, 343–350 (1966).

29. Elgjo, K. Epidermal cell population kinetics in chemically induced hyperplasia. Norwegian Monographs on Medical Science. Universitetsforalget, Oslo (1966).

30. Randers-Hansen, E. Mitotic activity in the oral epithelium of the rat. Variations according to age and the time of the day. Dept Periodontology and Dept Oral Pathology, The Royal Dental College, Copenhagen, Odont. T. 74, 196–201 (1966).

31. Iversen, O. H. Kinetics of epidermal reaction to carcinogens and other skin irritants. Adv. Biol. Skin 7, 37 (1966).

32. Leim, van du. The influence of the thickness of the epidermis on the latent time of ultraviolet erythema. Ultraviolet Erythema, Chap. 10, 126–135 Thesis. Univ Utrecht (1966).

33. Oehlert. W. Die Steuerung der Regeneration im mehrschichtigen plattenepithel. Verhandlungen der Deutschen Gesellschaften für Pathologie 50, 90–117 (1966).

34. Oehlert, W., Karasek, J. and Bertelmann, H. Untersuchungen zur normalen und gesteigerten zellneubildung im mehrschichtigen plattenepithel der schweineepidermis. Beitr. Path. Anat. 134, 395–417 (1966).

35. Bullough, W. S., Laurence, E. B., Iversen, O. H. and Elgjo, K. The vertebrate epidermal chalone. Nature 214, 578–580 (1967).

36. Giacometti, L. The healing of skin wounds in primates. I. The kinetics of cell proliferation. J. Invest. Dermatol. 48, 133–137 (1967).

37. Iversen, O. H. Simulering av det interne system for vekstkontroll i epidermis. Tidsskr. Norsk Laegefor. 87, 1831–1835 (1967).

38. Iversen, O. H. The growth regulation in epidermis. Acta Path. Microbiol. Scand. Suppl. 187, 44 (1967).

39. Iversen, O. H. and Elgjo, K. The effect of chalone on the mitotic rate and on the mitotic duration in hairless mouse epidermis, in Control of Cellular Growth in Adult Organisms, a Sigrid Juselius Foundation Symposium (Eds. Teir, H. and Rytomaa, T.) Academic Press, London and New York, pp. 88–91 (1967).

40. Baden, H. P. and Sviokla, S. Effect of chalone on epidermal DNA synthesis. Exp. Cell Res. 50, 644–646 (1968).

41. Bullough, W. S. and Laurence, E. B. The role of glucocorticoid hormones in the control of epidermal mitosis. Cell and Tissue Kinetics 1, 5–10 (1968).

42. Bullough, W. S. and Laurence, E. B. Epidermal chalone and mitotic control in the V × 2 epidermal tumor. Nature 220, 134–135 (1968).

43. Born, W. and Bickhardt, R. Zur regelung des zellnachschubs in der epidermis. Klin. Wochenschrift 46, 1312–1314 (1968).

44. Frankfurt, O. S. Effect of hydrocortisone, adrenalin, and actinomycin D on transition of cells to the DNA synthesis phase. Exp. Cell Res. 52, 220–232 (1968).

45. Hondius-Boldingh, W. H. and Laurence, E. B. Extraction, purification, and preliminary characterization of the epidermal chalone: a tissue-specific mitotic inhibitor obtained from vertebrate skin. Europ. J. Biochem. 5, 191–198 (1968).

46. Iversen, O. H. Effect of epidermal chalone on human epidermal mitotic activity in vitro. Nature 219, 75 (1968).

47. Iversen, O. H. Growth regulation in epidermis. Dermatol. Digest 7, 80 (1968).

48. Iversen, O. H., Bjerknes, R. and Devik, F. Kinetics of cell renewal, cell migration, and cell loss in the hairless mouse dorsal epidermis. Cell Tissue Kinet. 1, 351–367 (1968).

49. Elgjo, K. The stability of the epidermal mitosis inhibiting factor (chalone) in water solution. Acta Path. Microbiol. Scand. 76, 31–34 (1969).

50. Hennings, H., Iversen, O. H. and Elgjo, K. Delayed inhibition of epidermal DNA

synthesis after injection of an aqueous skin extract (chalone). Virchows Arch. Abt. B Zellpath. 4, 45–53 (1969).

51. Elgjo, K. Epidermal cell proliferation during the first 24 hours after injection of an aqueous skin extract (chalone). Virchows Arch. Abt. B Zellpath. 4, 119–125 (1969).

52. Hall, Jr., R. G. DNA synthesis in organ cultures of the hamster cheek pouch. Inhibition of a homologous extract. Exp. Cell Res. 58, 429–431 (1969).

53. Kierny, C. E. and Rothberg, S. In vitro DNA synthesis in chick embryonic skin: a sensitive indicator for testing mitotic stimulatory or inhibitory actions. J. Invest. Dermatol. 53, 351–355 (1969).

54. Schellander, F. Reaktion von epidermis und subepidermalen bindegewebe auf hornschichtabrisse. Arch. Klin. Exp. Derm. 234, 158–167 (1969).

55. Bullough, W. S. The rejuvenation of the skin. J. Soc. Cosmet. Chem. 21, 503–520 (1970).

56. Bullough, W. S. and Laurence, E. B. Chalone control of mitotic activity in sebaceous glands. Cell Tissue Kinet. 3, 291–300 (1970).

57. Hell, Elizabeth. A stimulant to DNA synthesis in guinea pig ear epidermis. Br. J. Derm. 83, 632–636 (1970).

58. Stastny, M. and Cohen, S. Epidermal growth factor. IV. The induction of ornithine decarboxylase. Biochem. Biophys. Acta 204, 578–589 (1970).

59. Bishai, I. S. M., Moscarello, M. A. and Ritchie, A. C. Dimethylbenzanthracene binding to epidermal chalone. Nature 232, 114–116 (1971).

60. Brønstad, G. O., Elgjo, K. and Øye, I. Adrenalin increases cyclic 3′5′-AMP formation in hamster epidermis. Nature New Biol. 233, 78–79 (1971).

61. Bullough, W. S. and Deol, J. U. R. Über die regelung von gewebeersatz in der haut. Der Hautarzt 22, 174–180 (1971).

62. Bullough, W. S. and Deol, J. U. R. Chalone-induced mitotic inhibition in the Hewitt keratinising epidermal carcinoma of the mouse. Europ. J. Cancer 7, 425–431 (1971).

63. Elgjo, K. and Hennings, H. Epidermal chalone and cell proliferation in a transplantable squamous cell carcinoma in hamsters. I. In Vivo Results. Virchows Arch. Abt. B Zellpath. 7, 1–7 (1971).

64. Laurence, E. B. and Elgjo, K. Epidermal chalone and cell proliferation in a transplantable squamous cell carcinoma in hamsters. II. In vitro results. Virchows Arch. Abt. B Zellpath. 7, 8–15 (1971).

65. Elgjo, K. and Hennings, H. Epidermal mitotic rate and DNA synthesis after injection of water extracts made from mouse skin treated with actinomycin D: two or more growth-regulating substances. Virchows Arch. Abt. B Zellpath. 7, 342–347 (1971).

66. Elgjo, K., Laerum, O. D. and Edgehill, W. Growth regulation in mouse epidermis. I. G_2 inhibitor present in the basal cell layer. Virchows Arch. Abt. B Zellpath. 8, 277–283 (1971).

67. Frankfurt, O. S. Epidermal chalone. Effect on cell cycle and on development of hyperplasia. Exp. Cell Res. 64, 140–144 (1971).

68. Froese, G. Regulation of growth in hamster cells by a local inhibitor. Exp. Cell Res. 65, 297–306 (1971).

69. Gerstein, W. Cell proliferation in human fetal epidermis. J. Invest. Dermatol. 57, 262–265 (1971).

70. Hennings, H. and Elgjo, K. Hydrocortisone: inhibition of DNA synthesis and mitotic rate after local application to mouse epidermis. Virchows Arch. Abt. B Zellpath. 8, 42–49 (1971).

71. Laurence, E. B. and Randers-Hansen, E. An in vitro study of epidermal chalone and stress hormones on mitosis in tongue epithelium and ear epidermis of the mouse. Virchows Arch. Abt. B Zellpath. 9, 271–279 (1971).

72. Loebbecke, E. A. and Grundmann, E. Versuche zur ermittlung der proliferation der epithels von hauttransplantaten. Virchows Arch. Abt. B Zellpath. 9, 135–144 (1971).

73. Marks, F. Direct evidence of two tissue-specific chalone-like factors regulating mitosis and DNA synthesis in mouse epidermis. Hoppe-Seyler's Z. Physiol. Chem. Bd. 352, 1273–1274 (1971).

74. Marks, R., Fukui, K. and Halprin, K. The application of an in vitro technique to the study of epidermal replication and metabolism. Br. J. Derm. 84, 453–460 (1971).

75. Marrs, J. M. and Voorhees, J. J. A method for bioassay of an epidermal chalone-like inhibitor. J. Invest. Dermatol. 56, 174–181 (1971).

76. Marrs, J. M. and Voorhees, J. J. Preliminary characterization of an epidermal chalone-like inhibitor. J. Invest. Dermatol. 56, 353–358 (1971).

77. Potten, C. S. Tritiated thymidine incorporation into hair follicle matrix and epidermal basal cells after stimulation. J. Invest. Dermatol. 56, 311–317 (1971).

78. Potten, C. S., Jessup, B. A. and Croxson, M. B. Incorporation of tritiated thymidine into the skin and hair follicles. I. Oscillatory changes through the hair growth cycle. Cell Tissue Kinet. 4, 241–254 (1971).

79. Rothberg, S. and Ekel, T. M. Variation of DNA synthesis with age in chick embryo skin. Nature 229, 341–342 (1971).

80. Voorhees, J. J. and Duell, E. A. Psoriasis as a possible defect of the adenyl cyclase-cyclic AMP cascade: a defective chalone mechanism? Arch. Dermatol. 104, 352–358 (1971).

81. Bullough, W. S., Deol, J. U. R. Chalone control of mitotic activity in the eccrine sweat glands. Br. J. Derm. 86, 586–592 (1972).

82. Bullough, W. S. The control of epidermal thickness. Parts I and II. Br. J. Derm. 87, 187–199 (1972).

83. Chopra, D. P., Ruey, J. Y. and Flaxman, B. A. Demonstration of a tissue-specific inhibitor of mitosis of human epidermal cells in vitro. J. Invest. Dermatol. 59, 207–210 (1972).

84. Dahl, M. C. Y. and Shuster, S. A rapid in vitro assay of epidermal chalone. J. Invest. Dermatol. 58, 253 (1972).

85. Deleschuse, C., Regmier, M. and Prunieras, M. Inhibition specifique de la synthese de DNA dans des cultures primaires de cellules epidermiques. Ann. Der. Syph. (Paris) 99, 291–293 (1972).

86. Delescluse, C., Regnier, M. and Prunieras, M. L. Specific effect of epidermal extract on DNA synthesis in tissue culture. J. Invest. Dermat. 58, 253–254 (1972).

87. Elgjo, K. Chalone inhibition of cellular proliferation. J. Invest. Dermatol. 59, 81–83 (1972).

88. Elgjo, K., Laerum, O. D. and Edgehill, W. Growth regulation of mouse epidermis II. G_1 inhibitor present in the differentiating cell layer. Virchows Arch. B. Zellpath. 10, 229–236 (1972).

89. Flaxman, B. A., Chopra, D. P. Cell cycle of normal and psoriatic epidermis in vitro. J. Invest. Derm. 59, 102–105 (1972).

90. Laurence, E. B., Christophers, E., Randers-Hansen, E. and Rytomaa, T. Systemic factors influencing epidermal mitosis. Europ. J. Clin. Biol. Res. 17, 133–139 (1972).

91. Laurence, E. B. and Randers-Hansen, E. Regional specificity of the epidermal

chalone extracted from two different body sites. Virchows Arch. Abt. B. Zellpath. 11, 34–42 (1972).

92. Marks, R. The role of chalones in epidermal homeostasis. Br. J. Derm. 86, 543–548 (1972).

93. Rohrbach, R., Elgjo, K., Iversen, O. H. and Sandritter, W. Effects of methyl-cholanthrene on epidermal growth regulators. I. Variations in the M-factor. Beitr. Path. 147, 21–27 (1972).

94. Rowe, L. and Dixon, W. J. Clustering and control of mitotic activity in human epidermis. J. Invest. Dermatol. 58, 16–23 (1972).

95. Elgjo, K. Epidermal chalone: cell cycle specificity of two epidermal growth inhibitors. Natl. Cancer Inst. Monogr. 38, 71–76 (1973).

96. Elgjo, K. and Edgehill, W. Epidermal growth inhibitors (chalones) in dermis and serum. Virchows Arch. B. Zellpath. 13, 14–23 (1973).

97. Laurence, E. B. Experimental approach to the epidermal chalone. Nat. Cancer Inst. Monogr. 38, 37–46 (1973).

98. Laurence, E. B. The epidermal chalone and keratinizing epithelia. Nat. Cancer Inst. Monogr. 38, 61–68 (1973).

99. Marks, F. A tissue-specific factor inhibiting DNA synthesis in mouse epidermis. Nat. Cancer Inst. Monogr. 38, 79–90 (1973).

100. Rothberg, S. and Arp, B. C. Epidermal chalone and inhibition of DNA synthesis. Nat. Cancer Inst. Monogr. 38, 93–98 (1973).

101. Voorhees, J. J., Duell, E. A., Bass, L. J. and Harrell, E. R. Role of cyclic AMP in the control of epidermal growth and differentiation Nat. Cancer Inst. Monogr. 38, 47–60 (1973).

102. Yradwohl, P. Tissue-unspecificity of skin extracts tested for the presence of chalones. Experientia 29, 772 (1973).

103. Wright, R. K., Mandy, S. H., Haprin, K. M. and Hsia, S. L. Defects and deficiency of adenyl cyclase in psoriatic skin. Arch. Dermatol. 107, 47 (1973).

104. Bertsch, S. and Marks, F. Lack of an effect of tumor promoting phorbol esters and of epidermal G_1 chalone on DNA synthesis in the epidermis of newborn mice. Cancer Res. 34, 3283–3288 (1974).

105. Elgjo, K. Reversible inhibition of epidermal G_1 cells by repeated injections of aqueous skin extracts (chalone) Virchows. Arch. Abt. B. Zellpath, 15, 157–163 (1974).

106. Elgjo, K. Evidence for presence of the epidermal G_2 inhibitor ('epidermal chalone') in dermis. Virchows. Arch. B. Zellpath. 16, 243–247 (1974).

107. Iversen, O. H., Bhangoo, K. S. and Hansen, K. Control of epidermal cell renewal in the fat web. A study of the cell number, cell size and mitotic rate in the epidermis on both sides of the web after the removal of the epidermis on the ventral side only, w/special emphasis on growth control theories. Virchows Arch. B. Zellpath. 16, 157–179 (1974).

108. Krieg, L., Kuhlmann, I. and Marks, F. Effects of tumor-promoting phorbol esters and of acetic acid on mechanisms controlling DNA synthesis and mitosis (chalones) and on the biosynthesis of histidine-rich protein in mouse epidermis. Cancer Res. 34, 3135–3146 (1974).

109. Marks, F. Attempts to purify and characterize a factor inhibiting epidermal DNA synthesis ('G_1 chalone'). Hoppe-Seylers Z. Physiol. Chem. 355, 1228 (1974).

110. Nome, O. Tissue-specificity of the epidermal chalones. M. D. Thesis, University of Oslo. (1974).
111. Rohrbach, R., Laerum, O. D. Variations of mitosis-inhibiting chalone activity in epidermis and dermis after carcinogen treatment Cell Tissue Kinet. 7, 251–257 (1974).
112. Yamaguchi, T., Hirobe, T., Kinjo, Y. and Manaka, K. The effect of chalone on the cell cycle in the epidermis during wound healing. Exp. Cell Res. 89, 247–254 (1974).
113. Elgjo, K. Epidermal chalone and cyclic AMP: An in vivo study. J. Invest. Dermat. 64, 14–18 (1975).

Granulocytes

1. Rytomaa, R. and Kiviniemi, K. Control of DNA duplication by means of the granulocyte chalone. Europ. J. Cancer 4, 595–606 (1968).
2. Rytomaa, T. and Kiviniemi, K. Control of granulocyte production. I. Chalone and antichalone, two specific humoral regulators. Cell Tissue Kinet. 1, 329–340 (1968).
3. Rytomaa, T. and Kiviniemi, K. Control of granulocyte production. II. Mode of action of chalone and antichalone. Cell Tissue Kinet. 1, 341–350 (1968).
4. Kiviniemi, K. and Rytomaa, T. Control of cell production in rat chloroleukemia by means of the granulocyte chalone. Nature 220, 136–137 (1968).
5. Paran, M., Ichikawa, Y. and Sachs, L. Feedback inhibition of the development of macrophage and granulocyte colonies. II. Inhibition by granulocytes. Proc. Nat. Acad. Sci. 62, 81–87 (1969).
6. Rytomaa, T. Granulocytic chalone and antichalone. Hemic cells in vitro. In Vitro 4, 47–57 (1969).
7. Rytomaa, T. and Kiviniemi, K. Chloroma regression induced by the granulocytic chalone. Nature 222, 995–996 (1969).
8. Rytomaa, T. and Kiviniemi, K. The role of stress hormones in the control of granulocyte production. Cell and Tissue Kinet. 2, 263–268 (1969).
9. Rytomaa, T. and Kiviniemi, K. Regression of generalized leukemia in rat induced by the granulocyte chalone. Europ. J. Cancer 6, 401–410 (1970).
10. Paukovits, W. R. Control of granulocyte production: separation and chemical identification of a specific inhibitor (chalone). Cell and Tissue Kinetics 4, 539–547 (1971).
11. Lozzio, B. B., Lozzio, C. B. and Bamberger, E. G. Human spleen inhibitor of leukemic cell growth. Experientia 15, 87–89 (1973).
12. Paukovits, W. R. Granulopoiesis-inhibing factor: demonstration and preliminary chemical and biological characterization of a specific polypeptide (chalone). Nat. Cancer Inst. Monogr. 38, 147–155 (1973).
13. Rytomaa, T. Chalone of the granulocyte system. NCI Monogr. 38, 143–146 (1973).
14. Laerum, O. D. and Maurer, H. R. Proliferation kinetics of myelopoietic cells and macrophages in diffusion chambers after treatment with granulocyte extracts (chalone). Virchows Arch. B. Zellpath. 14, 293–305 (1973).
15. Bateman, A. E. Cell specificity of chalone-type inhibitors of DNA synthesis released by blood leucocytes and erythrocytes. Cell. Tissue Kinet. 7, 451–461 (1974).
16. Lord, B., Cercek, L., Cercek, B., Shah, G., Dexter, T. and Lajtha, L. Inhibitors of hemopoietic cell proliferation?: specificity of action within the hemopoietic system. Br. J. Cancer 29, 168–175 (1974).

17. Metcalf, D. Regulation by colony-stimulating factor of granulocyte and macrophage colony formation in vitro by normal and leukemic cells, in Control of Proliferation in Animal Cells (Eds. Clarkson, B. and Baserga, R.) New York: Cold Spring Harbor Laboratory, 887–907 (1974).
18. Paukovits, W. R. and Paukovits, J. B. Separation, identification and mechanism of action of the granulocyte chalone. Boll. 1st. Sieroter. Milan. 54, 177–187 (1975).
19. Rytömaa, T. and Kiviniemi, K. Cyclic adenosine 3′, 5′-monophosphate and inhibition of deoxyribonucleic acid synthesis in vitro. In Vitro 11, 1–5 (1975).

Inhibition of cultured cells

1. Simms, H. S. and Stillman, N. P. Substances affecting adult tissue in vitro. II. A growth inhibitor in adult tissue. J. Gen. Physiol. 20, 621–629 (1936–37).
2. Bischoff, R. Inhibition of mitosis by homologous tissue extracts. J. Cell Biol. 23, 10A–11A (1964).
3. Freed, J. J. and Sorof, S. Reversible inhibition of cell multiplication by a small class of liver proteins. Biochem. and Biophys. Res. Comm. 22, 1–5 (1966).
4. Nilsson, G. and Philipson, L. Cell growth inhibition of human cell lines. Exp. Cell Res. 51, 275–290 (1968).
5. Garcia-Giralt, E., Berumen, L. and Macieira-Coelho, A. Growth inhibitory activity in the supernatants of nondividing WI-38 cells. JNCI 45, 649–655 (1970).
6. Froese, Y. Regulation of growth in Chinese hamster cells by a local inhibitor. Exp. Cell Res. 65, 297–306 (1971).

Kidney

1. Goss, R. J. Mitotic response of the compensating rat kidney to injections of tissue homogenates. Cancer Res. 23, 1031–1035 (1963).
2. Saetren, H. The organ-specific growth inhibition of the tubule cells of the rat's kidney. Acta Chem. Scand. 17, 889 (1963).
3. Reiter, R. J. Cellular proliferation deoxyribonucleic acid synthesis in compensating kidneys of mice and the effect of food and water restriction. Lab. Invest. 14, 1636–1643 (1965).
4. Kurnick, N. B. and Lindsay, P. A. Compensatory renal hypertrophy in parabiotic mice. Lab. Invest. 19, 45–48 (1968).
5. Chopra, D. P. and Simnett, J. D. Demonstration of an organ-specific mitotic inhibitor in amphibian kidney. The effect of adult xenopus tissue extracts on the mitotic rate of embryonic tissue (in vitro). Exp. Cell Res. 58, 319–322 (1969).
6. Scaife, J. F. Mitotic inhibition induced in human kidney cells by methylglyoxal and kethoxal. Experimentia 25, 178–179 (1969).
7. Simnett, J. D. and Chopra, D. P. Organ-specific inhibitor of mitoses in the amphibian kidney. Nature 222, 1189–1190 (1969).
8. Chopra, D. P. and Simnett, J. D. Stimulation of mitosis in amphibian kidney by organ-specific antiserum. Nature 225, 657–658 (1970).
9. Saetren, H. The first mitotic wave released among rat kidney tubule cells by partial nephrectomy. Acta Path. Microbiol. Scand., Section A, Pathology, Vol. 78A, Fasc. 1 (1970).

10. Chopra, D. P. and Simnett, J. D. Tissue-specific mitotic inhibition in the kidneys of embryonic grafts and partially nephrectomized host xenopus laevis. J. Embryol. Exp. Morphol. 25 (3), 321–329 (1971).

11. Chopra, D. P. Regulation of mitosis in the embryonic kidney (Xenopus laevis) by kidney growth inhibitor (chalone). Nat. Cancer Inst. Monogr. 38, 189–196 (1973).

12. Dicker, S. E. and Morris, C. A. Investigation of a substance of renal cortex explant in vitro. J. Embryol. Exp. Morph. 31, 655–665 (1974).

Liver

1. Saetren, H. A principle of autoregulation of growth. Exp. Cell Res. 11, 229–232 (1956).

2. Lahtiharju, A. Influence of autolytic and necrotic liver tissue on liver regeneration in rat. Suppl., Acta Pathol. et Microbiol. Scand. 150, 1–99 (1961).

3. Rosens, Jr., G. L. Alteration of tumor cell and hepatic parenchymal cell mitotic rates in tumor-injected partially hepatectomized mice. Cancer Res. 28, 1469–1477 (1968).

4. Helpap, B. and Cremer, H. Kurze Mitteilung – Proliferationsvorgaenge in der traumatisch geschaedigten leber. Virchows Arch. Abt. B Zellpath. 6, 365–366 (1970).

5. Henderson, I. W. D. Growth retardant properties of liver extract. J. Surg. Oncol. 2, 221–229 (1970).

6. Scaife, J. F. Liver homeostasis: an in vitro evaluation of a possible specific chalone. Experientia 26, 1071–1072 (1970).

7. Miyamoto, M. and Terayama, H. Nature of rat liver cell sap factors inhibiting the DNA synthesis in tumour cells. Biochim. Biophys. Acta 228, 324–330 (1971).

8. Spielhoff, R. The specificity of the regulation of organ growth: the effect of tissue extracts on the incorporation of tritiated thymidine in liver and kidney. Proc. Soc. Exp. Biol. and Med. 138, 43–46 (1971).

9. Verly, W. G., Deschamps, Y., Pushpathadam, J. and Desrosiers, M. The hepatic chalone. I. Assay method for the hormone and purification of the rabbit liver chalone. Canadian J. Biochem. 49, 1376–1383 (1971).

10. Aujard, C., Chany, E. and Frayssinet, C. Inhibition of DNA synthesis of synchronized cells by liver extracts acting in vitro. Exp. Cell Res. 78, 476–478 (1973).

11. Brugal, G. Effects of adult intestine and liver extracts on the mitotic activity of corresponding embryonic tissues of Pleurodeles waltlii. Michah. (Amphibia, Urodela) Cell. Tissue. Kinet. 6, 519–524 (1973).

12. Hrachovec, J. P. Chalone-like substances inhibitory for hepatoma growth and for protein synthesis by liver ribosomes. Fed. Proc. 32, 858 (Abs. No. 3612) (1973).

13. Nadal, C. Synchronization of baby rat hepatocytes: a new test for the detection of factors controlling DNA synthesis in rat hepatic cells. Cell Tissue Kinet. 6, 437–446 (1973).

14. Verly, W. Y. The hepatic chalone. Nat. Cancer Inst. Monogr. 38, 175–184 (1973).

15. Volm, M., Ho, A. D., Mattern, J. and Wayss, K. Non-existence of tissue-specific growth inhibitors in the liver supernatant ('hepatic chalone') Exp. Path. 8, 341–348 (1973).

16. Simard, A., Corneille, L., Deschamps, Y. and Verly, W. Y. Inhibition of cell proliferation in the livers of hepatectomized rats by a rabbit hepatic chalone. Proc. Nat. Acad. Sci. U.S. 71, 1763–1766 (1974).

17. Deschamps, Y. and Verly, W. Y. The hepatic chalone. II. Chemical and biological properties of the rabbit liver chalone. Biomedicine 22, 195–208 (1975).
18. Molimard, R., Pieter, Y., Chany, E., Trineal, Y. and Frayssinet, C. An inhibitor of hepatoma cell multiplication in the efferent fluid from isolated perfused rat livers. Biomedicine (1975).

Lung

1. Simnett, J. D., Fisher, J. M. and Heppleston, A. G. Tissue-specific inhibition of lung alveolar cell mitosis in organ culture. Nature 223, 944–946 (1969).

Lymphocytes

1. Moorhead, J. F., Paraskova-Tchernozenska, E., Pirrie, A. J. and Hayes, C. Lymphoid inhibitor of human lymphocyte DNA synthesis and mitosis in vitro. Nature 224, 1207–1208 (1969).
2. Bullough, W. S. and Laurence, E. B. The lymphocyte chalone and its antimitotic action on a mouse lymphoma in vitro. Europ. J. Cancer 6, 525–531 (1970).
3. Lasalvia, E., Garcia-Giralt, E. and Macieira-Coelho, A. Extraction of an inhibitor of DNA synthesis from human peripheral blood lymphocytes and bovine spleen. Rev. Europ. Etudes Clin. et Biol., XV 789–792 (1970).
4. Jones, J., Paraskova-Tchernozenska, E. and Moorhead, J. In vitro inhibition of DNA synthesis in human leukemic cells by a lymphoid cell extract. Lancet, March 28, p. 654 (1970).
5. Garcia-Giralt, E., Lasalvia, E., Florentin, I. and Mathe, G. Evidence for a lymphocyte chalone. Europ. J. Clin. Biol. Res. 15, 1012–1015 (1970).
6. Houck, J. C., Irausquin, H. and Leikin, S. Lymphocyte DNA synthesis inhibition. Science 173, 1139–1141 (1971).
7. Houck, J. C., Irausquin, H. and Leikin, S. The lymphocyte chalone. Clin. Proc. Children's Hospital 28, 130–137 (1972).
8. Garcia-Giralt, E., Morales, V. H., Lasalvia, E. and Mathe, G. Suppression of graft-vs-host reaction by spleen extract. J. Immunol. 109, 878–880 (1972).
9. Kiger, N. Isolation and immunological study of thymic lymphocytic inhibitory factors. Eur. Etud. Clin. Biol 16, 566–572, 1971.
10. Kiger, N. et Florentin, I. Isolement et purification de substances thymiques lympho-cyto-inhibitrices. Ann. Inst. Pasteur 122, 707, 1972.
11. Kiger, N., Florentin, I. et Mathe, G. Some effects of a partially purified lymphocyte inhibiting factor from calf thymus. Transplantation 14, 448–454, 1972.
12. Chung, A. C. and Hufnagel, C. A. Some in vivo effects of chalone (mitotic inhibitor) obtained from lymphoid tissues. Nat. Cancer Inst. Monogr. 38, 131–134 (1973).
13. Florentin, I., Kiger, N. and Mathe, G. T lymphocyte specificity of a lymphocyte inhibiting factor (chalone) extracted from the thymus. Eur. J. Immunol. 3, 624–627 (1973).
14. Garcia-Giralt, E., Rella, W., Morales, V. H., Diaz-Rubio, E. and Richard, F. Extraction from bovine spleen of immunosuppressant with no activity on hemato-poietic spleen colony formation. Nat. Cancer Inst. Monogr. 38, 125–131 (1973).

15. Houck, J. C., Attallah, A. M. and Lilly, J. R. Some immunosuppressive properties of lymphocyte chalone. Nature 245, 148–150 (1973).
16. Kiger, N., Florentin, I., Mathe, G. A lymphocyte inhibiting factor (chalone?) extracted from thymus: immunosuppressive effects. Nat. Cancer Inst. Monogr. 38, 135–143 (1973).
17. Attallah, A. M. Partial purification and characterization of lymphocyte chalone. Ph.D. thesis in Genetics, George Washington University (1974).
18. Garcia-Giralt, E. and Macieira-Coelho, A. Differential effect of a lymphoid chalone on the target and non-target cells in vitro, in Lymphocyte Recognition and Effector Mechanisms. (Eds. K. Lindahl-Kiessling and D. Osobu) Academic Press, New York, p. 457–474 (1974).
19. Hersh, E. M., McCredie, K. B. and Freireich, E. J. Mechanism of production of inhibitor of lymphocyte blastogenic response to mitogens by cultured lymphoblastoid cell line cells. Transplantation 17, 221–227 (1974).
20. Lord, B., Cercek, L., Cercek, B., Shah, G., Dexter, T. and Lajtha, L. Inhibitors of hemopoietic cell proliferation?: specificity of action within the hemopoietic system. Br. J. Cancer 29, 168–175 (1974).
21. Papageorgien, P. S., Tibbetts, L., Sorokin, C. F. and Glade, P. R. Presence of a reversible inhibitor(s) for human lymphoid cell RNA, protein and DNA synthesis in the extracts of established human cell lines. Cell. Immunol. 11, 354–366 (1974).
22. Tanapatchaiyapong, P. and Zolla, S. Humoral Immunosuppressive substance in mice bearing plasma cytomas. Science 186, 748–750 (1974).
23. Zolla, S., Naor, D. and Tanapatchaiyapong, P. Cellular basis of immunodepression in mice with plasmacytomas. J. Immunology. 112, 2068–2076 (1974).
24. Attallah, A. M., Sunshine, G., Hunt, C. V. and Houck, J. C. The specific and endogenous mitotic inhibitor of lymphocytes (chalone). Exp. Cell Res. 93, 283–292 (1975).
25. Attallah, A. M. and Houck, J. C. Lymphocyte chalone concentrates and their effects upon leukemic cells in vitro. Proceedings of International Symposium of Haematology, Milan, Italy, September 1975. Boll. Ist. Sieroter. Milan. 54, 227–235 (1975).

Ascites

1. Bichel, P. Tumor growth inhibiting effect of JB-1 ascit fluid I. Europ. J. Cancer 6, 291–296 (1969).
2. Bradshaw, J. L. and Webb, D. R. Inhibition of Ehrlich ascites tumor growth by nucleoprotein. II. In vivo fate of the tumor cells. JNCI 43, 527–532 (1969).
3. Bichel, P. Feedback regulation of growth of ascites tumors in parabiotic mice. Nature 231, 449–450 (1971).
4. Bichel, P. Autoregulation of ascites tumor growth by inhibition of the G_1 and G_2 Phase. Europ. J. Cancer 7, 349–355 (1971).
5. Bichel, P. Specific growth regulation in three ascitic tumors. Europ. J. Cancer 8, 167–173 (1972).
6. Bichel, P. and Dombernowsky, P. On the resting stages of the JB-1 ascites tumor. Cell. Tiss. Kinet. 6, 359–367 (1973).

7. Dombernowsky, P., Bichel, P. and Hartmann, N. R. Cytokinetic analysis of the JB-1 ascites tumor at different stages of growth Cell Tiss. Kinet. 6, 347–357 (1973).
8. Bichel, P. Self-limitation of ascites tumor growth: a possible chalone regulation. Nat. Cancer Inst. Monogr. 38, 197–203 (1973).
9. Bichel, P. Further studies on the self-limitation of growth of JB-1 ascites tumours. Europ. J. Cancer 9, 133–138 (1973).
10. Dombernowsky, P., Bichel, P. and Hartmann, N. R. Cytokinetic studies of the regenerative phase of the JB-1 ascites tumour cell. Tiss. Kinet 7, 47–60 (1974).
11. Tanapatchaiypong, P. and Zolla, S. Humoral immunosuppressive substance in mice bearing plasmacytomas. Science 186, 748 (1974).

Erythrocytes

1. Kivilaakso, E. and Rytomaa, T. Erythrocyte chalone, a tissue-specific inhibitor of cell proliferation in the erythron. Cell Tissue Kinet. 4, 1–9 (1971).
2. Bateman, A. E. Cell specificity of chalone-type inhibitors of DNA synthesis released by blood leucocytes and erythrocytes. Cell. Tissue Kinet. 7, 451–461 (1974).
3. Lord, B., Cercek, L., Cercek, B., Shah, G., Dexter, T. and Lajtha, L. Inhibitors of hemopoietic cell proliferation?: specificity of action within the hemopoietic system. Br. J. Cancer 29, 168–175 (1974).

Fibroblasts

1. Njeuma, D. L. Mitosis and population density in cultures of embryonic chick and moust fibroblasts. Exp. Cell Res. 66, 237–243 (1971).
2. Njeuma, D. L. Non-reciprocal density-dependent mitotic inhibition in mixed cultures of embryonic chick and mouse fibroblasts. Exp. Cell Res. 66, 244–250 (1971).
3. Salas, J. and Green, H. Proteins binding to DNA and their relation to growth in cultured mammalian cells. Nature New Biol. 229, 165–169 (1971).
4. Houck, J. C., Weil, R. L. and Sharma, V. K. Evidence for a fibroblast chalone. Nature New Biol. 240, 210–211 (1972).
5. Houck, J. C., Sharma, V. K. and Cheng, R. F. Fibroblast chalone. Nat. Cancer Inst. Monograph. 38, 161–171 (1973).
6. Houck, J. C., Sharma, V. K. and Cheng, R. F. Fibroblast chalone and anti-chalone. Nature New Biol. 246, 111–113 (1973).

Melanocyte

1. Bullough, W. S. and Laurence, E. B. Control of mitosis in mouse and hamster melanomata by means of the melanocyte chalone. Europ. J. Cancer 4, 607–615 (1968).
2. Dewey, D. L. The melanocyte chalone. Nat. Cancer Inst. Monogr. 38, 213–216 (1973).
3. Seiji, M., Nakano, H., Akiba, H. and Kato, T. Inhibition of DNA and protein synthesis in melanomata by a melanoma extract. J. Invest. Dermat. 62, 11–19 (1974).

Intestine

1. Brugal, G. Effects of adult intestine and liver extracts on the mitotic activity of corresponding embryonic tissues of pleurodeles waltlii Michah. (Amphibia, Urodela). Cell Tissue Kinet. 6, 519–524 (1973).
2. Tutton, P. J. M. Control of epithelial cell proliferation in the small intestinal crypt. Cell Tissue Kinet. 6, 211–216 (1973).
3. Brugal, G. and Pelmont, J. Presence, dans l'intestin du Triton adulte pleurodeles waltlii Michah, de deux facteurs antimitotiques naturels (chalones) actifs sur la proliferation cellulaire dans l'intestin embryonnaire. C.R. Acad. Sc. Paris. 278D, 2831–2834 (1974).
4. Clarke, R. M. Control of intestinal epithelial replacement: lack of evidence for a tissue-specific blood-borne factor. Cell Tissue Kinet. 7, 241–250 (1974).
5. Brugal, G. and Pelmont, J. Existence of two Chalone-like substances in intestinal extracts from the adult newt, inhibiting embryonic intestinal cell proliferation. Cell. Tissue Kinet. 8, 171–187 (1975).

HeLa

1. Volm, M., Wayss, K. and Kinderer, H. A new model of growth regulation. Cell-specific inhibition of DNA synthesis in HeLa cells by endometrium extract. Die Naturwissenschafter, 56, 566–567 (1969).
2. Hinderer, H., Volm, M. and Wayss, K. Spezifische hemmung der DNA synthese von HeLa zellen durch endometrium extrakt. Exp. Cell Res. 59, 464–468 (1970).
3. Nilsson, G. Thymidine and uridine metabolism at cell growth inhibition of HeLa cells by human liver extract. Exp. Cell Res. 59, 207–216 (1970).

Lens

1. Voaden, M. J. Mitotic inhibitors in the rabbit lens: sulphydryl groups and the effect of heat on the lens protein. Exp. Eye Res. 7, 326–331 (1968).
2. Voaden, M. J. A chalone in the rabbit lens? Exp. Eye Res. 7, 326–331 (1968).

Stomach

1. Philpott, G. W. Tissue-specific inhibition of cell proliferation in embryonic stomach epithelium in vitro. Gastroenterology 61, 25–34 (1971).

Muscle

1. Florentin, R. A., Nam, S. C., Janakidevi, K., Lee, K. T., Reiner, J. M. and Thomas, W. A. Population dynamics of arterial smooth muscle cells. II. In vivo inhibition of entry into mitosis of swine arterial smooth muscle cells by aortic tissue extracts. Arch. Path. 95, 317–320 (1973).

2. Nam, S. C., Florentin, R. A., Janakidevi, K., Lee, K. T., Reiner, J. M. and Thomas, W. A. Population dynamics of arterial smooth muscle cells. III. Inhibition by aortic tissue extracts of proliferative response to internal injury in hypercholesterolemic swine. Exp. Mol. Path. 21, 259–267 (1974).

Uterus

1. Chevalier, S. and Verly, W. Y. About the existence of an endometrial chalone. Euro. J. Cancer, (1975).

Cheek pouch

1. Teel, R. W. Inhibition of DNA synthesis in hamster cheek pouch tissue in organ culture by dibutyryl cyclic AMP and a homologous extract. Biochem. Biophys. Res. Comm. 47, 1010–1014 (1972).

Sperm

1. Clermont, Y. and Mauger, A. Existence of a spermatogonical chalone in the rat testis. Cell Tissue Kinet, 7, 165 (1974).

Subject index